Medical Radiology

Diagnostic Imaging

Series Editors

Hans-Ulrich Kauczor
Paul M. Parizel
Wilfred C. G. Peh

The book series *Medical Radiology – Diagnostic Imaging* provides accurate and up-to-date overviews about the latest advances in the rapidly evolving field of diagnostic imaging and interventional radiology. Each volume is conceived as a practical and clinically useful reference book and is developed under the direction of an experienced editor, who is a world-renowned specialist in the field. Book chapters are written by expert authors in the field and are richly illustrated with high quality figures, tables and graphs. Editors and authors are committed to provide detailed and coherent information in a readily accessible and easy-to-understand format, directly applicable to daily practice.

Medical Radiology – Diagnostic Imaging covers all organ systems and addresses all modern imaging techniques and image-guided treatment modalities, as well as hot topics in management, workflow, and quality and safety issues in radiology and imaging. The judicious choice of relevant topics, the careful selection of expert editors and authors, and the emphasis on providing practically useful information, contribute to the wide appeal and ongoing success of the series. The series is indexed in Scopus.

Mohamed Fethi Ladeb
Filip Vanhoenacker
Editors

Imaging of Primary Tumors of the Osseous Spine

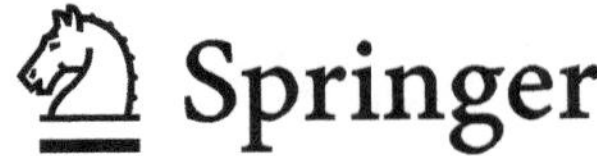

Editors
Mohamed Fethi Ladeb
Department of Radiology
M Kassab Orthopedic Institute
Tunis, Tunisia

Filip Vanhoenacker
Department of Radiology
AZ Sint-Maarten Mechelen
Mechelen, Belgium

ISSN 0942-5373 ISSN 2197-4187 (electronic)
Medical Radiology
ISSN 2731-4677 ISSN 2731-4685 (electronic)
Diagnostic Imaging
ISBN 978-3-031-56885-5 ISBN 978-3-031-56886-2 (eBook)
https://doi.org/10.1007/978-3-031-56886-2

This Springer imprint is published by the registered company Springer Nature Switzerland AG
The registered company address is: Gewerbestrasse 11, 6330 Cham, Switzerland

Paper in this product is recyclable.

Preface

Soon after the completion of our previous book *Imaging of Synovial Tumors and Tumor-Like Conditions*, Professor Mohamed Fethi Ladeb invited me again to collaborate on a book project *Imaging of Primary Tumors of the Osseous Spine*.

Because our collaboration on the previous book went very smoothly, I accepted immediately. The concept, contents of the book, and the choice of authors for the separate chapters were finalized within weeks following his invitation.

This book contains five major parts. The first part is related to epidemiology, classification, pathology, genetics, and molecular biology of tumors of the osseous spine. Part II discusses the basic imaging semiology, imaging modalities, staging, and imaging-guided biopsy. Part III provides an up-to-date systematic review of all primary bone tumors of the spine and its mimics, with emphasis on the imaging findings. Part IV focusses on surgical and interventional treatment. Finally, the subject of Part V is posttreatment evaluation.

We are incredibly grateful that the series editors of Medical Radiology-Diagnostic Imaging (Springer) Professor Wilfred Peh and Professor Paul Parizel entrusted us with the task to edit this book. We have been very fortunate to work with very talented and outstanding experts in the field of musculoskeletal imaging from the school of Tunis and from all Flemish University Hospitals: Antwerp, Ghent, Brussels, and Leuven, supplemented by excellent contributions from highly esteemed researchers from the UK, France, Spain, Germany, Greece, Macedonia, Italy, Turkey, Singapore, and Canada. It is exciting that so many talented radiologists from different universities we are currently affiliated with contributed to our book.

We particularly want to thank our trainers and mentors in musculoskeletal (MSK) radiology. We are also deeply indebted to the technicians and colleagues in our respective departments for providing us with high-quality images. We would like to express our special thanks to Springer-Verlag for the opportunity to edit this book. Last but not least, we want to thank our families for their constant support while we were working on this amazing project.

We hope that this work becomes a valuable and practical resource for graduated clinical radiologists, orthopedic surgeons, oncologists, pathologists as well as residents and researchers of these disciplines.
We hope you enjoy reading it.

Mechelen, Belgium
Tunis, Tunisia
January 2024

Filip M. Vanhoenacker
Mohamed Fethi Ladeb

Contents

Part I

Epidemiology, Classification, Pathology, Genetics and Molecular Biology

Epidemiology of Primary Tumors of the Osseous Spine

Klaas De Corte and Vasiliki Siozopoulou

Contents

K. De Corte
University Hospital Antwerp, Antwerp, Belgium
e-mail: klaas.decorte@uza.be

V. Siozopoulou (✉)
Cliniques Universitaire Saint-Luc,
Bruxelles, Belgium
e-mail: vasiliki.siozopoulou@saintluc.uclouvain.be

Abstract

Primary tumors of the osseous spine, though rare, pose significant diagnostic and therapeutic challenges. This comprehensive text offers an in-depth analysis of the pathologic and histologic features, epidemiology, clinical presentation, and management strategies of these tumors, aimed at enhancing the radiologist's role in multidisciplinary care. Through a synthesis of global data, this book delineates the incidence, prevalence, and regional variations of spinal tumors, underscoring the importance of a nuanced approach to patient care.

Advancements in imaging techniques—conventional radiography, computed tomography (CT), magnetic resonance imaging (MRI), and nuclear medicine—form the backbone of the diagnostic process, providing detailed insights into tumor morphology and guiding subsequent interventions. The text emphasizes the integration of imaging findings with clinical and pathological data to refine differential diagnoses and therapeutic decisions.

Management strategies are discussed with a focus on the latest surgical, radiotherapeutic, and chemotherapeutic approaches, highlighting the need for individualized treatment plans. This book also addresses the prognostic factors influencing patient outcomes, offering a valuable resource for evidence-based practice.

Med Radiol Diagn Imaging (2024)
https://doi.org/10.1007/174_2024_475,
Published Online: 28 March 2024

In conclusion, this text serves as a critical resource for radiologists, facilitating a deeper understanding of primary osseous spinal tumors. It advocates for ongoing research and technological innovation to improve diagnostic precision and expand treatment options, ultimately aiming to enhance patient survival and quality of life.

1 Introduction

Though comprising a small fraction of oncological research, mainly due to their relative rarity, the study of primary tumors of the osseous spine plays a crucial role in optimizing diagnoses and treatment modalities within this complex clinical niche (Chi et al. 2008; Dang et al. 2015; Dreghorn et al. 1990). The anatomical intricacies of the spinal column and its consequent implications linked to tumor manifestation and management render these entities particularly challenging to tackle. Because of the diverse range of histologic subtypes, their incidence and prevalence exhibit marked global variation as well (Fenoy et al. 2006; Kelley et al. 2007; Laubscher et al. 2015; Mukherjee et al. 2011). Therefore, a thorough exploration of their epidemiology is of paramount importance.

Epidemiological study delineates the distribution, determinants, and frequency of diseases within populations, thereby informing, guiding, and ultimately shaping evidence-based interventions for disease control and management (Dreghorn et al. 1990). With respect to tumors of the osseous spine, a comprehensive understanding of their epidemiology is crucial in providing radiologists and other healthcare professionals with insights into their geographical, demographical, anatomical, and chronological distribution. Such insights can significantly enhance diagnostic accuracy, prognostic prediction, and therapeutic interventions (Chi et al. 2008; Dang et al. 2015; Dreghorn et al. 1990).

Even though osseous spine tumors constitute a minor proportion of all bone tumors, their clinical significance cannot be overstated (Laubscher et al. 2015). Presenting with a variety of symptoms ranging from localized pain to neurological complications, their management requires a deep understanding of the implications of tumor location and the degree of spinal cord or nerve root involvement (Fenoy et al. 2006; Mukherjee et al. 2011; Munoz-Bendix et al. 2015).

A critical aspect of understanding these tumors involves investigating their global epidemiology. This includes prevalence, incidence, and variations across different regions (Wewel and O'Toole 2020; Wilartratsami et al. 2014). Documented variations in incidence and tumor type among different regions and between pediatric and adult populations exemplify the need for geographical analysis in osseous spine tumor epidemiology (Wilartratsami et al. 2014; Zhou et al. 2017). Tumor types such as chordoma, Ewing's sarcoma, and osteosarcoma commonly occur, albeit with variations in frequency and spinal location (Munoz-Bendix et al. 2015; Wewel and O'Toole 2020; Wilartratsami et al. 2014; Zhou et al. 2017).

Furthermore, the exploration of demographic and risk factors associated with osseous spine tumors is essential for a complete understanding of these neoplasms. Factors such as age, gender, and genetic predispositions significantly impact the incidence and manifestation of these tumors (Kelley et al. 2007; Munoz-Bendix et al. 2015). Insight into these variables contributes to patient management strategies and provides potential avenues for preventive measures.

Given the dynamic nature of the global health landscape, forward-looking analysis is an integral part of epidemiology. Projections for future trends in osseous spine tumor epidemiology are influenced by a plethora of factors, including demographic shifts, environmental changes, and developments in diagnostic and therapeutic technologies (Dang et al. 2015; Kelley et al. 2007).

This chapter aims to provide a concise and integrative summary of the key aspects of the epidemiology of primary tumors of the osseous spine, drawing from various global studies. By bringing together the findings from these studies, we aim to equip radiologists and other healthcare professionals with a more nuanced understanding of these tumors, providing them with robust handholds to navigate the challenges posed by these entities in their clinical practice.

2 Global Epidemiology

The global epidemiology of primary osseous spinal tumors presents a complex landscape marked by a rich tapestry of varying incidence and prevalence rates, common tumor types, regional predilections, and temporal trends. A deeper dive into these patterns provides invaluable insights not only for the clinical understanding of these conditions but also for informing research and policy decisions in healthcare planning and resource allocation.

Primary osseous spinal tumors, although rare, represent a significant subset of bone tumors with substantial clinical impact (Fenoy et al. 2006; Mukherjee et al. 2011). They account for a range between 2.8% and 13% of all bone tumors, depending on the region and population studied (Wilartratsami et al. 2014; Zhou et al. 2017). These variations may be attributed to numerous factors including population demographics, genetic predispositions, environmental factors, and healthcare systems' capacity for early detection.

An examination of the global data reveals complex patterns. In a comprehensive review of the Siriraj Bone Tumor Registry, which amassed data from 1996 to 2010, 85 out of 1679 investigated primary bone tumors were identified as primary spinal tumors (Wilartratsami et al. 2014). This equates to a prevalence rate of approximately 5.1% within the investigated sample, underscoring the clinical importance of these conditions given their potential severity. In this series, several tumor types emerged with prominence.

Chordoma, the most common tumor type in this series, accounted for nearly a third (32.9%) of all primary spinal tumors (Wilartratsami et al. 2014). Chordomas are malignant tumors that arise from remnants of the notochord, a structure present in embryonic development. They are slow growing but locally aggressive and are often challenging to treat due to their proximity to critical structures such as the spinal cord and major blood vessels. Chordomas most commonly occur at the ends of the axial skeleton, particularly the sacrum and base of the skull.

The next most common tumors identified are hemangiomas. These tumors are described in up to 26% as an incidental radiological finding (Peckham and Hutchins 2019), and they are also incidentally found in almost 11% of autopsies (Doppman et al. 2000). Hemangiomas, on the other hand, are benign vascular tumors. Spinal hemangiomas are usually asymptomatic and often discovered incidentally. However, in rare cases, they can expand and cause compression of the spinal cord or nerve roots, leading to pain or neurological symptoms.

Giant cell tumors account for 17.6% of cases (Wilartratsami et al. 2014). Giant cell tumors are generally benign but can be locally aggressive. They are composed of multiple cell types, including the characteristic osteoclast-like giant cells.

In contrast, a survey of the Leeds Regional Bone Tumor Registry in the United Kingdom found a lower incidence of primary osseous tumors (Zhou et al. 2017). Out of 1950 cases, only 2.8% were identified as primary tumors of the axial skeleton (Zhou et al. 2017). However, despite this regional variation, chordomas again emerged as the most prevalent tumor type, reinforcing their global significance.

Osteosarcoma, the second most common tumor in the Leeds Registry, is a malignant bone-forming tumor. It is typically associated with long bones, particularly around the knee, but it can occur in the spine. Spinal osteosarcomas are rare and can be challenging to diagnose due to their infrequency and the complexity of spinal anatomy. When present, they often require aggressive treatment due to their malignant nature (Zhou et al. 2017).

When considering the tumors' anatomical distribution, further patterns emerge. Malignant lesions, for instance, appear to predominate in certain regions, particularly the sacrum, accounting for 60% of all tumors in this region (Zhou et al. 2017). This information not only assists in formulating a differential diagnosis based on the patient's symptoms and tumor location, but it also indicates potential underlying etiologies related to the embryology or biomechanics of these specific spinal regions.

Moreover, these prevalence rates bear significant implications for healthcare planning and resource allocation. Regions with higher incidence of these tumors, such as those suggested by the Siriraj Bone Tumor Registry, might need to place greater emphasis on improving diagnostic and therapeutic capabilities to manage these conditions more effectively (Wilartratsami et al. 2014). Conversely, regions with lower prevalence rates, such as those suggested by the Leeds Registry, might focus resources on conditions with a higher local impact (Zhou et al. 2017).

Temporal trends in the epidemiology of osseous spine tumors also warrant consideration. In the Siriraj Bone Tumor Registry study, the number of malignant spinal tumors identified was approximately double that of benign tumors (Wilartratsami et al. 2014). This could indicate an increasing trend of malignant tumors over the study period, or it might reflect improvements in diagnostic technologies, leading to the detection of more malignant conditions (Wilartratsami et al. 2014).

Furthermore, it is crucial to recognize the importance of regional variations. As evident in the contrasting data from Thailand and the United Kingdom, we see two regions with distinctly different prevalence rates and common tumor types (Wilartratsami et al. 2014; Zhou et al. 2017). These differences underscore the importance of considering regional variations in the context of local healthcare practices and patient demographics.

In conclusion, understanding the global epidemiology of primary osseous spinal tumors is a complex but vital task. It requires a comprehensive and nuanced perspective that considers variations in prevalence, common tumor types, regional predilections, and temporal trends. This understanding will undoubtedly influence healthcare planning, research directions, and development of therapeutic strategies. As our world continues to change, the epidemiology of these conditions may shift, warranting continual surveillance and analysis. This information empowers us in our mission to enhance patient outcomes and advance the field of spine oncology.

3 Demographic and Risk Factors

Primary osseous spine tumors, a complex and varied group of neoplasms, present unique challenges in diagnosis and treatment. A nuanced understanding of their epidemiology, including the influence of demographic and risk factors, is indispensable for managing these conditions. As we delve into the intricate interplay of these variables, it becomes clear that the epidemiology of spinal tumors mirrors the diverse and multifaceted nature of these neoplasms themselves.

The influence of age on the incidence and type of primary spinal tumors cannot be overstated. Analysis of multiple registries reveals an average age ranging from 38.9 to 44.68 years among patients (Kelley et al. 2007; Mukherjee et al. 2011; Wilartratsami et al. 2014). However, this average belies a broad age spectrum, encompassing both pediatric and adult populations (Zhou et al. 2017). A striking manifestation of this age-dependent variation is seen in the types of tumors prevalent among different age groups. While benign tumors such as aneurysmal bone cyst and osteoblastoma were most common among children, adults were more likely to be diagnosed with malignant tumors like osteosarcoma and chordoma (Kelley et al. 2007; Zhou et al. 2017). Furthermore, the most prevalent tumor in children was Ewing's sarcoma, emphasizing the marked age-related tumor type variations (Dang et al. 2015; Dreghorn et al. 1990). Figure 1 shows the overall ratio between benign and malignant tumors of the osseous spine.

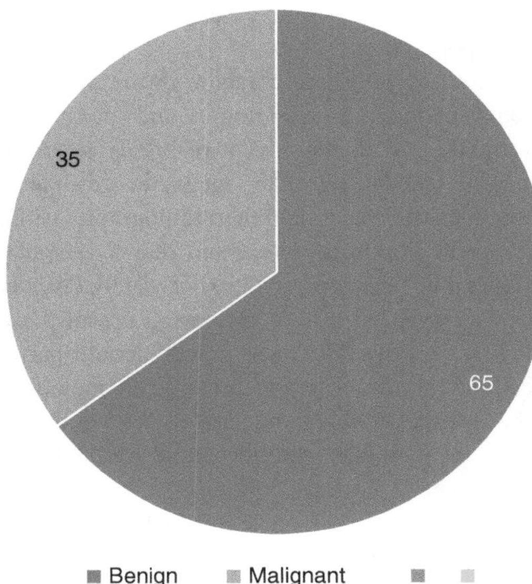

Fig. 1 Overall ratio between benign and malignant tumors of the osseous spine

Gender is another demographic variable influencing the occurrence of primary osseous spine tumors. Some registries suggest a marginal male predominance, while others indicate an almost even distribution between genders (Kelley et al. 2007; Munoz-Bendix et al. 2015; Wilartratsami et al. 2014; Zhou et al. 2017). A more detailed breakdown of the data reveals notable gender-based patterns, with certain tumor types displaying a clear gender predilection. In a study from the Leeds Regional Bone Tumor Registry, malignant lesions showed a male-to-female ratio of 2.1:1, while benign tumors occurred more frequently in women (Zhou et al. 2017). These data highlight the potential impact of gender on the biological behavior of these tumors.

Geographical location and ethnicity are further demographic factors shaping the landscape of primary spinal tumor epidemiology. According to the Surveillance, Epidemiology, and End Results (SEER) database in the United States, non-Hispanic whites exhibited a higher incidence rate compared to other ethnic groups (Fenoy et al. 2006). However, it is crucial to consider potential confounding factors such as disparities in healthcare access and socioeconomic status when interpreting these results.

In addition to demographic influences, a range of risk factors play a critical role in the incidence of primary osseous spine tumors. Prominent among these are certain genetic conditions, including neurofibromatosis type 2 and Paget's disease, which have been identified as significant risk factors for the development of these tumors (Laubscher et al. 2015; Zhou et al. 2017). In the Leeds study, a striking 63% of osteosarcomas, the second most common tumor type, were linked to preexisting Paget's disease (Zhou et al. 2017). This underlines the fundamental role of genetic predisposition in the pathogenesis of these neoplasms.

Moreover, environmental factors have been identified as influential contributors to the development of primary spinal tumors. For instance, radiation exposure has been linked to an increased risk of malignant spinal tumors (Chi et al. 2008; Fenoy et al. 2006). This highlights the need for continued vigilance regarding the potential impacts of environmental hazards, particularly in at-risk populations.

The complex interplay of demographic factors and risks paints a multifaceted picture of the epidemiology of primary osseous spine tumors. Age, gender, ethnicity, genetic predisposition, and environmental factors all play a role in determining the incidence and nature of these neoplasms. The detailed understanding of these factors is crucial in guiding the diagnosis, treatment, and ultimately prognosis of patients suffering from these conditions.

Our understanding of these factors will evolve as the field develops. The ongoing research promises to provide further insights into the biology and epidemiology of spinal tumors, potentially unveiling new therapeutic targets and improving patient outcomes. In the meantime, a comprehensive understanding of these demographic and risk factors provides a solid foundation for managing these challenging conditions.

The main risk factors are summarized in Table 1.

Table 1 Summary of the most common risk factors for the development of a bone tumor of the spine

Demographic and risk factors	Most quoted
Age	Benign tumors more common in pediatric population (aneurysmal bone cyst, osteoblastoma)
	Malignant tumors: Osteosarcoma and Ewing's sarcoma: more prevalent in pediatric population Chordoma: more common in adults
Gender	Benign tumors: more frequent in women (specific types not specified)
	Malignant lesions showed a male-to-female ratio of 2.1:1 (osteosarcoma, chordoma)
Geographical location and ethnicity	Non-Hispanic whites exhibited a higher incidence rate (specific types not specified)
Genetic conditions	Osteosarcomas linked to Paget's disease
Environmental factors	Radiation exposure (osteosarcoma, chordoma)
Multifactorial conditions	Combination of genetic predisposition and environmental exposures (specific types not specified)

4 Projections and Trends

When we consider the future of osseous spine tumor epidemiology, it is essential to consider the myriad factors that have shaped, and continue to shape, its trajectory. Projections and trends in the field are driven by a variety of influences, from changing demographics and environmental factors to advances in diagnosis and treatment.

One of the most apparent trends has been an increase in the incidence of these tumors. From the 1980s to the 2000s, the reported incidence rates rose from 5.6 to 8.7 per million (Fenoy et al. 2006; Mukherjee et al. 2011). This upward trend may be attributed to a combination of demographic shifts and advancements in diagnostic techniques. Our populations are growing older, and the incidence of spinal tumors increases with age (Kelley et al. 2007; Wilartratsami et al. 2014). As life expectancies rise around the globe, we can expect an increase in cases simply due to the aging population.

Another contributing factor is the advancements in imaging technologies and their wider availability. With the advent of highly sensitive imaging modalities like magnetic resonance imaging (MRI) and computed tomography (CT), we are now able to detect and diagnose spinal tumors much earlier and more accurately (Wewel and O'Toole 2020). The increasing use of these diagnostic tools in clinical practice could partly account for the observed increase in incidence rates. Moreover, this trend is likely to continue as these technologies become more refined and accessible.

Furthermore, environmental factors also play a significant role in shaping future projections. For instance, the association between radiation exposure and an increased risk of malignant spinal tumors may have far-reaching implications in our increasingly nuclear age (Chi et al. 2008; Fenoy et al. 2006). Moreover, industrialization and urbanization are associated with increased exposure to a variety of potential carcinogens. Therefore, environmental risk factors could potentially drive an increase in the incidence of these tumors in the future.

However, it is essential to recognize that our ability to manage spinal tumors is also evolving rapidly. Advancements in surgical techniques, radiation therapy, and chemotherapy have improved patient survival and quality of life (Wewel and O'Toole 2020). In the coming years, novel therapeutic approaches, such as targeted therapies and immunotherapies, hold promise for even better outcomes.

Furthermore, a better understanding of the genetic and molecular underpinnings could guide the development of personalized therapies. In this regard, the identification of specific genetic predispositions, such as neurofibromatosis type 2 and Paget's disease, may not only enable early detection but also pave the way for targeted interventions (Laubscher et al. 2015; Zhou et al. 2017).

Therefore, while we may anticipate an increase in the incidence of osseous tumors of the spine due to demographic and environmental changes, advancements in our ability to diagnose and treat these tumors may mitigate the associated morbidity and mortality.

In conclusion, the field of osseous spine tumor epidemiology is dynamic and influenced by numerous interrelated factors. Although projecting future trends is challenging, understanding these influences can guide our preparations and responses. As we look forward, our primary goal remains improving the prognosis and quality of life for individuals affected by these complex conditions.

5 Epidemiology of Metastatic Spine Disease: A Brief Overview

Indeed, while our primary focus throughout this book is on primary osseous spine tumors, it is crucial not to overlook the significant prevalence and impact of metastatic spine disease. The spine, as an anatomical and physiological hub, presents a site of considerable interest for metastatic disease, particularly from certain malignancies such as lung, breast, and prostate cancer (Fenoy et al. 2006). These secondary neoplasms carry profound implications for patients' quality of life and disease management, necessitating a comprehensive understanding of their epidemiology and behavior (Fenoy et al. 2006).

When considering the global epidemiology of spinal metastases, substantial variation is observed. This disparity may partially be attributable to differences in the prevalence of the associated primary malignancies, as well as the availability and utilization of advanced diagnostic modalities (Dreghorn et al. 1990). The higher incidence reported in developed nations like the United States could potentially be skewed by underreporting in resource-constrained regions, although this remains speculative (Dreghorn et al. 1990).

Considering demographic influences, the incidence of spinal metastases intrinsically aligns with the epidemiology of the primary malignancies from which they originate. As such, variables such as age, gender, and lifestyle factors (including smoking and alcohol consumption) play a crucial role. In essence, the demographic profile of spinal metastases will tend to reflect that of the primary cancers known for their propensity to metastasize to the bone, such as prostate and breast cancers, which are predominant in older adults (Wilartratsami et al. 2014).

In terms of clinical presentation, metastatic disease of the spine carries certain nuances that distinguish it from primary tumors. While primary tumors generally exhibit a proclivity toward a specific region of the spine, presenting with local pain or neurological symptoms secondary to neural compression (Mukherjee et al. 2011), metastases typically adopt a more diffuse pattern, with potential involvement of multiple vertebral bodies (Munoz-Bendix et al. 2015). Interestingly, they may remain asymptomatic until achieving a substantial size or precipitating pathological fractures (Munoz-Bendix et al. 2015).

A comprehensive management strategy for spinal metastases necessitates a multidisciplinary approach, which includes systemic therapies targeting the primary malignancy, as well as localized interventions such as surgical resection or radiation therapy, aimed at symptom relief and maintaining spinal stability (Laubscher et al. 2015).

Yet, despite significant progress in therapeutic options, the prognosis of patients with spinal metastases is frequently dismal, with survival often limited to a matter of months (Wewel and O'Toole 2020). This stark reality underscores the pressing need for continued research to develop more effective therapeutic strategies.

Trends in the epidemiology of spinal metastases in the future are likely to shadow the trajectories of the primary cancers. Any advancements in the early detection and management of these malignancies may, theoretically, lead to a reduction in the incidence of spinal metastases (Zhou et al. 2017). However, this assertion must be tempered by the understanding that extended survival from the primary cancers may conversely amplify the cumulative risk of metastatic disease development (Zhou et al. 2017).

In closing, although our focus in this book is primarily directed toward primary tumors of the osseous spine, this brief detour into the landscape of spinal metastases underscores its relevance in the clinical context. A clear understanding of the epidemiology of spinal metastases is fundamental for clinicians, researchers, and policymakers alike, offering invaluable insights that guide clinical decision-making, research priorities, and healthcare resource allocation. Nevertheless, it is equally important to acknowledge the complexities of this disease entity, encouraging continued exploration within this field to ultimately enhance patient outcomes.

6 Conclusion

Understanding the epidemiology of osseous spine tumors is not merely an academic pursuit; it holds profound implications for clinicians, researchers, and policymakers alike. The trends and projections we have discussed provide a crucial context that can inform the development of medical practices, research agendas, and healthcare policies.

For clinicians, the increasing incidence rates and age-related patterns underscore the need for heightened awareness and vigilance (Fenoy et al. 2006; Mukherjee et al. 2011; Wilartratsami et al. 2014). The high prevalence of pain and neurological symptoms as presenting symptoms emphasizes the necessity for clinicians to consider osseous spine tumors in their differential diagnoses when encountering these presentations, particularly in older adults (Zhou et al. 2017). Furthermore, with the identification of certain genetic predispositions, healthcare providers may be able to identify high-risk individuals for earlier detection and intervention (Laubscher et al. 2015).

Researchers are presented with a host of opportunities and challenges by these epidemiological trends. The rising incidence rates signal a pressing need for ongoing research to understand the etiological factors underpinning this increase, which may span from changes in environmental exposures to advances in diagnostic capabilities (Chi et al. 2008; Fenoy et al. 2006; Wewel and O'Toole 2020). Further research into the genetic and molecular mechanisms of these tumors can also open doors for the development of targeted therapies and personalized treatment strategies (Laubscher et al. 2015; Zhou et al. 2017).

For policymakers, these trends underscore the importance of allocating adequate resources toward the diagnosis and treatment of osseous spine tumors. As the population ages and incidence rates rise, the burden of these tumors on healthcare systems is likely to increase (Wilartratsami et al. 2014). Ensuring the accessibility and affordability of diagnostic modalities and treatments is a pressing concern. Furthermore, given the association between radiation exposure and certain malignant spinal tumors, policies related to radiation safety and monitoring are pertinent (Chi et al. 2008; Fenoy et al. 2006).

In conclusion, the epidemiological landscape of osseous spine tumors presents both challenges and opportunities. By continuing to track and analyze these trends, we can better understand these complex conditions and, ultimately, improve the prognosis and quality of life for individuals affected by them. The interplay of research, clinical practice, and policy will continue to shape this field, informing our collective response to these formidable health challenges.

7 Key Points

1. Understanding the epidemiology of osseous spine tumors is crucial for clinicians, researchers, and policymakers to guide clinical decision-making, research priorities, and healthcare resource allocation.
2. Demographic and risk factors, such as age, gender, and genetic predispositions, significantly impact the incidence and manifestation of primary spinal tumors.
3. The incidence rates and age-related patterns of osseous spine tumors highlight the need for heightened awareness and vigilance among clinicians, particularly in older adults.

4. The identification of specific genetic predispositions can enable early detection and targeted interventions for osseous spine tumors.
5. Continual surveillance and analysis of the epidemiology of primary tumors of the osseous spine are necessary due to the dynamic nature of the global health landscape.

References

Chi JH, Bydon A, Hsieh P et al (2008) Epidemiology and demographics for primary vertebral tumors. Neurosurg Clin N Am 19:1–4

Dang L, Liu X, Dang G et al (2015) Primary tumors of the spine: a review of clinical features in 438 patients. J Neurooncol 121:513–520. https://doi.org/10.1007/s11060-014-1650-8

Doppman JL, Oldfield EH, Heiss JD (2000) Symptomatic vertebral hemangiomas: treatment by means of direct intralesional injection of ethanol. Radiology 214:341–348. https://doi.org/10.1148/radiology.214.2.r00fe46341

Dreghorn CR, Newman RJ, Hardy GJ, Dickson RA (1990) Primary tumors of the axial skeleton. Experience of the Leeds Regional Bone Tumor Registry. Spine (Phila Pa 1976) 2:137–140. https://doi.org/10.1097/00007632-199002000-00018

Fenoy AJ, Greenlee JDW, Menezes AH et al (2006) Primary bone tumors of the spine in children. J Neurosurg 105(4 Suppl):252–260

Kelley SP, Ashford RU, Rao AS, Dickson RA (2007) Primary bone tumours of the spine: a 42-year survey from the Leeds Regional Bone Tumour Registry. Eur Spine J 16:405–409. https://doi.org/10.1007/s00586-006-0188-7

Laubscher M, Held M, Dunn RN (2015) Primary bone tumours of the spine: presentation, surgical treatment and outcome. SA Orthop J 14:22–28

Mukherjee D, Chaichana KL, Gokaslan ZL et al (2011) Survival of patients with malignant primary osseous spinal neoplasms: results from the Surveillance, Epidemiology, and End Results (SEER) database from 1973 to 2003. J Neurosurg Spine 14:143–150. https://doi.org/10.3171/2010.10.SPINE10189

Munoz-Bendix C, Slotty PJ, Ahmadi SA et al (2015) Primary bone tumors of the spine revisited: a 10-year single-center experience of the management and outcome in a neurosurgical department. J Craniovertebr Junction Spine 6:21–29. https://doi.org/10.4103/0974-8237.151587

Peckham ME, Hutchins TA (2019) Imaging of vascular disorders of the spine. Radiol Clin North Am 57:307–318

Wewel JT, O'Toole JE (2020) Epidemiology of spinal cord and column tumors. Neurooncol Pract 7:I5–I9. https://doi.org/10.1093/nop/npaa046

Wilartratsami S, Muangsomboon S, Benjarassameroj S et al (2014) Prevalence of primary spinal tumors: 15-year data from Siriraj Hospital. J Med Assoc Thai 97(Suppl 9):S83–S87

Zhou Z, Wang X, Wu Z et al (2017) Epidemiological characteristics of primary spinal osseous tumors in Eastern China. World J Surg Oncol 15:73. https://doi.org/10.1186/s12957-017-1136-1

Classification, Pathology, Genetics, and Molecular Biology of Primary Tumors of the Osseous Spine

Klaas De Corte and Vasiliki Siozopoulou

Contents

Abstract

Primary tumors of the osseous spine represent a diverse group of entities with varying prognostic and therapeutic implications. This chapter provides an exhaustive review of their classification, pathology, genetics, and molecular biology, as per the latest World Health Organization (WHO) guidelines. It delineates the categorization of these neoplasms into benign, intermediate, and malignant classes, each with distinct biological behaviors and clinical outcomes.

Radiological staging, a cornerstone of diagnostic accuracy, is discussed with an emphasis on the integration of computed tomography (CT), positron emission tomography (PET)/CT, and meticulous biopsy techniques. Such approaches are critical for the precise localization and characterization of spinal lesions, guiding therapeutic decision-making.

Pathological assessment distinguishes between benign and malignant tumors, underscoring the prognostic and management nuances. Genetic profiling, including the identification of pathognomonic markers such as the EWSR1-FLI1 fusion in Ewing's sarcoma, provides insights into tumor pathogenesis and potential avenues for targeted therapy.

Molecular diagnostics emerge as a transformative tool, enabling the subclassification of histopathologically similar tumors, which

K. De Corte
University Hospital Antwerp, Edegem, Belgium
e-mail: klaas.decorte@uza.be

V. Siozopoulou (✉)
Cliniques Universitaire Saint-Luc,
Bruxelles, Belgium
e-mail: vasiliki.siozopoulou@saintluc.uclouvain.be

Med Radiol Diagn Imaging (2024)
https://doi.org/10.1007/174_2023_474,
Published Online: 21 March 2024

is essential for individualized patient management. The chapter advocates for a multidisciplinary strategy, incorporating pathology, genetics, molecular biology, and imaging to optimize patient care.

This chapter aims to provide clinicians and researchers with a thorough understanding of the complexities of spinal tumors, supporting the advancement of diagnostic and therapeutic modalities in spinal oncology.

1 Classification

Comprehensive understanding and classification of primary osseous tumors of the spine are of paramount importance.

Spinal tumors are broadly classified according to their anatomical location into intramedullary, intradural extramedullary, and extradural including osseous tumors (Das et al. 2023; Kumar et al. 2020). These extradural tumors, being the most prevalent, often present significant risks such as spinal cord compression, necessitating meticulous management (Kumar et al. 2020).

The World Health Organization (WHO) (WHO Classification of Tumours Editorial Board 2020) has provided a histological classification for bone tumors, which are primarily divided into benign, intermediate (locally aggressive), intermediate (rarely metastasizing), and malignant categories based on their biological potential (WHO Classification of Tumours Editorial Board 2020). This classification applies well to the spinal location of osseous tumors.

In the radiological examination of spinal lesions, accurate staging is crucial. When a solitary spinal lesion is identified, local and systemic staging should be undertaken to determine the origin and extent of the lesion. The staging process often incorporates computed tomography (CT) scans of the chest, abdomen, and pelvis, alongside whole-body MRI. Positron emission tomography (PET)/CT is also increasingly utilized for this purpose (Charest-Morin et al. 2019) (see also chapters "PET and PET/CT and Local and Distant Staging"). Following appropriate staging, a well-coordinated biopsy is essential to confirm the diagnosis. This biopsy should be performed in the center where the patient will receive definitive treatment to ensure proper orientation and minimize the risk of tumor recurrence (Charest-Morin et al. 2019) (see also chapter "Imaging-Guided Biopsy").

Over the years, the adoption of Enneking's principles (see also chapter "Local and Distant Staging"), originally designed for the appendicular musculoskeletal tumors, has significantly contributed to the classification of primary bone tumors of the spine (Charest-Morin et al. 2019). According to Enneking's classification, benign tumors are subdivided into S1 (latent), S2 (active), and S3 (aggressive) stages. For latent lesions, observation is usually recommended, while active or aggressive lesions may necessitate aggressive curettage or wide/marginal resection. On the other hand, malignant tumors are categorized based on the grade (low vs. high), local extension (intra- vs. extracompartmental), and presence or absence of metastasis. In cases where metastasis is absent, a wide resection is typically advocated (Charest-Morin et al. 2019).

The integration of the WHO classification and Enneking's principles not only guides diagnostic and therapeutic strategies but also enhances the understanding of tumor biology, thereby aiding radiologists and other medical professionals in tailoring management plans and prognosticating the disease course (Charest-Morin et al. 2019). Continuous collaborative research is imperative to further refine these classification systems to mirror the evolving understanding of tumor biology and behavior, which in turn can significantly contribute to improved patient care and outcomes.

2 Pathology, Genetics, and Molecular Biology

2.1 Introduction

Primary osseous tumors of the spine can be either benign or malignant (WHO Classification of Tumours Editorial Board 2020; Charest-Morin et al. 2019). Benign lesions, often characterized

Table 1 Overview of benign and malignant bone tumors involving the spine

Benign tumors
Hibernoma
Chondromyxoid fibroma
Vertebral hemangioma
Osteoid osteoma/osteoblastoma
Osteochondroma
Giant cell tumor
Malignant tumors
Osteosarcoma
Ewing's sarcoma
Chondrosarcoma
Chordoma
Undifferentiated pleomorphic sarcoma
Fibrosarcoma
Solitary bone plasmacytoma
Lymphoma
Metastatic disease

by a limited potential for local recurrence, stand in contrast to the malignant tumors, known for their aggressive behavior and propensity for metastasis. We aim to elucidate the histological, genetic, and molecular intricacies of these tumors, which is pivotal for accurate diagnosis and effective management.

Benign and malignant tumors of the osseous spine discussed in this chapter are summarized in Table 1.

2.2 Benign Tumors

2.2.1 Introduction

The categorization and understanding of benign tumors, whether arising from the vertebral body, neural arches, or other bone structures, are crucial for effective clinical management. These tumors, while distinct in their origins and behaviors, share certain traits that often dictate their clinical course and the therapeutic strategies employed.

2.2.2 Osteochondroma

2.2.2.1 Pathology

Osteochondromas exhibit a three-layered structure, consisting of a perichondrium, cartilage, and bone. The outermost layer is a fibrous perichondrium, which seamlessly continues with the periosteum of the bone below. The middle layer is a cartilage cap resembling disorganized growth plate cartilage, with superficial chondrocytes appearing clustered, while those closer to the bone transition become larger, resembling hypertrophic cells of the growth plate (Fig. 1). Over time, cellularity within this layer diminishes, sometimes with extensive coarse and irregular calcification. Observations of binucleated cells, calcification, focal necrosis, nodularity, and degenerative cystic/mucoid changes do not indicate malignancy as nuclear atypia, and mitoses are absent (WHO Classification of Tumours Editorial Board 2020). The histological arrangement of chondrocytes in an orderly columnar fashion within the cartilage cap differentiates osteochondromas from potential malignancies, which may exhibit a thicker cartilaginous cap, irregular cartilaginous surface, or spindle cell proliferation at the cartilage-bone interface (Kim et al. 2009).

2.2.2.2 Genetics and Molecular Biology

The pathogenesis of osteochondromas is rooted in the biallelic inactivation of either the EXT1 or the EXT2 gene. In instances of multiple osteochondromas, heterozygous germline alterations in either EXT1 or EXT2 gene, coupled with somatic loss of the remaining wild-type allele within the cartilage cap of osteochondromas, are observed. On the other hand, solitary sporadic osteochondromas predominantly exhibit homozygous deletions of EXT1 in about 80% of the cases. Both EXT1 and EXT2 genes encode for glycosyltransferases crucial for heparan sulfate biosynthesis (WHO Classification of Tumours Editorial Board 2020). The cartilage cap of osteochondroma harbors a mix of wild-type (normal heparan sulfate) and mutated (heparan sulfate-deficient) cells. Heparan sulfate proteoglycans play a vital role in modulating endochondral ossification by forming an osmotic gradient around chondrocytes and controlling signal transduction. Loss of heparan sulfate may provide a proliferative advantage to the mutated chondroprogenitor cells, causing a loss of

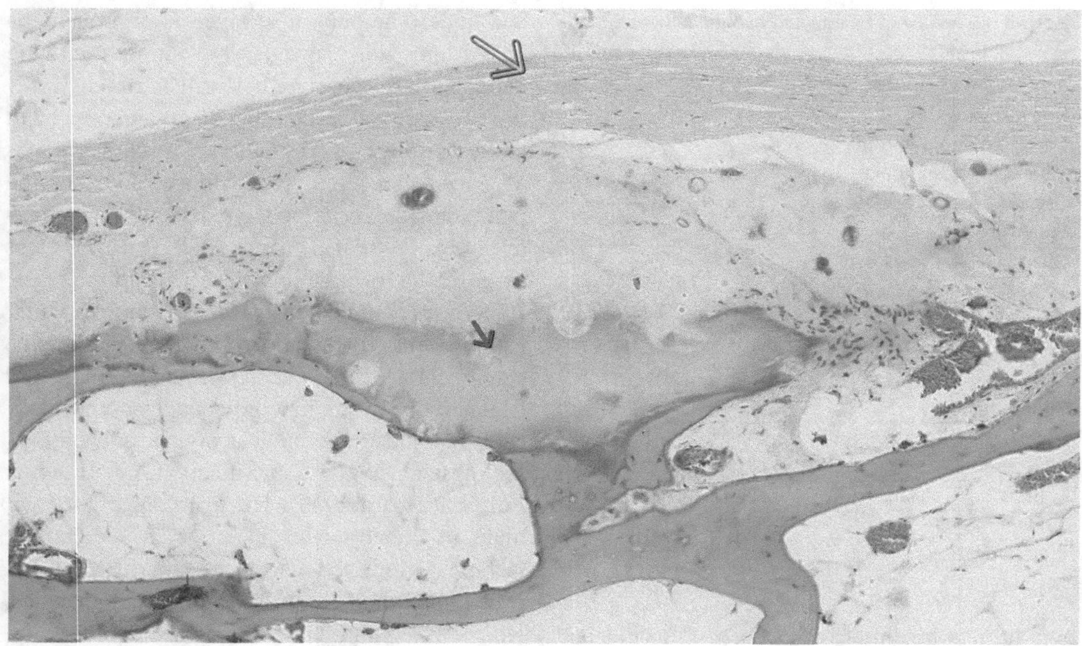

Fig. 1 Osteochondroma. Cap composed of mature hyaline cartilage (blue arrow) with overlying fibrous perichondrium (red arrow), H&E

polarity. This defective heparan sulfate affects multiple signaling pathways including those involving hedgehog, BMP, FGFR3, and WNT/β-catenin, prompting EXT-mutated cells to grow out of the bone, recruiting normal cells to form an osteochondroma (WHO Classification of Tumours Editorial Board 2020).

2.2.3 Giant Cell Tumor

Giant cell tumor of bone (GCTB) is a unique osteolytic tumor that typically arises in the metaphysis of long bones, with the potential to extend into the epiphysis, mainly affecting individuals in their third to fifth decades of life, and slightly more common in females. While the majority of GCTBs develop in the long bones, about 7–15% occur in the spine, where they preferentially affect the sacrum, making them the most common benign sacral tumors (WHO Classification of Tumours Editorial Board 2020). Patients often experience local pain, and those with spinal GCTBs may also suffer from neurological symptoms due to compression or invasion of neural structures.

2.2.3.1 Pathology

Histologically, GCTBs are characterized by a rich blend of osteoclast-like giant cells and mononuclear stromal cells, with the latter believed to be the neoplastic component of the tumor. These tumors exhibit aggressive local behavior with a potential for recurrence, especially when incomplete resection occurs (Kumar et al. 2020). Despite being classified as benign, GCTBs may undergo malignant transformation, estimated at about 10% in spinal occurrences, and can metastasize, albeit rarely, to the lungs (WHO Classification of Tumours Editorial Board 2020). The characteristic imaging features include a lytic, expansile lesion without matrix mineralization, displaying low-to-intermediate signal intensity on T1-weighted and T2-weighted MR images (WHO Classification of Tumours Editorial Board 2020).

The microscopy of giant cell tumor is illustrated in Fig. 2a.

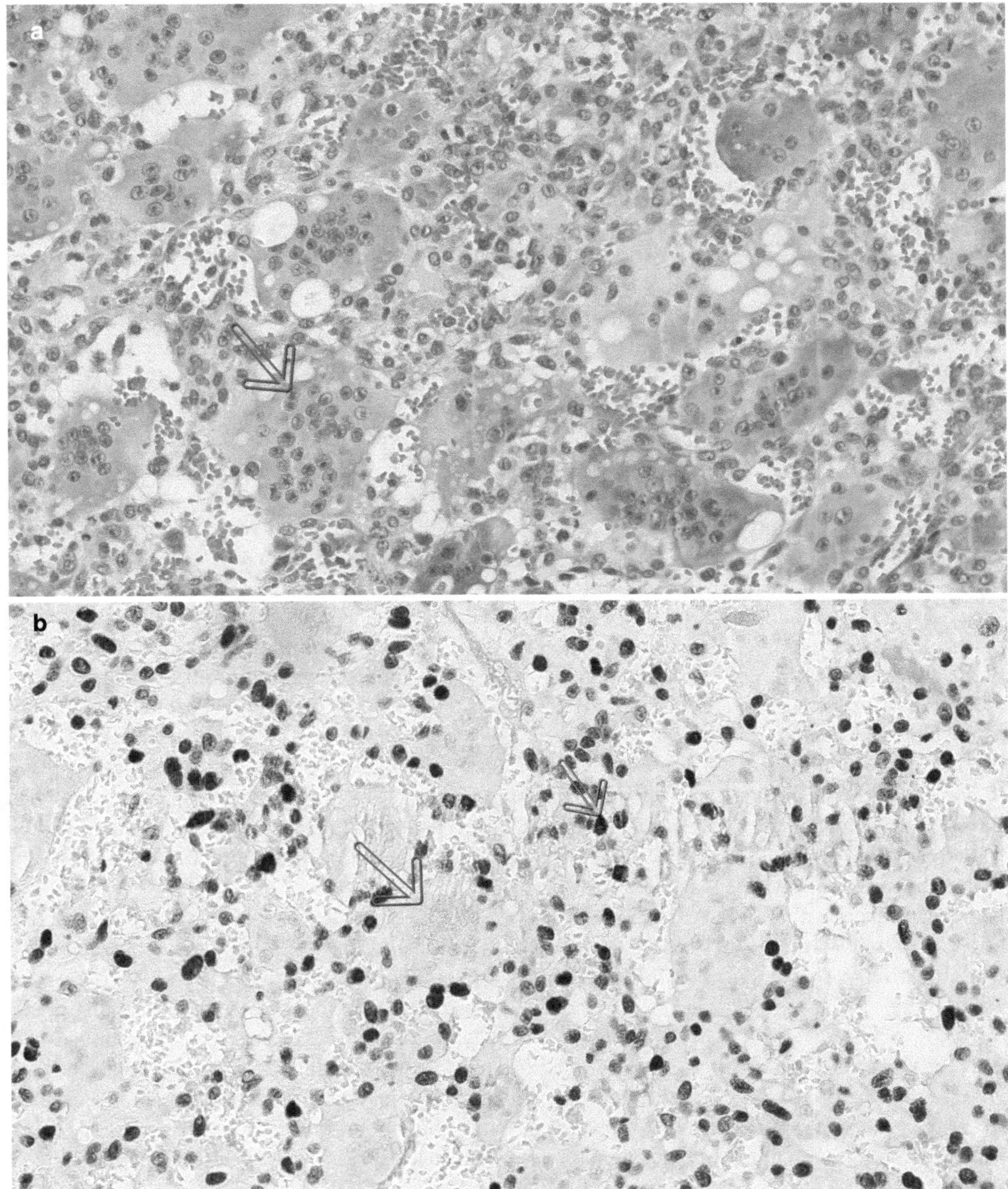

Fig. 2 Giant cell tumor of the bone. (**a**) The lesion is characterized by a large number of nonneoplastic osteoclast-like giant cells (blue arrow), and in between small round mononuclear cells, H&E. (**b**) The mononuclear cells (red arrow), but not the osteoclast-like giant cells (blue arrow), typically express the histone 3G34W. This helps in the differentiation of GCT from other bone tumors that contain osteoclast-like giant cells, H3G34W, DAB

2.2.3.2 Genetics and Molecular Biology

Molecularly, GCTBs are primarily driven by mutations in the H3-3A (H3F3A) gene, with approximately 95% of the tumors harboring pathogenic H3-3A gene mutations, the majority being H3.3 p.Gly34Trp mutations (WHO Classification of Tumours Editorial Board 2020). These mutations influence the behavior of neoplastic stromal cells, which are of osteoblastic lineage, and their interaction with osteoclast-like giant cells. The RANK ligand inhibitor, denosumab, has shown promise in maturing the mutant cells and forming bone, though further studies are needed to establish the long-term efficacy and safety of this treatment (WHO Classification of Tumours Editorial Board 2020). Mutation-specific immunohistochemistry for histone 3G34W is highly specific for GCTB (Schaefer 2018) (Fig. 2b).

GCTBs have also been associated with other genetic syndromes and conditions like Paget's disease of bone and the pheochromocytoma-paraganglioma syndrome, which are characterized by early postzygotic H3.3 mutations. The molecular mechanism driving the neoplasm, particularly how mutant H3.3 contributes to the tumor's aggressive behavior, remains undefined. The mechanism underlying malignant transformation is also not fully elucidated, although mutations in TP53 and HRAS genes have been identified in some malignant GCTBs not associated with prior irradiation (WHO Classification of Tumours Editorial Board 2020).

2.2.4 Osteoid Osteoma/Osteoblastoma

Osteoid osteoma and osteoblastoma are benign osteogenic tumors characterized by their bone-forming nature; however, they possess distinct pathological, genetic, and molecular features that set them apart.

2.2.4.1 Pathology

Osteoid osteoma is typically smaller in size, with a diameter less than 2.0 cm, and often characterized by a central nidus of vascular fibrous connective tissue surrounded by an osteoid matrix. The surrounding bone shows sclerosis. The central nidus contains differentiated plump osteoblasts present as a single layer around trabeculae of unmineralized or mineralized woven bone. Multinucleated giant cells and osteoclasts are frequently observed within the lesions (Fig. 3). Lesions larger than 1.5 cm are usually categorized as osteoblastoma (Van Goethem et al. 2004; WHO Classification of Tumours Editorial Board 2020).

On the other hand, osteoblastoma, morphologically similar to osteoid osteoma, is larger with a general size greater than 2 cm in dimension. Its pathology is marked by interconnecting delicate woven bone trabeculae, usually rimmed by a single layer of polygonal osteoblasts within a richly vascularized stroma. These trabeculae may display different levels of mineralization, from osteoid to densely mineralized woven bone, sometimes exhibiting a pagetoid appearance. Osteoclast-like giant cells are scattered throughout the tumor, and the borders are usually well defined, often showing peripheral bone maturation toward lamellar bone. Despite the morphological similarities, osteoblastomas possess a growth potential unlike osteoid osteomas, and they tend to be more aggressive, especially when they permeate the host bone (WHO Classification of Tumours Editorial Board 2020).

2.2.4.2 Genetics and Molecular Biology

The genetic underpinnings and molecular biology of both tumors have been linked to rearrangements of the FOS gene, which has been identified in both osteoid osteomas and osteoblastomas, shedding light on a potential common genetic etiology. This rearrangement is present in a significant portion of the cases and can be detected at the protein level using anti-FOS (c-FOS) N-terminus immunohistochemistry, resulting in nuclear immunoreactivity in the osteoblastic cells. The FOS gene is a member of the AP-1 family of transcription factors, which when increased can promote cell growth. The rearrangement in FOS leads to a loss of regulatory elements, similar to the v-Fos retroviral oncogene. Additionally, prostaglandins, especially PGE2, PGI2, and COX-2, have been impli-

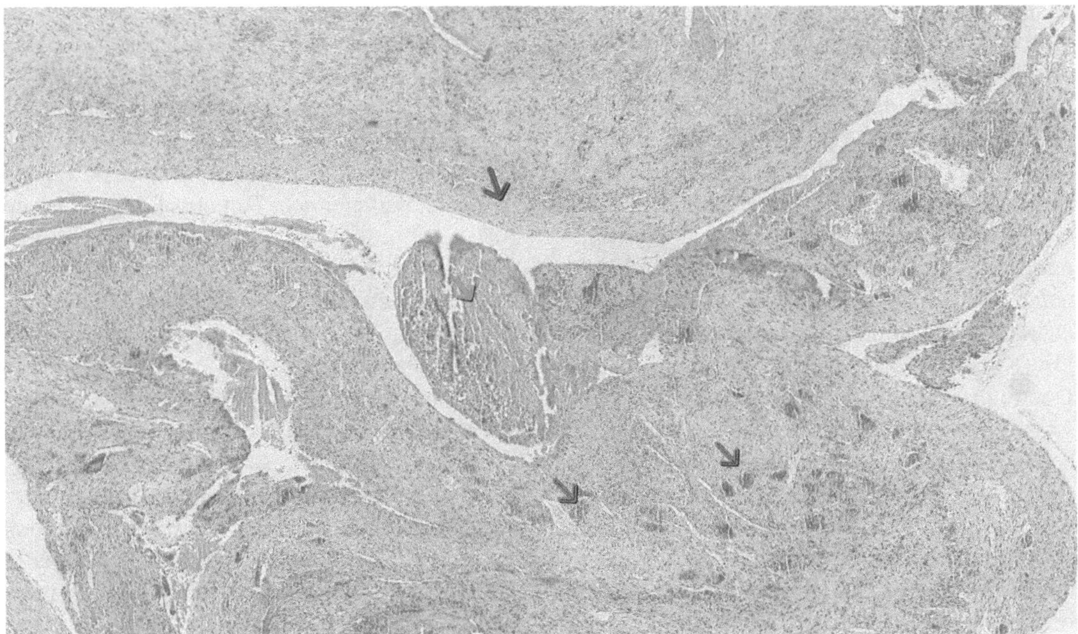

Fig. 3 Osteoid osteoma. Dense calcified, non-lamellar bone tissue separated by interstitial tissue, containing osteoblastic cells (blue arrow) and few osteoclastic cells (red arrow), H&E

cated in the characteristic pain syndrome of osteoid osteoma and may explain the exquisite sensitivity to NSAIDs (WHO Classification of Tumours Editorial Board 2020).

In a smaller percentage of osteoblastoma cases, FOSB rearrangement has been detected. Whole-genome DNA sequencing analysis performed in osteoblastomas shows diploid tumor cells with few other somatic alterations. Previously, karyotypic abnormalities such as rearrangement of chromosome 13 and deletions on chromosome 22 have been reported; these activate the WNT/β-catenin signaling pathway (WHO Classification of Tumours Editorial Board 2020).

The pathological, genetic, and molecular biology analyses of osteoid osteomas and osteoblastomas demonstrate their unique characteristics while also highlighting a shared genetic etiology indicative of these osteogenic tumors. The study of their genetic and molecular biology sheds light on the oncogenetic mechanisms of these tumors. This knowledge is critical for developing more effective diagnostic and therapeutic strategies. Specifically, both tumors exhibit novel histomorphological and immunohistochemical features, including areas of lesional non-osteoblastic stroma and presence of scattered large cells with smudged/degenerate nuclei. These shared features question the rationale behind their separate classification and suggest a common pathogenetic origin, despite their clinical and radiological differences. Additionally, the identification of FOS gene rearrangement and significant expression of c-FOS in these tumors underscores their distinct yet related nature, assisting in differentiating them from osteosarcomas for diagnostic purposes (Amary et al. 2019).

2.2.5 Vertebral Hemangioma

2.2.5.1 Pathology

Hemangiomas, predominantly found in the vertebral column, are benign vasoformative neoplasms characterized by the proliferation of vascular channels of varying calibers within the bone (WHO Classification of Tumours Editorial Board 2020; Cocco et al. 2018; Acosta et al. 2006).

Histologically, they exhibit a range of features with capillary and cavernous hemangiomas being composed of thin-walled, blood-filled vessels lined by a single layer of flat, cytologically banal endothelial cells (WHO Classification of Tumours Editorial Board 2020). These vessels intricately permeate the marrow and surround preexisting trabeculae. In vertebral hemangiomas, they consist of a collection of irregular vascular spaces lined by bland endothelial cells and can manifest capillary, cavernous, or venous origin (Kim et al. 2009; Van Goethem et al. 2004). Due to the tumor's presence, there is a tendency for the bone trabeculae to thicken because of some level of destruction caused by the tumor (Van Goethem et al. 2004). Macroscopically, hemangiomas appear as soft, well-demarcated, dark-red masses, sometimes displaying a honeycomb appearance due to intralesional sclerotic bone trabeculae and scattered blood-filled cavities (WHO Classification of Tumours Editorial Board 2020). Radiologically, the thickened vertical trabeculae of hemangiomas cause parallel linear densities described as having a "jail bar" or "corduroy" appearance or may show lytic foci with honeycomb trabeculations (Kim et al. 2009; Cocco et al. 2018). The immunohistochemical profile of hemangiomas is also distinct, with reactive new bone formation being prominent and the tumor cells staining for endothelial markers such as CD31, ERG, FLI1, CD34, and factor VIII-related antigen, emphasizing their vascular nature (WHO Classification of Tumours Editorial Board 2020).

2.2.5.2 Genetics and Molecular Biology

Despite their benign nature, hemangiomas have shown some genetic underpinnings. A fusion gene EWSR2-NFATC1 due to the translocation t(18;22)(q23;q12) has been reported in one case, hinting at a potential genetic aspect related to the development of this benign tumor (Cocco et al. 2018). In terms of molecular biology, the complete understanding surrounding hemangiomas is yet to be fully elucidated. The reported fusion gene EWSR2-NFATC1 is a molecular aspect that has come to light (Cocco et al. 2018). However, no consistent chromosomal changes have been identified, which leaves a considerable gap in understanding the complete molecular biology underpinning hemangiomas (Cocco et al. 2018). This gap extends to the unclear etiology and pathogenesis of hemangiomas, which have both developmental and neoplastic origins postulated (WHO Classification of Tumours Editorial Board 2020).

2.2.6 Aneurysmal Bone Cyst (ABC)

2.2.6.1 Pathology

Aneurysmal bone cysts (ABCs) are benign osseous neoplasms, distinguished by their multiloculated blood-filled spaces. These cysts frequently occur in the metaphyseal regions of long bones and can affect the posterior elements of vertebral bodies. Patients with ABCs typically experience pain and swelling, and vertebral involvement may lead to neurological deficits due to nerve or spinal cord compression (WHO Classification of Tumours Editorial Board 2020).

Histologically, ABCs are well circumscribed, featuring blood-filled cystic spaces. These spaces are separated by fibrous septa populated by fibroblasts and multinucleated osteoclast-type giant cells, alongside reactive woven bone (Fig. 4). The fibrous septa often shape the contours of the woven bone, which is sometimes basophilic, known as "blue bone." The cellular components within these septa, while dense and mitotically active, do not exhibit atypical features, aligning with the benign nature of ABCs (WHO Classification of Tumours Editorial Board 2020). On morphology, ABCs can mimic giant cell tumor, especially in cases of numerous giant cells. In these instances, the clinical image along with immunohistochemistry and the molecular analysis can help in the right diagnosis.

2.2.6.2 Genetics and Molecular Biology

On a molecular level, ABCs harbor cytogenetic rearrangements in the USP6 gene, located at chromosome band 17p13.2. The most prevalent rearrangement is the translocation t(16;17)(q22;p13), leading to upregulation of USP6 transcription. Such rearrangements, found in about 70% of ABCs, are not associated with any dis-

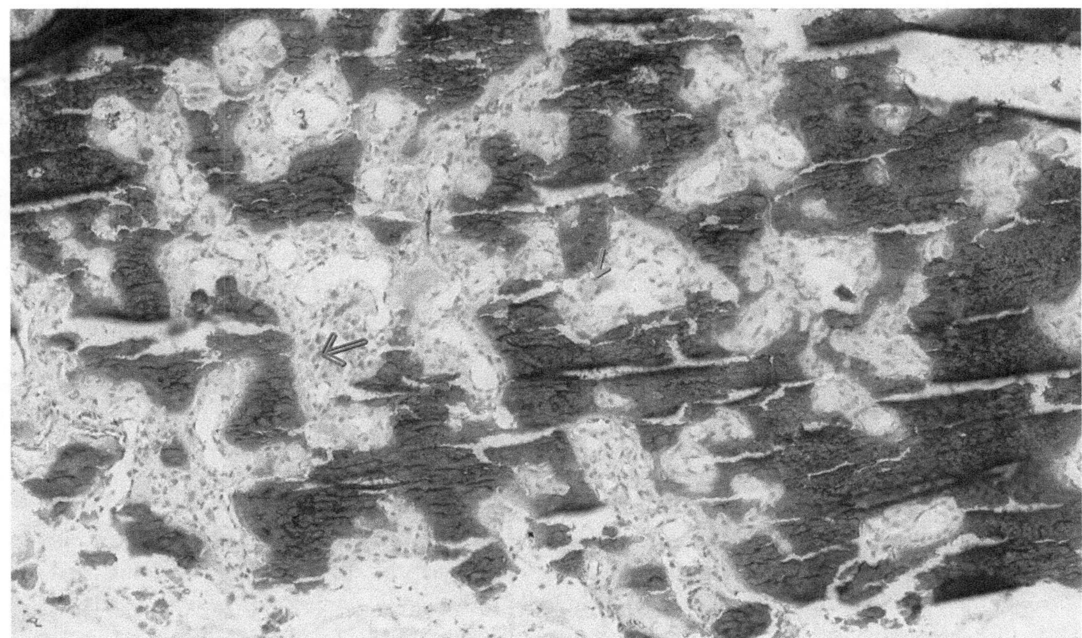

Fig. 4 Aneurysmal bone cyst (ABC). Fibrous wall (blue arrow), presence of giant cells (red arrow), and hemorrhage (green arrow), H&E

tinct biological behavior. The neoplastic component of ABCs, characterized by USP6 rearrangements, comprises a spindle cell population indistinguishable from normal fibroblasts and myofibroblasts. The other cellular elements within the cyst, such as inflammatory and endothelial cells, do not show USP6 rearrangements, suggesting their reactive nature (WHO Classification of Tumours Editorial Board 2020).

Detection of the USP6 gene rearrangement, which is essential for the diagnosis of ABC, can be achieved using fluorescence in situ hybridization (FISH). This test confirms the presence of the rearrangement, even though the percentage of affected cells may be low (WHO Classification of Tumours Editorial Board 2020).

2.2.7 Chondromyxoid Fibroma

Chondromyxoid fibroma (CMF) is a benign lobulated cartilaginous neoplasm exhibiting a distinct zonal architecture comprising chondroid, myxoid, and myofibroblastic areas (WHO Classification of Tumours Editorial Board 2020). This neoplasm mostly occurs in the long bones, particularly the proximal tibia and distal femur.

2.2.7.1 Pathology

The histopathological hallmarks of CMF are sharply demarcated lobules of tumor tissue from the surrounding bone. These lobules manifest a characteristic pattern with stellate or spindle-shaped cells in a myxoid background. The centers of the lobules closely resemble hyaline cartilage both in extracellular matrix and cell composition. Unique features like hypocellular centers, hypercellular peripheries, and sometimes calcification, predominantly in older patients and in flat-bone tumors, are noted. Hyaline cartilage is found in about 19% of cases. Occasionally, microscopic cystic or liquefactive changes are evident. The morphology sometimes presents challenges in differential diagnosis with high-grade central chondrosarcoma, although the clinicoradiological features and histology are quite distinct between these entities (WHO Classification of Tumours Editorial Board 2020).

2.2.7.2 Genetics and Molecular Biology

The pathogenesis of CMF is primarily driven by a series of genetic events involving the glutamate receptor gene GRM1. The recombination of GRM1 with various 5′ partner genes through promoter swapping and gene fusion events leads to the upregulated expression of transcripts encompassing the entire GRM1 coding region. This upregulation is highly specific to CMF, distinguishing it from other cartilaginous neoplasms. These genetic alterations are brought about by complex rearrangement processes, predominantly chromoplexy, but also chromothripsis. However, it is noted that around 10% of CMF cases do not exhibit upregulated GRM1 expression, suggesting that a different genetic pathway may be operative in this subset of tumors (WHO Classification of Tumours Editorial Board 2020).

On a molecular level, the immunohistochemistry of CMF reflects its cartilaginous nature through immunopositivity for S100. The ultrastructural features observed under electron microscopy reveal the stellate cells having irregular cell processes, scalloped cell membranes, cytoplasmic fibrils, and glycogen, exhibiting features of both chondroblastic and fibroblastic differentiation. Cells with classic features of chondrocytes, those with myofibroblastic features, and intermediate forms are described in CMF (WHO Classification of Tumours Editorial Board 2020).

In selected cases, the exceedingly specific upregulation of GRM1 expression in CMF can serve as a strong diagnostic adjunct, aiding in distinguishing this entity from its mimics. Nonetheless, molecular analysis is generally not deemed necessary for diagnosis (WHO Classification of Tumours Editorial Board 2020).

The amalgam of distinct pathological features, coupled with the underlying genetic and molecular mechanisms, plays a pivotal role in understanding, diagnosing, and managing CMF. Despite its benign nature, the elucidation of its pathogenetic mechanisms can significantly contribute to the precision in diagnosis and the effectiveness in treatment, fostering better clinical outcomes especially in cases where local recurrence occurs (WHO Classification of Tumours Editorial Board 2020).

2.2.8 Hibernoma

Hibernoma of bone is a rare benign adipocytic tumor characterized by brown fat differentiation, affecting the spine in 58% of cases (WHO Classification of Tumours Editorial Board 2020; Myslicki et al. 2019). The mean age at presentation is 59 years with female predominance (Myslicki et al. 2019). Hibernoma of bone is usually asymptomatic and detected incidentally (WHO Classification of Tumours Editorial Board 2020; Myslicki et al. 2019).

2.2.8.1 Pathology

The histopathological features of hibernomas include a rich capillary network and the presence of eosinophilic and pale, polygonal, multivacuolated, granular, brown fat cells, with a variable component of univacuolated white fat. The nuclei of the brown fat cells are small, round, centrally located with small nucleoli. Classic hibernomas contain more than 70% brown fat, with lipoma-like subtypes containing more white fat. There is no nuclear atypia or mitotic activity observed. The gross appearance of hibernomas is well circumscribed and vaguely lobular and ranges in color from brown to yellow (WHO Classification of Tumours Editorial Board 2020). These pathological characteristics are essential diagnostic criteria for identifying hibernomas, which are entirely benign and typically do not recur post-local excision (WHO Classification of Tumours Editorial Board 2020; Um et al. 2020).

2.2.8.2 Genetics and Molecular Biology

Cytogenetically, almost all hibernomas exhibit breakpoints in chromosome arm 11q, particularly clustering to 11q13. Various analyses have revealed complex genomic rearrangements involving translocations and interstitial deletions affecting both homologues of chromosome 11. These rearrangements result in deletions clustered to a 3 Mb region in 11q13, covering the tumor suppressor genes MEN1 and AIP. However, no somatic single-nucleotide variants in MEN1 and AIP have been detected in hibernoma. Hibernomas strongly express the brown fat marker gene UCP1, but there is no detected rearrangement, amplification, or increased expression of HMGA2, CDK4, or MDM2 (WHO Classification of Tumours Editorial Board 2020).

In addition to the molecular features, there is an observed association of hibernomas with multiple endocrine neoplasia type 1 (MEN1) (WHO Classification of Tumours Editorial Board 2020). Moreover, the imaging features observed from MRI and FDG PET, particularly the metabolic activity shown in FDG PET, further underline the molecular and metabolic activity of brown fat in hibernoma (WHO Classification of Tumours Editorial Board 2020).

The complex genomic rearrangements and the expression of the brown fat marker gene UCP1 indicate a sophisticated molecular biology underlying hibernoma, which along with its distinct pathological features contributes to its identification and understanding. The involvement of chromosome 11q and the expression of particular genes further hint at the genetic aspect of hibernoma. Although hibernomas are benign lesions, diagnosis on morphology can be challenging, especially in differentiating these tumors from other (malignant) entities. Knowledge of the molecular mechanism behind hibernomas will lead to accurate diagnosis and ultimately appropriate management of the lesion.

2.3 Malignant Tumors

2.3.1 Osteosarcoma

2.3.1.1 Pathology

Osteosarcoma, though primarily seen in the appendicular skeleton, can occasionally manifest in the vertebral column, accounting for less than 5% of all osteosarcomas. It typically presents as a large intramedullary mass, often with a destructive and permeative growth pattern, replacing marrow space and encasing preexisting trabeculae (WHO Classification of Tumours Editorial Board 2020). Histologically, osteosarcoma is a high-grade spindle cell neoplasm that forms osteoid (Fig. 5) and often has associated giant cells. The nature of the matrix can vary, leading to subtypes such as osteoblastic, fibroblastic, and chondroblastic osteosarcomas (Kim et al. 2009). Other subtypes like telangiectatic aneurysmal osteosarcoma (TAEOS) and small cell osteosarcoma (SCOS) have distinct histopathological features (WHO Classification of Tumours Editorial Board 2020).

2.3.1.2 Genetics and Molecular Biology

The genetic underpinnings of osteosarcoma encompass a broad spectrum of alterations. Although the etiology remains elusive, an increased incidence is noted in individuals with certain genetic syndromes like Li–Fraumeni syndrome and hereditary retinoblastoma due to inactivation of TP53 and RB1 genes, respectively (WHO Classification of Tumours Editorial Board 2020). Germline mutations in RECQ helicases have been associated with conventional osteosarcoma (COS) (WHO Classification of Tumours Editorial Board 2020).

Osteosarcoma is marked by complex chromosomal aneuploidy and significant intertumoral and intratumoral heterogeneity, attributed to chromosomal instability (WHO Classification of Tumours Editorial Board 2020). Key genomic alterations include amplifications in certain chromosome arms like 6p, 8q, and 17p, housing critical genes such as RUNX2, VEGFA, MYC, and CDC5L. TP53 antagonist MDM2 is amplified in about 10% of cases, suggesting a potential evolutionary pathway for the disease (WHO Classification of Tumours Editorial Board 2020).

The phenomenon of chromoanagenesis, encompassing chromothripsis and chromoplexy, leads to massive and chaotic chromosomal alterations through single catastrophic events (WHO Classification of Tumours Editorial Board 2020). Sequencing studies have identified chromoanagenesis as the molecular mechanism initiating chromosomal complexity in more than 90% of conventional osteosarcoma cases, with inactivating mutations of TP53 proposed as a potential trigger (WHO Classification of Tumours Editorial Board 2020).

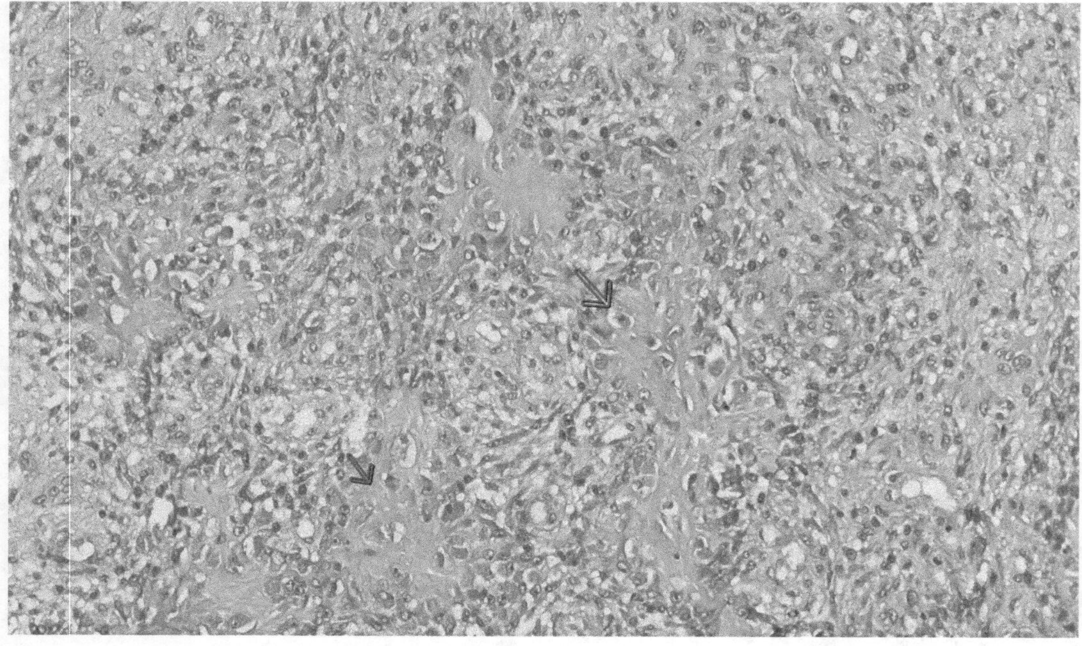

Fig. 5 Conventional osteosarcoma. Strong atypical, undifferentiated cells and immature bone (blue arrows), H&E

The molecular biology further identifies various driver genes, somatic alterations, and gene expression profiling, which have provided insights into the tumorigenesis and potential therapeutic targets. For instance, the hypermethylation of certain genes and the association of macrophage expression profiles with lack of metastases have been reported, indicating the intricate interplay of genetic and epigenetic factors in osteosarcoma pathology (WHO Classification of Tumours Editorial Board 2020).

2.3.2 Ewing's Sarcoma

2.3.2.1 Pathology

Histologically, ES consists mainly of uniform small round cells with round nuclei containing finely stippled chromatin and inconspicuous nucleoli, scant clear or eosinophilic cytoplasm, and indistinct cytoplasmic membranes, known as classic Ewing's sarcoma (Fig. 6). At times, cells may be larger with prominent nucleoli and irregular contours, referred to as atypical Ewing's sarcoma (WHO Classification of Tumours Editorial Board 2020). Previously, a higher degree of neuroectodermal differentiation was termed as primitive neuroectodermal tumor (WHO Classification of Tumours Editorial Board 2020). Immunohistochemically, about 95% of ES cases show strong, diffuse membranous expression of CD99, a cell surface glycoprotein, which is a relevant diagnostic marker. Other markers like NKX2-2, FLI1, and ERG are often expressed in cases with corresponding gene fusions. Some cases may also exhibit expression of neuroendocrine antigens and/or S100 (WHO Classification of Tumours Editorial Board 2020).

2.3.2.2 Genetics and Molecular Biology

The quintessential genetic characteristic of ES is chromosomal translocation t(11;22)(q24;q12), resulting in the EWSR1-FLI1 fusion transcript and protein, found in approximately 85% of cases. The second most common translocation is t(21;22)(q22;q12), culminating in EWSR1-ERG fusion in about 10% of cases. These translocations form FET-ETS fusion genes, pivotal in ES pathogenesis. These fusion genes encode chimeric transcription factors that serve as master regulators, activating and repressing thousands of

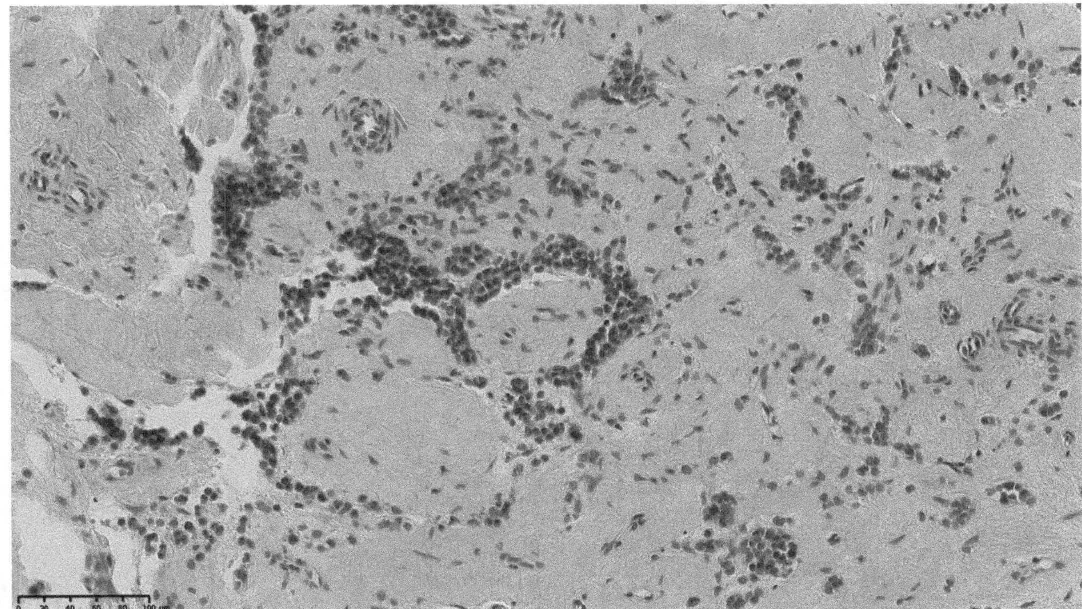

Fig. 6 Ewing's sarcoma. The lesion typically consists of small blue round cells. The cells have this characteristic color because of the hyperchromatic nucleus and the very limited, almost indistinguishable cytoplasm, H&E

genes (WHO Classification of Tumours Editorial Board 2020). The fusion proteins bind both GGAA microsatellites and canonical ETS-binding sites in the genome, establishing an oncogenic gene expression program underlying transformation and tumor initiation (WHO Classification of Tumours Editorial Board 2020).

2.3.3 Chondrosarcoma

2.3.3.1 Pathology

Chondrosarcomas (CSs) are a diverse group of malignant bone tumors characterized by the production of cartilage matrix by the tumor cells. They are categorized into several subtypes based on histological characteristics and location, including conventional, dedifferentiated, clear cell, and mesenchymal chondrosarcoma.

Primary chondrosarcomas, especially those of the mobile spine, are rare lesions. Two reviews documented 22 and 21 patients from two institutions (Instituto Rizzoli and University of Texas MD Anderson Cancer Center) over 59 and 43 years, respectively (Kim et al. 2009). Histologically, grade I chondrosarcomas are mild to moderately cellular neoplasms comprising neoplastic chondrocytes within lacunae in a chondroid matrix. With increasing grade, there is greater nuclear atypia (Fig. 7), cellularity, and often necrosis. A coexistent spindled morphologic pattern suggests a diagnosis of another more highly malignant tumor, like dedifferentiated chondrosarcoma (Kim et al. 2009). The histologic differential of low-grade chondrosarcomas includes chordoma, with immunohistochemical staining differentiating between the lesions; chondrosarcomas demonstrate immunoreactivity for S100 protein but not keratin, whereas chordomas are immunoreactive for both (Kim et al. 2009).

2.3.3.2 Genetics and Molecular Biology

The molecular and genetic underpinning of chondrosarcoma is complex, involving several mutations and molecular pathways:

1. *IDH1* and *IDH2* mutations: Common in conventional and dedifferentiated chondrosarcomas, these mutations lead to the production of 2-hydroxyglutarate, contributing to malignant

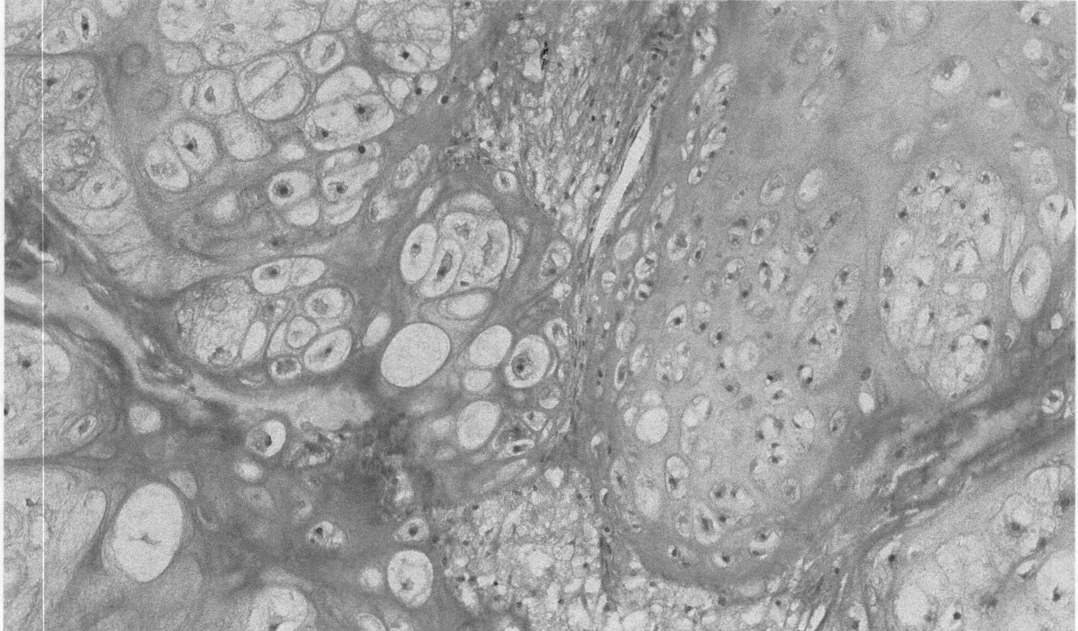

Fig. 7 Chondrosarcoma. Cartilage matrix wherein are embedded cells with variable sizes. The cells have a perinuclear halo, called lacuna. Usually, the cellularity increases by higher grade, H&E

cartilaginous matrix formation. These mutations could also be used as prognostic biomarkers for the prediction of patient outcome and the design of appropriate treatment plans (Vuong et al. 2021).

2. *EXT1* and *EXT2* mutations: These mutations predispose individuals to developing secondary peripheral chondrosarcoma, especially in cases of hereditary multiple exostoses (Wuyts et al. 1998).
3. *TP53* and *CDKN2A* mutations: Common in high-grade or dedifferentiated chondrosarcoma, these mutations result in a loss of function of tumor suppressor genes (Cross et al. 2022).
4. Collagen *COL2A1* mutations: These mutations are associated with chondrosarcoma formation, particularly during skeletal development and endochondral ossification (Tarpey et al. 2013).

Moreover, molecular pathways like Hedgehog signaling, essential for chondrocyte differentiation, are implicated in chondrosarcoma pathogenesis. Dysregulation of other pathways, including Wnt/β-catenin and growth factor signaling pathways like TGF-β and IGF, also plays significant roles in chondrosarcoma development and progression. Additionally, epigenetic changes, such as DNA methylation and histone modifications, have been associated with chondrosarcoma. Understanding these genetic and molecular aspects is critical as it provides a basis for targeted therapy approaches, moving toward better management and treatment of chondrosarcoma (WHO Classification of Tumours Editorial Board 2020).

2.3.4 Chordoma

2.3.4.1 Pathology

Chordoma is a malignancy that usually manifests in the axial skeleton, portraying a phenotype reminiscent of the notochord. Pathologically, conventional chordomas comprise large epithelioid cells with either clear or light eosinophilic cytoplasm. These cells, often referred to as physaliphorous cells (Fig. 8), are organized in lobules

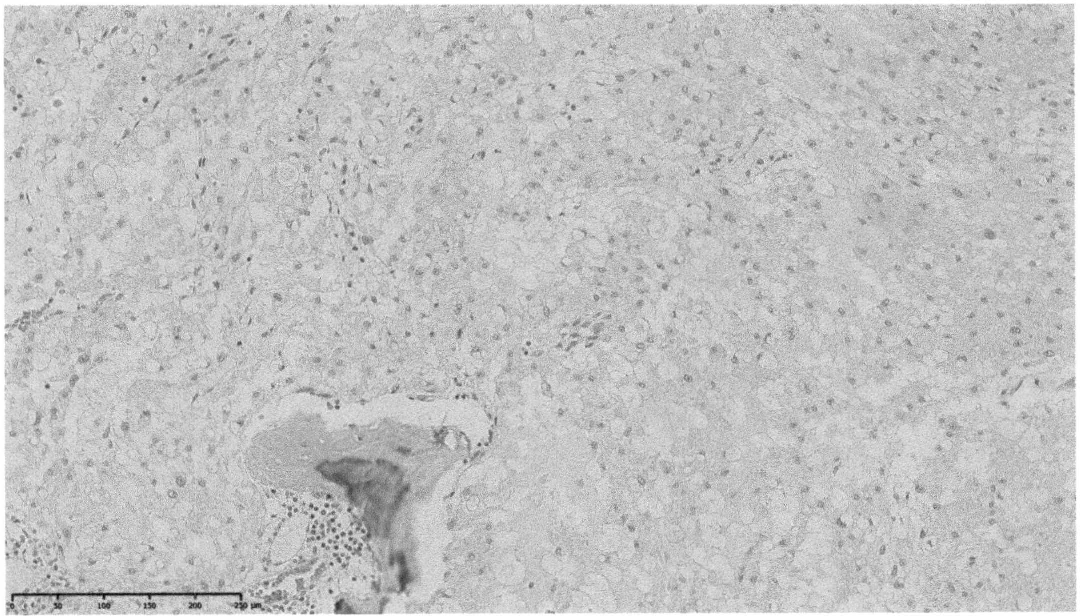

Fig. 8 Chordoma. Typically, large cells with light eosinophilic to clear cytoplasm, called physaliphorous cells, H&E

separated by fibrous septa. They may appear in cords and nests embedded within an extracellular myxoid matrix. The tumor often exhibits a substantial degree of intratumoral cytological heterogeneity, displaying features such as nuclear atypia and pleomorphism. The term "chondroid chordoma" is designated when a substantial area of the matrix mimics hyaline cartilaginous tumors (WHO Classification of Tumours Editorial Board 2020). Immunohistochemically, the tumor cells are diffusely immunoreactive for cytokeratin and EMA, with a variable positivity for S100. Still, the most specific immunohistochemical marker is the brachyury (Sangoi 2011) (Fig. 9). The diagnostic hallmark is the expression of brachyury, which helps to differentiate chordoma from other tumors like chondrosarcoma, carcinoma, and chordoid meningioma (WHO Classification of Tumours Editorial Board 2020).

2.3.4.2 Genetics and Molecular Biology

On a genetic and molecular basis, chordoma is characterized by the expression of brachyury, encoded by the TBXT gene. In approximately 27% of cases, this expression is correlated with a copy number gain of TBXT, a transcription factor crucial for notochordal development. The strong association of the SNP rs2305089 in TBXT with chordoma patients suggests a significant contribution to the tumor's development. Brachyury has also been identified as a master regulator of an oncogenic transcriptional network, impacting diverse signaling pathways including components of the cell cycle and extracellular matrix. Furthermore, silencing of TBXT in chordoma cell lines leads to growth arrest and senescence, highlighting the critical role of TBXT in chordoma pathology. Additionally, mutations in the PI3K signaling pathway have been reported in 16% of cases, while mutations (always inactivating) of LYST have been described in 10% of cases. EGFR (HER1) also appears to play a significant role in chordoma, with its inhibition reducing cell survival. In rare instances, chordoma has been associated with a germline tandem duplication of TBXT, and some rare cases of childhood chordoma occur in the setting of tuberous sclerosis, triggered by germline loss-of-function mutations in the tumor suppressor gene TSC1 or TSC2 (WHO Classification of Tumours Editorial Board 2020).

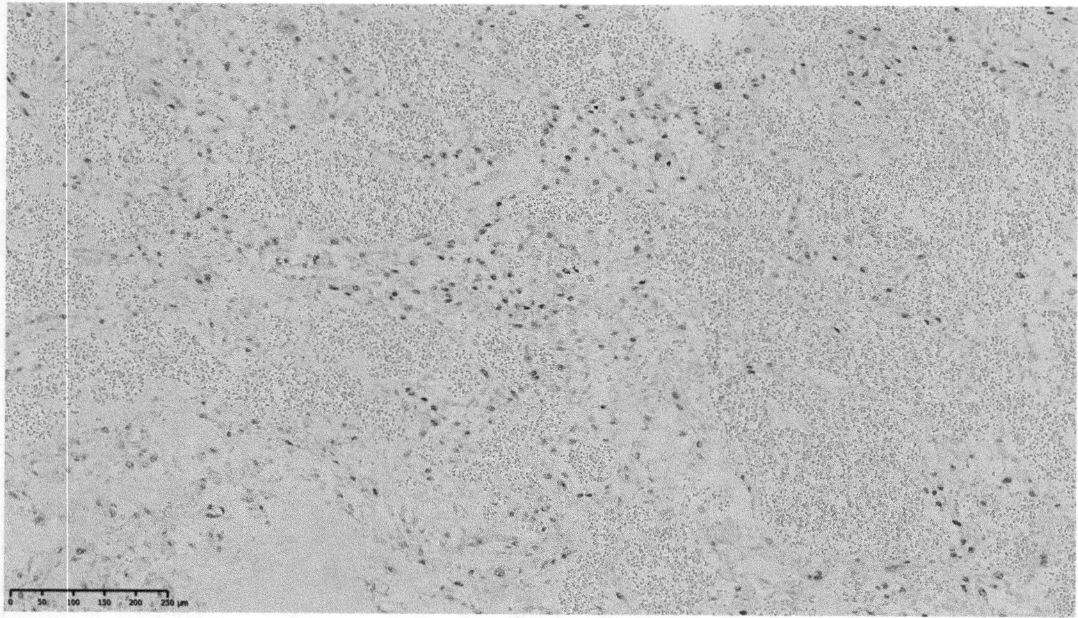

Fig. 9 Chordoma. Brachyury is typically expressed in chordomas showing a nuclear expression in the neoplastic cells. Brachyury, DAB

2.3.5 Undifferentiated Pleomorphic Sarcoma (Malignant Fibrous Histiocytoma)

2.3.5.1 Pathology

Undifferentiated pleomorphic sarcoma (UPS), formerly called malignant fibrous histiocytoma (MFH), is particularly rare in spinal location. The histological presentation of UPS is diverse, with four subtypes described, the most common being storiform-pleomorphic UPS. Histologically, UPS is a pleomorphic tumor chiefly comprised of pleomorphic mesenchymal cells arranged in a storiform pattern. These cells display notable atypia with the presence of giant cells and fibroblastic cells, alongside frequent mitosis, indicative of an active cell division process, which is a hallmark of malignancy (Kim et al. 2009).

Radiologically, osseous UPS exhibits aggressive characteristics such as bone lysis and a permeative or moth-eaten pattern on plain radiographic and CT findings. Moreover, on MRI, a low signal on T2-weighted images and intermediate signal intensity on T1-weighted images are observed (Kim et al. 2009).

2.3.5.2 Genetics and Molecular Biology

The exact genetic and molecular underpinnings of UPS remain to be fully elucidated. However, regarding the so-called MFH, it is posited that these tumors could originate from primitive mesenchymal cells capable of multidirectional differentiation, implying a level of cellular plasticity that might be underlined by genetic or molecular factors (Kim et al. 2009).

The ambiguity surrounding whether UPS represents a homogeneous entity or a collection of diverse types of sarcomas suggests a complex genetic and molecular background. The multidirectional differentiation potential of the implicated primitive mesenchymal cells hints at a sophisticated interplay of molecular signaling pathways and genetic controls that govern cellular differentiation and proliferation in UPS.

The diversity in histologic subtypes and the pleomorphic nature of the tumor cells in UPS further underscore the likelihood of complex genetic and molecular interactions contributing to the pathology of these tumors. There are some reports of USPs with H3-3A (H3F3A) or H3-3B (H3F3B) p.Gly34 mutation (Ogura et al. 2017).

This may indicate an association with giant cell tumor of the bone. Understanding these molecular and genetic bases could be pivotal for the development of targeted therapeutic strategies and better diagnostic tools for USP.

2.3.6 Fibrosarcoma

2.3.6.1 Pathology

Fibrosarcoma of bone is a rare spindle cell malignant neoplasm, which exhibits relatively monomorphic fibroblastic tumor cells and a characteristic fascicular, often herringbone, architecture (WHO Classification of Tumours Editorial Board 2020). It is typically associated with the bone, but can also occur in soft tissue, primarily within the deep musculature and often associated with adjacent fascia or periosteum (Kim et al. 2009). The most common clinical manifestations include local pain, swelling, limitation of motion, and pathological fractures. Radiologically, fibrosarcoma presents as eccentrically located, lytic lesions exhibiting a geographical, moth-eaten, or permeative pattern of destruction with frequent extension into surrounding soft tissues (WHO Classification of Tumours Editorial Board 2020). Histologically, it is recognized for its variability among malignant mesenchymal tumors. The tumor cells in fibrosarcoma of bone are described as polygonal cells arranged in a herringbone pattern, surrounded by dense collagenous stroma, infiltrating into surrounding cortical lamellar bone (Kim et al. 2009). This neoplasm requires a careful diagnostic approach as its histopathological features can be seen in a variety of bone tumors, making fibrosarcoma a diagnosis of exclusion (WHO Classification of Tumours Editorial Board 2020).

2.3.6.2 Genetics and Molecular Biology

The genetic landscape of fibrosarcoma is not well elucidated. However, some studies have indicated a high number of genomic imbalances, with common losses and gains in specific chromosomal regions. Notably, homozygous deletion of CDKN2A (Niini et al. 2010) and deletions in STARD13 were observed. A rare yet significant finding is a novel STRN-NTRK3 gene fusion in cases of primary fibrosarcoma of the radius, hinting at potential therapeutic avenues targeting NTRK (WHO Classification of Tumours Editorial Board 2020). Molecular genetics plays a pivotal role in the diagnostic process, helping to exclude tumor-specific aberrations and thus aiding in an accurate diagnosis (WHO Classification of Tumours Editorial Board 2020; Cocco et al. 2018). The molecular complexity indicated by these genetic findings suggests a convoluted pathogenesis and underscores the importance of molecular diagnostics in accurately categorizing fibrosarcoma amidst a spectrum of spindle cell neoplasms of bone and soft tissue (WHO Classification of Tumours Editorial Board 2020; Kim et al. 2009).

Both fibrosarcoma of bone and soft tissue reflect a complex interplay of pathological and molecular biological factors. The diagnostic challenge posed by its histopathological similarity to other neoplasms underscores the importance of advancing our understanding of its molecular biology to develop more precise diagnostic criteria and potentially unveil novel therapeutic targets.

2.4 Hematopoietic Neoplasms of the Spine

2.4.1 Solitary Bone Plasmacytoma

2.4.1.1 Pathology

Solitary bone plasmacytoma (SBP) is a localized intra-osseous neoplasm composed of clonal plasma cells, with no evidence of other bony lesions or plasma cell myeloma (PCM) (WHO Classification of Tumours Editorial Board 2020). This condition often manifests in the sixth decade of life, with a male predominance (Kim et al. 2009). Patients typically present with localized pain, and sometimes fractures, especially in cases of vertebral SBP, which can lead to spinal cord compression (WHO Classification of Tumours Editorial Board 2020). Histologically, SBP displays a monotonous collection of neoplastic plasma cells with various features including eccentric, round, moderately pleomorphic nuclei, alongside rich basophilic cytoplasm (Kim et al. 2009). In more detailed histopathological examination, SPB may exhibit sheets of neoplastic plasma cells, which could range from small and mature to enlarged, immature, and atypical. Rare occurrences of anaplastic morphology, amyloid deposition, and crystal-storing histiocytosis have also been noted (WHO Classification of Tumours Editorial Board 2020).

2.4.1.2 Genetics and Molecular Biology

The genetic and cytogenetic landscape of SBP is heterogeneous, resembling changes observed in PCM. Key features include clonal rearrangement of immunoglobulin (Ig) heavy- and light-chain genes, with a heavy load of mutations in the variable region of the Ig heavy-chain gene. Complex karyotypes are common in SBP, and FISH has been identified as a more sensitive technique for detecting cytogenetic abnormalities compared to routine karyotyping (WHO Classification of Tumours Editorial Board 2020). Diagnostic molecular pathology outlines the rearrangement of Ig heavy- and light-chain genes as a characteristic feature of SBP (WHO Classification of Tumours Editorial Board 2020). While the etiology remains unknown, the pathogenesis of SBP appears closely tied to genetic and cytogenetic abnormalities, with a significant emphasis on the clonal nature of plasma cells involved in the disease (WHO Classification of Tumours Editorial Board 2020). The genetic and molecular underpinnings of SBP provide an avenue for better understanding the pathology and potentially developing targeted therapeutic strategies for managing this rare disease.

2.4.2 Primary Spinal Lymphoma

Lymphomas are a heterogeneous group of malignancies of the lymphatic system, with two primary types being Hodgkin's lymphoma (HL) and non-Hodgkin's lymphoma (NHL). When lymphomas involve the osseous spine, they are often classified as primary bone lymphomas (PBLs), a rare condition constituting less than 5% of primary bone tumors (Sundaresan et al. 2009).

2.4.2.1 Pathology

The pathology of lymphoma in the osseous spine is characterized by the proliferation of lymphoid cells, which may lead to bone destruction and spinal complications. The tumor cells can infiltrate the bone marrow, erode the bone matrix, and potentially extend into the surrounding soft tissues and spinal canal. Imaging modalities like MRI and CT are useful in evaluating the extent of bone and soft tissue involvement. Histologically, the tumor cells in lymphomas can resemble normal lymphocytes but are usually larger with distinct nucleoli and a moderate amount of cytoplasm (Kim et al. 2009).

2.4.2.2 Genetics and Molecular Biology

The genetic underpinnings of lymphomas are complex with many subtypes having characteristic genetic alterations. For instance, B-cell lymphomas often harbor translocations involving the immunoglobulin heavy-chain locus, while T-cell lymphomas frequently have alterations in the T-cell receptor genes. Moreover, various genetic mutations and translocations have been associated with different subtypes of lymphomas, which play crucial roles in the pathogenesis and progression of the disease (Kim et al. 2009).

On a molecular level, lymphomas exhibit a range of abnormalities that contribute to their pathogenesis. These abnormalities may include overexpression of oncogenes, under-expression or deletion of tumor suppressor genes, and dysregulation of various signaling pathways. Additionally, epigenetic alterations and aberrant microRNA expression are also known to play significant roles in lymphomagenesis (Kim et al. 2009).

Mature B- and T-cell lymphomas, which could involve the osseous spine, are diverse in their biology and etiology, with distinctions in cell lineage and differentiation states. The molecular biology of these lymphomas often reflects the normal developmental biology of lymphocytes, with genetic lesions mimicking or exaggerating normal signaling events. Gene expression profiling has been crucial in understanding the biology of these lymphomas, revealing distinct molecular signatures associated with different stages of lymphocyte development, and in some instances, highlighting potential therapeutic targets (WHO Classification of Tumours Editorial Board 2020).

2.5 Bone Metastases

2.5.1 Pathology

Bone metastases occur when cancer cells spread from their primary location to bone through the bloodstream. These metastatic lesions can involve any bone but have a predilection for the axial skeleton and long bones, due to the higher blood flow in these regions (WHO Classification of Tumours Editorial Board 2020). The clinical presentation is typically pain, with pathological fractures often occurring. Radiographically, metastases may appear lytic, sclerotic, or mixed, depending on the type of primary cancer. Histologically, the metastases resemble the primary cancer, whether adenocarcinoma or squamous cell carcinoma, and are often accompanied by hemorrhage, fibrosis, and osteoclast-like giant cell reactions which can obscure the metastatic cells (WHO Classification of Tumours Editorial Board 2020).

2.5.2 Genetics and Molecular Biology

The molecular diagnostics of bone metastases depend on the primary tumor. Immunohistochemistry is instrumental in suggesting or confirming the primary origin, utilizing markers that are specific to the primary cancer (WHO Classification of Tumours Editorial Board 2020). The identification of metastatic cells can be supported by molecular diagnostics, which may provide diagnostic or prognostic insights. For instance, certain genetic alterations identified in the primary tumor can also be present in the metastatic lesions and can influence the prognosis and therapeutic response (WHO Classification of Tumours Editorial Board 2020). The survival rates for patients with bone metastases are largely dependent on the nature of the primary tumor, with some studies indicating a median survival of around 5.1 months for spinal metastases (WHO Classification of Tumours Editorial Board 2020).

3 Conclusion

The delineation between benign and malignant entities not only serves as a clinical guidepost but also underscores the nuanced approach required for the management of spinal tumors. Benign lesions, such as vertebral hemangiomas and osteogenic tumors like osteoid osteoma and osteoblastoma, present a clinical challenge in balancing intervention with the potential for morbidity associated with treatment, given their typically indolent behavior.

Malignant tumors, including lymphomas and chondrosarcomas, demand a more aggressive and nuanced approach, reflecting their complex genetic and molecular profiles that drive their pathogenesis. The genetic and molecular insights into these tumors, such as the EWSR1-FLI1 fusion in Ewing's sarcoma and the IDH mutations in chondrosarcomas, are pivotal in advancing diagnostic precision and therapeutic strategies. The role of molecular diagnostics is particularly emphasized, as it becomes increasingly clear that histopathological assessment alone may not suffice for the accurate categorization and prognostication.

4 Key Points

- Benign versus malignant differentiation: Understanding the distinction between benign and malignant spinal tumors is crucial for appropriate management and prognostication.
- Genetic insights: Genetic markers, such as the EWSR1-FLI1 fusion in Ewing's sarcoma, offer critical insights into tumor behavior and potential therapeutic targets.
- Molecular diagnostics: Advances in molecular diagnostics are essential for the precise classification of tumors, which may present similarly on histopathological examination.
- Collaborative approach: Effective patient care for spinal tumors requires a collaborative approach, integrating insights from pathology, genetics, and molecular biology with imaging features.
- Continued research: Ongoing research is imperative to refine classification systems and improve patient outcomes, reflecting the dynamic nature of tumor biology.

- Radiologists' role: Radiologists must integrate traditional imaging with emerging molecular diagnostic techniques to enhance the accuracy of diagnoses and contribute to personalized treatment plans.

Acknowledgments The images are made by scanned slides using the NDP viewer.

Special thanks to Professor Dr. Christine Galant, Pathology Department of Cliniques Universitaires Saint Luc/UCLouvain.

References

Acosta FL, Dowd CF, Chin C et al (2006) Current treatment strategies and outcomes in the management of symptomatic vertebral hemangiomas. Neurosurgery 58:287–295. https://doi.org/10.1227/01.NEU.0000194846.55984.C8

Amary F, Markert E, Berisha F et al (2019) FOS expression in osteoid osteoma and osteoblastoma. Am J Surg Pathol 43:1661–1667. https://doi.org/10.1097/PAS.0000000000001355

Charest-Morin R, Fisher CG, Sahgal A et al (2019) Primary bone tumor of the spine—an evolving field: what a general spine surgeon should know. Global Spine J 9:108S–116S

Cocco E, Scaltriti M, Drilon A (2018) NTRK fusion-positive cancers and TRK inhibitor therapy. Nat Rev Clin Oncol 15:731–747. https://doi.org/10.1038/s41571-018-0113-0

Cross W, Lyskjær I, Lesluyes T et al (2022) A genetic model for central chondrosarcoma evolution correlates with patient outcome. Genome Med 14:99. https://doi.org/10.1186/s13073-022-01084-0

Das JM, Hoang S, Mesfin FB (2023) Intramedullary spinal cord tumors. In: StatPearls. StatPearls Publishing, Treasure Island, FL

Kim DK, Chang UK, Kim SH, Bilsky MH (2009) Tumors of the spine. Am J Neuroradiol 30:E137. https://doi.org/10.3174/ajnr.A1719

Kumar N, Tan WLB, Wei W, Vellayappan BA (2020) An overview of the tumors affecting the spine—inside to out. Neurooncol Pract 7:I10–I17

Myslicki FA, Rosenberg AE, Chaitowitz I, Subhawong TK (2019) Intraosseous hibernoma: five cases and a review of the literature. J Comput Assist Tomogr 43(5):793–798. https://doi.org/10.1097/RCT.0000000000000912

Niini T, López-Guerrero JA, Ninomiya S et al (2010) Frequent deletion of CDKN2A and recurrent coamplification of KIT, PDGFRA, and KDR in fibrosarcoma of bone—an array comparative genomic hybridization study. Genes Chromosomes Cancer 49:132–143. https://doi.org/10.1002/gcc.20727

Ogura K, Hosoda F, Nakamura H et al (2017) Highly recurrent H3F3A mutations with additional epigenetic regulator alterations in giant cell tumor of bone. Genes Chromosomes Cancer 56:711–718. https://doi.org/10.1002/gcc.22469

Sangoi AR (2011) Specificity of brachyury in the distinction of chordoma from clear cell renal cell carcinoma and germ cell tumors: a study of 305 cases. Mod Pathol 24(3):425–429

Schaefer IM (2018) Immunohistochemistry for histone H3G34W and H3K36M is highly specific for giant cell tumor of bone and chondroblastoma, respectively, in FNA and core needle biopsy. Cancer Cytopathol 126(8):552–566. https://doi.org/10.1002/cncy.22000

Sundaresan N, Rosen G, Boriani S (2009) Primary malignant tumors of the spine. Orthop Clin N Am 40:21–36

Tarpey PS, Behjati S, Cooke SL et al (2013) Frequent mutation of the major cartilage collagen gene COL2A1 in chondrosarcoma. Nat Genet 45:923–926. https://doi.org/10.1038/ng.2668

Um M-K, Lee E, Lee JW et al (2020) Spinal intraosseous hibernoma: a case report and review of literature. J Korean Soc Radiol 81:965. https://doi.org/10.3348/jksr.2020.81.4.965

Van Goethem JWM, Van Den Hauwe L, Özsarlak Ö et al (2004) Spinal tumors. Eur J Radiol 50:159–176. https://doi.org/10.1016/j.ejrad.2003.10.021

Vuong HG, Ngo TNM, Dunn IF (2021) Prognostic importance of IDH mutations in chondrosarcoma: an individual patient data meta-analysis. Cancer Med 10:4415–4423. https://doi.org/10.1002/cam4.4019

WHO Classification of Tumours Editorial Board (2020) Soft tissue and bone tumours, 5th edn. International Agency for Research on Cancer, Lyon

Wuyts W, Van Hul W, De Boulle K et al (1998) Mutations in the EXT1 and EXT2 genes in hereditary multiple exostoses. Am J Hum Genet 62:346–354. https://doi.org/10.1086/301726

Part II

Basic Semiology, Imaging Modalities and Staging

Semiology of Primary Bone Tumors of the Spine Including Diagnostic Algorithm

Wiem Abid and Filip Vanhoenacker

Contents

W. Abid (✉)
Department of Radiology, University Hospital Brussel (Vrije Universiteit Brussel), Brussels, Belgium
e-mail: wiem.abid.pro@gmail.com

F. Vanhoenacker
General Hospital Sint-Maarten Mechelen, Mechelen, Belgium

Department of Radiology, University Hospital Antwerp, Edegem, Belgium

Faculty of Medicine and Health Sciences, University of Antwerp, Antwerp, Belgium

Faculty of Medicine and Health Sciences, University of Ghent, Ghent, Belgium

Faculty of Medicine, University of KU Leuven, Leuven, Belgium
e-mail: filip.vanhoenacker@telenet.be

Abstract

In this chapter, we present an overview of the clinical and radiologic semiology of the benign and malignant bone tumors of the osseous spine, and we propose an imaging algorithm using an analytical approach to facilitate the diagnosis.

Primary solitary osseous tumors of the spine are uncommon in comparison to metastases and myeloproliferative disorders such as multiple myeloma and lymphoma.

Many solitary primary lesions have characteristic radiologic features that help to make the diagnosis with confidence.

An analytic approach based on clinical information such as the age and the symptoms of the patient together with the radiologic semiology, the localization of the lesion within the spine segment and within the vertebra, and the multiplicity enables the radiologist to recognize tumors of the spine with characteristic features such as enostosis, osteoid osteoma, osteoblastoma, osteochondroma, chondrosarcoma, vertebral angioma, and aneurysmal bone cyst.

The differential diagnosis may include other primary spinal tumors, vertebral metastases, and tumor-like conditions mimicking a spinal tumor, such as Paget disease, spondylitis, aseptic osteitis, the unilateral arch hypertrophy, or microcrystalline arthropathies.

Conventional radiographs are the first step in the initial detection and characterization but

Med Radiol Diagn Imaging (2023)
https://doi.org/10.1007/174_2023_430,
Published Online: 31 May 2023

are limited because of the complex anatomy of the spine and superposition. CT and MRI are the imaging techniques of choice for further characterization, staging, and guiding biopsy.

The final diagnosis is based on the histopathological examination of the biopsy.

1 Introduction

Primary osseous tumors of the spine are uncommon lesions in comparison to metastases and myeloproliferative disorders such as multiple myeloma and lymphoma, accounting for only 3.4–9% of all primary skeletal neoplasms (Subbarao and Jacobson 1979; Masaryk 1991; Munday et al. 1994; Afshani and Kuhn 1991; Kozlowsi et al. 1984; Weinstein and McLain 1987; Levine et al. 1992; Bernard et al. 2013). Solitary bone lesions of the spine have a large differential diagnosis. Characterization of the lesions can be based on the age of the patient, the number of lesions, the location in the spinal segment, the location within the individual vertebra, the morphology, and the density or signal intensity with the enhancement pattern of the lesions on CT and MR, respectively (Khan and De Schepper 2007). In this chapter, we propose an imaging algorithm using an analytical approach to guide the radiologist to characterize osseous spine lesions with confidence and better accuracy. This is important to avoid unnecessary biopsies of benign lesions.

2 Characterization of Tumor or Tumor-Like Condition of the Osseous Spine

Characterization of tumor or tumor-like condition of the osseous spine is done by the analysis of multiple parameters, including non-imaging parameters and imaging parameters on different imaging modalities. It is of utmost importance that the radiologist considers the non-imaging parameters before he starts analyzing the imaging parameters.

2.1 Multiplicity

It is important to determine whether spinal lesions are solitary or multifocal as this may alter the differential diagnosis.

Bone metastases are the most common multiple lesions of the osseous spine (Fig. 1). Metastases of the osseous spine are the most common secondary to breast and lung cancers in women and prostate and lung cancers in men. Thirty percent of metastases are multifocal (Van Goethem et al. 2004). Lymphoproliferative lesions (multiple myeloma and lymphoma) are the most frequent multiple primary spinal tumors.

Benign lesions that may present as multifocal lesions are summarized in Table 1. Vertebral hemangiomas may be multiple in 25–30% of the cases (Ross et al. 1987; Orguc and Arkun 2014). Multiple dense bone islands aka enostosis may solitary or multiple. Multiplicity should raise the possibility of osteopoikilosis. Osteopathia striata rarely involves the spine and may manifest as multifocal streaks and stripes. Melorheostosis is another sclerosing bone disease that rarely involves the spine resulting with a typical dripping candle wax appearance (Orguc and Arkun 2014). Fibrous dysplasia and eosinophilic granuloma (EG), which need to be considered in children, are less commonly multifocal in the spine (Khan and De Schepper 2007).

2.2 Clinical Information

Age Age is one of the most important keys to the diagnosis because some tumors have a predilection for certain age groups (see chapter "Epidemiology").

Most primary bone tumors are seen in patients over 30 years of age. In this group of age, they are frequently malignant except for vertebral hemangiomas and bone islands. Metastases and myeloma

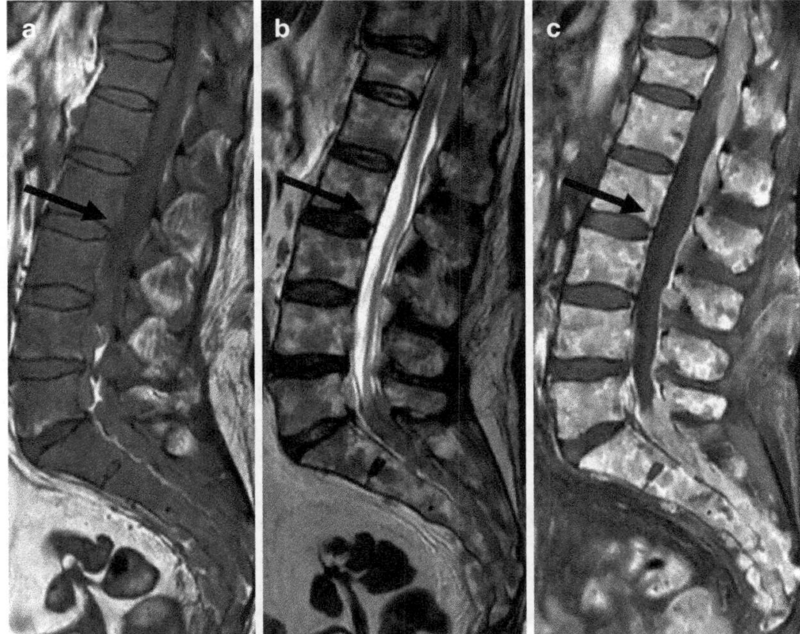

Fig. 1 (**a–c**) Multiple spine lesions. Multiple T1 hypointense (arrow on sagittal T1 image (**a**)) and T2 hyperintense (arrow on sagittal T2 image (**b**)) lesions in the lumbar spine with peripheral contrast enhancement (arrow on sagittal T1 after administration of contrast image (**c**)) suggesting diffuse bone metastases

Table 1 Most common multifocal tumors and tumorlike conditions of the osseous spine

Multiple benign lesions of the osseous spine	Multiple malignant lesions of the osseous spine
• Vertebral hemangiomas • Enostosis/osteopoikilosis • Fibrous dysplasia • Eosinophilic granuloma • SAPHO • Tuberculosis	• Metastases • Lymphoproliferative lesions (multiple myeloma and lymphoma)

should always be included in the differential diagnosis. Spinal bone tumors in patients under 30 years of age are uncommon and are generally benign except for Ewing's sarcoma and osteosarcoma (Greenspan 2004; Rodallec et al. 2008). Common tumors are osteoid osteoma, aneurysmal bone cyst (ABC), Ewing's sarcoma in a young patient, giant cell tumor in the middle-aged patient, and chordoma in the elderly (Khan and De Schepper 2007).

Table 2 summarizes the most common histological tumor types of the osseous spine according to their age distribution.

2.2.1 Clinical History

Multiple lesions seen in a patient with a prior oncologic history suggest metastatic bone disease.

A prior oncologic history with a history of radiotherapy suggests radiation-induced tumors (Khan and De Schepper 2007; Rodallec et al. 2008).

Fat-containing lesions with sharp demarcation corresponding to the radiotherapy field seen in a patient with an antecedent of radiotherapy for an oncologic disease suggest radiation-induced fatty replacement (Fig. 2).

2.2.2 Common Symptoms and Typical Presentations

As most tumors present with **nonspecific symptoms**, this parameter is of little help.

Eighty-five percent of **adult patients** complain of back pain (Orguc and Arkun 2014; Rodallec et al. 2008). Unlike adults, neurologic dysfunction caused by primary tumors of the spine is a common symptom in children (Murovic and Sundaresan 1992; Beer and Menezes 1997).

In children, according to the study of Beer and Menezes (1997), more than two-thirds of patients complained of back pain and neurologic deficit. Concern should be raised also in the group of age for underlying occult neoplasm in

Table 2 Most common histological tumor types of the osseous spine according to their age distribution

Age	<30 years	<30 years	>30 years	>30 years
Matrix	Benign	Malignant	Benign	Malignant
Histologic type				
Osteoid	Osteoid osteoma Osteoblastoma Enostoma	Osteosarcoma	Enostoma	Osteosarcoma
Cartilaginous				Chondrosarcoma
Mixed (osteoid + cartilaginous)	Osteochondroma		Osteochondroma	
Fibrous	Fibrous dysplasia			
Cystic/blood	ABC Hemangioma		Hemangioma	
Other cell types	GCT Eosinophilic granuloma	Ewing's sarcoma/ PNET	GCT	Chordoma
Lymphoproliferative				Multiple myeloma Plasmacytoma Lymphoma

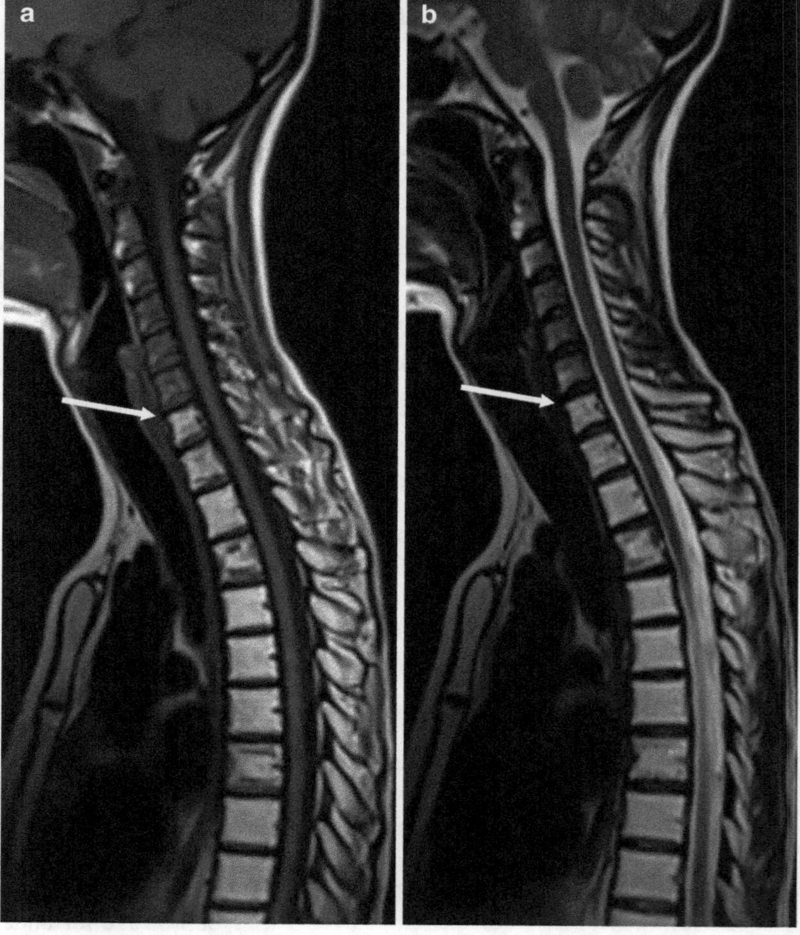

Fig. 2 (**a** and **b**) A previous history of radiation therapy for a lymphoma of the mediastinum in a 28-year patient. T1 (arrow on a sagittal T1 image (**a**)) and T2 (arrow on a sagittal T2 image (**b**)) high signal of the thoracic vertebral bodies corresponding to fat-containing lesions with sharp demarcation in the radiotherapy field suggesting radiation induced fatty replacement

the presence of painful scoliosis, especially at night (Bernard et al. 2013). Scoliosis or kyphosis may be an early manifestation of disease in the case of osteoid osteoma, neuroblastoma, aneurysmal bone cyst, giant cell tumor, and eosinophilic granuloma (Beer and Menezes 1997).

The clinical presentation can be highly suggestive of certain osseous spine tumors allowing the final diagnosis (Rodallec et al. 2008). Osteoid osteoma manifests typically with localized spinal pain, or radicular pain increasing in severity and frequency, worsening at night, and being relieved by aspirin/salicylates. Osteoblastoma manifests with a localized, moderately tender, and sometimes palpable mass. Osteogenic sarcoma and chordomas tend to involve the nerve roots and ganglia with pain localized according to the topographic location of the tumor (Beer and Menezes 1997; Menezes and Sato 1990, 1995). Aggressive hemangioma and malignancies are generally symptomatic (Khan and De Schepper 2007).

2.3 Topography

2.3.1 Location Within the Spinal Segment

The preferential location of a tumor in the spine within the spinal segment helps in the assessment of the nature of the lesion (Khan and De Schepper 2007). The lumbar and thoracic regions are more commonly involved than in the cervical spine (Weinstein and McLain 1987; Beer and Menezes 1997). Involvement of the sacrum in primary tumors is 1.3 to 4 times less frequent (Bernard et al. 2013). Some tumors are typically located at the ends of the spinal column. Chordoma is typically located at the clivus and craniocervical junction. At this level, the differential diagnosis should include pseudotumoral lesions of the foramen magnum such as calcium pyrophosphate dihydrate deposits (Fig. 3), synovial pannus, and craniovertebral junction tuberculosis. Chordomas that develop from remnants of the primitive noto-

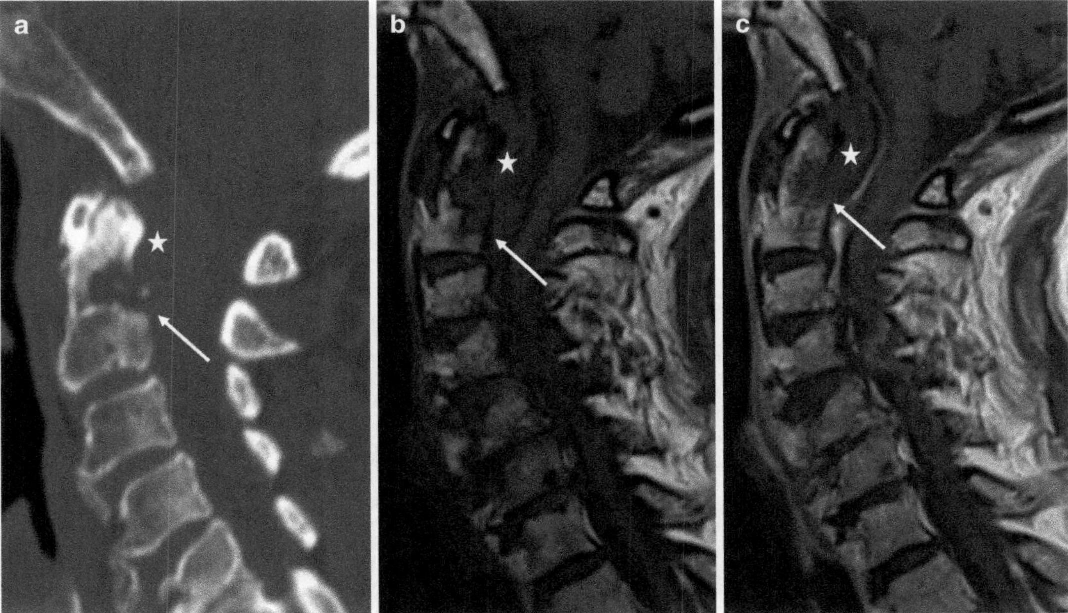

Fig. 3 Typical location of calcium pyrophosphate dihydrate deposits at the level of the C1-C2 joint. Note pressure erosion at the posterior aspect of the odontoid process of C2 (arrow on the sagittal CT image (**a**)) with subtle increased density within a soft tissue mass located posteriorly to the odontoid process of C2 (star on the sagittal CT scan image (**a**)), appearing hypointense on the sagittal T1-WI (star on the sagittal T1 image (**b**)) and non-enhancing on the sagittal T1-WI after administration of contrast (star) (**c**). This is a pseudotumoral lesion consisting of calcium pyrophosphate dihydrate deposits. It should be considered as a differential diagnosis for malignant lesions such as chordoma

chord are also frequently found in the sacrococcygeal region (Fig. 4a). Giant cell tumors are frequently seen in the sacrum (Fig. 4b) (Rodallec et al. 2008). A destructive lytic lesion of the sacrum suggests a giant cell tumor if it is eccentrically located in a middle-aged adult, and a chordoma if it is central with peripheral mineralization in an older patient (Bernard et al. 2013).

Table 3 summarizes the most common histological tumor types of the osseous spine according to their preferential location in the cervical, thoracic, lumbar, or sacral spine.

2.3.2 Location Within the Individual Vertebra

The site of origin of a lesion within a vertebra is another key to the correct characterization. The *posterior elements* can be involved in case of a mineralized tumor such as osteoid osteoma and osteoblastoma (Fig. 5a), seen in young patients, or in case of a non-mineralized expansile lesion with fluid-fluid levels such as the aneurysmal bone cyst (Fig. 5b, c) (Rodallec et al. 2008; Bernard et al. 2013). Benign tumors commonly affect the *body of the vertebra* such as hemangioma (Fig. 6), bone islands and GCT. Malignant tumors like chordomas and Ewing's sarcomas can also be seen in the vertebral body (Khan and De Schepper 2007).

Table 4 and Fig. 7 summarize the most common histological tumor types of the osseous spine according to their preferential location in the individual vertebra (either anterior or posterior elements).

The distribution of hematopoietic marrow is helpful to explain the occurrence of metastasis

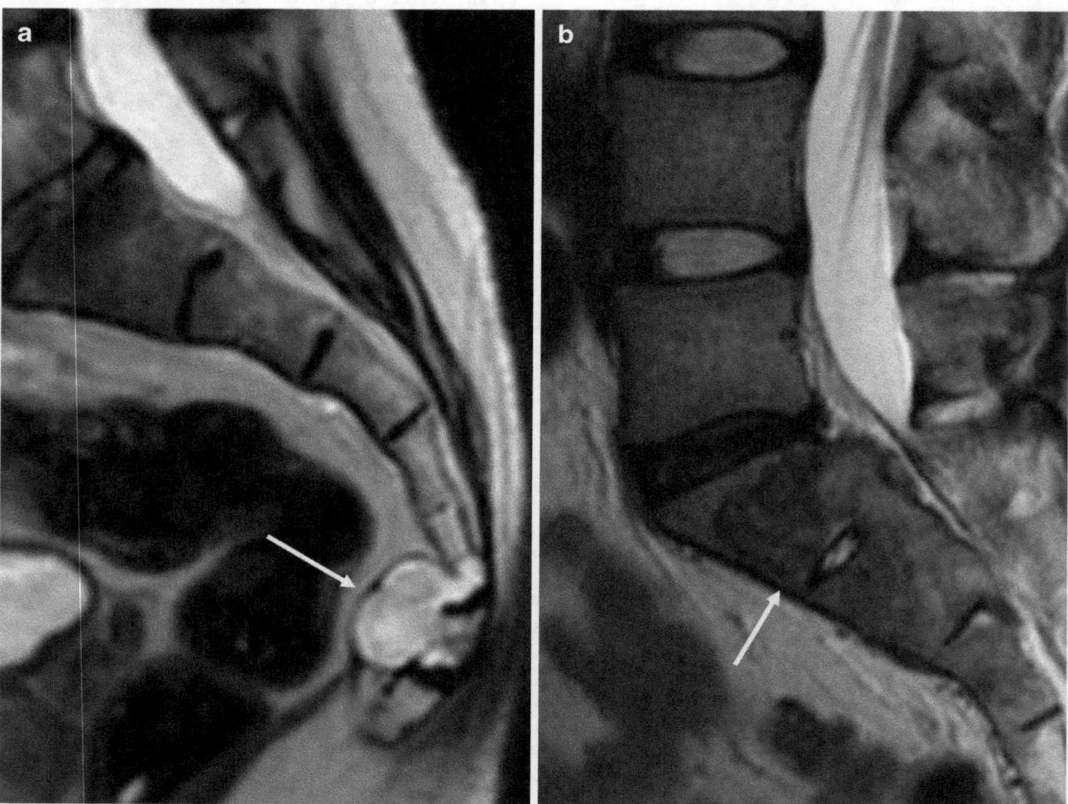

Fig. 4 (**a** and **b**) Lesions typically located within the sacrum. Chordoma with T2 hyperintensity (arrow on the sagittal T2 image (**a**)). Giant cell tumor with a typical relative low signal of the lesion on T2-weighted sequences, due to hemosiderin deposition (arrow on the sagittal T2 image (**b**))

and hematologic malignancies such as plasmacytoma, multiple myeloma, and lymphoma in the axial skeleton. The sacrum is the most common localization of hematologic malignancies because of the abundant hematopoietic or red marrow in adults (Fig. 8) (Rodallec et al. 2008).

2.4 Imaging Parameters

2.4.1 Margination

Benign tumors have on conventional radiography (CR) and CT scans sclerotic margins with geographic pattern and a narrow zone of transition (Fig. 9a), while malignant tumors have poorly defined margins with permeative bone destruction (Fig. 9b). A permeative appearance, with a broad zone of transition indicating aggressive biologic activity, is commonly present in malignant tumors such as osteosarcoma, Ewing's sarcoma, and metastatic disease. However, this appearance can also be depicted in an aggressive hemangioma.

Table 3 Most common histological tumor types of the osseous spine according to their location in the spinal segment

Preferential segmental location within the spine	Common tumors
Cervical spine	Osteoblastoma ABC Osteochondroma (C2)
Thoracic spine	Hemangioma Enostosis ABC Chondrosarcoma
Lumbar spine	Enostosis Osteoid osteoma
Sacral spine	Chordoma GCT Ewing's sarcoma Plasmacytoma Lymphoma Benign notochordal proliferation

Soft tissue extension suggests malignancy but can be seen in some benign tumors such as aneurysmal bone cyst, aggressive hemangioma, and eosinophilic granuloma (Rodallec et al. 2008).

Periosteal reaction is uncommon and difficult to assess in vertebral lesions. It can be seen in osteosarcoma (Khan and De Schepper 2007).

MR imaging can show associated nonspecific changes with sometimes a misleading aggressive appearance in the bone marrow and soft tissues (Davies et al. 2002; Assoun et al. 1994; Woods et al. 1993). Bone marrow edema can be seen either in aggressive malignant lesions or in benign lesions such as osteoid osteoma or osteoblastoma (Fig. 10a, b) (Riahi et al. 2018; Mechri et al. 2018; Rodallec et al. 2008).

2.4.2 Type of the Matrix

The type of tumor matrix can help the radiologist to suggest the correct diagnosis of the different bone-forming, cartilage-forming or fibrous tumors.

The most frequent bone-forming tumors are osteoblastic metastasis, bone island, lymphoma, and osteosarcoma. **Tumors with an osteoid**

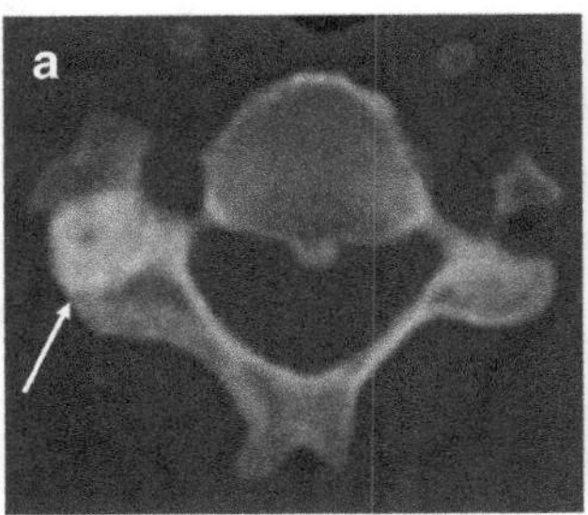

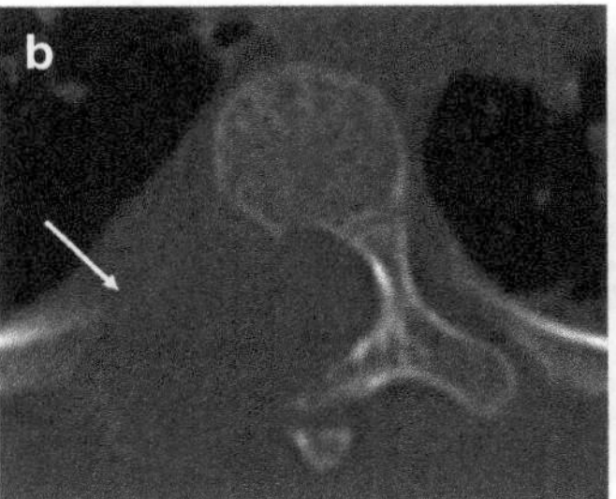

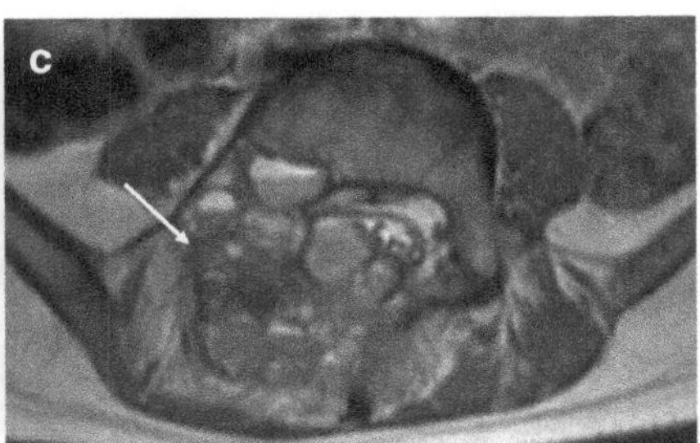

Fig. 5 (**a**–**c**) Typical localization of tumors in the posterior elements. (**a**) Mineralized tumor (arrow on the axial CT scan image) in the posterior elements suggesting an osteoblastoma. (**b**) Typical localization of a non-mineralized expansile tumor (arrow on the axial CT scan image) in the posterior elements suggesting an ABC. (**c**) Typical localization of a non-mineralized expansile tumor in the posterior elements of the same patient in (**b**) with fluid-fluid levels (arrow on the axial T2 image) suggesting an ABC (Courtesy of Dr Tim Vanderhasselt)

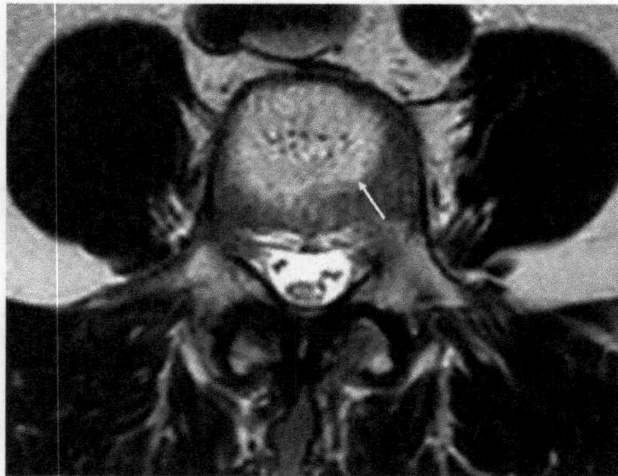

Fig. 6 Location within the vertebral body (arrow). A T2 hyperintense lesion within the vertebral body. Note the polka dot sign in the lesion on the axial T2-weighted image suggesting a hemangioma

Table 4 Most common histological tumor types of the osseous spine (**highlighted in bold**) according to their location in the individual vertebra (either anterior or posterior elements)

Topography within a vertebra	Vertebral body	Posterior elements
Benign	***Exceptions:*** • Hemangioma • EG • Enostosis • GCT	• **OO** • **Osteoblastoma** • **ABC** • **Exostosis**
Malignant	• **Metastasis** • **MM** • **Lymphoma** • **Chordoma**	***Exceptions:*** • Chondrosarcoma • Osteosarcoma • Ewing's sarcoma

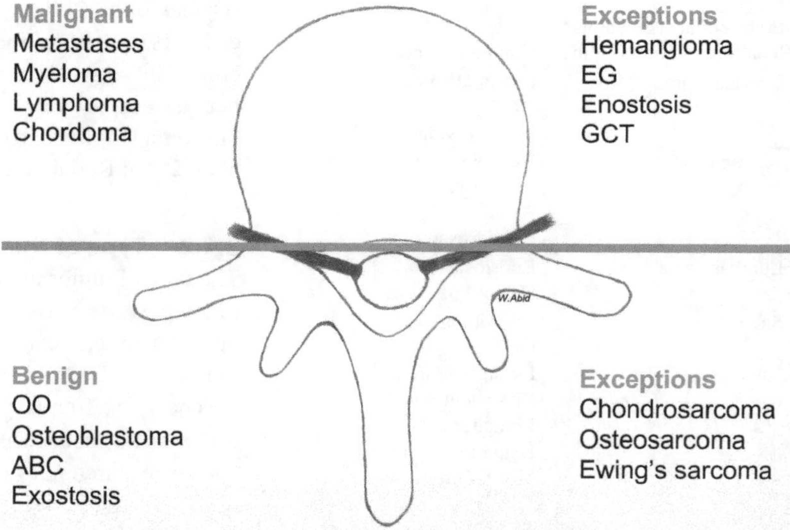

Fig. 7 Drawing with the preferential localizations of spine tumors in an axial image of a vertebra

matrix can manifest with a trabecular ossification pattern in benign bone-forming lesions and as a cloud-like or ill-defined amorphous pattern without an organized trabecular pattern in malignant tumors such as *osteosarcomas*.

Enostosis or dense bone island (Fig. 11a) which is one of the most frequent benign bone-forming tumors is characterized histologically by hamartomatous cortical bone embedded within the trabecular network of the medullary cavity (Shi et al. 2015; Riahi et al. 2018). Osteosarcomas present usually as mixed osteosclerotic-osteolytic lesions. Sclerosing osteoblastic osteosarcomas with marked mineralization presenting as an ivory vertebra are rare. A purely lytic pattern can be depicted in telangiectatic osteosarcoma with a cystic architecture simulating an aneurysmal bone cyst (Mechri et al. 2018).

Cartilage-forming tumors present punctate comma- or arc-like or annular calcifications on CR and CT (Fig. 11b). Cartilage matrix on Magnetic Resonance Imaging (MRI) is a high signal and a lobular morphology and ring and arc enhancement pattern (Fig. 11c, d) (Rodallec et al.

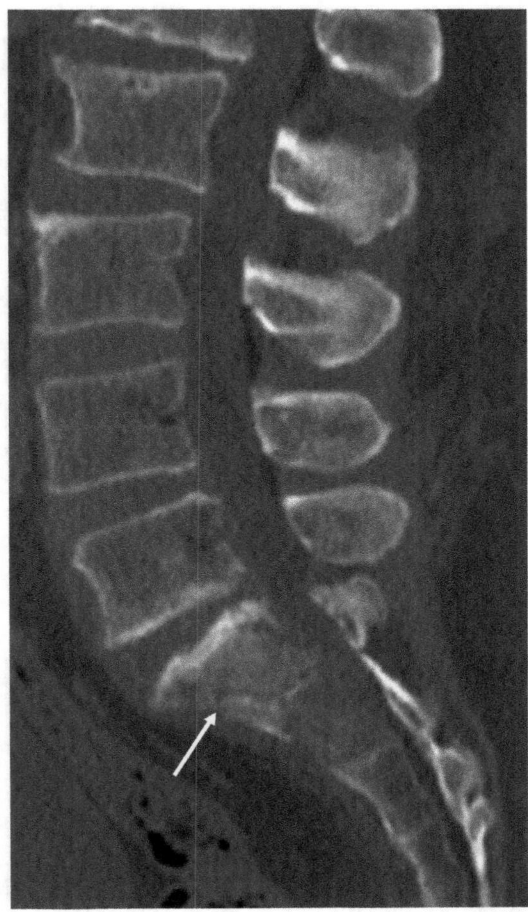

Fig. 8 The sacrum is a common localization of hematologic malignancy. This sagittal CT scan image shows a lymphoma with an associated pathological fracture (arrow)

2008). The most common cartilage-forming tumors are osteochondroma (Fig. 11e), chondroblastoma, and chondrosarcoma (Rodallec et al. 2008).

The diagnosis of fibrous dysplasia is made on CR or CT scan by identification of a ground-glass attenuation, which is indicative of a **fibrous matrix** (Fig. 12) (Rodallec et al. 2008).

2.4.3 Expansion

Bone expansion can be seen in benign conditions such as aneurysmal bone cyst, osteoblastoma, GCT, and occasionally in aggressive hemangioma. Bone expansion and destruction with soft tissue extension may be frequently encountered in malignant lesions like chordoma, Ewing's sarcoma, and chondrosarcoma (Khan and De Schepper 2007).

2.4.4 Locoregional Extension

Ewing's sarcoma (Fig. 13a) and chordoma commonly have an extensive **soft tissue component**. Soft tissue extension is not exclusively seen in malignant tumors but also in some benign lesions such as osteoblastoma (Fig. 13b, d) and less frequently aggressive hemangioma (Fig. 13c). Lesions with soft tissue extension are typically symptomatic (Khan and De Schepper 2007). Assessment of the possible extension of a cervical spine tumor to the supra-aortic trunks requires CT-angiographic or MR-angiographic evaluation. Tumors of the thoracic spine should be scrutinized for invasion of the pleura, mediastinum, or ribs. Tumors of the lumbar spine and of the sacrum warrant evaluation of the lesion's extension into the retroperitoneum, sacroiliac joints, and pelvis, respectively (Rodallec et al. 2008). It is important to assess for an associated epidural component. Some tumors such as vertebral metastasis or vertebral hemangioma may extend posteriorly to the anterior epidural space with sparing of the posterior longitudinal ligament, which is strongly attached to the posterior vertebral body cortex in the midline and is more loosely attached laterally, resulting in the "draped curtain sign" with a bilobular intraspinal aspect on the axial images (Shah and Salzman 2011). (Fig. 13c).

2.4.5 Other Differential Features and Typical Patterns

2.4.5.1 Fluid-Fluid Levels

Fluid-fluid levels (FFL) are due to sedimentation of blood degradation products (Fig. 14) (Hudson 1984; Beltran et al. 1986; Khan and De Schepper 2007). Van Dyck et al. in a large series of 700 bone and 700 soft tissue tumors demonstrated that FFL is a rare finding in bone and soft tissue tumors, with a prevalence of 2.7% and 2.9% in bone and soft tissue tumors, respectively. It is best seen on T2-weighted images. FFLs can present in benign and malignant bone and soft tissue

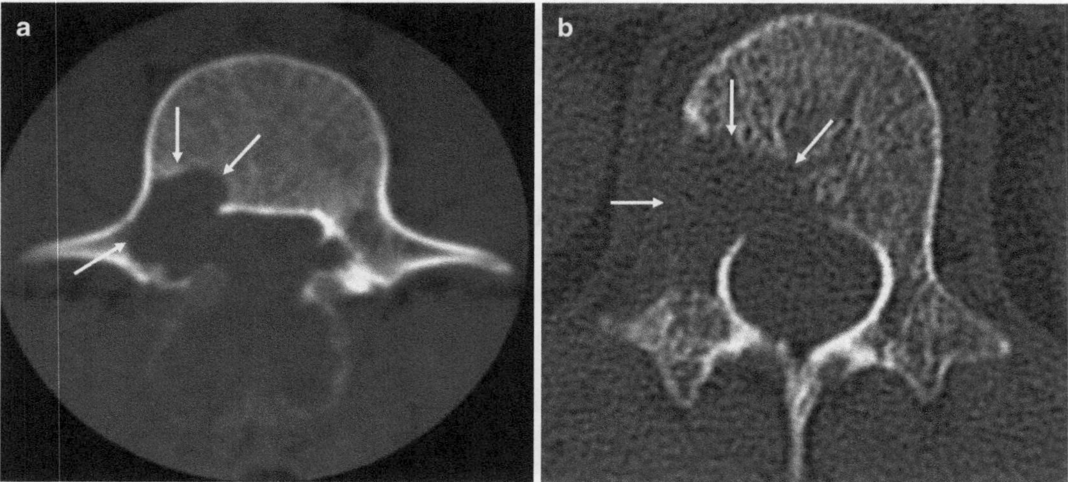

Fig. 9 (**a** and **b**) Margination. (**a**) Sclerotic margins with geographic pattern and a narrow zone of transition (arrows on axial CT scan image) in ABC. (**b**) Poorly defined margins with permeative bone destruction (arrows on axial CT scan image) in a metastasis

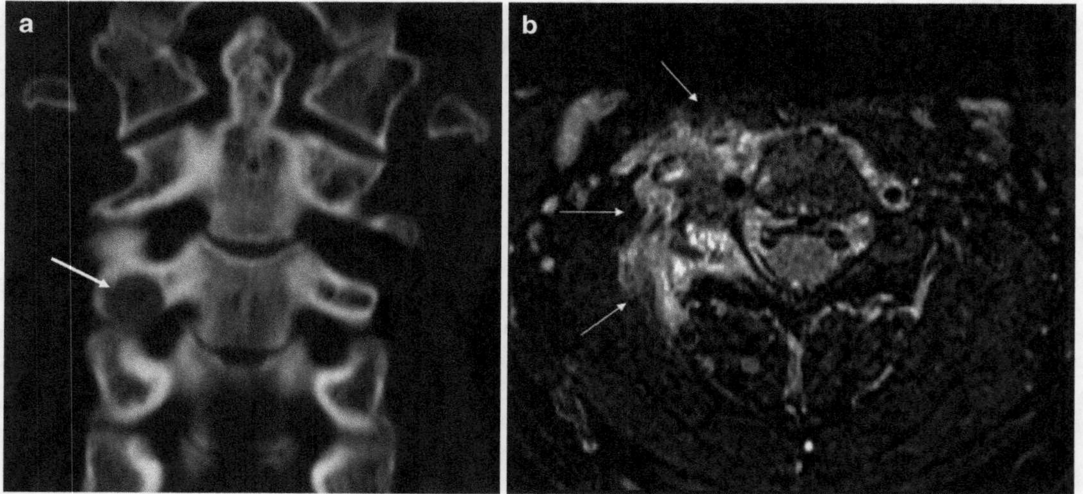

Fig. 10 (**a** and **b**) Associated nonspecific changes. (**a**) Tumor with an osseous matrix located in the posterior elements of C3 (arrow on a coronal CT image) suggestive for an osteoblastoma. (**b**) Important surrounding soft tissue edema (arrows on axial T2 fat saturated axial image). This axial T2 fat saturated axial image may have a misleading aggressive appearance

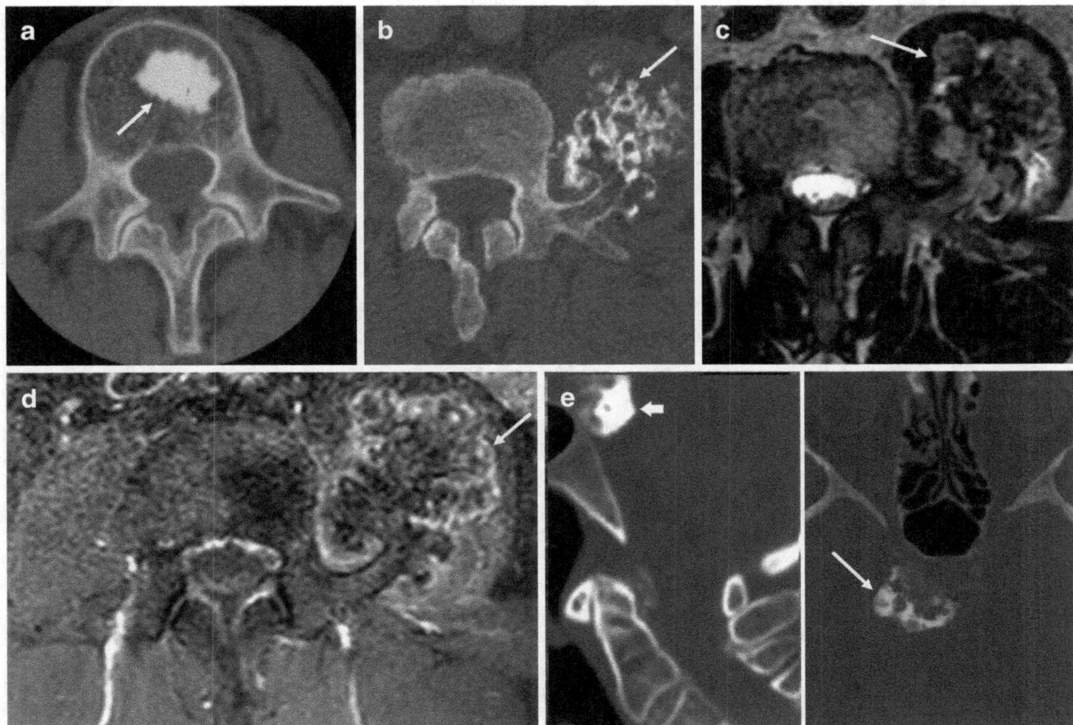

Fig. 11 (a–e) Type of the matrix. (**a**) Tumor with an osseous matrix located within the vertebral body (arrow on axial CT scan image of a vertebral body) suggesting enostosis or dense bone island. (**b**) Tumor with a chondroid matrix and typical punctate comma- or arc-like or annular calcifications (arrow on axial CT scan image of a lumbar vertebra) suggesting a chondrosarcoma. (**c**) Typical T2 high signal and a lobular morphology in a tumor with a cartilage matrix (arrow on axial T2 Fat Sat image) suggesting a chondrosarcoma. (**d**) Typical (osteochondroma) ring and arc enhancement pattern in a tumor with a cartilage matrix (arrow on axial T1 Fat Sat image after contrast administration) suggesting a chondrosarcoma. (**e**) Tumor with a chondroid matrix (osteochondroma) and typical punctate comma- or arc-like or annular calcifications located at the posterior aspect of the clivus (arrows on sagittal and axial CT scan images). It is characterized by a bony protrusion covered by a cartilaginous cap

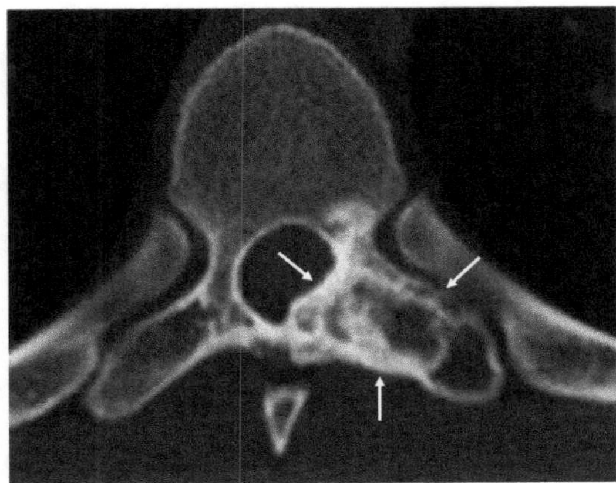

Fig. 12 Fibrous matrix. Typical ground-glass attenuation (arrows) in a tumor with a fibrous matrix: fibrous dysplasia of the left transverse process (arrows on axial CT scan image of a dorsal vertebra)

tumors (Van Dyck et al. 2006). This finding in a vertebral lesion may be encountered in primary or secondary aneurysmal bone cysts, in a coexisting benign tumor such as osteoblastoma, GCT, and fibrous dysplasia, but may also be seen in telangiectatic osteosarcoma (Ilaslan et al. 2004; Murphey et al. 2003; Khan and De Schepper 2007; Rodallec et al. 2008).

2.4.5.2 Nidus

A nidus is characteristic of osteoid osteoma (Fig. 15). Radiographically and on CT, it manifests with a lucent center which is the nidus, with variable central mineralization surrounded by extensive reactive sclerosis (Khan and De Schepper 2007). CT is the examination of choice to demonstrate the nidus and it is highly specific.

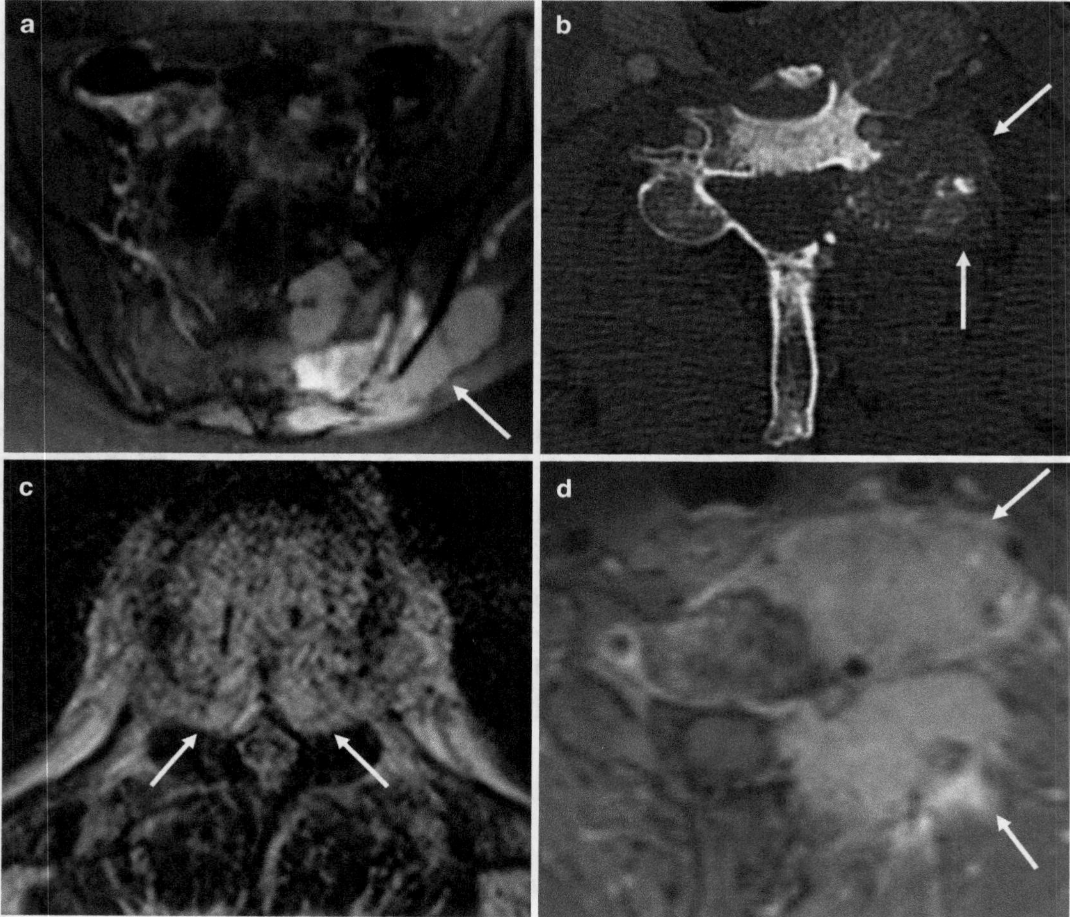

Fig. 13 (**a**–**d**) Soft tissue extension. (**a**) Enhancing extensive soft tissue component in Ewing's sarcoma (arrow on axial T1 Fat Sat image after administration of contrast). (**b**) Extensive soft tissue component in an osteoblastoma of the left transverse process (arrows on axial CT scan image). This soft tissue component enhances after administration of contrast on image (Courtesy of Dr Yannick De Brucker) (**d**) (arrows on axial T1 Fat Sat image (**d**) after administration of contrast) (Courtesy of Dr Yannick De Brucker). (**c**) Enhancing extensive soft tissue component to the epidural space causing a "*draped curtain sign*" in an aggressive hemangioma (axial T1 Fat Sat image (**d**) after administration of contrast)

MRI shows bone and soft tissue edema adjacent to the lesion, but the nidus is not always visible. Dynamic gadolinium enhanced MRI improves detection of the nidus. In the study of Zampa et al., dynamic MRI significantly increased nidus conspicuity compared to nonenhanced MRI and CT. In 31.6% of the cases, nidus was more clearly discernible at dynamic MRI compared to CT (Zampa et al. 2009). Dynamic contrast-enhanced imaging helps in the localization of the tumor nidus, especially in case of intra-articular osteoid osteoma mimicking arthritis. It is seen as an early arterial-phase focal enhancement after the gadolinium injection, with fast washout, as a result of its hypervascularity (Corrêa and Costa 2023).

2.4.5.3 Vertical Striations

Vertical striations or a "honeycomb" or "corduroy" patterns seen on conventional radiography (Fig. 16a) are typically seen in vertebral hemangioma. Vertebral hemangioma manifests also with the "polka-dot" appearance on axial CT scan (Fig. 16b) (Khan and De Schepper 2007; Rodallec et al. 2008).

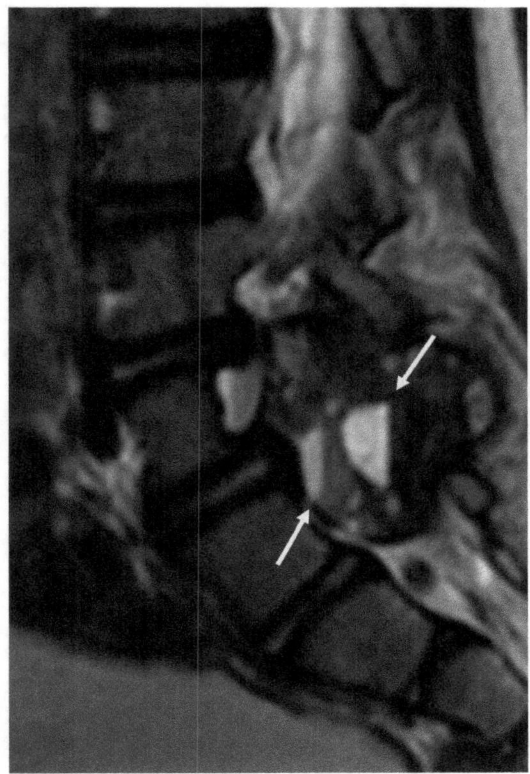

Fig. 14 Fluid-fluid levels. Sagittal T2-weighted image of the lumbar spine showing fluid-fluid levels (arrows) in an ABC of the posterior elements due to sedimentation of blood degradation products (Courtesy of Dr Tim Vanderhasselt)

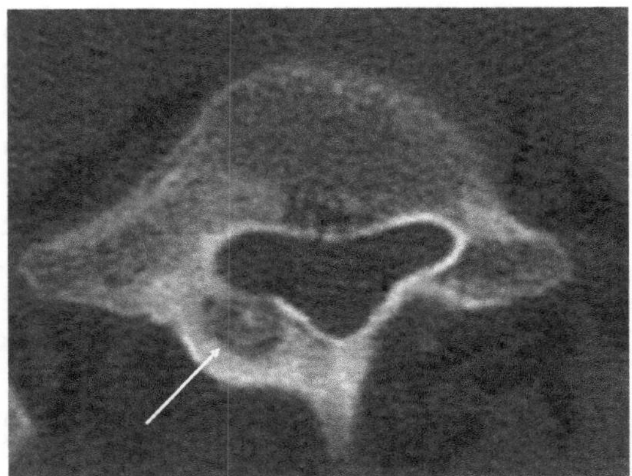

Fig. 15 Nidus (arrow) in an osteoid osteoma in the right lamina

2.4.5.4 Brush Border/Spiculated Margins

This sign is seen in dense bone islands or enostosis which is histologically composed of cortical bone (Fig. 17). Dense bone islands are commonly solitary but may be multiple, and this condition is seen in osteopoikilosis.

Enostosis are round to oval lesions, ranging in size between 2 mm to 2 cm in diameter, have commonly irregular spiculated or thornlike margins aka brush borders, that merge into the surrounding medullary or cancellous bone. This lesion is commonly located adjacent to the endosteal surface of the cortex. In some cases, especially in large lesions, distinguishing enostosis from some osteoblastic metastases may be equivocal. Imaging features like thornlike margins, the solitary occurrence, and the normal adjacent trabecular bone help to differentiate these lesions from osteoblastic metastasis, avoiding the need for biopsy (Vidal and Murphey 2007). CT attenuation threshold could serve as an additional tool in helping to make a diagnosis without additional tests or a biopsy. Ulano et al. showed in their study that CT attenuation measurements are reliable to distinguish untreated osteoblastic metastases from enostosis. A mean attenuation of 885 HU and a maximum attenuation of 1060 HU provide reliable thresholds. A metastatic lesion is favored below these thresholds (Ulano et al. 2016).

2.4.5.5 Vertebra Plana

This presentation is depicted typically in eosinophilic granuloma and to a lesser extent in giant cell tumor (Fig. 18) (Khan and De Schepper 2007).

2.4.5.6 Ivory Vertebra

It manifests with marked sclerosis involving the entire vertebral body. In this case, lymphoma (Fig. 19), Paget's disease, osteoblastic metastasis, tuberculosis, or SAPHO should be suggested (Khan and De Schepper 2007).

2.4.5.7 A "Mini-Brain" Appearance

Plasmacytoma can manifest with a "mini-brain" appearance mimicking the MR appearance of the brain surface (Major et al. 2000; Khan and De Schepper 2007).

A mini-brain appearance in an expansile lesion of the vertebral body, seen commonly on axial images, with a thickened cortical strut

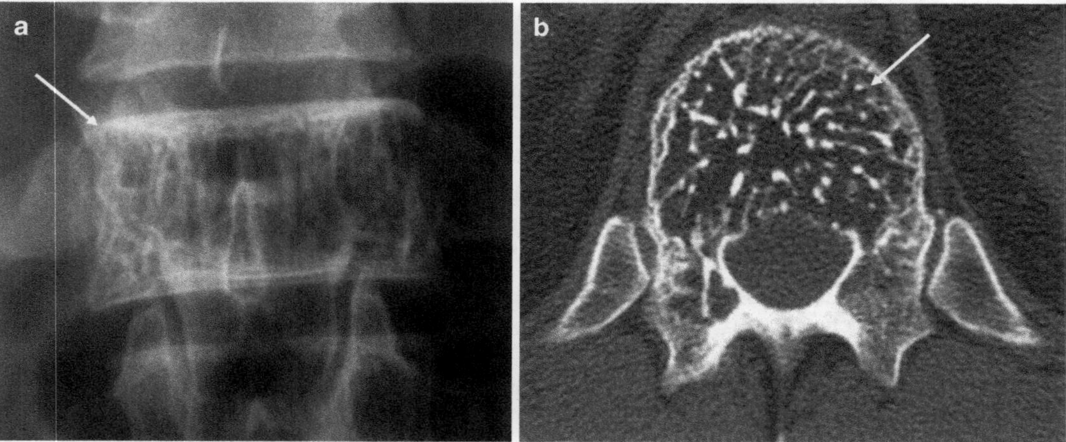

Fig. 16 (**a** and **b**) Thickened trabeculae in a hemangioma. (**a**) Conventional radiography showing vertical striations (arrow) resulting in a "jail *bar*" appearance on anteroposterior views. (**b**) On axial CT, this results in a "*polka dot sign*" (arrow)

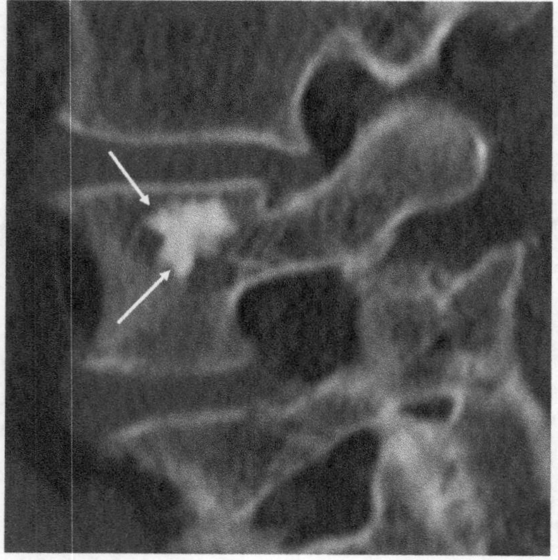

Fig. 17 Brush border/spiculated margins. Bone islands or enostosis with the typical irregular spiculated or thorn-like margins that merge into the surrounding cancellous bone (arrows) on sagittal CT scan image

and a characteristic low T1 and high T2 signals, is according to Major et al. highly suggestive of a solitary plasmacytoma. The cortical thickening is probably compensatory response from the lytic process of the plasmacytoma. This could be due to the less aggressive nature of plasmacytoma compared with other lytic primary bone or metastatic spine lesions (Major et al. 2000).

2.4.5.8 A "Dumbbell" or "Mushroom" Shape

This pattern may be seen in chordoma (Fig. 20) (Khan and De Schepper 2007). Chordomas are rare malignant primary bone arising from notochord remnants. They represent up to 20% of primary bone tumors of the spine (Muneer et al. 2019). Chordomas are destructive osseous masses with involvement of the adjacent soft tissues and indolent growth, leading to displacement of adjacent tissue rather than invade it (Farsad et al. 2009). This explains why chordomas can be large at the time of diagnosis. On MRI, they show a "dumbbell" or "mushroom" appearance with an expansile exophytic component adjacent to the vertebral body from which the tumor originates (Smolders et al. 2003). The paraspinal component can extend along the margins of the adjacent vertebral body but typically spares the intervertebral disc (Benson et al. 2020).

2.4.5.9 Relative Sparing of the Disc Space

This feature is commonly seen in chordoma in which a destructive lesion of the vertebral body extends over several segments with preservation of the disc space (Fig. 21) (Smolders et al. 2003; Rodallec et al. 2008). Disk spaces are also preserved in eosinophilic granuloma with the typical complete or incomplete collapse of the vertebral body (vertebra plana) (Rodallec et al. 2008). It can also be seen in ABC or multiple myeloma.

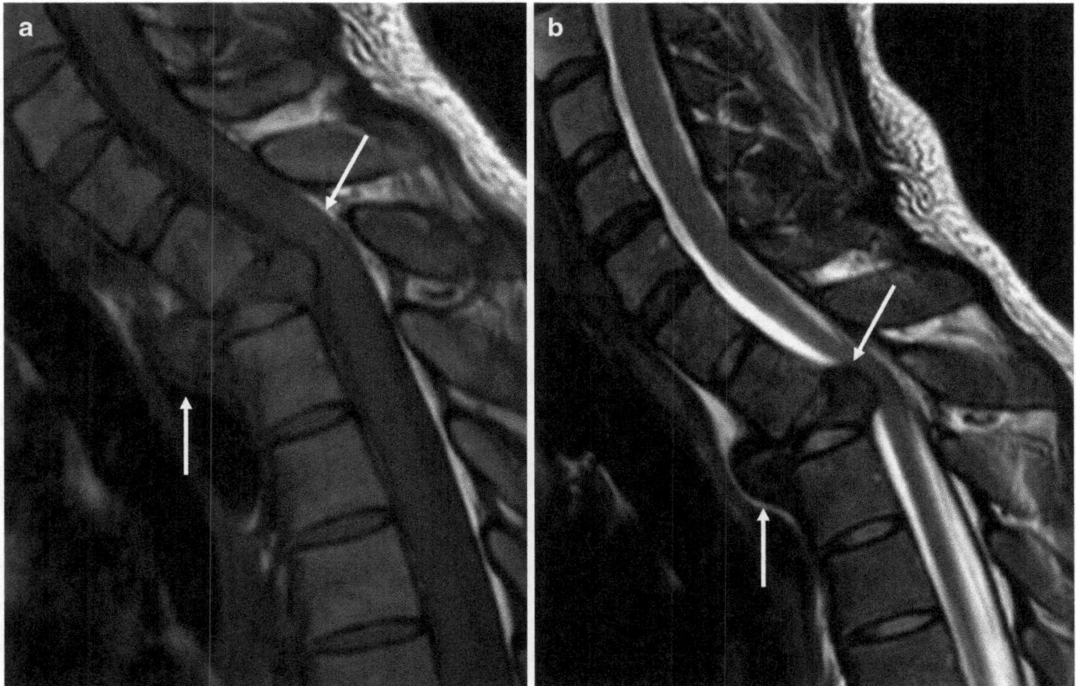

Fig. 18 (**a** and **b**) Vertebra plana in a giant cell tumor. (**a**) T1-WI (**b**) T2-WI showing collapse of Th2 (arrows). Note also relative sparing of the disc space and a low signal on T2-WI, in keeping with hemosiderin

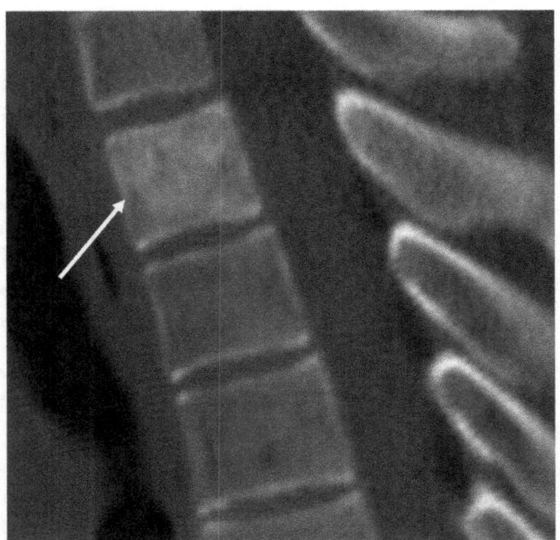

Fig. 19 Marked sclerosis involving the entire vertebral body (arrow) in lymphoma on sagittal CT scan image

2.4.5.10 Signal Intensity on MRI

Unfortunately, most tumors have a nonspecific signal, being low signal on T1-weighted images and high on T2-weighted images.

Some lesions, however, are of low signal on T2-weighted images, such as giant cell tumors due to the presence of hemosiderin or fibrous tissue (Fig. 22a).

Other lesions contain fat and are of high signal on T1-weighted images.

Vertebral hemangioma (Fig. 22b), fibrous dysplasia, Paget disease, and Schmörl's node commonly contain fat (Rodallec et al. 2008). In case of increased fatty contents in multiple vertebrae should raise the possibility of previous radiotherapy. The knowledge of a history of previous radiotherapy and the sharp demarcation of the lesion within the radiotherapy field are the clues to the correct diagnosis.

2.4.5.11 Contrast Enhancement Pattern and Degree of Enhancement

Cartilage matrix on Magnetic Resonance Imaging (MRI) displays a typical ring and arc enhancement pattern (Fig. 11d).

Distinguishing benign and malignant spine lesions can be challenging in some special cases

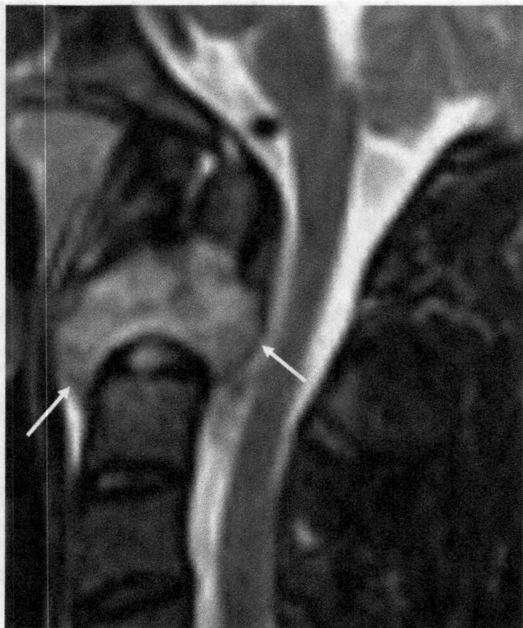

Fig. 20 Dumbbell sign in a chordoma. Sagittal T2-WI. Destructive osseous mass with soft tissues extension leading to displacement of adjacent tissue, resulting in a "dumbbell" or "mushroom" appearance (arrows) with an expansile exophytic component adjacent to the vertebral body from which the tumor originates

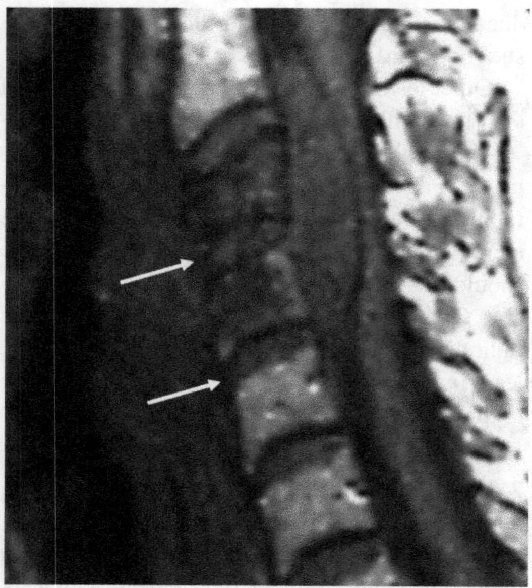

Fig. 21 Preservation of the disc space. Tumor extending over several segments with *preservation of the disc space* (arrows) suggestive of a chordoma on sagittal T1 image

such as differentiating atypical hemangiomas from vertebral malignant lesions.

Typical vertebral hemangiomas (VHs) have a fatty stroma with vascular components and are T1/T2 hyperintense, especially on Turbo Spin Echo sequences according to the amount of fat content, with a variable enhancement.

Atypical VHs have low-fat content and high vascularity and are T1 iso-/hypointense and T2 hyperintense and enhance after gadolinium contrast administration.

Atypical VHs may be aggressive if they have an increased vascular component and less fatty stroma showing potential cortical erosion, extradural soft tissue, expansion to the posterior elements, and even invasion of the spinal canal (Mcevoy et al. 2016). In addition, the vertical trabecular appearance can be more difficult to visualize making the diagnosis even more challenging (Gaudino et al. 2015). Their MRI appearance often mimics primary bone malignancies or metastatic lesions (Gaudino et al. 2015).

Atypical VHs and malignant lesions are commonly undistinguishable in routine spine MR imaging leading in some cases to more invasive examinations (Morales et al. 2018).

Dynamic contrast-enhanced (DCE) MR imaging perfusion is a noninvasive method that allows obtaining quantitative parameters representing the physiology of the microvascular environment of each lesion (Morales et al. 2018).

Morales et al. demonstrated that qualitative assessment of contrast-enhancement curves and quantitative analysis of perfusion parameters are able to differentiate atypical hemangiomas from vertebral metastatic lesions.

Atypical hemangioma time-intensity curves have a minimal and delayed enhancement, with no washout. Metastases have a rapid wash-in phase, higher peak, and clear washout, which is a common indicator of malignancy. Quantitative analysis of the perfusion parameters depicts lower perfusion values in atypical hemangiomas compared with metastatic lesions (Morales et al. 2018).

2.4.5.12 Diffusion-Weighted Imaging

The spine is the most common site of skeletal metastases, due to the abundant vascularization and

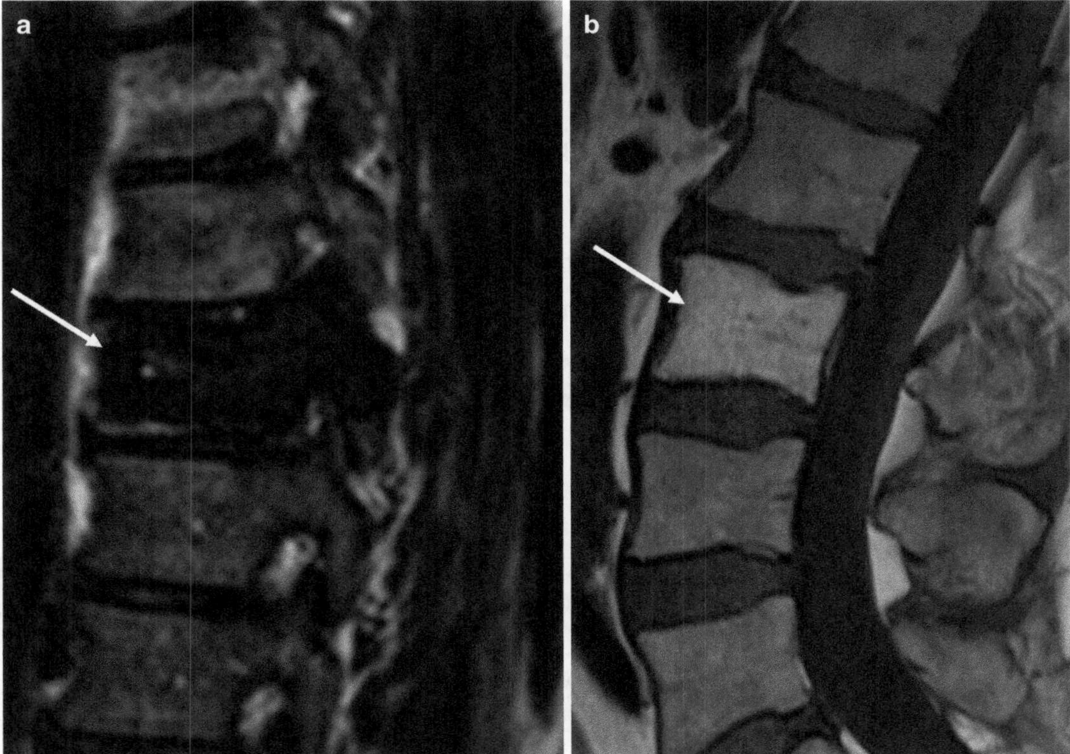

Fig. 22 (**a** and **b**) Signal intensity on MRI. (**a**) Sagittal T2-WI shows a low signal of the vertebral lesion due to the presence of hemosiderin or fibrous tissue in a giant cell tumor (arrow). (**b**) Sagittal T1-WI of the lumbar spine showing a hyperintense vertebral body (arrow) suggesting fatty tissue in a vertebral hemangioma

red bone marrow (Yuh et al. 1996). MRI is sensitive to detect them but edema in an acute fracture can mimic those lesions (Zhou et al. 2002). Metastases appear T1 hypointense, T2 hyperintense, and enhance following contrast administration (Gold et al. 1990). Conventional MR sequences may be nonspecific to distinguish benign from pathologic fracture (Karchevsky et al. 2008).

Diffusion-weighted imaging with ADC maps helps to distinguish benign versus malignant vertebral fractures. This was demonstrated in the meta-analysis of Karchevsky et al. (2008).

The meta-analysis concluded that the hypointense signal in fractured vertebrae on DWI with an increased ADC is in favor of a benign fracture (Karchevsky et al. 2008).

Hyperintense signal on DWI is due to the limited motion of water molecules in hypercellular lesions (Baur et al. 1998). The intracellular volume fraction is more important than the interstitial space in highly cellular metastatic lesions (Herneth et al. 2002). This lowers ADC values because the water diffusion coefficient is approximately ten times lower in the intracellular than in the extracellular space (Zhou et al. 2002). The interstitial space is increased in benign fractures because they are associated with edema in the acute phase. For this reason, the cellularity of benign fractures is lower than that of metastatic lesions with a significantly higher ADC than pathologic compression fractures (Zhou et al. 2002).

3 Imaging Algorithm

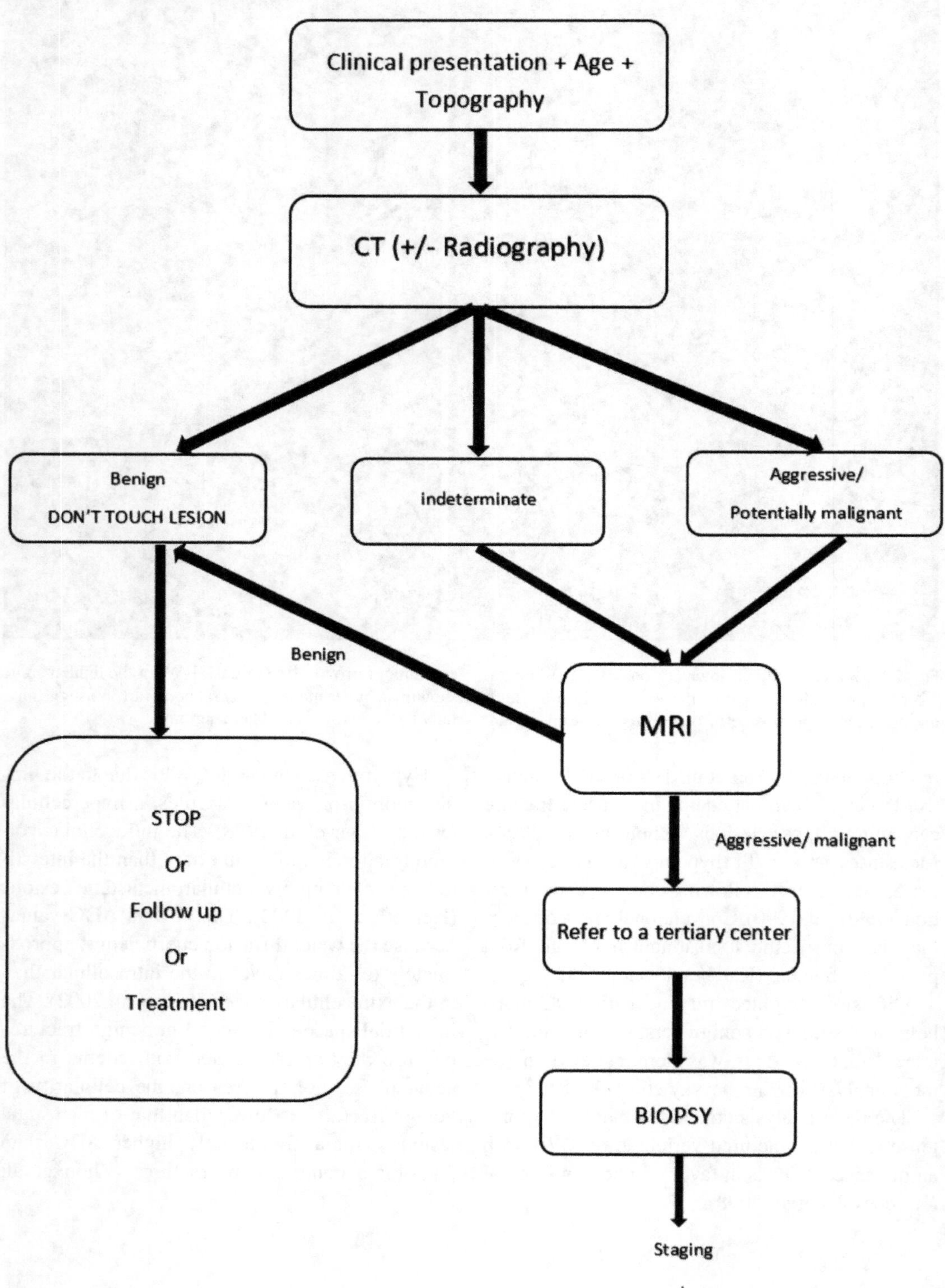

4 Conclusion

Variable lesions may affect the osseous spine. Lymphoproliferative disorders such as multiple myeloma and lymphoma represent the majority of extradural tumors. Bone metastases are the most frequent secondary extradural lesions. Solitary lesions are rare and have a wide differential diagnosis requiring a multimodality approach based on the knowledge of specific clinical and radiological parameters for each lesion to avoid unnecessary workups of benign lesions.

Initial imaging using radiography is not very sensitive because of the complex anatomy of the vertebrae. Cross-sectional imaging is important to characterize a spinal lesion, especially of the posterior elements. Magnetic resonance imaging (MRI) is the imaging modality of choice for local staging of those lesions to facilitate treatment and management of aggressive lesions.

It is also important to keep in mind the differential diagnosis of tumors of the osseous spine including tumor-like conditions such as infectious lesions, microcrystalline arthropathies, or Paget's disease.

5 Key Points

- Bone metastases are the most common multiple lesions of the osseous spine.
- Lymphoproliferative lesions (multiple myeloma and lymphoma) are the most frequent multiple primary tumors of the osseous spine.
- Benign lesions may also present as multifocal lesions (hemangiomas, enostosis).
- Solitary lesions are rare and have a wide differential diagnosis requiring a multimodality approach.
- Benign lesions often present as asymptomatic incidental findings.
- Malignant lesions are often symptomatic and present with either back pain, neurologic symptoms, or scoliosis particularly in children.
- Important semiological parameters for characterization to remember include the following:
  - Age and clinical information
  - Multiplicity
  - Topography in the spine
  - Imaging findings
    - Morphology: Margination—Matrix—Expansion—Locoregional Extension
    - Density/signal intensity/contrast enhancement
    - Specific patterns
- Imaging modalities:
  - Conventional radiography: not sensitive due to complex anatomy of the vertebrae and superposition.
  - Cross-sectional imaging (CT scan): important for detection and characterization of osseous spinal lesions, especially of the posterior elements.
  - Magnetic resonance imaging (MRI): imaging modality of choice for local staging.

References

Afshani E, Kuhn JP (1991) Common causes of low back pain in children. Radiographics 11:269–291

Assoun J, Richardi G, Railhac JJ et al (1994) Osteoid osteoma: MR imaging versus CT. Radiology 191(1):217–223

Baur A, Stabler A, Bruning R et al (1998) Diffusion-weighted MR imaging of bone marrow: differentiation of benign versus pathologic compression fractures. Radiology 207:349–356

Beer SJ, Menezes AH (1997) Primary tumors of the spine in children. Natural history, management, and long-term follow-up. Spine (Phila Pa 1976) 22(6):649–58; discussion 658–9

Beltran J, Simon DC, Levy M et al (1986) Aneurysmal bone cysts: MR imaging at 1.5 T. Radiology 158:689–690

Benson JC, Vizcaino MA, Kim DK et al (2020) Exophytic lumbar vertebral body mass in an adult with back pain. AJNR Am J Neuroradiol 41(10):1786–1790

Bernard SA, Brian PL, Flemming DJ (2013) Primary osseous tumors of the spine. Semin Musculoskelet Radiol 17(2):203–220

Corrêa DG, Costa FM (2023) Osteoid osteoma mimicking arthritis. J Clin Rheumatol 29(1):e1–e2

Davies M, Cassar-Pullicino VN, Davies AM et al (2002) The diagnostic accuracy of MR imaging in osteoid osteoma. Skeletal Radiol 31(10):559–569

Farsad K, Kattapuram SV, Sacknoff R et al (2009) Sacral chordoma. Radiographics 29:1525–1530

Gaudino S, Martucci M, Colantonio R et al (2015) A systematic approach to vertebral hemangioma. Skeletal Radiol 44:25–36

Gold RI, Seeger LL, Bassett LW et al (1990) An integrated approach to the evaluation of metastatic bone disease. Radiol Clin North Am 28:471–483

Greenspan A (2004) Radiologic evaluation of tumors and tumor-like lesions. In: Vives MJ (ed) Orthopedic imaging: a practical approach, 4th edn, Philadelphia, pp 529–570

Herneth AM, Philipp MO, Naude J et al (2002) Vertebral metastases: assessment with apparent diffusion coefficient. Radiology 225(3):889–894

Hudson TM (1984) Fluid levels in aneurysmal bone cysts: a CT feature. AJR Am J Roentgenol 142:1001–1004

Ilaslan H, Sundaram M, Unni KK et al (2004) Primary vertebral osteosarcoma: imaging findings. Radiology 230(3):697–702

Karchevsky M, Babb JS, Schweitzer ME (2008) Can diffusion-weighted imaging be used to differentiate benign from pathologic fractures? A meta-analysis. Skeletal Radiol 37(9):791–795

Khan SHM, De Schepper AM (2007) Primary tumors of the osseous spine. In: Van Goethem JWM, Van den Hauwe L, Parizel PM (eds) Spinal imaging. Medical radiology. Springer, Berlin, pp 475–500

Kozlowsi K, Beluffi G, Diard F et al (1984) Primary vertebral tumours in children: report of 20 cases with brief literature review. Pediatr Radiol 14:129–139

Levine AM, Boriani S, Donati D et al (1992) Benign tumors of the cervical spine. Spine 17:S399–S405

Major NM, Helms CA, Richardson WJ (2000) The "mini brain": plasmacytoma in a vertebral body on MR imaging. AJR Am J Roentgenol 175:261–263

Masaryk TJ (1991) Neoplastic disease of the spine. Radiol Clin North Am 29:829–845

McEvoy SH, Farrell M, Brett F et al (2016) Haemangioma, an uncommon cause of an extradural or intradural extramedullary mass: case series with radiological pathological correlation. Insights Imaging 7:87–98

Mechri M, Riahi H, Sboui I et al (2018) Imaging of malignant primitive tumors of the spine. J Belg Soc Radiol 102(1):56

Menezes AH, Sato Y (1990) Primary tumors of the spine in children-natural history and management. In: Marlin AE (ed) Concepts in pediatric neurosurgery, vol 10. Karger, Basel, pp 30–53

Menezes AH, Sato Y (1995) Primary tumors of the spine in children-natural history and management. Pediatr Neurosurg 23:101–114

Morales KA, Arevalo-Perez J, Peck KK et al (2018) Differentiating atypical hemangiomas and metastatic vertebral lesions: the role of T1-weighted dynamic contrast-enhanced MRI. AJNR Am J Neuroradiol 39(5):968–973

Munday TL, Johnson MH, Hayes CW et al (1994) Musculoskeletal causes of spinal axis compromise: beyond the usual suspects. Radiographics 14:1225–1245

Muneer M, Badran S, Al-Hetmi T (2019) A rare presentation of axial chordoma and the approach to management. Am J Case Rep 20:773–775

Murovic J, Sundaresan N (1992) Pediatric spinal axis tumors. Neurosurg Clin N Am 3:947–958

Murphey MD, Wan Jaovisidha S, Temple HT et al (2003) Telangiectatic osteosarcoma: radiologic-pathologic comparison. Radiology 229(2):545–553

Orguc S, Arkun R (2014) Primary tumors of the spine. Semin Musculoskelet Radiol 18(3):280–299

Riahi H, Mechri M, Barsaoui M et al (2018) Imaging of benign tumors of the osseous spine. J Belg Soc Radiol 102(1):13

Rodallec MH, Feydy A, Larousserie F et al (2008) Diagnostic imaging of solitary tumors of the spine: what to do and say. Radiographics 28(4):1019–1041

Ross JS, Masaryk TJ, Modic MT et al (1987) Vertebral hemangiomas: MR imaging. Radiology 165(1):165–169

Shah LM, Salzman KL (2011) Imaging of spinal metastatic disease. Int J Surg Oncol 2011:769753

Shi LS, Li YQ, Wu WJ et al (2015) Imaging appearance of giant cell tumor of the spine above the sacrum. Br J Radiol 88(1051):20140566

Smolders D, Wang X, Drevelengas A et al (2003) Value of MRI in the diagnosis of non-clival, non-sacral chordoma. Skeletal Radiol 32:343–350

Subbarao K, Jacobson HG (1979) Primary malignant neoplasms. Semin Roentgenol 14:44–57

Ulano A, Bredella MA, Burke P et al (2016) Distinguishing untreated osteoblastic metastases from enostoses using CT attenuation measurements. AJR Am J Roentgenol 207(2):362–368

Van Dyck P, Vanhoenacker FM, Vogel J et al (2006) Prevalence, extension and characteristics of fluid-fluid levels in bone and soft tissue tumors. Eur Radiol 16(12):2644–2651

Van Goethem JW, Van den Hauwe L, Ozsarlak O et al (2004) Spinal tumors. Eur J Radiol 50:159–176

Vidal JA, Murphey MD (2007) Primary tumors of the osseous spine. Magn Reson Imaging Clin N Am 15(2):239–255

Weinstein JN, McLain RF (1987) Primary tumors of the spine. Spine 12:843–851

Woods ER, Martel W, Mandell SH et al (1993) Reactive soft-tissue mass associated with osteoid osteoma: correlation of MR imaging features with pathologic findings. Radiology 186(1):221–225

Yuh WT, Quets JP, Lee JH et al (1996) Anatomic distribution of metastases in the vertebral body and modes of hematogenous spread. Spine 21:2243–2250

Zampa V, Bargellini I, Ortori S et al (2009) Osteoid osteoma in atypical locations: the added value of dynamic gadolinium-enhanced MR imaging. Eur J Radiol 71(3):527–535

Zhou XJ, Leeds NE, McKinnon GC et al (2002) Characterization of benign and metastatic vertebral compression fractures with quantitative diffusion MR imaging. AJNR Am J Neuroradiol 23:165–170

Conventional Radiography and Computed Tomography

Violeta Vasilevska Nikodinovska,
Simranjeet Kaur, and Radhesh Lalam

Contents

V. Vasilevska Nikodinovska
Medical Faculty, University "Ss. Cyril and Methodius", Skopje, Macedonia

Department of Radiology, University Surgical Clinic "St. Naum Ohridski", Skopje, Macedonia

S. Kaur · R. Lalam (✉)
Department of Radiology, The Robert Jones and Agnes Hunt Orthopaedic Hospital, Oswestry, Shropshire, UK
e-mail: Simranjeet.kaur5@nhs.net; radhesh.lalam@nhs.net

Med Radiol Diagn Imaging (2023)

https://doi.org/10.1007/174_2023_465,
Published Online: 26 November 2023

Abstract

Conventional radiography is the basic imaging modality for the diagnosis of primary bone tumors of the spine, readily available, often the first examination performed in patients presenting with spinal symptoms such as back pain, mass, or scoliosis. The major limitation is lesion identification in complex anatomy and superimposition.

Weight-bearing radiographs are key to assessing the alignment of the spine as this information is not provided by other imaging modalities. It may help the surgeon in making a decision regarding overall spinal balance and need for stabilization.

Multidetector CT allows precise anatomical delineation and evaluation of the lesions in complex anatomical locations, where radiographs are not sufficient. Visualization of minor bony changes, tumor mineralization, small calcifications, cortical changes, and periosteal reactions is best possible on CT scan. The lack of characterization of soft tissue along with the lack of precise extent of medullary involvement, which is important for staging, is a major limitation of CT for precise delineation of the lesion extent. MRI can overcome this problem. CT plays an important role in performing imaging-guided biopsy.

All three imaging modalities have complementary value with specific advantages for each modality and are often performed together in each individual patient with spinal tumor.

1 Introduction

Primary tumors of the vertebral column make up 10% of all spinal tumors (Hsu et al. 2009). Based on their anatomic locations, they are classified as extradural tumors, extramedullary intradural tumors, and intramedullary tumors. The majority of spine tumors are extradural in location, which can involve the bones, disks, and adjacent paraspinal soft tissues, presenting with a typical imaging appearance (Simmons and Zheng 2006). The World Health Organization has classified the primary bone tumors as osteogenic, chondrogenic, vascular, hematopoietic, notochordal, osteoclastic giant cell-rich, fibrogenic, and other mesenchymal tumors of the bone (Murphy and Kransdorf 2021; WHO 2020). Familiarity with the characteristic radiological imaging features can help the radiologist reach an accurate diagnosis in some cases.

Radiographs are the most crucial part of the initial diagnosis of primary bone tumors of the spine. However, there is one major limitation, lesion identification in complex anatomy, and superimposition (Riahi et al. 2018). CT scan with multiplanar reformations can be considered in those areas. Thus, a multimodality imaging approach for bone tumor evaluation such as conventional radiography (CR), CT, and MRI is needed for further tumor evaluation. Radiographs and CT are also important for staging and treatment planning of the disease (Goyal et al. 2019). A primary osseous vertebral tumor is often seen on MRI first but will still need radiography/CT for further assessment by providing additional, complementary information for further diagnostic and therapeutic workup of the patient (Fig. 1). CT provides superior cortical bony details compared to MRI. It is helpful in tumor matrix characterization, and it has a unique role in guiding biopsy (Riahi et al. 2018; Jarvik and Deyo 2002; Lateef and Patel 2009). CT is more rapidly acquired compared to MRI and therefore more favored in the acute setting.

1.1 What Can Be Analyzed on Initial Radiography and CT in a Patient Suspected of a Spinal Bone Tumor?

On initial radiography

- Alignment—look for scoliosis: it often points to the presence and location of the spine tumor
- Alteration of normal radiological anatomy of the spine
- Analysis of the lesion: determination of the risk of malignancy and assessment of internal tumor composition

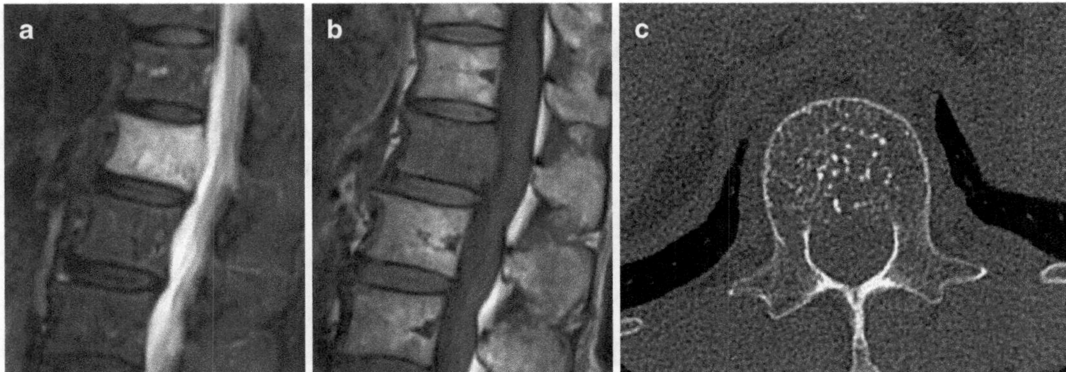

Fig. 1 Vertebral hemangioma. (**a**) Sagittal STIR. (**b**) Sagittal T1-weighted image (WI) depicts an expansile lesion in L1 occupying the entire vertebral body with bowing of the posterior vertebral body margin. There is replacement of marrow with a T1 hypointense and bright signal on the STIR sequences. The differential diagnosis is wide based on the MRI appearance. However, (**c**) axial CT depicts the typical polka-dot appearance representing the vertical sclerotic trabeculae, which is pathognomonic for hemangioma

On initial spine CT, what should be reported?

- Location of the lesion within the vertebra (body and posterior elements) and sacrum
- Structural changes of the bone
- Enhancing epidural mass associated with spinal canal narrowing with spinal cord compression at the level of the affected vertebral body
- Soft tissue mass extending into intervertebral foramina with distorted and compressed exiting nerve roots
- Paraspinal soft tissue component extending in continuation of the vertebral lesion
- Tumor matrix mineralization of the paravertebral, epidural, and intervertebral foraminal soft tissue components and its characteristics
- Height and symmetry of the intervertebral disk
- Structural changes of adjacent ribs

2 Conventional Radiography

CR is the basic imaging modality for the diagnosis of bone tumors, readily available, often the first examination performed in patients presenting with spinal symptoms such as back pain, mass, or scoliosis (Jarvik and Deyo 2002). The diagnostic principle is that it has relatively high sensitivity and relatively high spatial resolution in imaging bone tissues, based on the change in bone mineral density caused by the change in the concentration of calcium in the bone. It has limited use for chondromatous lesion examination and analysis.

Routine radiographic projections include anteroposterior (AP) and lateral projections. It is best for spinal radiographs to be centered at the level of the tumor location. Additional views of the spine such as double-oblique radiographs may be necessary sometimes for further clarification, but nowadays, these have been replaced by cross-sectional imaging such as CT or MRI.

Appropriate weight-bearing full-length spine radiographs can be obtained when evaluating a patient for suspected imbalance. Whole-spine radiographs must include cervico-occipital region and both femoral heads. Plain radiographs can be obtained either through a standardized method using long-film acquisitions with a radiographic source located 180 cm (72 in.) away from the subject or, more recently, through the use of an EOS™ system. This system is a slot-scanning device that allows the simultaneous acquisition of full-length spine radiographs, in the standing position, both in the PA (or AP) and in the lateral position with a significant dose reduction when compared with traditional digital radiography acquisitions (Dubousset et al. 2007).

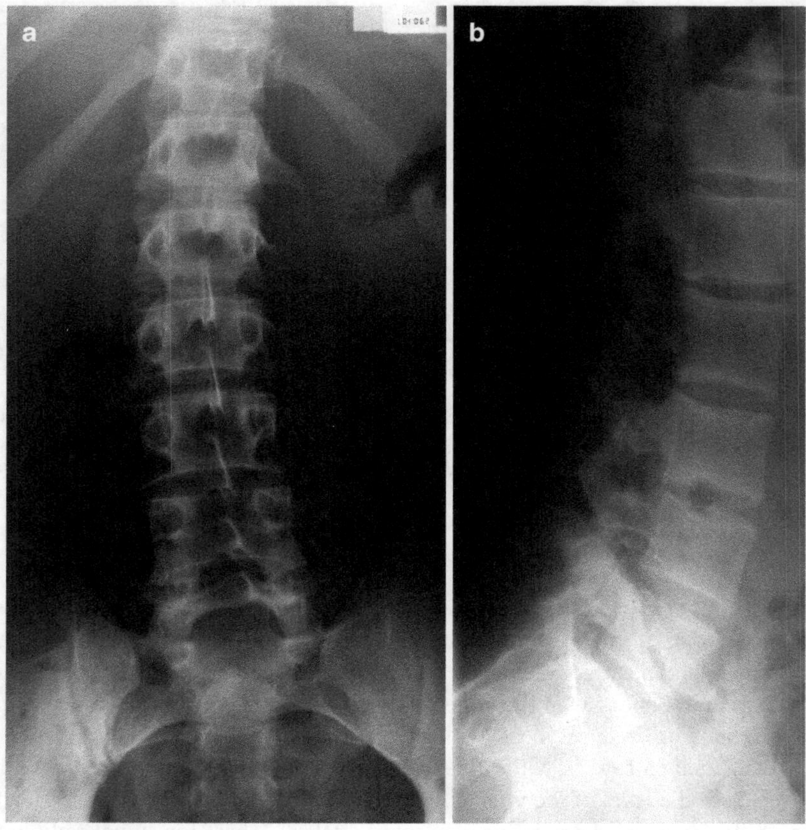

Fig. 2 Osteoid osteoma. (**a**) Anteroposterior and (**b**) lateral radiograph in a patient with osteoid osteoma involving the left pedicle of L1 vertebra. There is lumbar scoliosis with convexity toward the right and the apex of the scoliotic curve at L1. There is sclerosis of the left-sided pedicle with the osteoid osteoma being on the concave side of the curve

Whole-spine radiographs (AP and lateral, often standing/weight-bearing) are performed to assess the alignment of the spine before surgical treatment. Local scoliosis, rotational, due to muscular spasm, may raise suspicion of spine tumor even in the absence of clear visualization of the lesion at radiography (Riahi et al. 2018; McLeod et al. 1976) (Fig. 2). Weight-bearing radiographs are key to assessing the alignment of the spine as this information is not provided by other imaging modalities. It may help the surgeon in making a decision regarding overall spinal balance and need for stabilization.

2.1 Radiological Anatomy of the Spine

When analyzing radiographs of the spine, radiologists should be aware of the normal radiographic anatomy of the vertebral column. This is particularly difficult in the vertebral column because of the overlap of bowel and visceral structures. In addition, the vertebra has a complex anatomical morphology when compared to a long bone, and the complex posterior elements overlapping over the vertebral body on an AP radiograph can often be difficult to appreciate. However, subtle disruption of these normal anatomical landmarks may be the earliest sign of a spinal tumor. Some of the common landmarks to identify on a typical AP radiograph of the vertebra are noted in Fig. 3. Special care should be taken to carefully evaluate the circumferential symmetric cortical margin of the cortex around the pedicle on either side to identify any subtle disruption to this circumferential sclerotic border. The lateral radiograph may give more information when the lesion is located in the posterior elements due to less overlap of other structures.

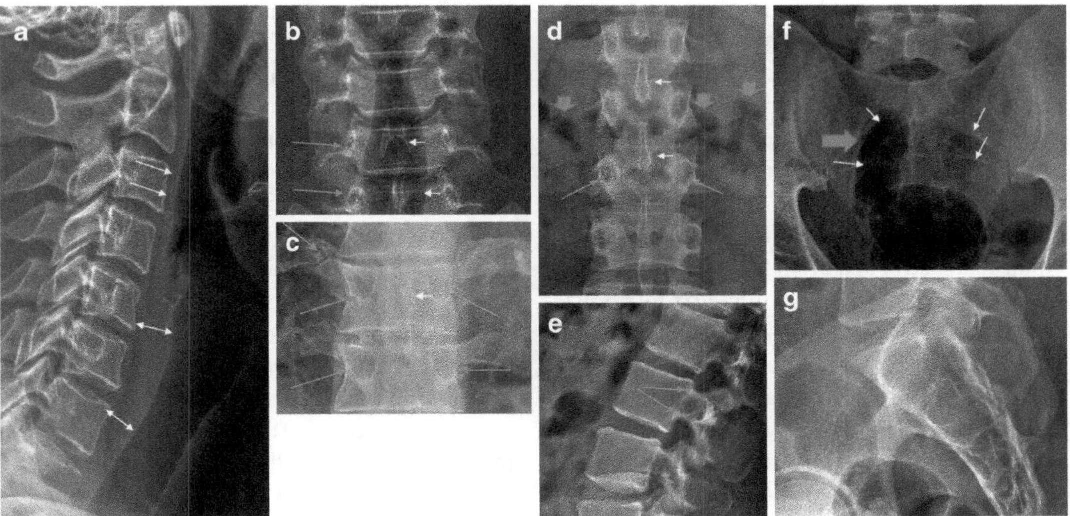

Fig. 3 Radiological anatomy of the spine. (**a**) Lateral (L) radiograph of the cervical spine presents the normal width of the prevertebral space (arrows); (**b**) anteroposterior radiograph of cervical spine AP; (**c**) anteroposterior radiograph of thoracic spine; (**d**, **e**) lumbar spine AP and L; radiography of sacral bone AP (**f**) and (**g**) L shows foramina (arrows). Pedicle (blue thin arrows), costovertebral articulation (red arrows), spinous process (short arrows), bowel gas translucency (thick blue arrows)

Prevertebral soft tissue analysis may give information about the presence of a soft tissue mass that extends along vertebral bodies.

2.2 Structural Changes of the Spine in Primary Spine Tumors

Initial evaluation of suspected bone tumor of the spine begins with orthogonal radiographs of the affected area, followed by cross-sectional imaging, such as CT and MRI. It is important to recognize early radiological signs of the presence of the bone tumor. The assessment of the tumor characteristic helps to predict benignity versus malignancy. Lesion margins, or zone of transition, described as narrow or wide, correlate with the rate of growth which are important radiographic features that form the basis of the grading system of lytic bone lesions (Lodwick classification; see chapter "Local and Distant Staging"). Further assessment of imaging findings will help in more specific diagnoses.

The radiographs in spine lesions will indicate structural changes and, in some cases, also sagittal imbalance (Azad et al. 2022). The size of the tumor, its density, internal matrix, and periosteal reaction can be assessed. Radiographs give valuable information about the nature of the tumor and the differentiation of lucent from sclerotic lesion (osteolytic vs. osteoblastic), which helps in differential diagnosis. When a lytic lesion has an expanded, remodeled "blown-out" or "ballooned" bony contour of the host bone, with a regular or a delicate trabeculated appearance, this may be a sign of lesions such as aneurysmal bone cyst or myeloma. The distribution of the tumor within the vertebral body can be central or eccentric. Some tumors are preferentially located at the midline of the spine (vertebra or sacrum). In eccentrically distributed lesions, bony septa can be seen, which may give a radiographic "soap bubble" appearance. Larger lesions at presentation may, however, appear central in location.

Tumor matrix mineralization is related to the tissue of origin of the tumor (bone- or cartilage-forming tumors and fibrogenic tumors). The internal matrix of a bone lesion is best evaluated on CR and CT and points to cell lineage (i.e., osteoid, chondroid, or fibrohistiocytic). On CR, due to complex anatomy and overlapping structures, the type of tumor matrix mineralization is a bit difficult to be seen and differentiated. Osteoblastic tumors can display amorphous or cloud-like matrix and often lack an organized trabecular pattern. The degree of matrix mineralization can be quite variable; thus, the radiographic appearance of osteoblastic tumors may range from densely blastic to nearly completely lytic. Cartilage-forming tumors typically exhibit punctate annular or commalike calcifications at radiography, which are better demonstrated on CT, whereas a ground-glass appearance is reserved for the fibrous stroma in fibrous dysplasia.

Benign tumors usually exhibit geographic bone destruction and sclerotic margins without soft tissue extension (except ABC, aggressive hemangioma, and eosinophilic granuloma). Malignant tumors usually have poorly defined margins, permeative bone destruction, and a soft tissue mass, often difficult to recognize at radiography. Radiographs demonstrate cortical/endplate destruction, expansion of the vertebra, and presence of reactive sclerosis. Trabecular preservation and its structural changes, thickened/sclerotic or destroyed, deserve careful observation since it can give valuable information about bone structure changes. Vertical striations or a "honeycomb" pattern, for example, is highly suggestive of hemangioma of the vertebral body (Fig. 4).

The pedicle of the vertebral arch and the sclerotic rim of the base of spinous process may show lytic or sclerotic changes, with or without expansion and destruction (Fig. 4b). The symmetry of the findings with the other pedicle can be assessed through a comparison of the same vertebra and with those of adjacent vertebra. Subtle asymmetry is especially important and can increase the suspicion of the presence of the lesion. Osteolysis of the pedicle may be evident in the anteroposterior view of the thoracolumbar spine as the so-called owl's-eye sign with loss of the typical elliptical appearance of the sclerotic rim of the pedicle on the affected side (Fig. 5). Also, trans-

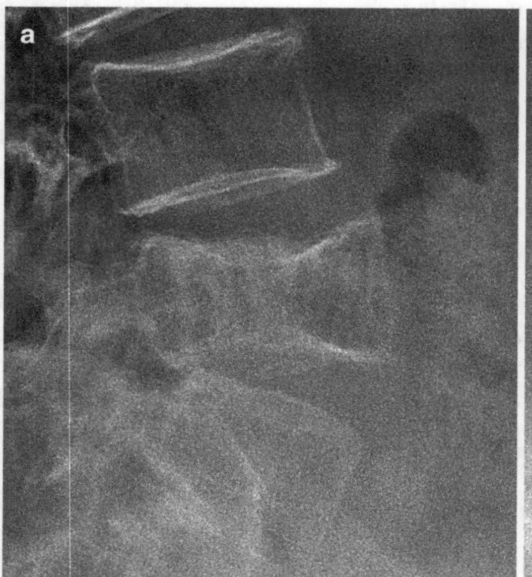

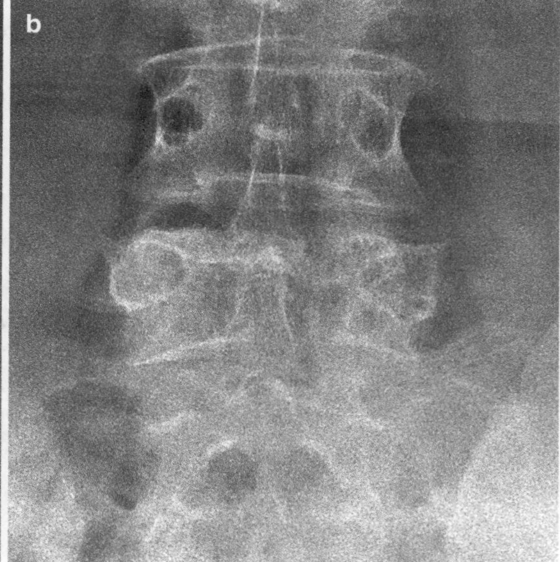

Fig. 4 Aggressive hemangioma. (**a**) Lateral radiograph of L4 vertebra with vertical striation of the vertebral body, which is highly suggestive for hemangioma. (**b**) Anteroposterior radiograph shows enlarged but preserved sclerotic margin of the pedicles. There are endplate depression and posterior cortical bowing without cortical disruption

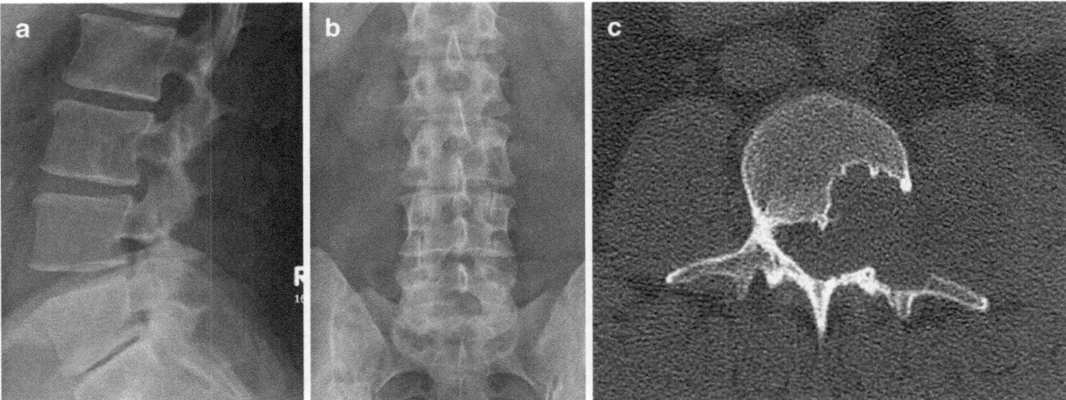

Fig. 5 Schwannoma. (**a**) Lateral and (**b**) anteroposterior radiograph of lumbosacral spine depicts a lobulated expansile lucent lesion involving the posterior body of L3 vertebra with extension into the pedicle. (**c**) Axial CT depicts a slow-growing well-marginated lesion characterized by well-defined sclerotic margins. Histology showed this lesion to be a benign schwannoma

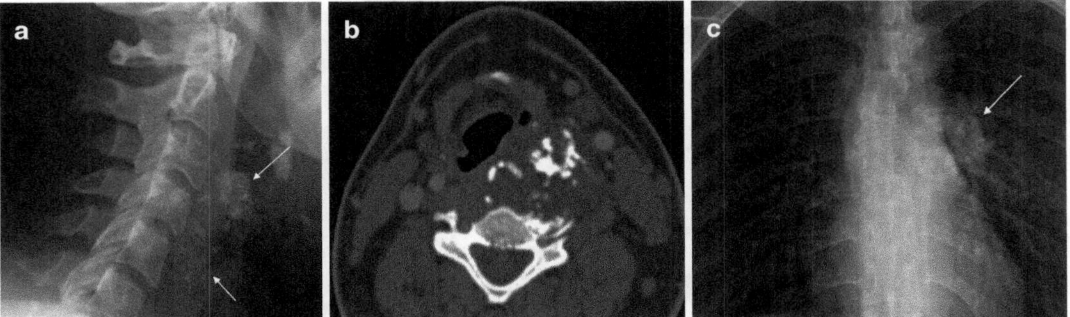

Fig. 6 Chondrosarcoma and osteosarcoma. (**a**) Cervical spine lateral radiograph presents prevertebral space widening in a patient with chondrosarcoma depicting calcification in front of C3 and C4 vertebral bodies with subtle contour abnormality and cortical erosion. The matrix mineralization is best depicted on (**b**) axial CT, which shows the typical ring and arc chondroid matrix (arrows). (**c**) Anteroposterior radiograph of thoracic spine depicts left-sided paravertebral soft tissue mass with calcification in patient with T6 osteosarcoma (arrow)

verse process hypertrophy on an AP radiograph, which can appear immediately adjacent to the lesion, may suggest osteoid osteoma (possibly as a result of local osseous hyperemia) (Williams et al. 2012).

Prevertebral soft tissue widening may suggest mass extension along vertebral bodies. The paravertebral soft tissues, particularly in the thoracic spine, are a good clue for the diagnosis of a vertebral tumor (Fig. 6). Tumor may extend through the vertebral articulation, costovertebral articulation, and intervertebral disk and into the adjacent vertebral segment.

On CR and CT, the compromised vertebral stability which may occur due to ballooning, a multilobulated lytic lesion that resembles a “soap bubble” with a “blown-out” appearance, can be assessed (Burch et al. 2008; Murphey et al. 1996). Primarily, lytic lesions may commonly cause pathological fractures seen as vertebral collapse (partial or complete). In incomplete vertebral collapse, anterior wedging of the vertebral body is

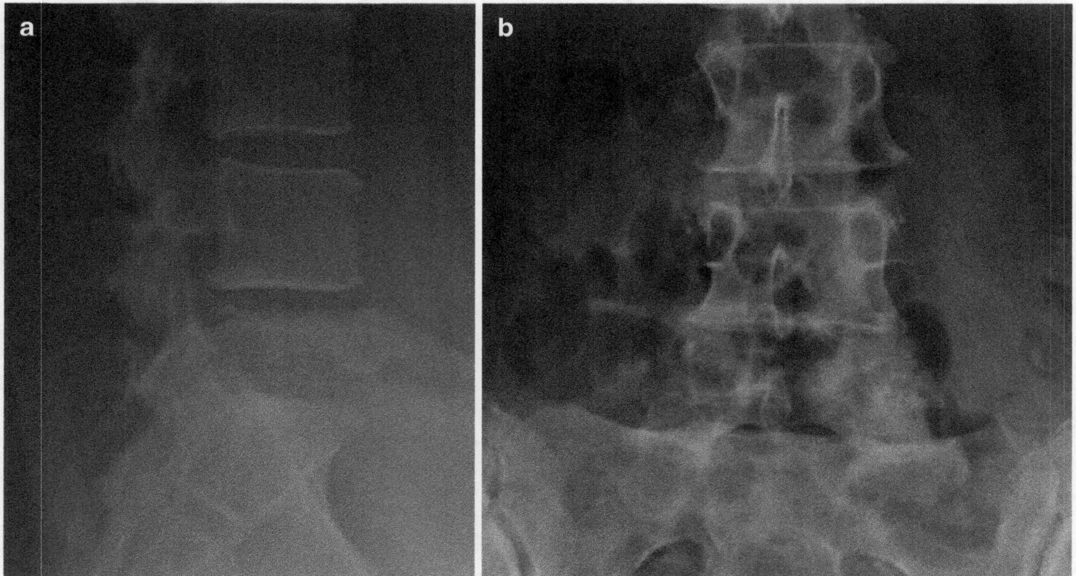

Fig. 7 Primary bone sarcoma. (**a**) Lateral and (**b**) anteroposterior radiograph of lumbosacral spine depicts complete collapse of L1 resulting in vertebra plana in a patient with primary bone sarcoma

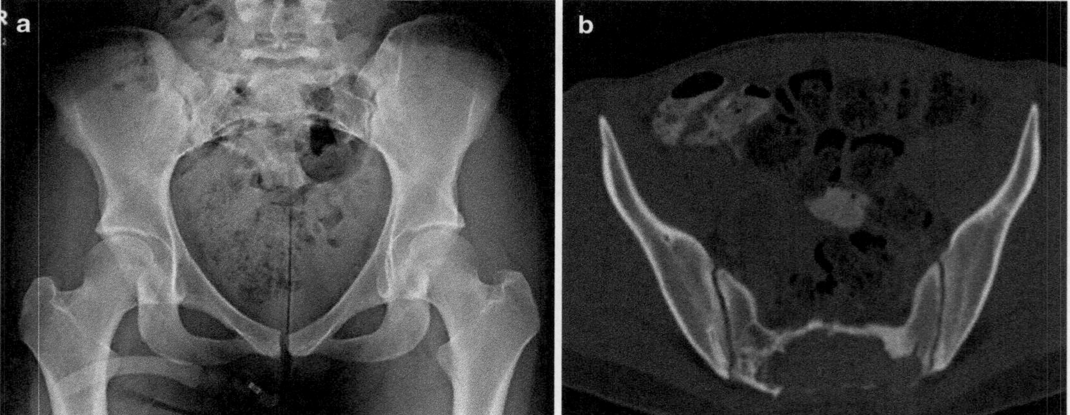

Fig. 8 Giant cell tumor. (**a**) Anteroposterior radiograph of pelvis in a patient with giant cell tumor of the sacrum appears unremarkable. The lesion detection is extremely difficult because of the overlapping gas-filled bowel shadows. (**b**) Axial CT however clearly depicts the lucent expansile lesion with exquisite cortical thinning

better observed on lateral radiographs. A complete vertebral body collapse is known as vertebra plana (Codd et al. 2006; Levin et al. 2006) (Fig. 7).

Sacral tumors are often not visible on radiography due to the flat nature of the sacral bone and the overlap of the sacrum by pelvic viscera (Figs. 8 and 9).

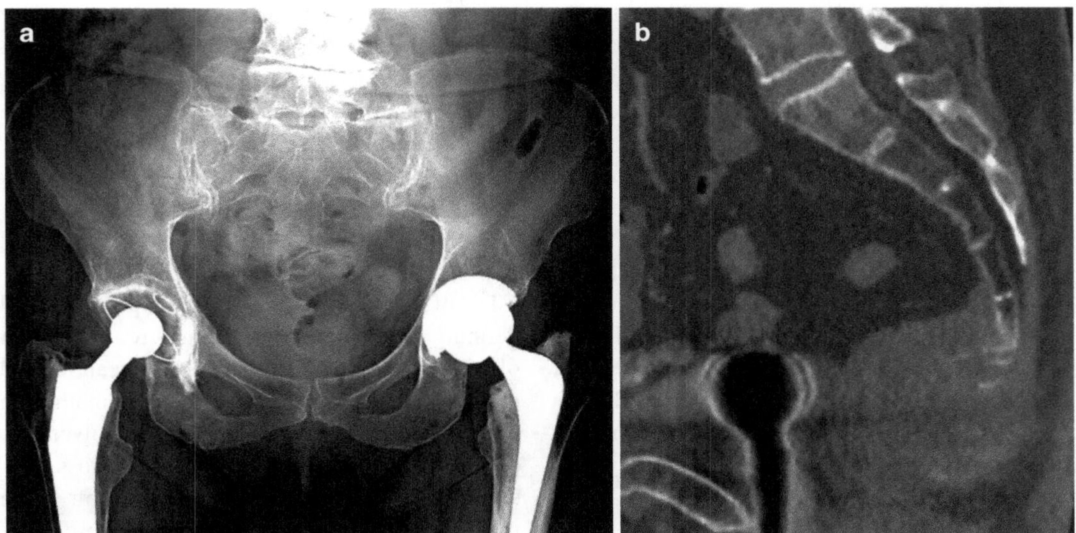

Fig. 9 Sacrococcygeal chordoma. (**a**) Anteroposterior radiograph of pelvis in a patient with chordoma. It is very difficult to diagnose the abnormality on the plain radiograph because of the complex anatomy and superimposition by bowel and urinary bladder. (**b**) Sagittal CT in the same patient depicts a large sacrococcygeal chordoma with associated extra-osseous soft tissue

2.3 Advantages and Disadvantages of Conventional Radiography

Advantages: Radiographs are easy to perform, excellent for initial examination of spinal tumors and for follow-up of some tumors and in postoperative follow-up. They are often diagnostic, accessible, inexpensive, and critical in evaluating bone tumors. For some tumors, the diagnosis can be reached on a radiograph. Radiographs are often complementary and contributory even when a lesion is first detected on MRI scan and are routinely required in this situation. CR provides information on calcifications, skeletal structure, and fractures. Whole-spine radiography gives valuable information about spine alignment.

Disadvantages: A complex and dense three-dimensional anatomical structure of the spine is difficult to appreciate on two-dimensional radiographs. Several overlapping structures such as the viscera, bowel and lungs, and their opacification or lucent appearance cause difficulties in the assessment of spine tumors on radiographs. In this context, the complexity and density of the vertebral bony structures make it difficult to identify and correctly interpret a spinal tumor. Small primary osseous tumors are therefore often missed on radiographs. This may lead to a considerable delay in diagnosis.

3 Computed Tomography

Cross-sectional imaging is considered essential for staging and treatment planning for vertebral lesions. Computed tomography (CT) is a technology using ionizing radiation to generate images resulting from different absorption of X-ray of the specific tissues examined. CT scanner with 16 slices and above produces good cross-sectional displays and allows multidimensional 2D and 3D reconstructions. The advantage of CT is the detailed assessment of bone and thus offers a great advantage in evaluating the osseous spine. With its higher contrast resolution, multidetector CT allows precise anatomical delineation and evaluation of the lesions in complex anatomical locations, where radiographs are not sufficient. Visualization of minor bony changes, tumor mineralization, small calcifications, cortical changes, and periosteal reactions are best seen on CT scans. However, CT scan is not sensitive to the microperiosteal reaction of the spinal osseous tumors, which may cause missed diagnosis or misdiagnosis (Yang et al. 2019; Sahinarslan et al. 2013). The lack of characterization of soft tissue along with the lack of precise extent of medullary involvement, which is important for staging, is a major limitation of CT for precise delineation of the lesion extent. MRI can overcome this problem. CT plays an important role in performing imaging-guided biopsy.

3.1 CT Examination of the Spine

Multidetector CT is performed in most cases with a large field of view without and with contrast medium application. With the use of an isotropic volume acquisition, it is possible to obtain axial, sagittal, and coronal reformatted images that are of the same quality as the source images. Two-dimensional multiplanar reformatted images are useful in the evaluation of cortical bone destruction and calcified tumor matrix. An optimal slice thickness depending on the spinal segment of interest is required. It is beneficial in spine CT examinations to review multiplanar reformations. The use of MDCT with thin slices (2–3 mm thickness) and small fields of view (12–20 cm) is recommended to maximize spatial resolution. However, thin slices mean increased radiation dose, so care must be taken to minimize it, especially in young patients. Images should be reviewed at window settings that are appropriate for demonstrating a range of display densities, including soft tissue and osseous abnormalities, in order to optimize spatial and contrast resolution.

CT angiography can be used to identify critical vascular structures that may be affected by a surgical approach. It is commonly used to depict the relationship of cervical spinal tumors to the supra-aortic trunks. In the thoracolumbar location of the tumor, CT angiography is useful in the evaluation of the artery of Adamkiewicz (Yoshioka et al. 2006, 2018). However, conventional angiography is superior in determining the precise relationship between the tumor and the spinal vessels.

3.2 Lesion Assessment on CT

CT is of immense help in delineating the site and defining the anatomic origin, nature, and extent of bone destruction and radiologic feature of a given lesion. CT is the most accurate method in depicting the extent of osseous involvement, degree of cancellous and cortical bone loss, preserved or interrupted cortex, and any soft tissue mineralization. It is less accurate for soft tissue extension of the lesion, with or without spinal canal narrowing.

CT can demonstrate if a lesion is centrally or eccentrically located (Fig. 10). Larger lesions at presentation often appear spuriously at a central location. CT gives information about locoregional tumoral extension as well. In thoracic spinal tumors, presurgical accurate delineation of the relationship of the lesion to the pleura, mediastinum, and ribs is needed (Fig. 11). In tumors of the lumbar spine, the involvement of the retroperitoneum should be assessed. Presence of a fat line between the lesion and the psoas muscle can be assessed for possible infiltration on CT.

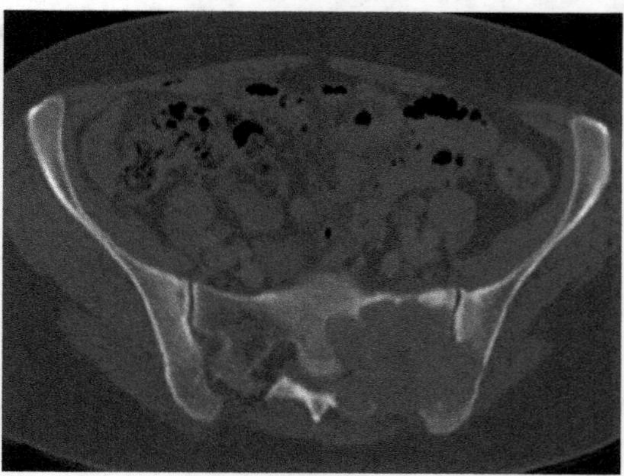

Fig. 10 Axial CT depicting a purely osteolytic expansile lesion of the sacral bone, with eccentric location and extension across the left sacroiliac joint

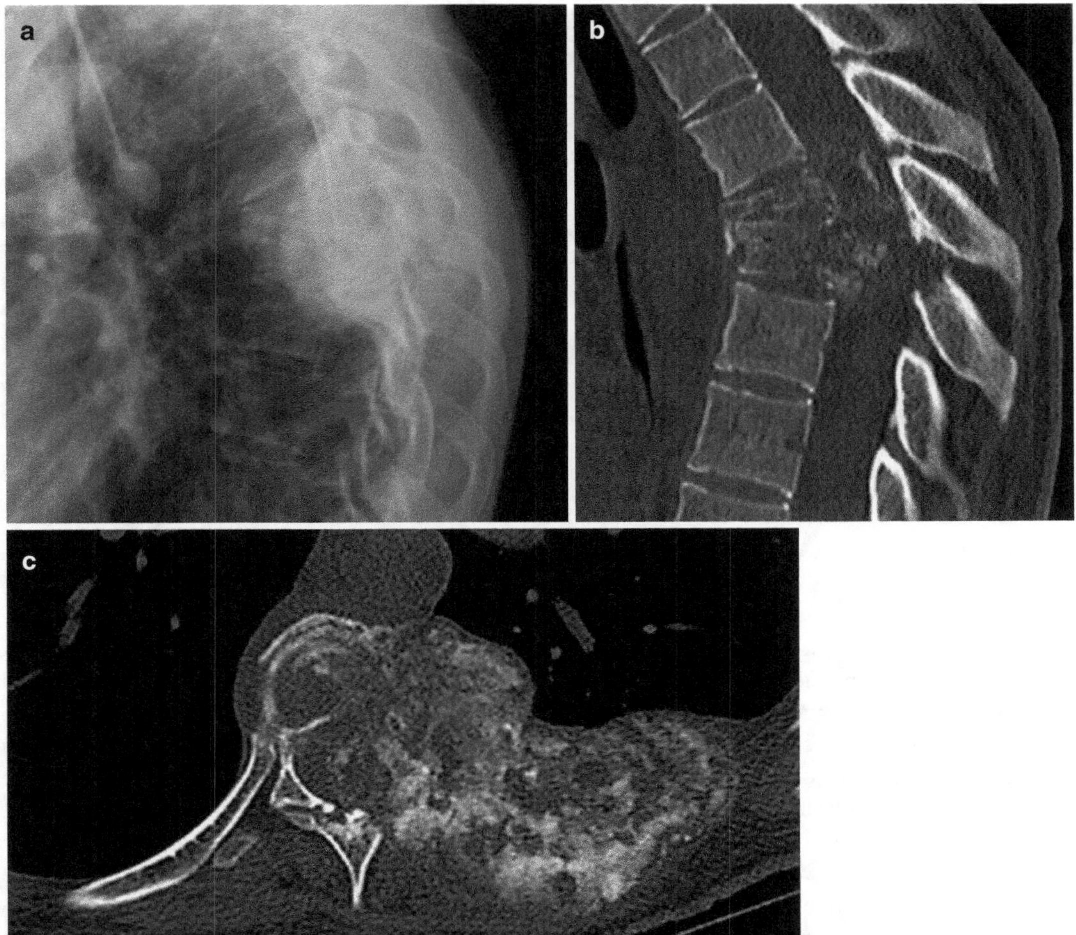

Fig. 11 Osteosarcoma. (**a**) Lateral radiograph depicts pathological collapse of T6 vertebral body with ill-defined sclerosis of T6 associated with a left-sided paravertebral soft tissue mass with calcification. (**b**) Sagittal and (**c**) axial CT demonstrates the collapse of T6 vertebral body with contiguous involvement of the T7 vertebra, which depicts permeative pattern of bone destruction. There is contiguous involvement of the left sixth rib with aggressive periosteal reaction and involvement of the spinal canal. There is a large associated paravertebral soft tissue with osteoid matrix consistent with the histological diagnosis of osteosarcoma

For sacral tumors, it is important to delineate lesion extension to the sacroiliac joints, iliac bone, and pelvis (Fig. 12). Post-processing, multiplanar reformatted images improve assessment of the localization, lesion size, shape, and extension.

Attenuation of the lesion, and its density, gives information about the tissue's cellularity. A lytic lesion usually demonstrates the same density as surrounding muscle on the native scan (Shi et al. 2016), with variable enhancement after contrast media application. Areas of hemorrhage or necrosis may create a heterogeneous density. Focal low-attenuation areas are seen in contrast-enhanced computed tomography presenting possible areas of necrosis. When the lesion is predominantly sclerotic, it can be of variable degree (subtle, mild, severe), which is suggestive of the osteoblastic activity of the tumor. Large foci of intratumoral fat within lesions can be identified on CT and can be found in vertebral

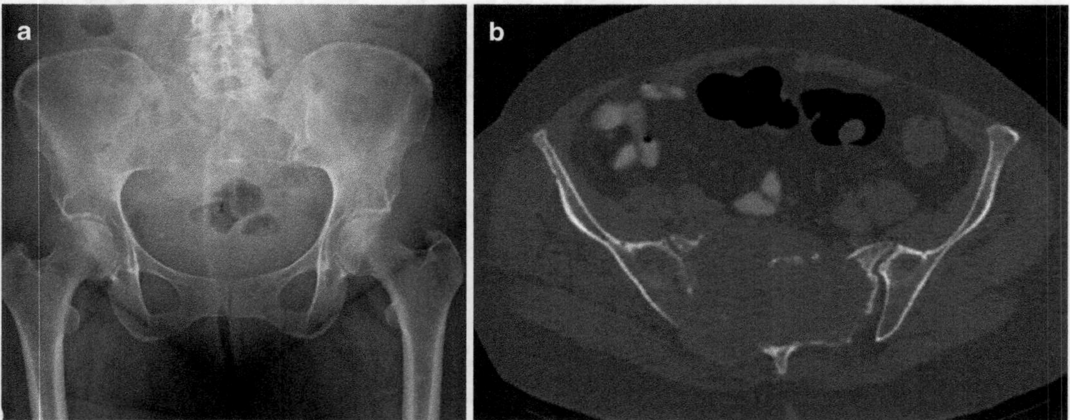

Fig. 12 (**a**) Plain radiograph in a patient depicts a lucent lesion involving the sacrum. (**b**) Axial CT in the same patient depicts the expansile destructive lesion with cortical destruction and associated extra-osseous soft tissue

hemangioma, fibrous dysplasia, Paget's disease, and Schmorl's node.

CT scans may show fluid-fluid levels and internal septations (Fig. 13), better demarcated after contrast administration. These fluid levels are more suggestive for ABC but have also been described in multiple spine lesions including telangiectatic osteosarcoma (giant cell tumor, osteoblastoma, chondroblastoma, solitary bone cysts, fibroxanthoma, or brown tumor) (Murphey et al. 2003; Ilaslan et al. 2004). However, this feature is better demonstrated on MRI (Fig. 13).

CT precisely gives the degree of trabecular and cortical bone destruction in areas at risk of impending fracture. Endplate preservation or its destruction can be depicted on CT. The cortex around the lytic areas may become thin or get penetrated or may disappear with an associated soft tissue mass. CT is performed additionally to MRI in a lytic lesion of the vertebra, for better assessment of cortical interruption indicating pathologic fracture (Vielgut et al. 2017).

In primarily lytic lesions, pathological fractures are common (Medow et al. 2007) that can be depicted earlier on CT (Rodallec et al. 2008). An anterior wedging of the vertebral body in incomplete vertebral collapse and vertebra plana can be better observed on sagittal reformatted CT images.

Vertical striations or a "honeycomb" pattern is highly suggestive of hemangioma of the vertebral body (Fig. 14). Multiplanar reformatted images improve detection of vascular grooves diagnostic for osteoid osteoma.

On radiography and CT, compromised vertebral stability can be suspected by ballooning and multilobulated lytic lesion that resembles a "soap bubble" with a "blown-out" appearance (Burch et al. 2008; Murphey et al. 1996), which can be seen in ABC, giant cell tumor, plasmacytoma, fibrous dysplasia, and chordoma.

CT plays a key role in demonstrating evidence of mineralized matrix. Its appearance is related to the tissue of origin of the tumor and is important for tumor characterization. CT is highly sensitive for detecting punctate annular or commalike calcifications and enhancing rings and arcs within the lesion, which are suggestive of cartilage-forming tumors (differential diagnosis of cartilage-forming tumors includes osteochondroma, chondroblastoma and chondrosarcoma, ABC, and chordoma). CT can display amorphous or cloud-like ossification in osteoblastic tumors much more clearly compared to radiography (Fig. 15). Fibrous dysplasia is easily diagnosed with CT, manifesting as ground-glass attenuation with sclerotic margins, whereas MRI has a nonspecific appearance.

CT gives more specific information about the delineation of the lesion from the surrounding unaffected bone, thereby depicting the nature of the margins of the tumor. In benign tumors, the

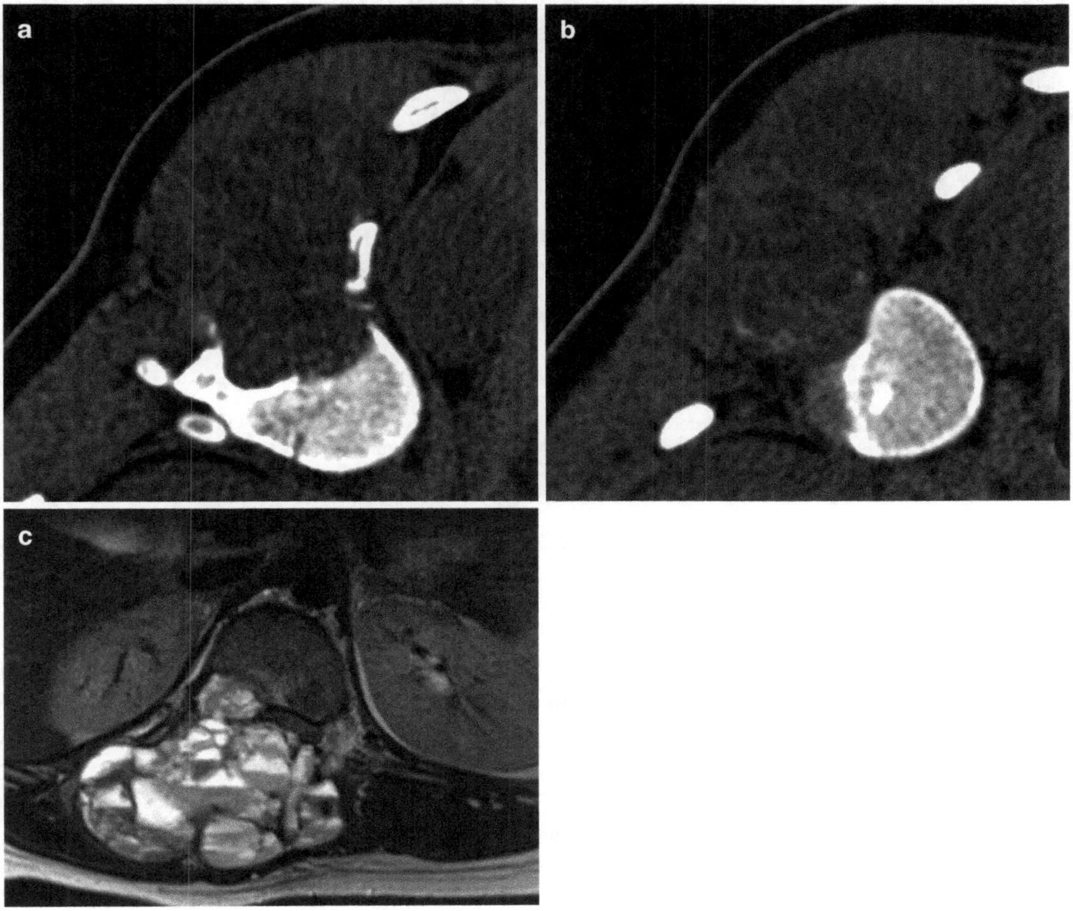

Fig. 13 (a) Axial CT at the time of biopsy depicts a large expansile lytic lesion with associated extra-osseous soft tissue component. (b) Axial CT at another level depicts the fluid-fluid levels based on the small differences in the fluid attenuation. (c) Axial T2 MRI depicting the multiple locules with fluid-fluid levels

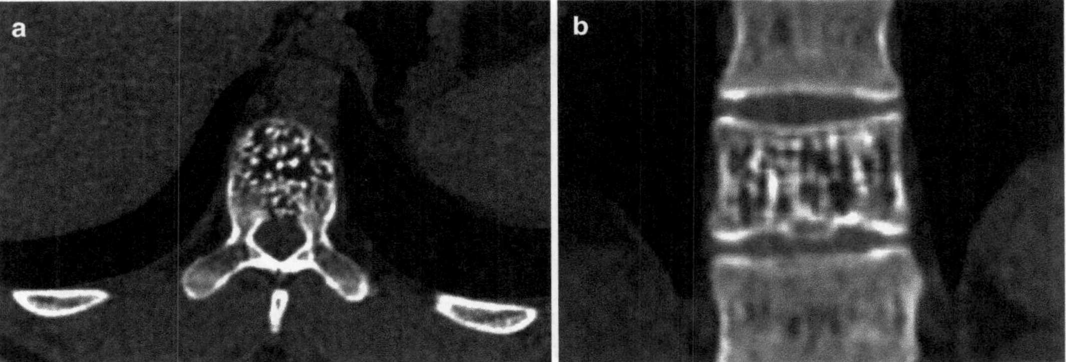

Fig. 14 Vertebral hemangioma. (a) Axial CT depicts the typical polka-dot appearance representing the thickened vertical trabeculae surrounded by fatty marrow or vascular lacunae in vertebral hemangioma. (b) Coronal reformats depicting the thickened vertical trabeculae giving rise to the jail bar sign, which is the coronal equivalent of the polka-dot sign on axial images

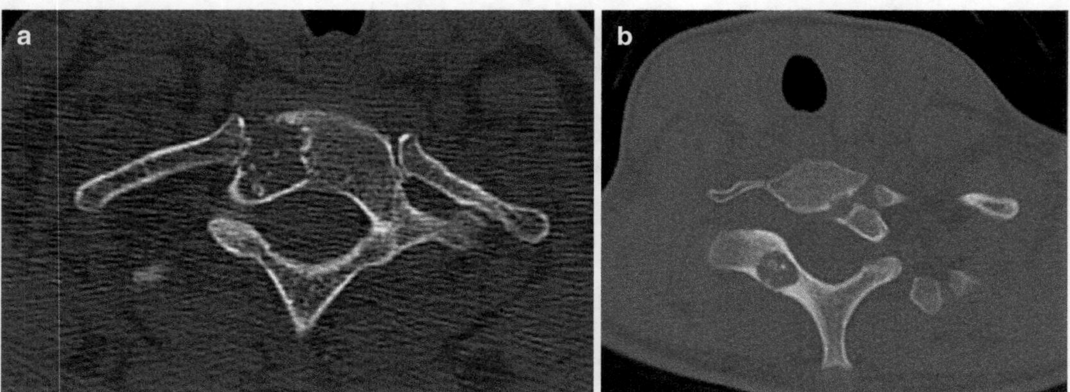

Fig. 15 Chondrosarcoma and osteoid osteoma. (**a**) Axial CT in a patient with chondrosarcoma depicts the typical ring and arc matrix mineralization. (**b**) Axial CT depicting the amorphous calcification within the lytic nidus with surrounding mild sclerosis in a patient with osteoid osteoma

margins are usually clearly demarcated, without or with a sclerotic rim of varying thicknesses. Exceptions are ABC, aggressive hemangioma, and eosinophilic granuloma, which may show aggressive pattern and poor margins despite being benign in nature. On the other hand, in malignant tumors which have poorly defined margins, the true extension of permeative bone destruction, preserved/destroyed trabeculae, and tumoral mass extension can be better assessed on CT compared to radiographs. For evaluation of the peritumoral edema including bone marrow edema and soft tissue edema, MRI is generally the method of choice.

CT gives information about the lesion extension from the vertebral body to the pedicle of the vertebral arch (lytic/sclerotic expansion, destruction, symmetry of the findings with the other pedicle), and articular facet, costovertebral articulation (Fig. 11c), adjacent vertebral segment, and spinous process (lytic/sclerotic expansion, destruction). Spinal canal can be compromised (mild, moderate, severe). Extension into the spinal canal may cause spinal cord and/or nerve root compression at the level of intervertebral foramina as well.

Although the differential diagnosis of sacral tumors is extensive, various primary neoplasms have characteristic features on CT scans. Sacrococcygeal CT scan may reveal the heterogeneity of the mass, location (upper, lower part), eccentrical or central invasion of the bone, extension to the coccyx, iliac bone, and gluteal muscles posteriorly, with extension to the pelvic cavity without rectal invasion.

CT is an ideal technique for the analysis of cortical destruction, foraminal disruption in the sacrum, and extension through sacroiliac joints. Extension across the sacroiliac joint is typical for GCT (Chhaya et al. 2005), but it can be seen in primary malignant tumors of the sacrum (chordoma, chondrosarcoma, plasmacytoma, Ewing's sarcoma). Preservation of the posterior cortex or sacral neural foramina destruction is a crucial information for treatment planning. CT can often identify small sacral tumors at a much early stage, thereby offering better chances of radical treatment (Figs. 8 and 9).

In preoperative planning of sacral tumors, if the upper border of the tumor is below the S1–S2 level, with less than 50% involvement of the sacroiliac joint, no stabilization device is needed since the stability of the spine will be preserved (Keykhosravi Otomo et al. 2022).

3.3 Advantages and Disadvantages of CT

One of the main advantages of CT scan is the ability to display lesions with complex structure, located in areas with complex anatomy and overlapping structures compared to radiography. The three-dimensional capacity of CT provides better information than radiographs.

CT demonstrates exquisite bony detail including the trabecular architecture, end plates and cortical bony details, and cortical integrity. Complications like compression fracture of the superior or inferior end plate, with CT, can be detected earlier in lytic lesions. CT precisely assesses the degree of trabecular and cortical bone destruction in areas at risk of impending fracture.

It can depict the bony tumoral matrix, anatomical origin of the lesion, paravertebral extension of the tumor, displacement and potential infiltration of the adjacent structures, and involvement of adjacent vertebrae.

CT enables the analysis of tumor margins (sclerotic rim) and the encroachment on the spinal canal.

MDCT provides an excellent 3D evaluation of lesions and bone, together with reformatted images in all planes, and can be used for accurate measurements required for surgery.

Due to higher contrast resolution, it can show tiny lesions clearly, thus allowing early detection of primary spinal osseous tumors and effectively avoiding the shortcomings of radiographs. CT is the preferred modality to guide a biopsy.

Disadvantages CT is not accurate for characterization of non-mineralized matrix, soft tissue involvement, medullary involvement, and degree of epidural extension/spinal canal compromise, all of which are better assessed on MRI imaging. Conventional CT is also poor at the evaluation of peritumoral edema, including marrow/soft tissue edema. CT scan is not sensitive to the microperiosteal reaction of the spinal osseous tumors. A further limitation of CT is the exposure to ionizing radiation during the examination.

3.4 CT in Presurgical Planning, Navigation System, and Postoperative Follow-Up

The possibility of tumor excision depends often on tumor extension in the bone, soft tissue, and involvement of neurological structures. Special emphasis should be placed on the invasion of the spinal canal, intra-osseous spread of the tumor, and extra-osseous spread to adjacent critical structures. All this information is needed for determining the possibility of wide marginal resection. Surgical planning in patients with malignant bone tumor of the spine is challenging for both orthopedic surgeons and neurosurgeons.

In treatment planning, CT plays an important role in showing spine anatomy and for measurements of the pedicle diameter at adjacent levels, which is important for selecting appropriate size and levels of pedicle screw placement.

3.4.1 Role of CT for Preoperative Planning for En Bloc Resection

Longitudinal and transverse extension of the tumor, neural structure involvement (cord and nerve roots), involvement of vascular structures, and stability of the vertebra must be commented in CT report. Stability assessment is dependent on the extent of bony invasion, especially the breakdown of cortical structures of the affected vertebra but also to the vertebral levels above and below. Any loss of vertebral height should be noted. The degree of kyphosis or other alteration in the general alignment of the vertebral column should be noted. However, CT is generally performed in a supine position, and additional weight-bearing radiographs of the whole vertebral column are needed for accurate assessment of alignment. This will assist the surgeon in planning the surgical approach and help to predict any intraoperative complications (Smith et al. 2022).

Preoperative CT can be used to create a three-dimensional model to aid in surgical planning and navigation during surgery.

Three-dimensional CT imaging allows the construction of a virtual anatomic overview enhancing the visualization of spinal disease. CT-based 3D printing technology enables the personalization of products to solve unconventional problems in spinal surgery. The surgeon may appreciate the anatomical details better on the printed model. Biomodeling accurately reproduces the morphology of a biologic structure from CT scans by using image processing software and rapid prototyping apparatus to produce a physical copy in acrylate (Izatt et al. 2007; Li et al. 2017).

Intraoperative computed tomography-based navigation system enables adequate neural decompression and maximal tumor resection (Konakondla et al. 2019). They improve the safety, accuracy, and reliability of pedicle screw placement (Uehara et al. 2017; Knez et al. 2019) and enable a lower rate of malpositioned hardware (Ouchida et al. 2020). Conventional navigation systems, which are based on reconstructions obtained using preoperative CT images, do not always accurately reproduce the intraoperative patient positioning. The intraoperative CT-based navigation system overcomes these problems, and it is now becoming the mainstay of navigated spine surgery (Otomo et al. 2022). The navigation systems help the surgeon direct the screw according to the patient's anatomical features, bypass the hidden nerves and blood vessels, avoid damage with almost 100% accuracy, and reduce the radiation dose for the surgeon and patient (Mukhametzhanov et al. 2019). Moreover, it is important to realize that the anatomic alignment changes between preoperative supine and intraoperative prone imaging, especially when multiple levels are involved. The recently introduced elastic imaging fusion software provides high registration accuracy and represents a considerable step toward efficiency and safety in CT-based image-guided surgery (Schmidt et al. 2021).

Postoperative spinal CT, with the use of optimized protocols and advanced metal artifact reduction techniques, is an important modality for evaluating the success of spinal instrumentation surgery and detecting postoperative complications. CT is accurate for determining the location and integrity of implants and identifying peri-implant changes (Ghodasara et al. 2019). Dual-energy CT is useful in metal artifact reduction, and it can assist to evaluate the spinal canal and detect possible tumor recurrence.

4 Multimodality Approach for Diagnosis of Primary Spine Tumors

There is an obvious difference in diagnosing primary spinal osseous tumors between radiography and cross-sectional imaging, both CT and MRI, with relatively low consistency. CT scan has the advantages of rapid scanning speed, even faster than radiography but at the expense of higher radiation dose. Multidetector row CT scan reduces the scanning time further, thereby leading to motion artifact reduction. MRI is even better at diagnosing and characterizing vertebral tumors due to its excellent contrast resolution (Yang et al. 2019).

However, all these three imaging modalities have complementary value with specific advantages for each modality as described earlier and are often performed together in each individual patient with spinal tumor.

5 Tumor Characterization by Radiography and CT

5.1 Benign Tumors

5.1.1 Osteoid Osteoma

Spinal osteoid osteoma should be suspected in any case of painful scoliosis in a young person seen at radiography (Kransdorf et al. 1991). The tumor is usually located at the concavity of the apex of the scoliosis, and this area should be carefully analyzed, particularly for asymmetry to the opposite side of the vertebra and the adjacent vertebra (Fig. 2). Regional osteoporosis may be seen. Radiography often shows sclerosis that obscures the oval lytic nidus or rarely only subtle sclerosis of the pedicle, in comparison with the opposite side. CT is the most accurate imaging tool to detect a lucent nidus of osteoid osteoma within the surrounding perinidal dense sclerosis and define the exact bony location and cortical thickening, which is not appreciated on other imaging modalities (Riahi et al. 2018; Erlemann 2006; Orguc and Arkun 2014; Ropper et al. 2011; Patnaik et al. 2016) (Fig. 15b) (see chapter "Osteoid Osteoma and Osteoblastoma" for further discussion). Radiolucent grooves (vascular groove sign) seen as thin lucent bands (approximately 1 mm in diameter), that course in oblique pathways through the bone, tracking toward the nidus, correspond to the enlarged arterioles that deliver blood from the periosteum to the hypervascular tumor nidus. This sign is a highly specific sign (moderately sensitive) for distinguishing osteoid osteoma from other radiolucent bone lesions on CT (Liu et al. 2011). However, the vascular groove sign is not pathognomonic of OO. It has also been described in chronic osteomyelitis.

5.1.2 Osteoblastoma

Osteoblastoma has similar radiological and histological appearance to osteoid osteoma, differentiated only in size (>1.5 cm) and less reactive sclerosis (Fig. 16). Osteoblastomas are often seen as an expansile lesion with variable matrix mineralization and a peripheral sclerotic rim and sclerosis (Murphey et al. 1996; Patnaik et al. 2016; Kumar et al. 1988; Galgano et al. 2016). In more aggressive forms of osteoblastomas, there are osseous expansion, bone destruction, infiltrating surrounding soft tissue, and variable intermixed matrix calcification (Murphey et al. 1996; Kumar et al. 1988; Galgano et al. 2016) (Fig. 17). In some cases, central cortical expansion, demarcated by a thin shell of bone and a paravertebral extension, may mimic an aneurysmal bone cyst (Ghodasara et al. 2019). CT is the method for differentiation of the type of osteoblastoma, whereas epidural extension in aggressive osteoblastoma can be better detected on MRI (Galgano et al. 2016) (see chapter "Osteoid Osteoma and Osteoblastoma" for further discussion).

5.1.3 Aneurysmal Bone Cyst

In cases of aneurysmal bone cyst, CT findings depend on the stage of the ABC. In the active growth phase, it shows a subperiosteal blowout pattern, and the mature stage has a soap bubble appearance with a distinct peripheral bony shell and internal bony septa and trabeculae, whereas the healing phase is characterized by progressive calcification and ossification of the cyst (Rajasekaran et al. 2019). Although commonly centered in the posterior elements, 75–90% of cases extend into the vertebral body (Orguc and Arkun 2014; Kransdorf and Sweet 1995). The cortical thinning with "eggshell cortex" is without disruption, which is better demonstrated on CT scan. Multiple fluid levels, within the lytic lesion, represent hemorrhage with sedimentation (Beltran et al. 1986). CT scans with narrow window settings can be performed to identify small differences in fluid attenuation. Supine positioning for around 10 min may be necessary to detect fluid levels (Orguc and Arkun 2014; Vidal and Murphey 2007). In sacral ABC at the sacroiliac joint, CT may show thinning and bulging of the cortex, within the time cortical disruption may appear, without crossing the sacroiliac joint (Llauger et al. 2000) (see chapter "Aneurysmal Bone Cyst and Other Cystic Lesions" for further discussion).

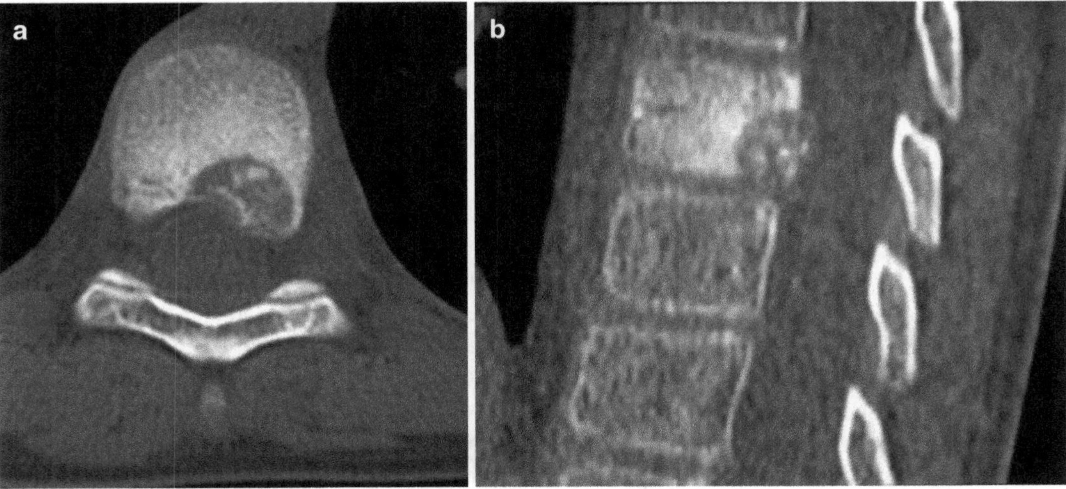

Fig. 16 Osteoblastoma. (**a**) Axial and (**b**) sagittal reformatted CT in a patient with osteoblastoma depicting the lucent lesion with imperceptible posterior cortex and central osteoid matrix mineralization with surrounding sclerosis

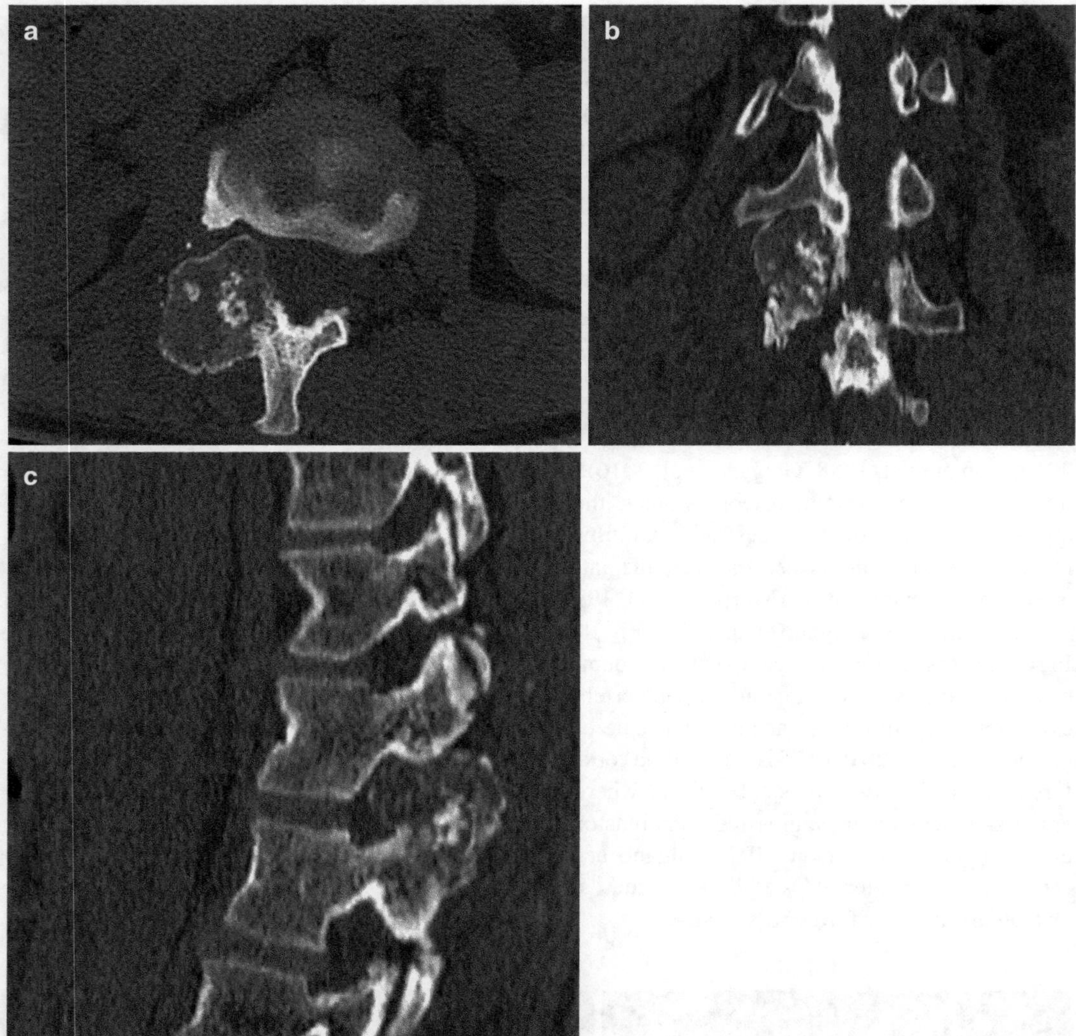

Fig. 17 Osteoblastoma. (**a**) Axial CT with (**b**) coronal and (**c**) sagittal reformats in a patient with osteoblastoma depicts a large expansile lesion in the right lamina of L1 vertebra. There is intralesional osteoid matrix and a well-defined peripheral rim

5.1.4 Hemangioma

Vertical striations, or coarse honeycomb appearance of the vertebral body, with preserved size is a typical appearance of hemangioma, better visualized on lateral plain film (Fig. 4a). It can be presented as a "mottled" appearance on X-ray and CT as well (Ropper et al. 2011). On axial CT, multiple dots (polka dots) representing a cross section of reinforced trabeculae are also suggestive of the diagnosis of hemangioma (Riahi et al. 2018; Murphey et al. 1996; Patnaik et al. 2016) (Figs. 1c and 14a). However, in some cases, a biopsy is necessary, since coarse vertical striations have been reported in GCT (Shi et al. 2016) and lymphangioma (Patnaik et al. 2016). An aggressive variant of vertebral hemangioma involves the entire vertebral body, with cortical expansion/destruction, irregular honeycombing, and soft tissue mass with extension into the neural arch (Patnaik et al. 2016) (Fig. 18) (see chap-

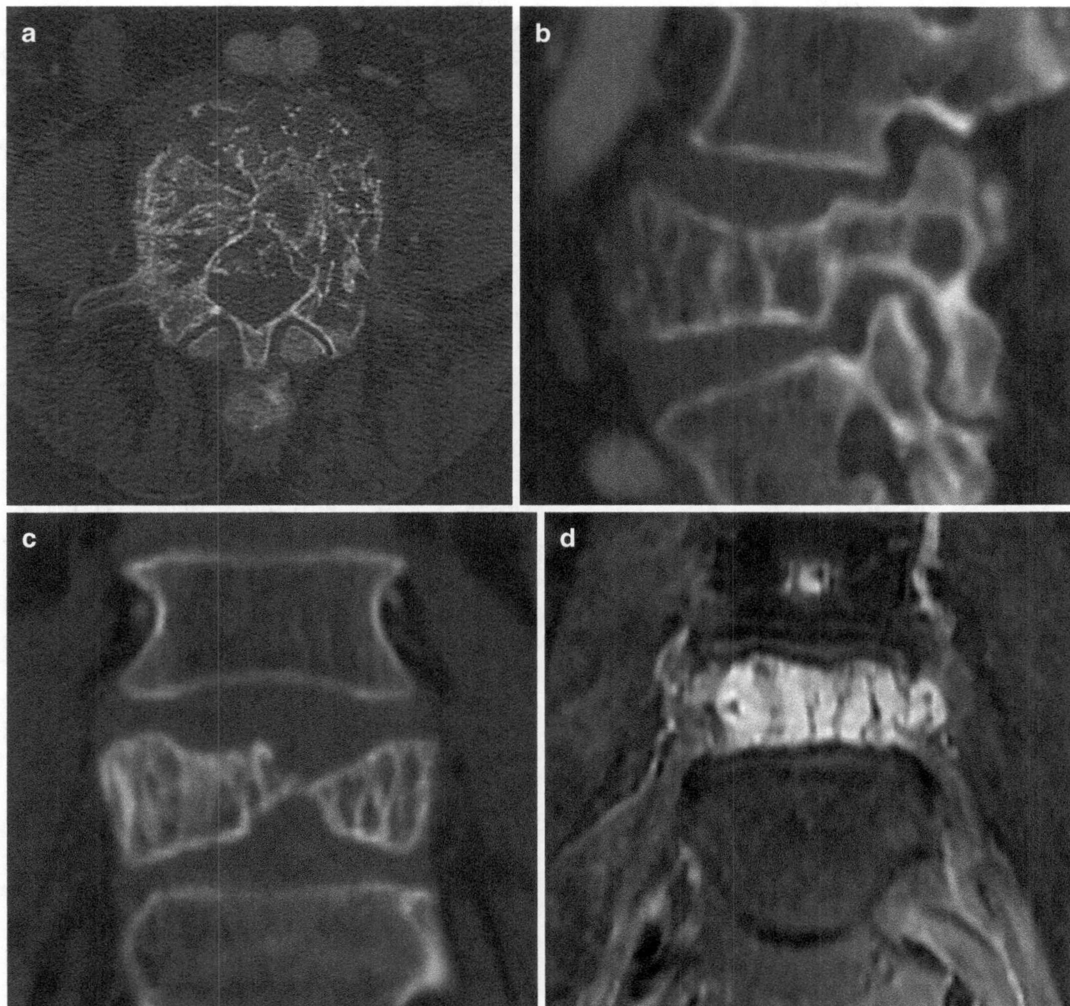

Fig. 18 Aggressive hemangioma. (**a**) Axial CT depicts coarse polka-dot appearance of the entire vertebral body and posterior elements on the left, with posterior extension into the spinal canal. On sagittal (**b**) and coronal (**c**) reconstruction, cortical depression/destruction of both end plates is seen with vertical sclerotic trabeculae that are presented on (**d**) coronal T2-WI MRI

ter "Vertebral Hemangioma and Angiomatous Neoplasms" for further discussion). These radiological findings can also be seen in lymphoma, but there is cortical permeation depicted on CT (Leong et al. 2016).

5.1.5 Giant Cell Tumor

Giant cell tumor can present as an expansile purely lytic lesion without matrix calcification (Fig. 19). It may have sclerotic rim that involves the vertebral body with extension into posterior elements, paraspinal tissue, adjacent disk, costovertebral articulation, and adjacent vertebrae in up to 79% of cases (Erlemann 2006; Orguc and Arkun 2014; Murphey et al. 2001; Hart et al. 1997; Shi et al. 2015). Vertebral collapse is often apparent with the destruction of cortical bone (Leong et al. 2016). In the thoracic spine, GCT may simulate posterior mediastinal mass on radiograph. Fluid-fluid levels, cystic areas, and

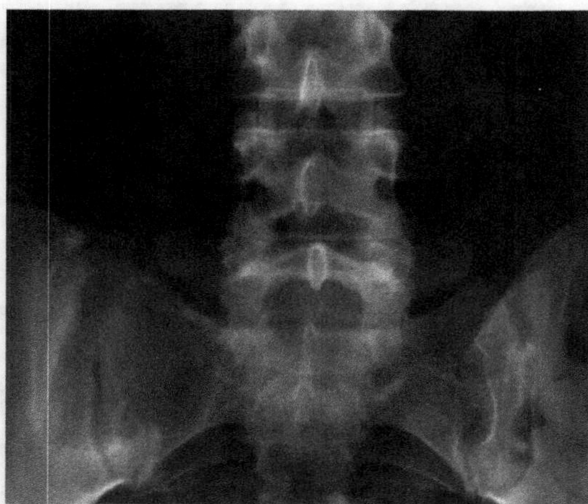

Fig. 19 Giant cell tumor. Anteroposterior plain radiograph depicts a lucent expansile lesion in the right hemisacrum with extension across the SI joint into the ilium in a patient with giant cell tumor

foci of hemorrhage may be observed on CT. Destruction of the sacral foraminal lines and extension across the sacroiliac joint are best evaluated on CT (Kwon et al. 2007) (Fig. 12). If the lesion grows eccentrically, the thin sclerotic rim in GCT usually appears opposite to the eccentric growing side (70%) (Shi et al. 2016); thus, on one side of the tumor, there is an expansile remodeling and breakthrough of the cortex, while on the other side of the tumor, there is a sclerotic border. This paradoxical appearance is helpful in diagnosing GCT. Bony septa can be seen extending from the border of the lesion extending to the inside of the mass, best seen on CT axial image. It may give a radiographic "soap bubble" appearance (Si et al. 2014) (see chapter "Giant Cell Tumors" for further discussion).

5.1.6 Osteochondroma

Osteochondroma has a mixed appearance on radiography. When lesions protrude on the tip of the spinous process and transverse process, it may be more obvious for the diagnosis even on plain film (Riahi et al. 2018). The continuity of the marrow and cortical portions of the bone from which it originates is pathognomonic and best evaluated with thin-section multiplanar CT images. Cartilaginous cap thicker than 1.5 cm in adults suggests sarcomatous degeneration (Orguc and Arkun 2014; Patnaik et al. 2016). CT enables the assessment of tumor relationship to the adjacent structures such as neuroforamina and central canal (Riahi et al. 2018) (see chapter "Cartilaginous Tumors" for further discussion).

5.1.7 Enostosis

CT is a method for diagnosis of enostosis (bone island) presented as a homogeneously dense, oval sclerotic focus of cancellous bone, with distinctive radiating spiculations or thornlike appearance at their periphery ("brush border"), which blend into the surrounding normal trabecular bone that confirms the diagnosis despite the lesion size (Fig. 20). Furthermore, CT density measurement (HU) may be helpful to differentiate bone island from osteoblastic metastasis (see chapter "Bone Island"). A mean attenuation of greater than 885 HU is a reliable method of differentiating enostosis from metastases. Due to the marked increased density, enostosis is also well seen on radiography (Riahi et al. 2018; Nguyen et al. 2020).

5.1.8 Ivory Vertebra

The ivory vertebra sign is indicative of diffuse sclerosis of a vertebral body when the trabecular pattern of normal bone is replaced by a dense, confluent chalkiness reflecting the activation of osteoblasts by the local pathologic process. A CT scan shows diffusely increased opacity, with unaffected size and margins of the vertebral body (Matthews and Dyer 2017) (Fig. 21). There are many causes of ivory vertebra appearing including lymphoma, osteosarcoma, and osteoblastoma in adults and in pediatrics, and in adults, this appearing can be seen in hemangioma, chordoma, Paget's disease of bone (Fig. 22), SAPHO syndrome, osteoblastic metastases, tuberculous spondylitis, sarcoidosis, and systemic mastocytosis.

5.1.9 Fibrous Dysplasia

Fibrous dysplasia can be seen on a radiograph with decreased height of the vertebral body and an expansile osteolytic lesion with faint ground-

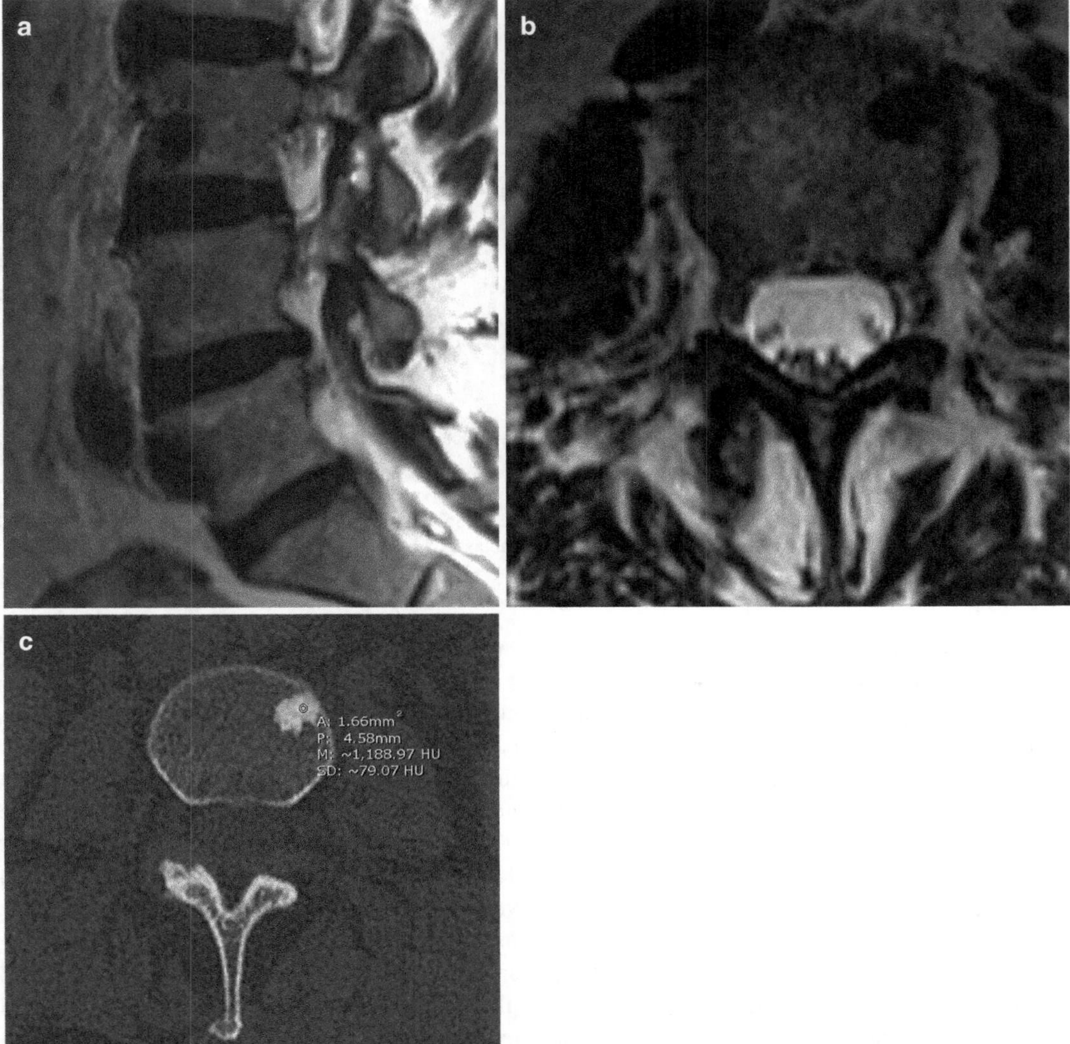

Fig. 20 Bone island. (**a**) Sagittal T2-WI and (**b**) axial T2-WI MRI depicting a low-signal-intensity lesion in the L3 vertebral body. The differential diagnosis includes sclerotic metastasis, bone island, and healed fibro-osseous lesion. (**c**) Axial CT depicts the densely sclerotic lesion having an attenuation of approximately 1188 HU with radiating spiculations blending into the normal surrounding trabecular bone, thereby confirming the diagnosis of bone island (enostosis)

glass opacity of the matrix. However, CT shows a mildly expansile lesion with a "blown-out" cortical shell or a lytic lesion with a sclerotic rim in the vertebral body with posterior element extension of the lesion. Reformatted sagittal CT scans will show contour deformities with bone remodeling due to the expansile nature of compression, as well as pathological fracture if present, which can also be seen on radiography (Riahi et al. 2018; Ropper et al. 2011; Park et al. 2012) (see chapter "Fibrous Dysplasia" for further discussion).

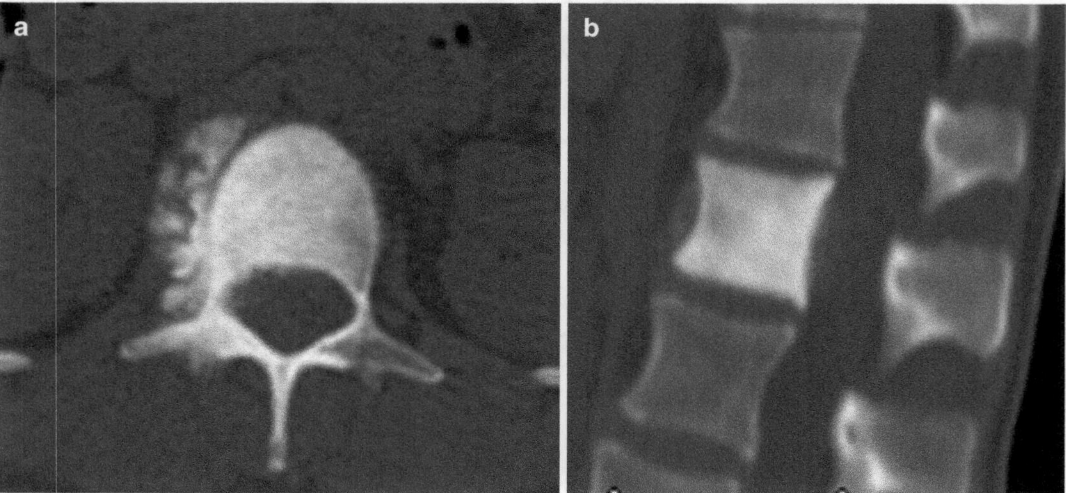

Fig. 21 Osteosarcoma. (**a**) Axial and (**b**) sagittal CT depicts dense diffuse sclerosis of L1 vertebral body resulting in ivory vertebra with aggressive associated periosteal reaction in a patient with pelvic osteosarcoma with spinal metastasis

5.1.10 Eosinophilic Granuloma/ Langerhans Cell Histiocytosis

Typical radiological appearance of spinal eosinophilic granuloma/Langerhans cell histiocytosis consists of incomplete or complete collapse of the vertebral body (vertebra plana) with increased opacity on plain film (see chapter "Langerhans Cell Histiocytosis"). Pedicles, posterior elements, and disk are preserved, which is better shown with CT. Epidural soft tissue extension is better depicted on MRI. Some cases may have asymmetrical one-sided vertebral collapse and affection of posterior elements (Khung et al. 2013).

5.2 Malignant Tumors

5.2.1 Chordoma

Chordoma is usually seen in the axial skeleton as a midline lytic expansile lesion, consistent with well-circumscribed soft tissue mass due to its slow growth with a "mushroom" appearance. When two adjacent vertebrae are involved without disk involvement, it may appear as a dumbbell-shaped tumor (Patnaik et al. 2016). Chordoma could enlarge the neuroforamen, giving a dumbbell appearance and mimicking a neurogenic tumor on CT axial images (Smolders et al. 2003). CT is more sensitive to amorphous calcifications. Amorphous and irregular calcifications are often seen at the periphery of the lesion, noted in 40% of the mobile spine and in up to 90% of sacrococcygeal lesions (Murphey et al. 1996). A lytic vertebral body lesion with partial vertebral collapse can be associated with the presence of prevertebral soft tissue swelling spanning a few levels that can be noted on lateral plain film (Lee et al. 2022). Tumoral epidural extension may cause cord compression indicating aggressiveness of the lesion.

In sacral lesions, frontal radiographs may have limited roles in the early stages due to overlapping bowel gas lucency in the pelvic region (Fig. 9). A lateral view would better demonstrate early destructive changes. Sacral chordoma may invade the piriformis muscle posterolaterally and gluteus maximus directly, whereas anteriorly, it can bulge the mesorectum, but usually, there is no invasion of the rectum since the presacral fascia limits the spread (Keykhosravi et al. 2022; Pillai and Govender 2018; Elafram et al. 2023) (Fig. 23) (see chapter "Notochordal Tumors" for further discussion).

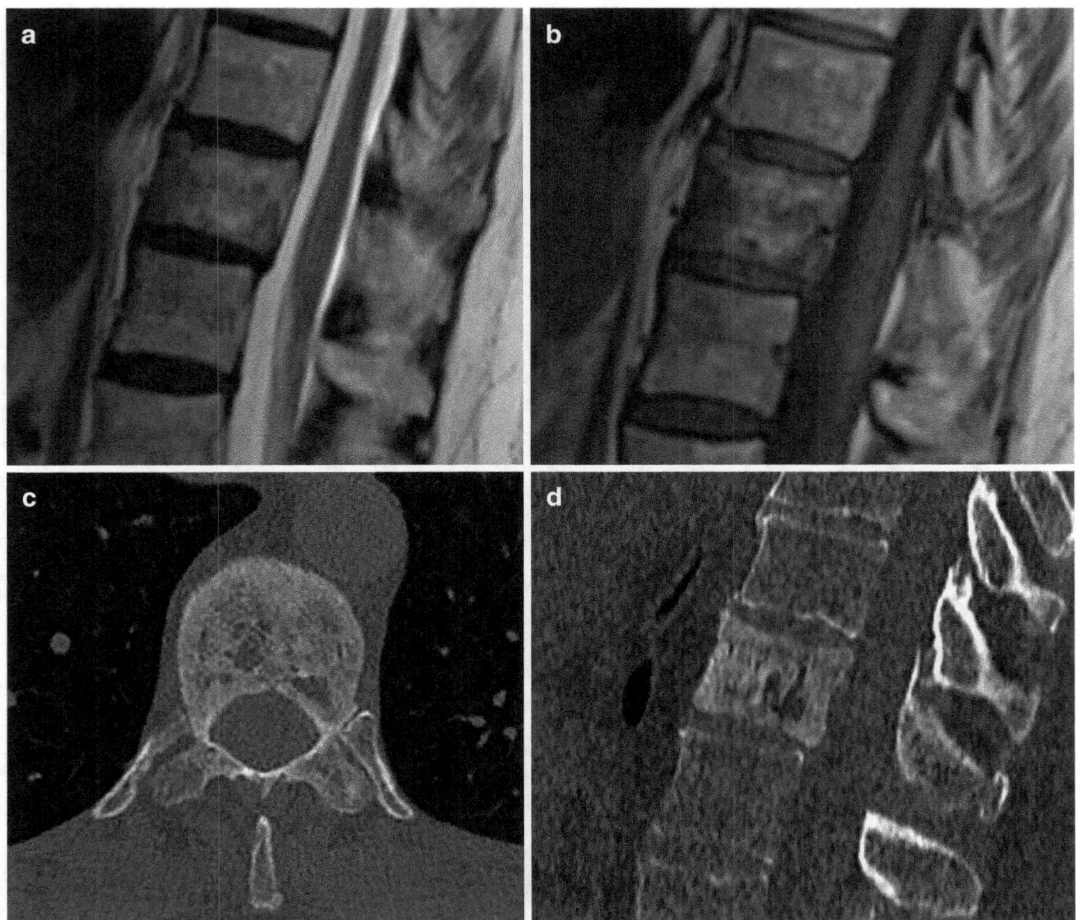

Fig. 22 Paget's disease. (**a**) Sagittal T2-WI and (**b**) sagittal T1-WI depict altered signal within T1 vertebral body with slight expansion. There is patchy low signal on T1-WI with interspersed foci of normal marrow fat. (**c**) Axial and (**d**) sagittal CT depicts the mixed lucent sclerotic appearance of the vertebral body with extension into the posterior elements and transverse processes with preserved cortical outline and coarsened trabecular pattern typical for Paget's disease

5.2.2 Osteosarcoma

Vertebral osteosarcoma at radiography and CT is usually seen as a mixed but predominantly osteosclerotic lesion due to the production of varying amounts of osteoid, cartilage, and fibrous tissue (Fig. 11). On CT, imaging can be seen as a moth-eaten, destructive, and expansile lesion often with a wide zone of transition (Katonis et al. 2011). In some cases, marked sclerosis of posterior elements, and body, can completely obscure normal bony outlines (Liu et al. 2023). In predominantly ossified lesions, the presence of patchy ossification within the paravertebral, intervertebral foramina, and epidural soft tissue mass that occupies the spinal canal can be assessed on CT. Rarely, tumors may have an "ivory vertebra" appearance (sclerosing osteoblastic osteosarcoma) (Khin et al. 2018). On the other hand, telangiectatic osteosarcoma is a purely lytic lesion, with cortical destruction and disappearance of posterior elements, which can be seen even on lateral radiographs of the spine. In partial vertebral collapse, the vertebral disk is usually spared (Murphey et al. 1996). Spinal

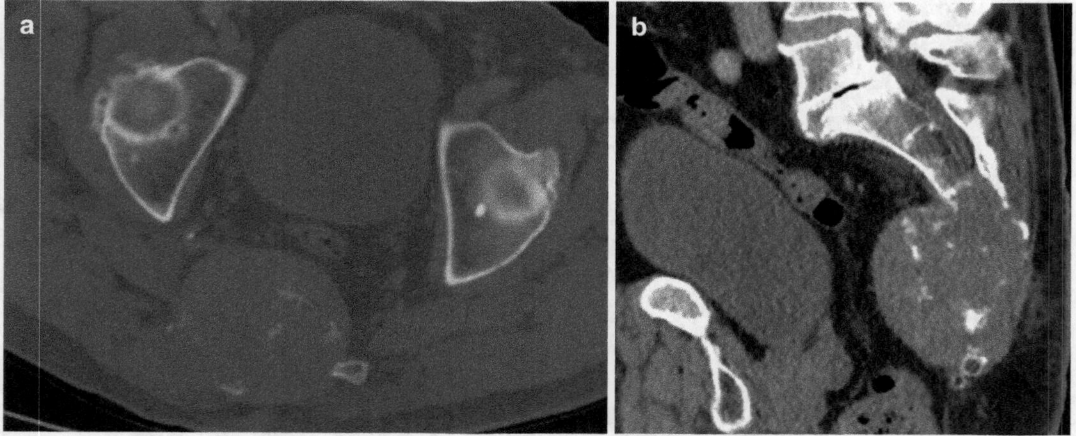

Fig. 23 Chordoma. (**a**) Axial CT in a patient with histologically proven chordoma depicts a large destructive sacral lesion with associated extra-osseous soft tissue and internal calcification. (**b**) Sagittal CT depicts the craniocaudal extent of the lesion with associated presacral soft tissue extension

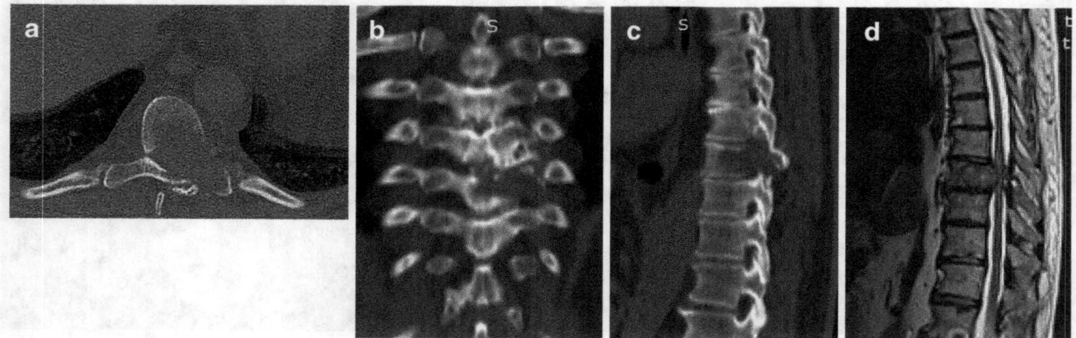

Fig. 24 Chondrosarcoma. CT axial (**a**), coronal (**b**), and sagittal (**c**) reformats in a patient with dedifferentiated chondrosarcoma at posterior aspect of T9 vertebral body extending to the left posterior elements, presented as purely lytic lesion without matrix mineralization, with sparing of the disk. On MRI sagittal T2-WI (**d**), posterior extension of the lesion and spinal canal compromise is better appreciated

osteosarcoma can be associated with some destruction of the transverse process and pedicle (7%) and extension to adjacent vertebrae in 17% of the cases, associated with intraspinal extension with invasion of the spinal canal in 84% of the cases (Ilaslan et al. 2004; Patnaik et al. 2016; Das et al. 2017; Katonis et al. 2013) (see chapter "Osteosarcoma" for further discussion).

5.2.3 Chondrosarcoma

Radiographs of spinal chondrosarcoma typically show lytic, expansile osseous destruction (Fig. 24) with intralesional irregular calcifications (ring-arc-shaped calcifications) and chondroid matrix mineralization better seen on CT when present (Fig. 15a). A geographic osteolytic mass with a sclerotic border can be seen on CT (Rodallec et al. 2008), associated with soft tissue mass in 70–80% (Patnaik et al. 2016; Nguyen et al. 2020; Katonis et al. 2011), which has lower attenuation than that of surrounding muscle reflecting high water content of hyaline cartilage. The soft tissue mass has "mushroom" appearance, often spanning several segments, with sparing the disks. The prevertebral soft tissue mass may cause widening of the prevertebral space.

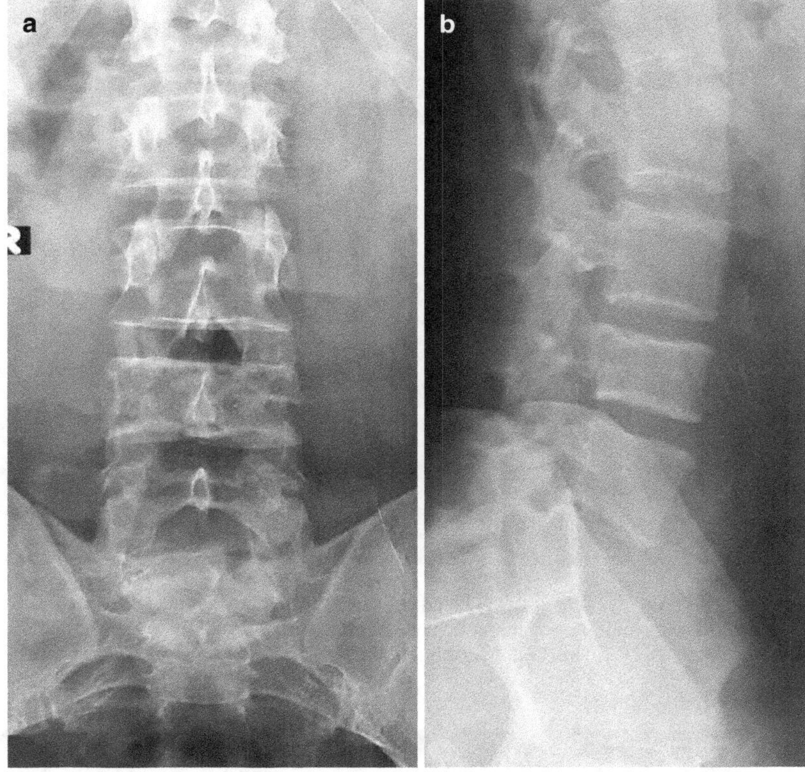

Fig. 25 Lymphoma. (**a**) Anteroposterior and (**b**) lateral plain radiograph shows decreased height of the vertebral body L4 with osteolytic destruction of the pedicles and posterior aspect of the vertebral body due to lymphoma

Adjacent vertebra and adjacent rib may be involved in 35% of the cases (Patnaik et al. 2016; Nguyen et al. 2020). Rarely, bony sequestra can be present, and in some cases, sclerosis may dominate, even with an "ivory" vertebra appearance (Mechri et al. 2018). In the sacrum, it can cross the sacroiliac joint which can be appreciated on CT (Mechri et al. 2018). Chondrosarcoma may arise from solitary osteochondroma. CT may provide the clue for malignant transformation (Riuvo and Hopper 2014) (see chapter "Cartilaginous Tumors" for further discussion). When chondroid calcification has an amorphous appearance, it is challenging to distinguish from osteoblastic calcifications such as those seen in osteosarcoma or Ewing's sarcoma (Nguyen et al. 2020).

5.2.4 Lymphoma

Lymphoma should be considered in the differential diagnosis of any sclerotic vertebral lesion. Bony sequestra may be seen as well. Radiologically, the lesions are lytic (Fig. 25), mixed, or rarely sclerotic causing ivory vertebra (Moussaly et al. 2015; Weber et al. 2019) (see chapter "Lymphoma" for further discussion).

5.2.5 Multiple Myeloma and Plasmacytoma

Ten to 20% of patients with multiple myeloma have a normal appearance on radiography (Lasocki et al. 2017). A pure lytic lesion can be seen on radiographs and CT with pathological compression fractures of the vertebral bodies due to the lesion or osteopenia, with cortical breakthrough, vertebral collapse, and soft tissue mass better presented (Fig. 26). Plasmacytoma is a clinical variant considered to represent an early stage of multiple myeloma, with stages of transition existing between the localized and the disseminated types (Knoeller et al. 2008). The radiographic appearance is less characteristic (Fig. 27).

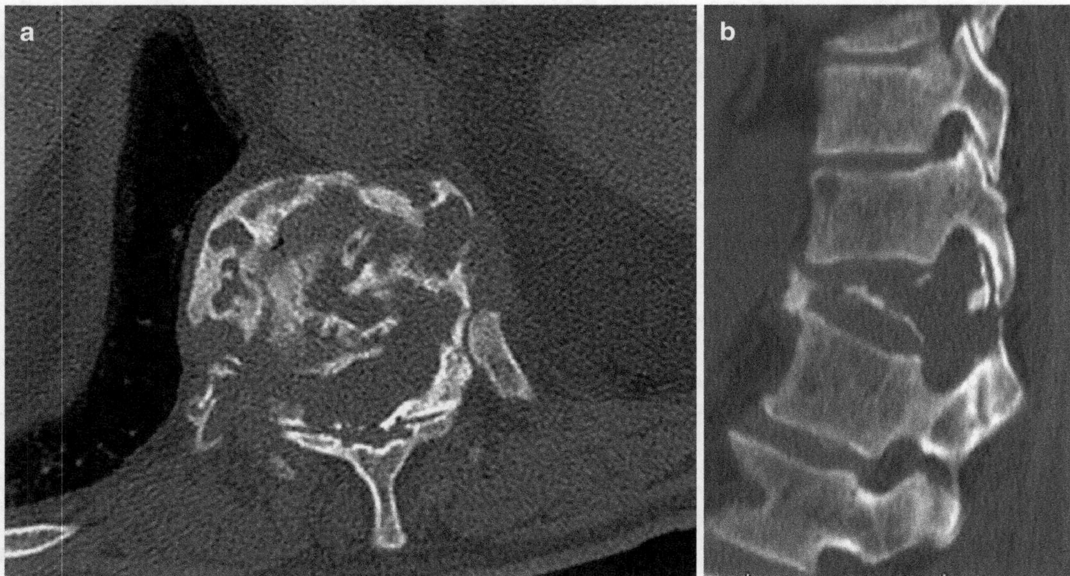

Fig. 26 Multiple myeloma. (**a**) Axial and (**b**) sagittal CT in a patient with multiple myeloma depicts pathological fracture of the T12 vertebral body with vertebra plana, and involvement and extension into the posterior elements. There is another small well-defined punched-out lytic lesion in the anterosuperior corner of T11 vertebral body

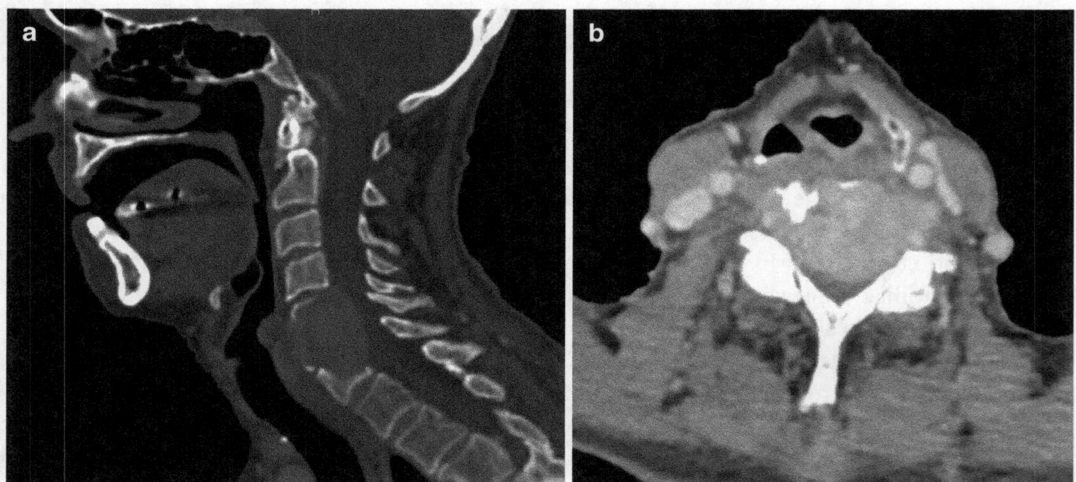

Fig. 27 Plasmacytoma. (**a**) Sagittal CT cervical spine shows a large expansile lytic lesion without any matrix mineralization involving C5–C7 vertebral bodies with extension across the disk spaces in a patient with plasmacytoma. (**b**) Axial CT angiography in the same patient depicts the mass to be homogeneously enhancing with spinal canal encroachment. There is encasement of both vertebral arteries with loss of fat planes but preserved blood flow

It can present with a multicystic "soap bubble" appearance involving the vertebral body. CT scan shows the mini-brain sign created by purely lytic vertebral lesion with cortical preservation. Solitary sclerotic plasmacytoma is rare (see chapter "Plasmacytoma" for further discussion).

5.3 Pseudotumors of the Osseous Spine

Pseudotumors of the spine may mimic primary bone tumor on radiographs and CT. They can be discovered incidentally or may be symptomatic. In most of the pseudotumors such as spondylolysis, sacral insufficiency fractures, Schmorl's node, inflammatory lesions of the costovertebral articulation, and crystal deposition, CT may give crucial information to narrow the differential diagnosis. For other entities such as red marrow normal variant, spondylodiscitis, hydatidosis, and post-traumatic/osteoporotic vertebral collapse, MRI is the method of choice for final differentiation. Degenerative and metabolic diseases may present as a mass lesion. Discrimination between bone tumors and bone tumor mimickers is of utmost importance in order to avoid inappropriate treatment (see chapter on "Pseudotumors" for further discussion).

6 Conclusion

Radiography and CT play a crucial role in the diagnosis and management of spinal tumors. While MRI is nowadays often performed as an initial test for spinal problems, the presence of a tumor of the osseous spine necessitates further evaluation of radiographs and/or CT subsequently, for further characterization and assessment of general spinal alignment, guiding biopsy and operative planning.

7 Key Points

- Conventional radiography (CR) is the basic imaging modality for the diagnosis of primary bone tumors of the spine.
- In some scenarios, weight-bearing radiographs may be useful for assessing the alignment of the spine.
- CR is easy to perform, accessible, and inexpensive. Due to the complex anatomy of the spine with overlapping structures, CR is less sensitive for the detection of tumors of the osseous spine.
- Multidetector CT allows precise anatomical delineation and evaluation of the lesions in complex anatomical locations, where radiographs are not sufficient.
- Minor bony changes, tumor mineralization, small calcifications, cortical changes, and periosteal reactions are best seen on CT scan.
- A major limitation of CT is difficulty of making precise assessment of medullary involvement. MRI can overcome this problem.
- CT plays an important role in performing imaging-guided biopsy.

References

Azad H, Ahmed A, Zafar I et al (2022) X-ray and MRI correlation of bone tumors using histopathology as gold standard. Cureus 14(7):e27262. https://doi.org/10.7759/cureus.27262

Beltran J, Simon DC, Levy M et al (1986) Aneurysmal bone cysts: MR imaging at 1.5 T. Radiology 158(3):689–690. https://doi.org/10.1148/radiology.158.3.3945739

Burch S, Hu S, Berven S (2008) Aneurysmal bone cysts of the spine. Neurosurg Clin N Am 19(1):41–47. https://doi.org/10.1016/j.nec.2007.09.005

Chhaya S, White LM, Kandel R et al (2005) Transarticular invasion of bone tumours across the sacroiliac joint. Skeletal Radiol 34(12):771–777. https://doi.org/10.1007/s00256-005-0016-x

Codd PJ, Riesenburger RI, Klimo P Jr et al (2006) Vertebra plana due to an aneurysmal bone cyst of the lumbar spine: case report and review of the literature. J Neurosurg 105(6 Suppl):490–495. https://doi.org/10.3171/ped.2006.105.6.490

Das S, Islam M, Mahbub H et al (2017) A case report of vertebral osteosarcoma: and appraisal. J Med Sci Health 3(3):26–28

Dubousset J, Charpak G, Skalli W et al (2007) EOS stereo-radiography system: whole-body simultaneous anteroposterior and lateral radiographs with very low radiation dose. Rev Chir Orthop Reparatrice Appar Mot 93:141–143. https://doi.org/10.1016/s0035-1040(07)92729-4

Elafram R, Abcha O, Romdhane MB et al (2023) Chordoma of the lumbar spine—a potential diagnosis not to be forgotten. Radiol Case Rep 18(2):506–510. https://doi.org/10.1016/j.radcr.2022.10.037

Erlemann R (2006) Imaging and differential diagnosis of primary bone tumors and tumor-like lesions of the spine. Eur J Radiol 58(1):48–67. https://doi.org/10.1016/j.ejrad.2005.12.006

Galgano MA, Goulart CR, Iwenofu H et al (2016) Osteoblastomas of the spine: a comprehensive review. Neurosurg Focus 41(2):E4. https://doi.org/10.3171/2016.5.FOCUS16122

Ghodasara N, Yi PH, Clark K et al (2019) Postoperative spinal CT: what the radiologist needs to know. Radiographics 39:1840–1861. https://doi.org/10.1148/2019190050

Goyal N, Kalra M, Soni A et al (2019) Multi-modality imaging approach to bone tumors—state-of-the art. J Clin Orthop Trauma 10(4):687–701. https://doi.org/10.1016/j.jcot.2019.05.022

Hart RA, Briana S, Biagini R et al (1997) A system for surgical staging and management of spine tumors: a clinical outcome study of giant cell tumors of spine. Spine 22(15):1773–82; discussion 1783. https://doi.org/10.1097/00007632-199708010-00018

Hsu W, Kosztowski TA, Zaidi HA (2009) Multidisciplinary management of primary tumors of the vertebral column. Curr Treat Options Oncol 10(1–2):107–125. https://doi.org/10.1007/s11864-009-0102-8

Ilaslan H, Sundaram M, Unni KK, Shives TC (2004) Primary vertebral osteosarcoma: imaging findings. Radiology 230(3):697–702. https://doi.org/10.1148/radiol.2303030226

Izatt MT, Thorpe PLPJ, Thompson RG et al (2007) The use of physical biomodellig in complex spinal surgery. Eur Spine J 16(9):1507–1518. https://doi.org/10.1007/s00586-006-0289-3

Jarvik JG, Deyo RA (2002) Diagnostic evaluation of low back pain with emphasis on imaging. Ann Intern Med 137(7):586–597. https://doi.org/10.7326/0003-4819-137-7-200210010-00010

Katonis P, Alpantaki K, Michail K et al (2011) Spinal chondrosarcoma: a review. Sarcoma 2011:378957. https://doi.org/10.1155/2011/378957

Katonis P, Datsis G, Karantanas A (2013) Spinal osteosarcoma. Clin Med Insight Oncol 7:199–208. https://doi.org/10.4137/CMO.S10099

Keykhosravi E, Rezaee H, Tavallaii A et al (2022) A giant sacrococcygeal chordoma: a case report. Brain Tumor Res Treat 10(1):29–33. https://doi.org/10.14791/btrt.2022.10.e12

Khin YT, Peh WCG, Chang KTE, Mya SN (2018) High-grade primary osteosarcoma of the thoracic spine presenting as an ivory vertebra. Int J Cancer Clin Res 10:23937/2378–3419/1410099

Khung S, Budzik JF, Amzalliag-Bellenger EA et al (2013) Skeletal involvement in Langerhans cell histiocytosis. Insights Imaging 4(5):569–579. https://doi.org/10.1007/s13244-013-0271-7

Knez D, Nahle IS, Vrtovec T et al (2019) Computer-assisted pedicle screw trajectory planning using CT-inferred bone density: a demonstration against surgical outcomes. Med Phys 46(8):3543–3554. https://doi.org/10.1002/mp.13585

Knoeller SM, Uhl M, Gahr N et al (2008) Differential diagnosis of primary malignant bone tumors in the spine and sacrum. The radiological and clinical spectrum: mini review. Neoplasma 55(1):16–22. PMID: 18190235.

Konakondla S, Albers JA, Li X et al (2019) Maximizing sacral chordoma resection by precise 3-dimensional tumor modeling in the operating room using intra-operative computed tomography registration with preoperative magnetic resonance imaging fusion and intraoperative neuronavigation: a case series. World Neurosurg 125:e1125–e1131. https://doi.org/10.1016/j.wneu.2019.01.257

Kransdorf MJ, Sweet DE (1995) Aneurysmal bone cyst: concept, controversy, clinical presentation, and imaging. AJR Am J Roentgenol 164(3):573–580. https://doi.org/10.2214/ajr.164.3.7863874

Kransdorf MJ, Stull MA, Gilkey FW, Moser RP Jr (1991) Osteoid osteoma. Radiographics 11(4):671–696. https://doi.org/10.1148/radiographics.11.4.1887121

Kumar R, Guinto FC, Madewell JE et al (1988) Expansile bone lesions of the vertebra. Radiographics 8(4):749–769. https://doi.org/10.1148/radiographics.8.4.3175086

Kwon JW, Chung HW, Cho EY et al (2007) MRI findings of giant cell tumors of the spine. AJR Am J Roentgenol 189(1):246–250. https://doi.org/10.2214/AJR.06.1472

Lasocki A, Gaillard F, Harrison SJ (2017) Multiple myeloma of the spine. Neuroradiol J 30(3):259–268. https://doi.org/10.1177/1971400917699426

Lateef H, Patel D (2009) What is the role of imaging in acute low back pain? Curr Rev Musculoskelet Med 2(2):69–73. https://doi.org/10.1007/s12178-008-9037-0

Lee SH, Kwok KY, Wong SM et al (2022) Chordoma at the skull base, spine, and sacrum: a pictorial essay. J Clin Imaging Sci 5(12):44. https://doi.org/10.25259/JCIS_62_2022

Leong S, Kok HK, Delaney H et al (2016) The radiologic diagnosis and treatment of typical and atypical bone hemangiomas: current status. Can Assoc Radiol J 67(1):2–11. https://doi.org/10.1016/j.carj.2014.07.002

Levin DA, Hensinger RN, Graziano GP (2006) Aneurysmal bone cyst of the second cervical vertebrae causing multilevel upper cervical instability. J Spinal Disord Tech 19(1):73–75. https://doi.org/10.1097/01.bsd.0000172073.38814.f9

Li X, Wang Y, Zhao Y et al (2017) Multilevel 3D printing implant for reconstructing cervical spine with metastatic papillary thyroid carcinoma. Spine 42(22):E1326–E1330. https://doi.org/10.1097/BRS.0000000000002229

Liu PT, Kujak JL, Roberts CC, de Chadarevian JP (2011) The vascular groove sign: a new CT finding associated with osteoid osteomas. AJR Am J Roentgenol 196(1):168–173. https://doi.org/10.2214/AJR.10.4534

Liu C, Qiu Y, Li T, Wang F (2023) Primary osteosarcoma of the thoracic vertebrae: a case report and literature review. Asian J Surg 46(6):2337–2339. https://doi.org/10.1016/j.asjsur.2022.11.140

Llauger J, Palmer J, Amores S et al (2000) Primary tumors of the sacrum: diagnostic imaging. AJR Am J

Roentgenol 174(2):417–424. https://doi.org/10.2214/ajr.174.2.1740417

Matthews G, Dyer RB (2017) The "ivory vertebra" sign. Abdom Radiol (NY) 42(1):334–336. https://doi.org/10.1007/s00261-016-0866-9

McLeod RA, Dahlin DC, Beabout JW (1976) The spectrum of osteoblastoma. AJR Am J Roentgenol 126(2):321–325. https://doi.org/10.2214/ajr.126.2.321

Mechri M, Riahi H, Sboui I et al (2018) Imaging of malignant primitive tumors of the spine. J Belg Soc Radiol 102(1):56. https://doi.org/10.5334/jbsr.1410

Medow JE, Agrawal BM, Resnick DK (2007) Polyostotic fibrous dysplasia of the cervical spine: case report and review of the literature. Spine J 7(6):712–715. https://doi.org/10.1016/j.spinee.2006.10.023

Moussaly E, Nazha B, Zaarour M, Atallah JP (2015) Primary non-Hodgkin's lymphoma of the spine: a case report and literature review. World J Oncol 6(5):459–463. https://doi.org/10.14740/wjon947w

Mukhametzhanov K, Mukhametzhanov DZ, Karibaev BM et al (2019) Using an intraoperative computed tomography scanner with a navigation station for spinal surgery. Electron J Gen Med 16(6):em182. https://doi.org/10.29333/ejgm/115859

Murphey MD, Andrews CL, Flemming DJ et al (1996) From the archives of the AFIP. Primary tumors of the spine: radiologic pathologic correlation. Radiographics 16(5):1131–1158. https://doi.org/10.1148/radiographics.16.5.8888395

Murphey MD, Nomikos GC, Flemming DJ et al (2001) From the archives of AFIP. Imaging of giant cell tumor and giant cell reparative granuloma of bone: radiologic-pathologic correlation. Radiographics 21(5):1283–1309. https://doi.org/10.1148/radiographics.21.5.g01se251283

Murphey MD, wan Jaovisidha S, Temple HT et al (2003) Telangiectatic osteosarcoma: radiologic-pathologic comparison. Radiology 229(2):545–553. https://doi.org/10.1148/radiol.2292021130

Murphy MD, Kransdorf MJ (2021) Staging and classification of primary musculoskeletal bone and soft-tissue tumors according to the WHO 2020 update, from the AJR special series on cancer staging. AJR Am J Roentgenol 217(5):1038–1052. https://doi.org/10.2214/AJR.21.25658

Nguyen TT, Thelen JC, Bhatt AA (2020) Bone up on spinal osseous lesions: a case review series. Insights Imaging 11(1):80. https://doi.org/10.1186/s13244-020-00883-6

Orguc S, Arkun R (2014) Primary tumors of the spine. Semin Musculoskelet Radiol 18(3):280–299. https://doi.org/10.1055/s-0034-1375570

Otomo N, Funao H, Yamanouchi K et al (2022) Computed tomography-based navigation system in current spine surgery: a narrative review. Medicina (Kaunas) 58(2):241. https://doi.org/10.3390/medicina58020241

Ouchida J, Kanemura T, Satake K et al (2020) True accuracy of percutaneous pedicle screw placement in thoracic and lumbar spinal fixation with a CT-based navigation system: intraoperative and postoperative assessment of 763 percutaneous pedicle screws. J Clin Neurosci 79:1–6. https://doi.org/10.1016/j.jocn.2020.07.012

Park SK, Lee IS, Chou YO et al (2012) CT and MRI of fibrous dysplasia of the spine. Br J Radiol 85(1015):996–1001. https://doi.org/10.1259/bjr/81329736

Patnaik S, Jyotsnarani Y, Uppin SG, Susarla R (2016) Imaging features of primary tumors of the spine: a pictorial essay. Indian J Radiol Imaging 26(2):279–289. https://doi.org/10.4103/0971-3026.184413

Pillai S, Govender S (2018) Sacral chordoma: a review of literature. J Orthop 15(2):679–684. https://doi.org/10.1016/j.jor.2018.04.001

Rajasekaran S, Aiyer SN, Shetty AP et al (2019) Aneurysmal bone cyst of C2 treated with novel anterior reconstruction and stabilization. Eur Spine J 28(2):270–278. https://doi.org/10.1007/s00586-016-4518-0

Riahi H, Mechri M, Barsaoui M et al (2018) Imaging of benign tumors of the osseous spine. J Belg Soc Radiol 102(1):13. https://doi.org/10.5334/jbsr.1380

Riuvo C, Hopper MA (2014) Spinal chondrosarcoma arising from a solitary lumbar osteochondroma. JBR-BTR 97(1):21–24. https://doi.org/10.5334/jbr-btr.743

Rodallec MH, Feydy A, Larousserie F et al (2008) Diagnostic imaging of solitary tumors of the spine: what to do and say. Radiographics 28(4):1019–1041. https://doi.org/10.1148/rg.284075156

Ropper AE, Cahill KS, Hanna JW et al (2011) Primary vertebral tumors: a review of epidemiologic, histological, and imaging findings, Part I: Benign tumors. Neurosurgery 69(6):1171–1180. https://doi.org/10.1227/NEU.0b013e31822b8107

Sahinarslan A, Erbas G, Kocaman SA et al (2013) Comparison of radiation-induced damage between CT angiography and conventional coronary angiography. Acta Cardiol 68(3):291–297. https://doi.org/10.1080/ac.68.3.2983424

Schmidt FA, Mullally M, Lohmann M et al (2021) With intraoperative computed tomography data for image-guided spinal surgery. Int J Spine Surg 15(2):295–301. https://doi.org/10.14444/8039

Shi LS, Li YQ, Wu WJ et al (2015) Imaging appearance of giant cell tumour of the spine above the sacrum. Br J Radiol 88(1051):20140566. https://doi.org/10.1259/bjr.20140566

Shi Z, Zhou H, Yang B et al (2016) Giant cell tumor of thoracic spine misdiagnosed as hemangioma: report of a case and review of literature. Int J Clin Exp Med 9(8):16831–16839

Si MJ, Wang CG, Wang CS et al (2014) Giant cell tumours of the mobile spine: characteristic imaging features and differential diagnosis. Radiol Med 119(9):681–693. https://doi.org/10.1007/s11547-013-0352-1

Simmons ED, Zheng Y (2006) Vertebral tumors: surgical versus nonsurgical treatment. Clin Orthop Relat Res 443:233–247. https://doi.org/10.1097/01.blo.0000198723.77762.0c

Smith E, Hegde G, Czyz M et al (2022) A radiologists' guide to en bloc resection of primary tumors in the spine: what does the surgeon want to know? Indian J Radiol Imaging 32(2):205–212. https://doi.org/10.1055/s-0042-1744162

Smolders D, Wang X, Drevelengas A et al (2003) Value of MRI in the diagnosis of non-clival, non-sacral chordoma. Skeletal Radiol 32(6):343–350. https://doi.org/10.1007/s00256-003-0633-1

Uehara M, Takahashi J, Ikegami S et al (2017) Optimal cervical screw insertion angle determined by means of computed tomography scans pre- and postoperatively. Spine J 17(2):190–195. https://doi.org/10.1016/j.spinee.2016.08.025

Vidal JA, Murphey MD (2007) Primary tumors of the osseous spine. Magn Reson Imaging Clin N Am 15(2):239–55, vii. https://doi.org/10.1016/j.mric.2007.05.003

Vielgut I, Liegl-Atzwanger B, Bratschitsch G et al (2017) Langerhans-cell histiocytosis of the cervical spine in an adult patient: case report and review of the literature. J Orthop 14(2):264–267. https://doi.org/10.1016/j.jor.2017.03.010

Weber MA, Papakonstantinou O, Vasilevska Nikodinovska V, Vanhoenacker FM (2019) Ewing's sarcoma and primary osseous lymphoma: spectrum of imaging appearances. Semin Musculoskelet Radiol 23(1):36–57. https://doi.org/10.1055/s-0038-1676125

WHO (ed) (2020) WHO classification of tumours of soft tissue and bone, 5th edn. WHO. https://publications.iarc.fr/Book-And-Report-Series/Who-Classification-Of-Tumours/Soft-Tissue-And-Bone-Tumours-2020

Williams R, Foote M, Deverall H (2012) Strategy in the surgical treatment of primary spinal tumors. Global Spine J 2(4):249–266. https://doi.org/10.1055/s-0032-1329886

Yang L, Zhang S, Gu R et al (2019) Imaging features of primary spinal osseous tumors and their value in clinical diagnosis. Oncol Lett 17(1):1089–1093. https://doi.org/10.3892/ol.2018.9659

Yoshioka K, Niinuma H, Ehara S et al (2006) MR angiography and CT angiography of the artery of Adamkiewicz: state of the art. Radiographics 26(Suppl 1):S63–S73. https://doi.org/10.1148/rg.26si065506

Yoshioka K, Tanaka R, Takagi H et al (2018) Ultra-high-resolution CT angiography of the artery of Adamkiewicz: a feasibility study. Neuroradiology 60(1):109–115. https://doi.org/10.1007/s00234-017-1927-7

Magnetic Resonance Imaging of Primary Bone Tumors of the Spine

Hend Riahi, Mokhtar Mars, Mohamed Chaabouni, Mouna Chelli Bouaziz, and Mohamed Fethi Ladeb

Contents

H. Riahi (✉) · M. Chaabouni · M. Chelli Bouaziz
M. F. Ladeb
Department of Radiology, Institut Mohamed Kassab d'orthopédie, Ksar Said, Tunisia

M. Mars
Research Laboratory, ISTMT, Tunis, Tunisia
e-mail: mokhtar.mars@mms.tn

Abstract

Magnetic resonance imaging (MRI) is a non-invasive diagnostic tool that is commonly used for the evaluation of spinal bone tumors. This imaging modality provides detailed information about the location, size, extent, and characteristics of the tumor, as well as its relationship to adjacent structures. MRI is particularly useful for identifying soft tissue involvement and is more sensitive than other imaging modalities in detecting metastatic spinal tumors. In addition, MRI can be used to monitor tumor response to therapy and to guide biopsies or surgical planning. However, there are certain limitations to MRI, such as its inability to distinguish between benign and malignant tumors solely based on imaging characteristics. Nevertheless, MRI remains an important tool for the evaluation of spinal bone tumors, and its use can help guide treatment decisions and improve patient outcomes.

Abbreviations

BW	Bandwidth
CP	Circularly polarized
CT	Computed tomography
DWI	Diffusion-weighted imaging
EPI	Echo-planar spin-echo sequence

Med Radiol Diagn Imaging (2023)
https://doi.org/10.1007/174_2023_441,
Published Online: 10 August 2023

ETL	Echo train length
FO	Fat-only
FOV	Field of view
FS	Fat-suppressed
IP	In phase
IV	Intravenous
mADC	Mean apparent diffusion coefficient
MRI	Magnetic resonance imaging
OP	Out of phase
SAR	Specific absorption rate
STIR	Short tau inversion recovery
T1-WI	T1-weighted image
T2-WI	T2-weighted image
TE	Echo time
TR	Repetition time
WB-MRI	Whole-body MRI
WO	Water-only

1 Introduction

Primary tumors of the spine are infrequent lesions, representing less than 5% of all bone tumors (Murphey et al. 1996). Clinical manifestations and symptom of spinal bone tumors can vary, from asymptomatic to severe back pain, including mass effect with epidural or paravertebral soft tissue involvement.

Imaging features of the primary spinal bone tumors are often nonspecific. Imaging modalities can provide useful tools for narrowing the differential diagnosis and directing biopsy (Garcia et al. 2017).

Radiography has a limited role because of the complex anatomy of the spine. CT scan is suited to evaluate the lesion extent, delineate cortical outline, and know matrix calcification/ossification (see chapter "Radiology and CT"). MRI is the method of choice. The extent of lesion whether osseous or extra-osseous, marrow infiltration, epidural, nerve, and cord involvement can be better depicted in MRI (Patnaik et al. 2016).

2 MRI Technique

2.1 Patient Positioning

Patients can be positioned headfirst or feetfirst. The advantage of headfirst is the accurate calculation of SAR by the MR system, whereas the feetfirst position reduces the claustrophobic feelings. A knee support accessory is used for patient comfort (Van Goethem 2010).

We routinely use headfirst position (Fig. 1).

2.2 Coils

Coils play a major role in the overall image quality. They are the fundamental magnetic interface between the MR imaging system and the human subject. Coils are now routinely designed to match the anatomical regions of interest and optimized for the pulse sequences used in each application (Asher et al. 2010).

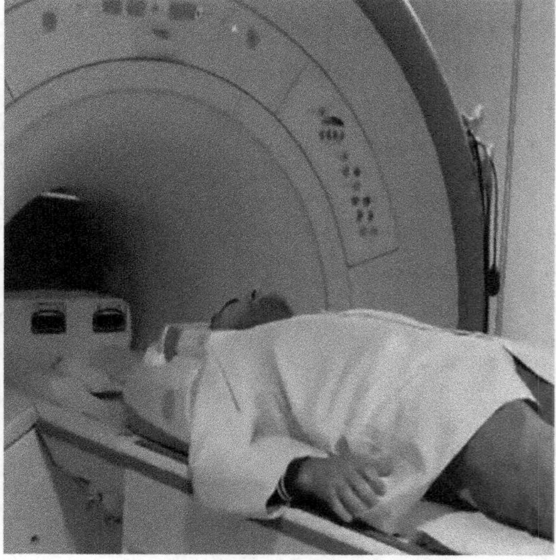

Fig. 1 Headfirst position for MRI of the spine

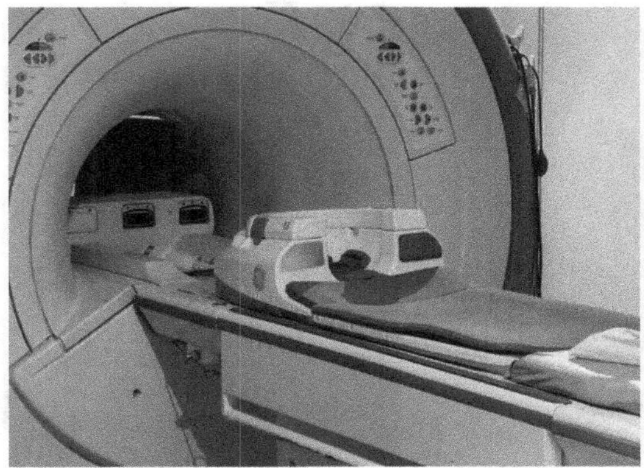

Fig. 2 Coil used for MRI of the spine

Many types of coils are used in spine imaging: linearly polarized, circularly polarized (CP), phase array, and matrix coils.

Coils for thoracic and lumbar spine examinations consist of a flat box incorporated in a lumbar (or thoracic) support or directly into the patient's table. A cervical spine coil is made of anterior and posterior part, and it is usually more raised providing better support for the patient's neck. The cervical spine coil can be combined with the head coil for some manufacturers (Van Goethem 2010) (Fig. 2).

2.3 Pulse Sequences

After positioning the patient, we start the protocol with midsagittal and coronal localizer images. Their field of view (FOV) should be larger than the FOV of the images desired. Coronal localizers are positioned so that they intersect the spine (Fig. 3). Sagittal sequences are positioned parallel to the spine on coronal localizers. Axial images are positioned on sagittal localizers, orthogonal to the spinal canal (Van Goethem 2010).

2.4 T1-Weighted Sequence

T1-weighted images (WI) (Figs. 4 and 5) are the best choice for evaluating anatomy (Gebauer et al. 2008) and are the most important sequence for the evaluation of bone marrow invasion (O'Flanagan et al. 1991; Onikul et al. 1996). T1-weighted imaging mediates better guidance of resection. There is a strong correlation of radiological lesion size on T1-WI with size on gross pathology for primary osseous malignancies.

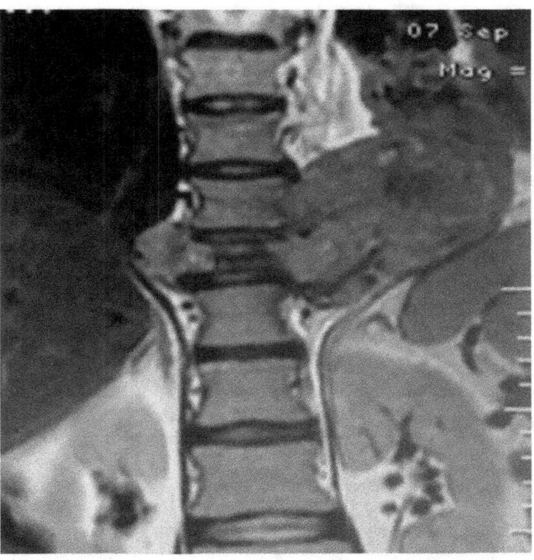

Fig. 3 Giant-cell tumor of D11. Coronal FSE T2 is the best sequence showing soft tissue extension

T1-WI also provides excellent contrast between the cortical bone, bone marrow, and surrounding tissues (Davies et al. 2009). Most bone tumors will be evident as lesions with low signal against a background of surrounding fatty marrow.

2.5 T2-Weighted Sequence

The T2-WI (Figs. 3, 4, and 5) has a long TR and long TE. T2-WI is sensitive to pathologic changes in tissue, including any process in which cells and extracellular matrix have an increased water content. T2-WI is a crucial factor in delineating extra-osseous tumors, peritumoral edema, and surrounding normal tissues (Bohndorf et al. 1986). In fact, when MR imaging is used, biological tissues and fluids with excess amounts of free water have long T2 values and, therefore, tend to be the most conspicuous on T2-WI.

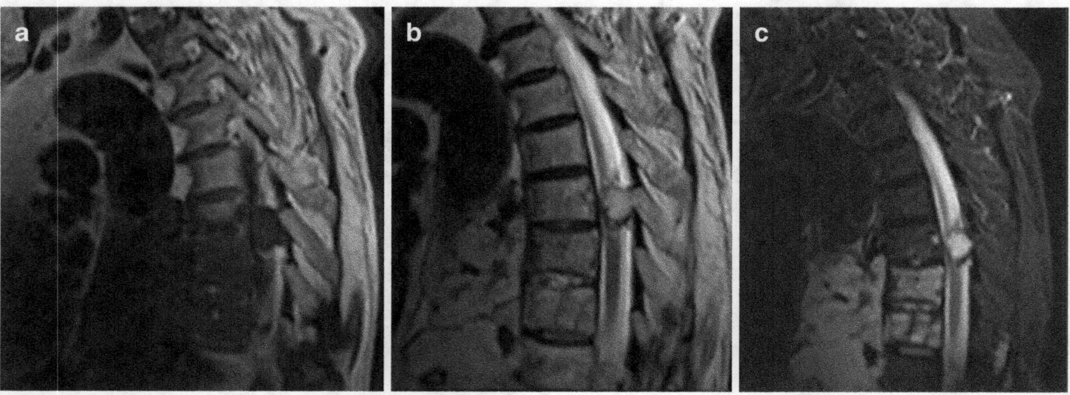

Fig. 4 Chondrosarcoma of D7, D8, and D9. Sagittal T1-WI (**a**), T2-WI (**b**), and STIR (STIR) (**c**) MR images show low T1 and high T2 signal of cartilaginous matrix, which is better seen on STIR

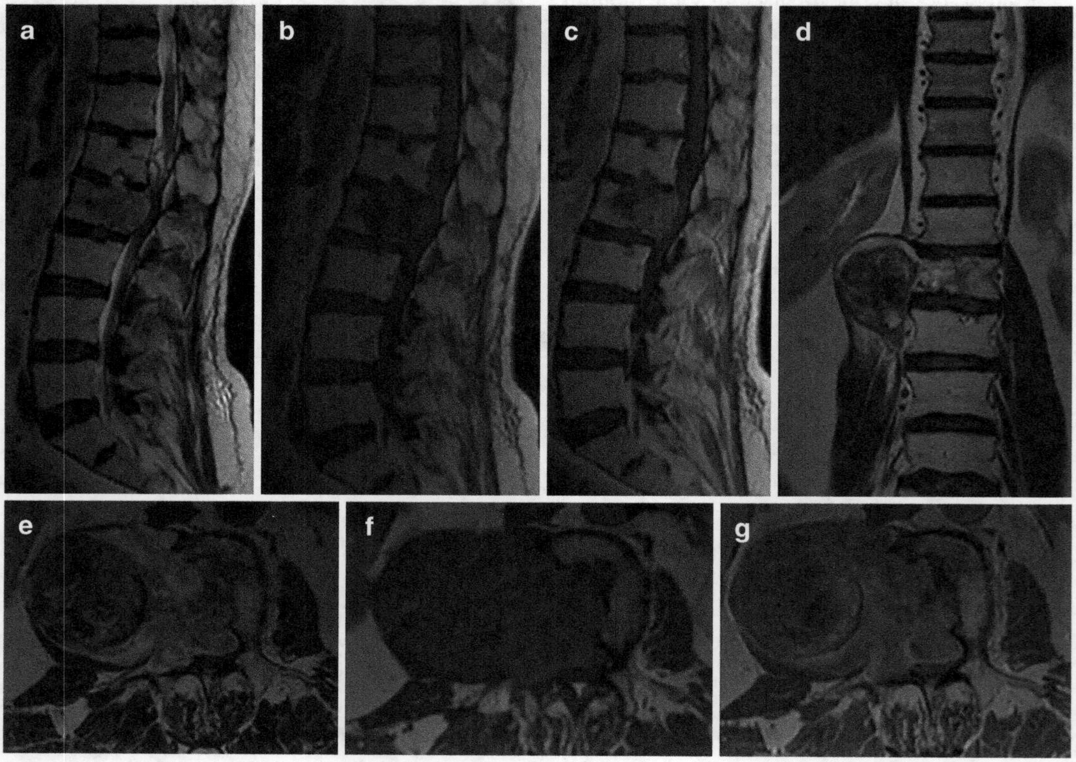

Fig. 5 Chondroma of L2. Sagittal T2-WI (**a**), T1-WI (**b**), T1-WI postcontrast (**c**), coronal T2-WI (**d**), axial T2-WI (**e**), T1-WI (**f**), T1-WI postcontrast (**g**). Coronal and axial planes are best suited to delineate soft tissue extension and contact to blood vessels

Water shows higher signal than fat on T2-WI, but suppressing the fat signal can allow an even better evaluation of the extent of bone marrow edema, which is seen in nearly 70% of musculoskeletal malignancy (Hanna et al. 1991).

This bone marrow edema is common in both benign and malignant lesions (Alyas et al. 2007).

STIR and T2-WI provide the best means of evaluating neural compression (Rodallec et al. 2008).

2.6 Fat Suppression Technique

The use of fat suppression (FS) in MRI can confirm or exclude the presence of fat in a lesion. There are five techniques for fat saturation including spectral fat sat, SPAIR, Dixon, water excitation, and STIR.

Short TI inversion recovery (STIR) sequence (Fig. 6) is very efficient in difficult regions such us the cervical spine. It provides a homogeneous suppression of fat signals with an inverted T1 contrast. Liquid and tissues with T1 signal similar to or greater than that of water are of hyperintense signal. This can lead to overestimation of the tumoral extension and compromise its characterization (Nascimento et al. 2014).

2.7 Dixon

Dixon imaging consists of the acquisition of in-phase and out-of-phase images, from which water-only (WO) and fat-only (FO) images are reconstructed, producing four sets of images per acquisition, which simplifies and shortens the acquisition protocols (Guerini et al. 2015) (Fig. 7).

It provides fat-suppressed images that are more robust against field inhomogeneities than chemical shift selective techniques. In addition, it presents a higher signal-to-noise ratio than STIR (Omoumi 2022).

Fat-only (FO) images are not only sensitive, but also specific to the signal of fat. Therefore, the interpretation of FO images is more straightforward than that of T1-WI (Fig. 8). FO images are not subject to potential false negatives in detecting marrow-replacing lesions, as would be the case with T1-WI for lesions containing short T1 substances other than fat, such as melanin, methemoglobin, proteinaceous fluid, or paramagnetic substances (Maeder et al. 2018). Qualitative analysis of FSE T2-W Dixon sequence provides high diagnostic performance and high interobserver agreement for the differentiation between benign and malignant spinal

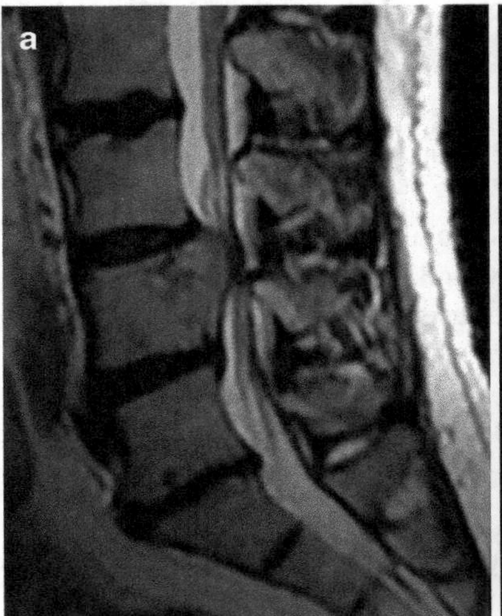

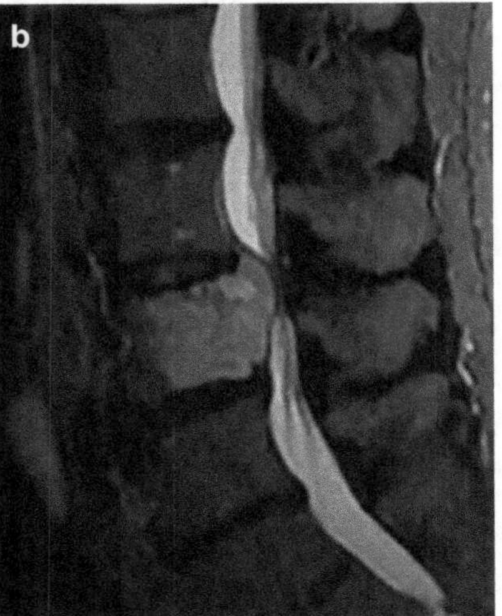

Fig. 6 Chordoma of L4. Sagittal STIR (**b**) delineates the process better than the FSE T2-WI (**a**)

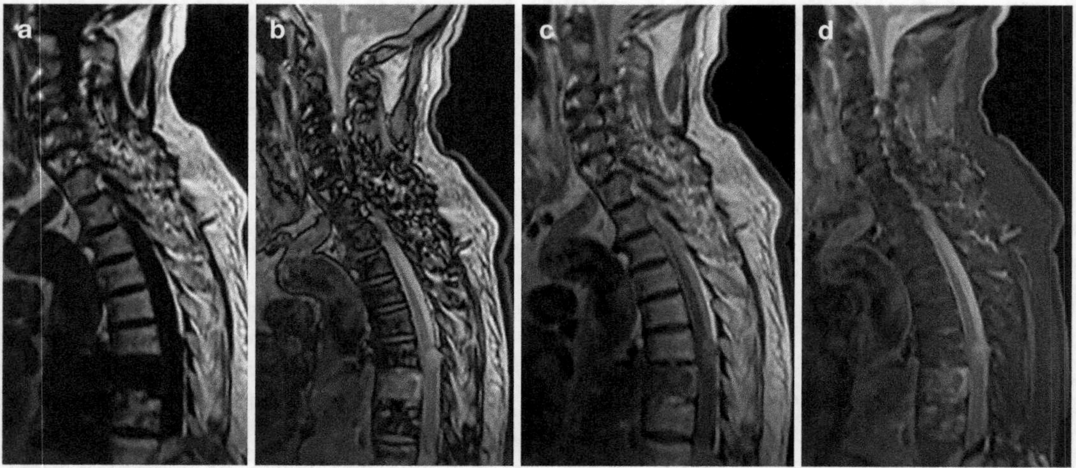

Fig. 7 Chondrosarcoma (same patient). T1 Dixon postcontrast sequence. (**a**) Fat only, (**b**) out of phase. (**c**) in phase (IP). (**d**) water only (WO)

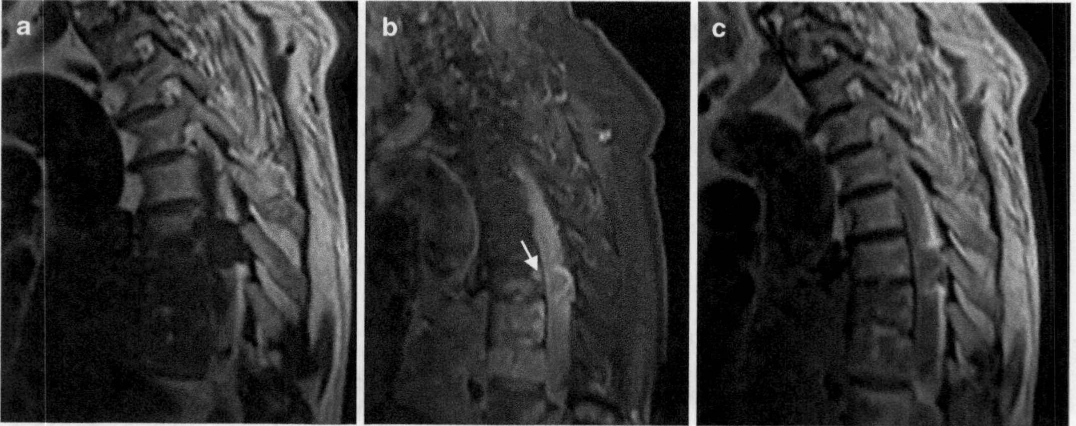

Fig. 8 Chondrosarcoma (same patient). Sagittal T1-WI (**a**), Dixon T1-WI postcontrast WO (**b**), and Dixon T1-WI postcontrast IP (**c**): note the high contrast between the lesions (arrow) and surrounding tissues

tumors and fractures. The same sequence allows quantitative analysis assessment with high diagnostic performance, which may be useful in doubtful cases (Bacher et al. 2021).

2.8 Diffusion-Weighted Imaging

An echo-planar spin-echo sequence (EPI) is the most commonly applied DWI sequence in clinical routine imaging owing to the ability to rapidly acquire data within one time frame (Subhawong et al. 2014).

Diffusion-weighted imaging (DWI) reflects the random motion of water molecules in intracellular and extracellular spaces, providing useful information regarding tumor cellularity. DWI with mean apparent diffusion coefficient (mADC) quantification is a reproducible tool to differentiate benign from malignant solid tumors of the spine with 76% accuracy. The mADC values of benign bone tumor were statistically higher than those of malignant tumors. However, the large overlap between cases may make mADC not helpful in a specific patient such as giant cell tumors with low mADC values due to their high cellularity and chondrosarcoma that may have high mADC values (Pozzi et al. 2018).

2.9 DCE

Conventional morphologic MRI is often insufficient for precise noninvasive characterization of musculoskeletal tumors (Wu and Hochman 2009).

Gadolinium-based contrast helps distinguish solid from necrotic areas and edema from viable tumors. It allows an accurate determination of the degree of vascularization. It also allows depiction of extra-osseous extension and differentiation of recurrent tumor vs. postoperative fibrosis (Vanhoenacker et al. 2010).

Fast acquisition techniques after gadolinium-based contrast medium injection, at a dose of 0.1–02 mmol/kg with the speed of 2–3 mL/s, allow contrast-enhanced dynamic imaging (DCE) (Fig. 9). Kinetic enhancement of the tissue during and after injection consisted of repeated 10–12 images, and the duration of the sequence is about 300 s (Guan et al. 2020). DCE determines time to peak, maximum enhancement, slope (degree of enhancement during the first pass), washout rate, and shape of the signal enhancement time curve. Additionally, some evidence suggests that time to peak of the postcontrast T1-weighted signal can distinguish benign from malignant lesions in almost 80% of cases (Nascimento et al. 2014).

In DCE, the first pass of the contrast agent serves to evaluate tissue vascularization and tumor perfusion (Fig. 9). Enhancement occurs earlier and is more marked in tissues characterized by an abundant vasculature and high capillary permeability. However, overlap occurs between highly vascular benign tumors and poorly vascularized malignant tumors (Verstraete and Lang 2000).

Dynamic imaging can also provide a more accurate determination of the tumor contours and identify well-vascularized areas of viable tumor tissue to select the biopsy site (Vanhoenacker et al. 2010).

Dynamic perfusion MRI makes a major contribution to patient follow-up during chemotherapy. Its diagnostic accuracy for differentiating good and poor responders has ranged from 85.7% to 100% (Drapé 2013).

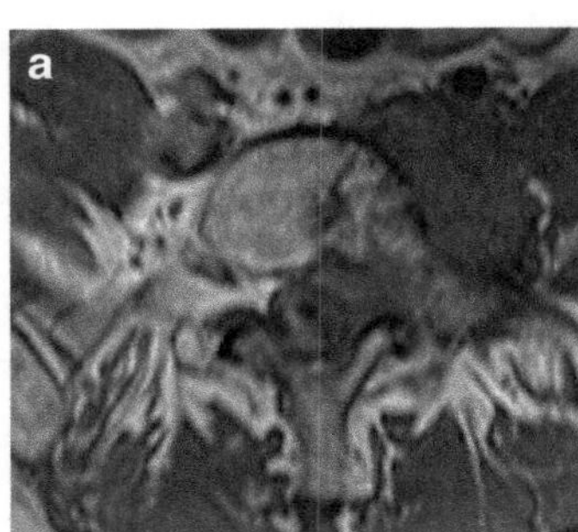

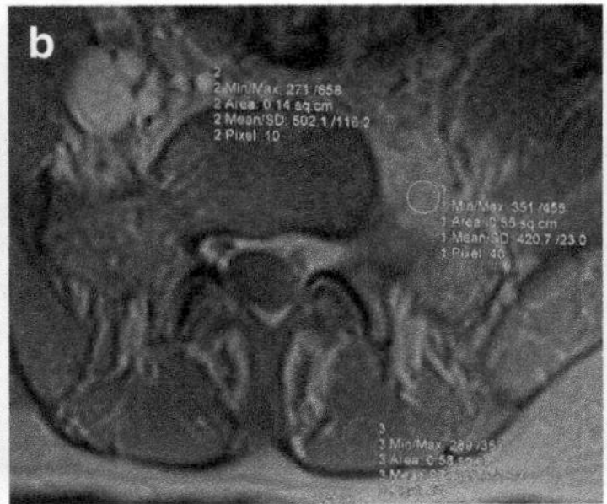

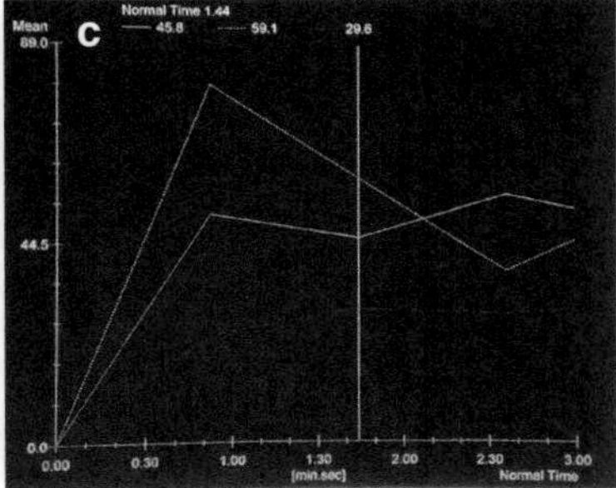

Fig. 9 Ewing's sarcoma of L4. Axial T1-WI; (**a**) T1 after dynamic injection of gadolinium contrast (**b**) and DCE signal intensity time curve; (**c**) the upper curve corresponds to vessel, and the lower to the lesion: showing a lesion in the left vertebral body of L4 with low T1-WI signal, and DCE-MRI enhancement kinetics shows the persistent enhancement pattern

3 MRI of Spinal Tumor

MRI is mandatory for preoperative workup and therapeutic follow-up of patients with musculoskeletal tumors. Morphological sequences assess tumor spread to the bone and to soft tissues and evaluate neural compression. Typically, neoplastic processes are of low signal on T1-WI and are hyperintense on STIR and fat-suppressed T2-WI relative to the adjacent disk and paravertebral muscles (Hanrahan and Shah 2011).

Diffusion-weighted images show restriction to the diffusion of water molecules in malignant tumors. A favorable therapeutic response is associated with a decrease in the signal intensity in high *b* values (Nascimento et al. 2014).

However, the use of DWI is still not included in the guidelines for routine evaluation of malignant tumors (American College of Radiology 2011).

Functional MRI improves tissue characterization and staging of spinal tumors. Perfusion imaging provides information on vascularization and perfusion. DCE identifies viable tumor sites to guide the biopsy. It is used to monitor preoperative chemotherapy and to differentiate residual tumors from scarring (Drapé 2013).

3-T MRI improves visualization of anatomic structures over 1.5-T MRI. Using a quantitative approach, skeletal muscle and non-degenerative disk can still be used as internal reference standards at 3 T to differentiate normal and neoplastic bone marrow, with superior results found for muscle at 3 T compared with 1.5 T (Zhao et al. 2009).

4 MRI Protocols and Parameters

The entire spine must always be imaged in bone tumors of the spine. Whole-body MRI may be used in multiple tumor disease such as Langerhans cell histiocytosis and hereditary multiple exostoses syndrome. WB-MRI could also be considered as reliable diagnostics in the staging of malignant lesions. Tables 1, 2, and 3 summarize MRI parameters that could be used in exploring primary bone tumors of the spine.

Table 1 Cervical spine

Sequence	Plane	TR (ms)	TE (ms)	Flip angle (°)	ETL	Slice thickness (mm)	Interslice gap (mm)	Matrix	FOV (mm)	BW (Hz/Px)	No of acq.
T1-W	Sag	600	10	150	3	3	0.3	256	220	191	2
T2-W	Sag	3800	86	150	16	3	0.3	320	220	191	2
STIR	Sag	3800	37	150	9	3	0.3	256	220	190	2
DW	Sag	2680	59	180	70	3	0.3	160	220	679	4
DCE	Sag	4.6	1.79	15	–	3	0.6	192	220	300	1
T1-W Gado	Sag	600	10	150	3	3	0.3	256	220	191	2
DIXON T1	Sag	600	14	140	2	3	0.3	256	220	206	2
DIXON T2	Sag	3500	93	150	15	3	0.3	320	220	260	2
T1-W	Ax	600	10	150	3	3	0.3	256	180	190	2
T2-W	Ax	5950	80	150	13	3	0.3	256	180	190	2
T1-W Gado	Ax	600	10	150	3	3	0.3	256	180	190	2

Table 2 Thoracic spine

Sequence	Plane	TR (ms)	TE (ms)	Flip angle (°)	ETL	Slice thickness (mm)	Inter-slice gap (mm)	Matrix	FOV (mm)	BW (Hz/Px)	No of acq.
T1-W	Sag	700	11	150	3	4	0.8	384	340	221	2
T2-W	Sag	4000	104	150	19	4	0.8	448	340	199	2
STIR	Sag	3800	37	150	9	4	0.8	256	340	190	2
DW	Sag	2680	59	180	70	4	0.8	160	340	679	4
DCE	Sag	4.6	1.79	15	–	4	0.8	192	340	300	1
T1-W Gado	Sag	700	11	150	3	4	0.8	384	340	221	2
DIXON T1	Sag	550	13	150	2	4	0.8	320	340	279	2
DIXON T2	Sag	4000	95	150	16	4	0.8	384	340	260	1
T1-W	Ax	580	10	150	3	3.5	0.35	256	190	250	2
T2-W	Ax	4770	89	150	13	3.5	0.35	320	190	191	2
T1-W Gado	Ax	580	10	150	3	3.5	0.35	256	190	250	2

Table 3 Lumbar spine

Sequence	Plane	TR (ms)	TE (ms)	Flip angle (°)	ETL	Slice thickness (mm)	Inter-slice gap (mm)	Matrix	FOV (mm)	BW (Hz/Px)	No of acq.
T1-W	Sag	600	9.7	150	3	4	0.8	320	260	200	3
T2-W	Sag	3600	99	150	17	4	0.8	384	260	197	2
STIR	Sag	3800	37	150	9	4	0.8	256	340	190	2
DW	Sag	2680	59	180	70	4	0.8	160	340	679	4
DCE	Sag	4.6	1.79	15	–	4	0.8	192	340	300	1
T1-W Gado	Sag	600	9.7	150	3	4	0.8	320	260	200	3
DIXON T1	Sag	743	13	150	3	4	0.8	256	260	283	2
DIXON T2	Sag	3800	95	150	15	4	0.8	320	260	200	2
T1-W	Ax	550	11	150	3	4	0.4	256	200	206	2
T2-W	Ax	4500	78	150	15	4	0.4	384	220	191	2
T1-W Gado	Ax	550	11	150	3	4	0.4	256	200	206	2

5 MRI Pitfalls

5.1 Macro-Motion

Patient motion is often visible along the phase-encoding direction. The acquisition is repeated with different phase-encoding steps, which makes the phase-encoding data more susceptible to motion degradation (Roth et al. 2016).

Examples of motion range from patient fidgeting to involuntary physiologic motion of respiration, bowel activity, and vascular pulsations. Different techniques can be used to minimize the impact of motion on the diagnostic quality of the final image such as selecting faster imaging techniques, selection of the optimum phase-encoding direction, use of saturation band as well as flow compensation (Morelli John et al. 2011), and utilizing non-Cartesian sampling. By using radial filling of the k-space, artifacts will be less pronounced.

5.2 Pulsation

If a pulsating vessel is imaged axially, the pulsating structure may result in a series of displaced "ghost" replicas of the primary vessel in the phase-encoding direction. One option used in the setting of this pulsation is to switch the frequency and phase-encoding directions (Hashemi et al. 2010).

5.3 Susceptibility

Susceptibility effects from blood products, calculi, air, and small metal objects may result in misregistration, signal loss, and signal pileup artifacts (Roth et al. 2016).

Secondary magnetic fields are generated by the "susceptibility" of a given substance to become magnetized (Hoff et al. 2016).

These secondary fields cause local derangement of the main magnetic field, and the degree of derangement determines the extent of the subsequent susceptibility artifact. Most tissues are "diamagnetic" and have a secondary field that opposes and detracts from the existing magnetic field. Other substances generate secondary fields that align with and add to the existing field, mildly for "paramagnetic" substances, and strongly for "ferromagnetic" substances (Bushburg et al. 2012).

Conventional measures that are routinely used to minimize these artifacts include scanning on a low-field (1.5 T) rather than a high-field (3 T) magnet as variation in susceptibility will necessarily be accentuated at higher magnetic fields. Increasing the readout bandwidth will decrease the effect of field inhomogeneity at the cost of a slight loss in overall signal. Decreasing voxel size and increasing the acquisition matrix can also reduce artifact (Suh et al. 1998).

5.4 Truncation

Truncation is an artifact, which results from insufficient data sampling. This phenomenon is seen between the spinal cord and cerebral spinal fluid. Solutions are to either decrease the pixel size or increase the high-frequency sampling to account for and thus appropriately display more of the high frequencies needed to delineate strikingly different tissue types correctly (Stadler et al. 2007).

6 Conclusion

Primary bone spinal tumors are rare, and the diagnosis may be challenging. Early and accurate detection is critical for improved patient outcomes. Optimal MRI technique and protocol are pivotal for treatment planning by delineating tumor extent, involvement of adjacent structures, and potential spinal cord compression.

7 Key Messages

- MRI is the most sensitive technique for the detection of primary bone tumors of the spine.
- Magnetic resonance imaging (MRI) is the study of choice for local staging, as it provides

the best contrast resolution for the identification of the margins of the lesion.
- MRI is accurate in evaluating other important information regarding the local extent of the tumor such as bone invasion, extra-osseous, epidural, nerve, vessels, and cord involvement.

References

Alyas F, James SL, Davies AM et al (2007) The role of MR imaging in the diagnostic characterisation of appendicular bone tumours and tumour-like conditions. Eur Radiol 17:2675–2686

American College of Radiology (2011) ACR Appropriateness Criteria. Follow-up of malignant or aggressive musculoskeletal tumors. http://www.acr.org/~/media/ACR/Documents/AppCriteria/Diagnostic/FollowupMalignantOrAggressiveMusculoskeletalTumors.pdf. Accessed 9 Apr 2014

Asher KA, Bangerter NK, Watkins RD, Gold GE (2010) Radiofrequency coils for musculoskeletal magnetic resonance imaging. Top Magn Reson Imaging 21(5):315–323. https://doi.org/10.1097/RMR.0b013e31823cd184. PMID: 22129644; PMCID: PMC4400851

Bacher S, Hajdu SD, Maeder Y, Dunet V, Hilbert T, Omoumi P (2021) Differentiation between benign and malignant vertebral compression fractures using qualitative and quantitative analysis of a single fast spin echo T2-weighted Dixon sequence. Eur Radiol 31(12):9418–9427. https://doi.org/10.1007/s00330-021-07947-1. Epub 2021 May 26. PMID: 34041569; PMCID: PMC8589814

Bohndorf K, Reiser M, Lochner B, Faux de Lacroix W, Steinbrich W (1986) Magnetic resonance imaging of primary tumours and tumour-like lesions of bone. Skeletal Radiol 15(7):511–517

Bushburg JT, Seibert AJ, Leidholdt EM Jr, Boone JM (2012) The essential physics of medical imaging, 3rd edn. Lippincott Williams & Wilkins, pp 477–493

Davies AM, Sundaram M, James SLJ (2009) Imaging of bone tumors and tumor-like lesions (techniques and applications). Springer, Berlin

Drapé JL (2013) Advances in magnetic resonance imaging of musculoskeletal tumours. Orthop Traumatol Surg Res 99(1 Suppl):S115–S123. https://doi.org/10.1016/j.otsr.2012.12.005. Epub 2013 Feb 4. PMID: 23380432

Garcia DAL, Aivazoglou LU, Garcia LAL et al (2017) Diagnostic imaging of primary bone tumors of the spine. Curr Radiol Rep 5:30. https://doi.org/10.1007/s40134-017-0220-1

Gebauer GP, Farjoodi P, Sciubba DM, Gokaslan ZL, Riley LH, Wasserman BA, Khanna AJ (2008) Magnetic resonance imaging of spine tumors: classification, differential diagnosis, and spectrum of disease. J Bone Joint Surg Am 90(Suppl 4):146–162

Guan Y, Peck KK, Lyo J, Tisnado J, Lis E, Arevalo-Perez J, Yamada Y, Hameed MR, Karimi S, Holodny A (2020) T1-weighted dynamic contrast-enhanced MRI to differentiate nonneoplastic and malignant vertebral body lesions in the spine. Radiology 297(2):382–389. https://doi.org/10.1148/radiol.2020190553. Epub 2020 Sep 1. PMID: 32870135; PMCID: PMC7643814

Guerini H, Omoumi P, Guichoux F et al (2015) Fat suppression with Dixon techniques in musculoskeletal magnetic resonance imaging: a pictorial review. Semin Musculoskelet Radiol 19:335–347

Hanna SL, Fletcher BD, Parham DM et al (1991) Muscle edema in musculoskeletal tumors: MR imaging characteristics and clinical significance. J Magn Reson Imaging 1:441–449

Hanrahan CJ, Shah LM (2011) MRI of spinal bone marrow: Part 2, T1-weighted imaging-based differential diagnosis. AJR Am J Roentgenol 197(6):1309–1321. https://doi.org/10.2214/AJR.11.7420. PMID: 22109284

Hashemi RH, Bradley WG Jr, Lisanti CJ (2010) Artifacts in MRI. In: Mitchell CW (ed) MRI: the basics, 3rd edn. Lippincott Williams & Wilkins, Philadelphia, PA, pp 185–213

Hoff MN, Andre JB, Stewart BK (2016) Artifacts in MRI. In: Saba L (ed) Magnetic resonance imaging. Taylor and Francis, Oxford, UK

Maeder Y, Dunet V, Richard R, Becce F, Omoumi P (2018) Bone marrow metastases: T2-weighted Dixon spin-echo fat images can replace T1-weighted spin-echo images. Radiology 286:948–959

Morelli John JN, Runge VM, Ai F et al (2011) An image-based approach to understanding the physics of MR artifacts. Radiographics 31:849–866

Murphey M, Andrews C, Flemming D, Temple T, Smith S, Smirniotopoulos J (1996) Primary tumors of the spine. Radiographics 16:1131–1158

Nascimento D, Suchard G, Hatem M et al (2014) The role of magnetic resonance imaging in the evaluation of bone tumours and tumour-like lesions. Insights Imaging 5:419–440

O'Flanagan SJ, Stack JP, McGee HM et al (1991) Imaging of intramedullary tumour spread in osteosarcoma. A comparison of techniques. J Bone Joint Surg Br 73:998–1001

Omoumi P (2022) The Dixon method in musculoskeletal MRI: from fat-sensitive to fat-specific imaging. Skeletal Radiol 51(7):1365–1369. https://doi.org/10.1007/s00256-021-03950-1. Epub 2021 Dec 20. PMID: 34928411; PMCID: PMC9098547

Onikul E, Fletcher BD, Parham DM et al (1996) Accuracy of MR imaging for estimating intraosseous extent of osteosarcoma. AJR Am J Roentgenol 167:1211–1215

Patnaik S, Jyotsnarani Y, Uppin SG, Susarla R (2016) Imaging features of primary tumors of the spine: a pictorial essay. Indian J Radiol Imaging 26:279–289

Pozzi G, Albano D, Messina C, Angileri SA, Al-Mnayyis A, Galbusera F, Luzzati A, Perrucchini G, Scotto G,

Parafioriti A, Zerbi A, Sconfienza LM (2018) Solid bone tumors of the spine: diagnostic performance of apparent diffusion coefficient measured using diffusion-weighted MRI using histology as a reference standard. J Magn Reson Imaging 47(4):1034–1042. https://doi.org/10.1002/jmri.25826. Epub 2017 Jul 29. PMID: 28755383

Rodallec MH, Feydy A, Larousserie F et al (2008) Diagnostic imaging of solitary tumors of the spine: what to do and say. Radiographics 28:1019–1014

Roth E, Hoff M, Richardson ML, Ha AS, Porrino J (2016) Artifacts affecting musculoskeletal magnetic resonance imaging: their origins and solutions. Curr Probl Diagn Radiol 45(5):340–346

Stadler A, Schima W, Ba-Ssalamah A, Kettenbach J, Eisenhuber E (2007) Artifacts in body MR imaging: their appearance and how to eliminate them. Eur Radiol 17:1242–1255

Subhawong TK, Jacobs MA, Fayad LM (2014) Insights into quantitative diffusion-weighted MRI for musculoskeletal tumor imaging. AJR Am J Roentgenol 203(3):560–572. https://doi.org/10.2214/AJR.13.12165. PMID: 25148158

Suh JS, Jeong EK, Shin KH, Cho JH, Na JB, Kim DH, Han CD (1998) Minimizing artifacts caused by metallic implants at MR imaging: experimental and clinical studies. AJR Am J Roentgenol 171(5):1207–1213

Van Goethem JWM (2010) Magnetic resonance imaging of the spine. In: Reimer P et al (eds) Clinical MR imaging. Springer, Berlin, pp 147–172

Vanhoenacker FM, Van Dyck P, Gielen J, De Schepper AM, Parizel PM (2010) Musculoskeletal system. In: Reimer P et al (eds) Clinical MR imaging. Springer, Berlin, pp 345–348

Verstraete KL, Lang P (2000) Bone and soft tissue tumors: the role of contrast agents for MR imaging. Eur J Radiol 34(3):229–246

Wu JS, Hochman MG (2009) Soft-tissue tumors and tumorlike lesions: a systematic imaging approach. Radiology 253:297–316

Zhao J, Krug R, Xu D, Lu Y, Link TM (2009) MRI of the spine: image quality and normal-neoplastic bone marrow contrast at 3 T versus 1.5 T. AJR Am J Roentgenol 192(4):873–880. https://doi.org/10.2214/AJR.08.1750. PMID: 19304689

PET/CT in Primary Tumors of the Osseous Spine

Sarah K. Ceyssens

Contents

S. K. Ceyssens (✉)
Department of Nuclear Medicine, Antwerp University Hospital, Edegem, Belgium

University of Antwerp, Antwerp, Belgium
e-mail: Sarah.Ceyssens@uza.be

Abstract

Accurate differentiation between a benign or malignant lesion is crucial to define the best therapeutic strategy in general. The main role of the current imaging modalities is to recognize typically benign disease, in which further invasive staging can be omitted, and patients with a suspected malignancy, who should be referred for biopsy. In most cases, these questions can be answered by means of conventional radiography, computed tomography (CT), and magnetic resonance imaging (MRI). However, occasionally, the appearance of a lesion on these imaging techniques might be inconclusive. The role of ^{18}F-FDG-PET/CT in the diagnosis and characterization of bone lesions is not yet fully defined due to rather limited data.

Besides confirmation of malignancy, it is essential to know the exact histology and grading of the primary tumor. In the evaluation of a musculoskeletal mass, core needle biopsies are generally accepted as an appropriate alternative to open biopsy. However, since sarcomas tend to be heterogeneous with areas of necrosis, there is a risk of sampling error and underestimating true tumor grade, as well as a substantial risk of redo biopsy and complications. Thus, a growing interest in using imaging modalities to guide biopsies toward the biologically most active zone seems logical. By identifying the metabolically most active portion of a tumor mass,

Med Radiol Diagn Imaging (2023)
https://doi.org/10.1007/174_2023_434,
Published Online: 18 May 2023

^{18}F-FDG-PET can guide biopsy to that tumoral part with most likely the highest histological grade.

In the diagnostic workup of malignancy, the strength of ^{18}F-FDG-PET/CT lies in its ability to detect metastases outside the standard field of view of CT and MRI, and in the exclusion of disease in equivocal results on conventional imaging. With regard to treatment monitoring, ^{18}F-FDG-PET/CT seems promising with a good correlation between an early and significant decline in metabolic activity and response to therapy in various tumors. Finally, ^{18}F-FDG-PET/CT is a useful tool for the detection of local recurrences and metastases after therapy.

1 Introduction

Radioisotopes of natural elements, oxygen-15, carbon-11, nitrogen-13, and fluorine-18, can be easily inserted into physiologic compounds in the human body without disrupting their characteristics ("physiologic labeling"). After administration of only small quantities of these positron-emitting radiopharmaceuticals, the biodistribution of these tracers can be revealed by positron emission tomography (PET) (Jones 1996).

The most commonly used tracer in PET is the glucose analogue fluorine-18-labeled 2-fluoro-2-deoxy-D-glucose, [^{18}F]FDG. Similar to glucose, [^{18}F]FDG is transported into the cell by the glucose transporter proteins and subsequently rapidly phosphorylated to [^{18}F]FDG-6-phosphate. Yet, since a hydroxyl group in the 2-position is replaced by a positron-emitting ^{18}F, the latter is—in contrast to glucose-6-phosphate—not a substrate for the glucose phosphate isomerase and thus cannot be converted to the fructose analogue. Most cancer cells show an increased expression of glucose transporter proteins and an upregulation of hexokinase activity at one hand, but a low phosphatase activity at the other hand. As a sum of this, [^{18}F]FDG-6-phosphate will accumulate in the cell, resulting in the so-called metabolic trapping and an increased signal in malignant cells compared to normal surrounding tissue (Warburg et al. 1931). However, increased ^{18}F-FDG uptake is not specific for cancer cells. Since it is also seen in neutrophils, eosinophils, macrophages, and proliferating fibroblasts, sometimes even more intense than in malignant cells (Kubota et al. 1992), an increased FDG uptake can also be seen in some inflammatory conditions, as well as infectious foci (Yamada et al. 1995; Pijl et al. 2020). Therefore, the entire medical history of the patient should be taken into account to reduce the risk of a false-positive result.

Aiming at the development of more specific radiopharmaceuticals, there is an ongoing search for new PET tracers, as well as an exploration of possible new information in "older" tracers. Apart from cancer cells, also the stroma in tumors plays an important role in the growth and spread. In case of a malignancy with a strong desmoplastic reaction, such as breast, colon, and pancreatic carcinoma, more than 90% of the total mass may consist of stroma. Cancer-associated fibroblasts (CAFs), a subpopulation of fibroblasts, are known to be involved in tumor growth, migration, and progression. These CAFs can be distinguished from normal fibroblasts by an increased expression of fibroblast activation protein (FAP), a type II membrane-bound glycoprotein of the dipeptidyl peptidase-4 family. Although FAP plays a role in normal developmental processes during embryogenesis and in tissue modeling, it is hardly expressed on adult normal tissues. An overexpression can be seen in wound healing, arthritis, atheromas, fibrosis, and more than 90% of epithelial carcinomas. The latter and the fact that overexpression correlates with a worse prognosis in cancer patients indicate that FAP activity might be involved in cancer development, cancer cell migration, and cancer spread. Therefore, these cells might be an attractive target for imaging and subsequent antitumor therapy (Loktev et al. 2018).

Given that PET relies on the detection of metabolic alterations, these examinations deliver data independently of structural features as provided by computed tomography (CT) and magnetic resonance imaging (MRI).

Consequently, these metabolic data will allow detection or monitoring of specific changes which are not associated with or which precede the anatomical changes. Combining the anatomical information of CT or MRI and the metabolic information of PET improves diagnostic accuracy, provides surgery and radiation therapy planning, and can guide biopsies by merging the anatomic and metabolic information in one single procedure. Still, studies are required to evaluate the impact of combining these imaging techniques on the overall diagnostic performance in general.

2 FDG-PET/CT in the Evaluation of Tumors of the Osseous Spine

Several disorders can affect the osseous spine. Depending on the underlying etiology, these can be classified as inflammatory, infectious, and degenerative diseases; tumors; or tumorlike conditions. Accurate differentiation between a benign and malignant mass is crucial to define the best therapeutic strategy. ^{18}F-FDG-PET/CT is increasingly used to study infectious disease, including spondylodiscitis. Since symptoms and laboratory findings are quite often nonspecific, diagnosis of spondylodiscitis is not always straightforward. Studies have shown a comparable diagnostic value of the latter technique to that of MRI. An important advantage of ^{18}F-FDG-PET/CT is the large field of view allowing visualization of metastatic infectious foci. Moreover, metallic implants are not contraindicated, and this technique allows differentiation between infection and degeneration. On the other hand, MRI is more sensitive in detecting small epidural abscesses (Kouijzer et al. 2018; Altini et al. 2020).

In case of malignancy, it is essential to know the exact histology and grading of the lesion. Although in a plethora of cases this can be accomplished by means of conventional radiography, computed tomography (CT), and magnetic resonance imaging (MRI), in some cases, the appearance of these lesions on these imaging techniques is inconclusive.

The role of ^{18}F-FDG-PET/CT in the diagnosis and characterization of bone lesions has not been fully defined yet, mainly due to limited data. Several studies have shown a correlation between FDG uptake and histological grade of the tumor, with a significant higher tracer uptake in intermediate/high-grade tumors compared to low-grade tumors. This is more likely to apply when considering tumors of the same histologic type, for instance cartilage tumors, although there is some overlap. A high FDG uptake can also be seen in aggressive benign tumors, such as recurrent osteoblastoma, fibrous dysplasia, and fibromatosis. In these cases, ^{18}F-FDG-PET might be a reflection of the biologic activity and thus local aggressiveness rather than grade of malignancy prompting more aggressive therapeutic approach (Schulte et al. 2000; Parghane and Basu 2017; Dimitrakopoulou-Strauss et al. 2002).

In the diagnostic workup of malignancy, the strength of ^{18}F-FDG-PET/CT lies in its ability to detect metastases outside the standard field of view of CT and MRI, and in the exclusion of disease in equivocal results on conventional imaging. Regarding treatment monitoring, ^{18}F-FDG-PET seems promising in several tumors such as sarcoma, with a good correlation between an early and significant decline in metabolic activity and response to therapy. Although further studies are necessary, recent studies suggest a role for the use of ^{18}F-FDG-PET for detection of local recurrence of these tumors.

2.1 Vertebral Hemangioma, Epithelioid Hemangioendothelioma, and Angiosarcoma

There is a great variety of vascular tumors of the bone ranging from a completely benign tumor such as a hemangioma at one side of the scale to an intermediately aggressive epithelioid hemangioendothelioma and a highly malignant angiosarcoma at the opposite side of the spectrum (Lee et al. 2017).

Vertebral hemangioma is an essentially benign lesion which can be classified into typical, atypical, and aggressive hemangioma. Although the typical hemangioma is in general ametabolic on ^{18}F-FDG-PET and negative on Tc-99m methyl diphosphonate (MDP) bone scintigraphy, the FDG uptake in aggressive hemangioma seems to vary and is higher than in case of a typical hemangioma. This might be due to internal hemorrhage, inflammation, and remodeling secondary to bone destruction and fractures, all of which could lead to hypermetabolism on ^{18}F-FDG-PET (Solav et al. 2019; Ko and Park 2013; Song et al. 2020). However, combining the metabolic information of FDG-PET with the characteristic structural features of hemangioma on CT will help correct diagnosis. In case of atypical features leading to inconclusive results on these imaging techniques, there might be an added value of a Tc-99m red blood cell (RBC) scan. Due to the fact that hemangiomas are sinuses filled with blood, these lesions show an increased uptake of Tc-99m-labeled RBCs, allowing differentiation from malignant lesions (Elhelf et al. 2019).

In epithelioid hemangioendothelioma and angiosarcoma, FDG uptake is significantly higher than in hemangioma, suggesting FDG-PET/CT to be a helpful tool in identifying benign from malignant vertebral vascular lesions (Song et al. 2020).

2.2 Enostosis

An enostosis, also known as bone island, is considered a benign lesion that can be diagnosed based on clinical context and (structural) imaging features. FDG-PET is not recommended in the general workup. However, since they usually present as an incidental finding, there are some reports showing an increased FDG uptake probably due to an increased activity of osteoblasts as well as proliferating fibroblasts and an increased blood flow (Ulano et al. 2016; Ran et al. 2018).

2.3 Osteoid Osteoma

Osteoid osteoma is a benign bone lesion with a central core of unmineralized bone matrix surrounded by a sclerotic zone. Since osteoid osteoma is normally negative on FDG-PET, this technique is not recommended in the general workup of these lesions. Nevertheless, there are some reports showing an increased tracer uptake probably due to a strong inflammatory response (Lim et al. 2007; Ishikura et al. 2021).

2.4 Giant Cell Tumor

Giant cell tumors are typically benign lesions. Yet, they can be locally aggressive and local recurrences occur in about 25% following resection. Sporadically, a giant cell tumor can undergo malignant transformation (Palmerini et al. 2019). Despite the benign nature of most of these lesions, a high FDG uptake can be seen due to the presence of the osteoclast-like multinucleated giant cell; spindle-shaped, fibroblast-like mesenchymal stromal cell; and macrophage-like cell (Parghane and Basu 2017; Muheremu et al. 2017).

In case the giant cell tumor of the bone is unresectable or resection would be associated with severe morbidity, the monoclonal antibody denosumab with high affinity and specificity to RANKL is a relatively new treatment option. In these cases, a significant decrease in FDG uptake was found to be predictable of a favorable tumor response and sustained tumor control with denosumab treatment (van Langevelde and McCarthy 2020).

2.5 Fibrous Dysplasia

Fibrous dysplasia is a benign bone disorder characterized by immature woven bone and stroma. Malignant transformation is rare. It can present in a monostotic or polyostotic form. As mentioned above, high FDG uptake might be seen in aggressive benign tumors, such as fibrous dysplasia. In these cases, the increased PET signal is linked to the presence of fibroblasts and considered a reflection of the biologic activity and thus local aggressiveness rather than grade of malignancy. However, due to this local aggressiveness, a more aggressive therapeutic approach might be advised (Parghane and Basu 2017). Furthermore, these fibrous lesions are soft and stringy, which makes the bone more fragile and prone to fracture. Since the processes of bone healing and acute inflammation are biologically closely tied together, it is not surprising that these could give rise to an increased signal on FDG-PET (Loi et al. 2016). Fibrous dysplasia lesions change over time until they become inactive and regress in adulthood, resulting in sclerotic lesions. Thus, metabolic and structural findings might vary with different evolutionary stages (Pozzessere et al. 2022).

2.6 Aneurysmal Bone Cyst and Other Cystic Lesions

In general, aneurysmal bone cysts and other cystic lesions are negative on FDG-PET. Hence, this technique is not recommended in the general workup of these lesions.

2.7 Notochordal Tumors

Benign notochordal cell (BNCT) and chordomas are rare tumors arising from the remnants of the notochord. Several case reports suggest that BNCTs are capable of malignant transformation and may progress to chordoma (Nishiguchi et al. 2010; Kreshak et al. 2014).

To the best of my knowledge, there is no literature on the use of ^{18}F-FDG-PET/CT in BNCT. Since it consists of adipocyte-like polymorphic vacuolate cells, resembling normal fatty marrow (Nishiguchi et al. 2010), one would expect no increased FDG uptake in these lesions.

Chordoma on the other hand is a low-grade, locally invasive lesion with relatively low metastatic potential. Studies have shown a heterogeneously increased FDG uptake in these lesions, suggesting that FDG-PET might be a valuable tool for staging, evaluation of treatment response, and assessment of local recurrence (Olson et al. 2021; Park and Kim 2008; Cui et al. 2018).

2.8 Langerhans Cell Histiocytosis

Langerhans cell histiocytosis (LCH, formerly called histiocytosis X) is a rare disease characterized by the proliferation of Langerhans cells, antigen-presenting cells which originate from the myeloid progenitor cells of the bone marrow. It can affect one organ or system, or present as disseminated disease in which LCH can affect all organs. In case of an isolated lesion, prognosis is in general good, with sometimes even a spontaneous remission. However, widespread disease is associated with increased mortality. Since the choice of therapy relies on whether the disease is uni- or multifocal, there is a need for a reliable technique for identifying lesions (Huynh and Nguyen 2021). Studies have shown that FDG-PET outperforms other imaging techniques (including conventional radiography, bone scan, CT) in the overall evaluation of the extent of lesions in the diagnostic workup of LCH patients. However, in vertebral lesions, sensitivity of PET seems lower than that of MRI, mainly due to the higher spatial resolution of the latter technique. The most beneficial aspects of FDG-PET in this patient group are the assessment of treatment response, with a significant decrease of the signal in responders, and monitoring for relapse (Phillips et al. 2009; Mueller et al. 2013; Jessop et al. 2020; Ferrell et al. 2021).

2.9 Lymphoma

Although secondary involvement of the axial skeleton in disseminated lymphoma is not uncommon, primary bone lymphoma is a rare presentation of lymphoma. It comprises 2% at most of all bone tumors and 5% of all extranodal lymphomas. Non-Hodgkin's lymphoma and diffuse large B-cell lymphoma (DLBCL) in particular represent the majority of primary bone lymphomas (Barz et al. 2021). In Hodgkin's disease, primary involvement of the bone is extremely rare, occurring in less than 1% (Müller et al. 2020).

FDG-PET/CT is considered a valuable tool to define disease location and extent at initial staging and to provide a baseline against which response or disease progression can be compared during treatment follow-up. Since residual mass on CT after the end of treatment is not necessarily associated with treatment failure in lymphomas, the value of PET in this setting lies in its ability to differentiate viable tumor from necrosis or fibrosis in residual masses (Juweid et al. 2005, 2007; Cerci et al. 2010; Cashen et al. 2011).

In 2009, a visual five-point scale using mediastinum and liver as reference levels, named the Deauville score, was developed by a panel of hematologists and nuclear medicine specialists, offering simple and reproducible criteria for response assessment in Hodgkin's lymphoma and diffuse large B-cell lymphoma (DLBCL) (Barrington et al. 2010). A few years ago, the Deauville score was revised in the Lugano classification. In the latter, residual uptake lower or equivalent to liver background (Deauville scores 1–3) is considered as complete metabolic response, whereas residual uptake higher than liver background (Deauville scores 4–5) is considered no metabolic response (no change from baseline), partial metabolic response (decrease in uptake compared to baseline), or progressive metabolic disease (increased uptake or new lesion). Since this Lugano classification has demonstrated good prognostic value and excellent interobserver reproducibility, FDG-PET/CT was formally incorporated into standard staging and response assessment of routinely FDG-avid lymphomas, while CT scan was preferred in non-avid disease (Cheson et al. 2014).

2.10 Plasmacytoma

Plasma cell tumors consist of two main groups, multiple myeloma and solitary plasmacytoma. The latter can present either as solitary extramedullary plasmacytoma (EMP) or as solitary plasmacytoma of bone (SBP) (Zhang et al. 2018).

In contrast with multiple myeloma, only few and small studies have examined the role of ^{18}F-FDG-PET/CT in solitary plasmacytomas. Based on the available scientific resources, a panel of expert European hematologists formulated recommendations on the diagnosis and management of these patients. Since solitary plasmacytoma is defined by the absence of systemic spread, imaging is required not only to detect and localize the primary lesion, but also to exclude a multiple myeloma (Fig. 1). Based on small prospective studies, the panel recommends either an MRI or an ^{18}F-FDG-PET/CT in addition to the skeletal survey or CT. Given that PET relies on the detection of metabolic alterations, this technique delivers data independently of structural features as provided by magnetic resonance imaging (MRI). As a consequence of this, both ^{18}F-FDG-PET/CT and MRI may offer complementary information.

Solitary plasmacytoma of bone evolves into multiple myeloma more frequently than extramedullary plasmacytoma and thus demonstrates worse prognosis compared with EMP. Therefore, confirmation of minimal infiltration of the bone marrow by aberrant plasma cells, presence of extra-hypermetabolic lesions on ^{18}F-FDG-PET/CT, and an abnormal serum-free light-chain ratio, all contain prognostic information.

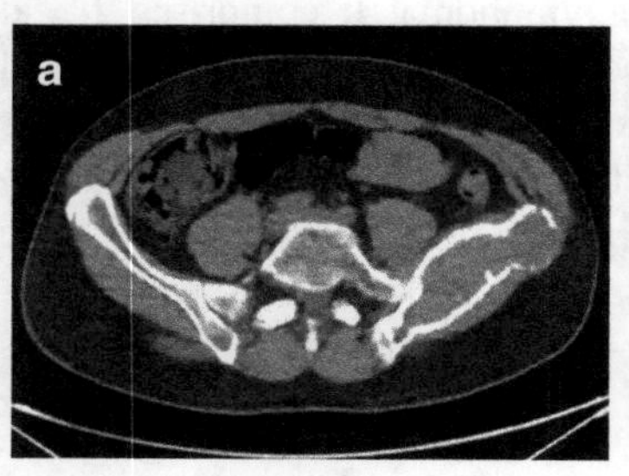

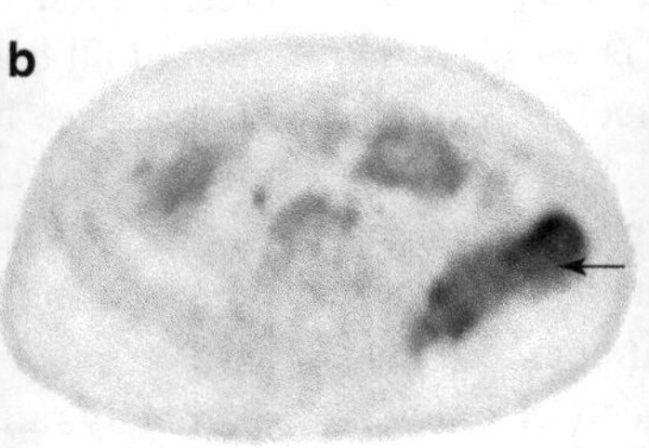

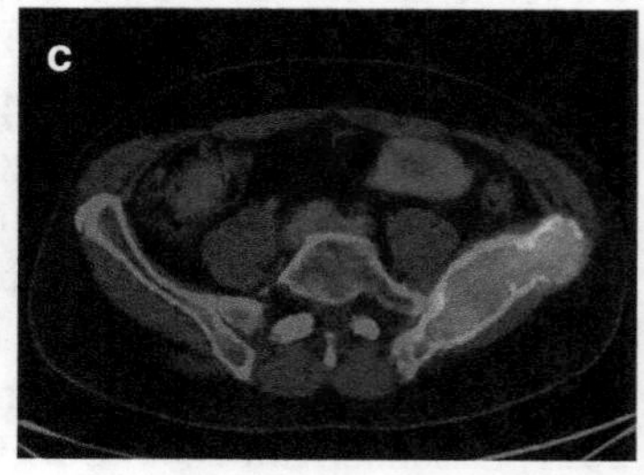

Fig. 1 Patient with a solitary plasmacytoma of the left hemipelvis with a moderate intense FDG uptake (arrow): CT (**a**), PET (**b**), and PET/CT fusion image (**c**)

Regarding response assessment, studies have demonstrated a higher sensitivity of ^{18}F-FDG-PET/CT compared to MRI. A persistent high tracer uptake during therapy is a sign of residual disease, while low FDG uptake after radiotherapy is most likely due to bone remodeling, which is not necessarily associated with poor prognosis. According to the expert panel, adjuvant chemotherapy can be considered in case of residual disease on ^{18}F-FDG-PET/CT after initial radiotherapy (Caers et al. 2018).

2.11 Paget's Disease

Paget's disease is characterized by an accelerated bone turnover due to an imbalance of osteoblastic and osteoclastic activity. It is often asymptomatic, and diagnosis can be incidental. In most cases, Paget's disease is a benign disorder. However, malignant transformation to sarcoma has been described in 1% of patients with longstanding Paget's disease.

In the majority of these patients, no abnormal ^{18}F-FDG is seen and ^{18}F-FDG-PET/CT can be a useful tool to discriminate typically benign disease from associated sarcoma. However, in patients with more active disease—measured by an elevated serum alkaline phosphatase—an increased tracer uptake can be seen, but lower than would be expected to be seen in case of malignancy. Moreover, complications due to the increased remodeling, such as fractures, may occur giving rise to an increased signal (Cook et al. 1997).

Regarding PET tracers other than ^{18}F-FDG, an incidental increase in Paget's disease has been reported in PSMA-PET probably related to bone remodeling and increased vascularization. Also using other tracers such as 11C-choline and 68Ga-DOTANOC, one must bear in mind that Paget's disease is a potential pitfall and the characteristic features on the CT portion should allow correct diagnosis and differentiation from malignant lesions (Leitch et al. 2017; Dondi et al. 2022) (Fig. 2).

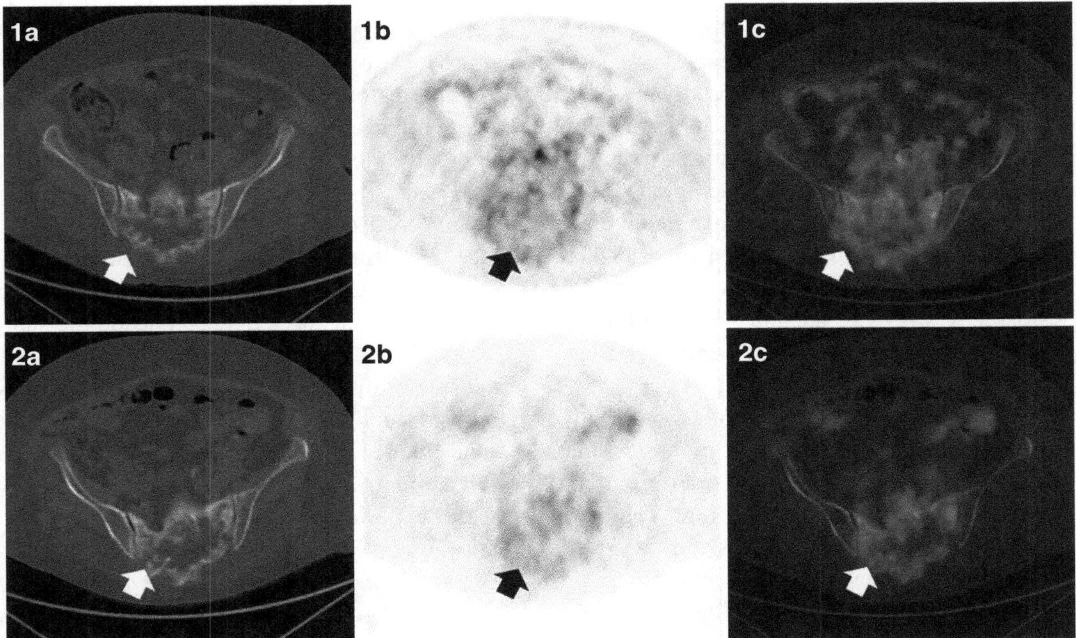

Fig. 2 Patient with Paget's disease of the sacrum with a discrete tracer uptake (arrow) on 18F-FDG-PET/CT ((row 1): CT (**1a**), PET (**1b**), and PET/CT fusion image (**1c**)) as well as on 68Ga-DOTANOC ((row 2): CT (**2a**), PET (**2b**), and PET/CT fusion image (**2c**))

Since ^{18}F-sodium fluoride reflects blood flow and osteoblastic activity, this tracer has great potential to detect Paget's disease as well as monitor noninvasively the efficacy of treatment with bisphosphonates in this patient population (Installé et al. 2005; Sang et al. 2021).

2.12 Sarcoma

2.12.1 Characterization and Grading of a Mass

With regard to the characterization and grading of soft tissue masses in general, a strong correlation between maximum tracer uptake (standardized uptake value, SUV) and mitotic count was found, as well as with the presence of tumor necrosis. Furthermore, several reports have shown a relation between tracer uptake and histological grade with a significantly higher ^{18}F-FDG uptake in intermediate/high-grade soft tissue sarcomas compared to low-grade tumors, although there is some overlap (Reyes Marlés et al. 2021). Considering other factors such as the difference in reaching peak activity concentration (a steady increase with a peak activity in FDG uptake around 4 h in high-grade malignant lesions versus a peak within 30 min followed by a washout in benign lesions) (Chen et al. 2020; Ferner et al. 2000; Lodge et al. 1999) or the uptake pattern (a more heterogeneous pattern in high-grade lesions versus a more homogeneous uptake in low-grade sarcoma) can help to distinguish intermediate/high-grade lesions from low-grade/benign lesions. However, adequate discrimination between low-grade tumors and benign lesions by ^{18}F-FDG-PET remains difficult (Lucas et al. 1999; Mayerhoefer et al. 2008). False-negative results can be seen in some low-grade sarcomas, while false-positive findings are seen in inflammatory lesions or lesions with high cellularity (e.g., giant cell tumor) (Ioannidis and Lau 2003).

In addition to confirmation of malignancy, it is essential to know the exact histology and grading of the primary tumor to define the best therapeutic strategy. The main role of the current imaging modalities is to recognize typically benign disease, in which further invasive staging can be omitted, and patients with a suspected malignancy, who should be referred for biopsy. In the evaluation of a musculoskeletal mass, core needle biopsies are generally accepted as an appropriate alternative to open biopsy. However, since sarcomas tend to be heterogeneous with areas of necrosis, there is a risk of sampling error and underestimating true tumor grade (Domanski et al. 2005). Additionally, since there is a risk of redo biopsy (in 15–20% of cases) and complications (20%), the growing interest in using imaging modalities to guide biopsies toward the biologically most active zone seems logical (Lucas et al. 1999). ^{18}F-FDG-PET is giving information on biological activity of different tumoral parts and on intratumoral heterogeneity, reflected as areas of high and low tracer uptake (Rakheja et al. 2012). By identifying the metabolically most active portion of a tumor mass, ^{18}F-FDG-PET can guide biopsy to that tumoral part most likely to contain tumor tissue of the highest grade present.

2.12.2 Evaluation of Disease Extent

Due to its clear, detailed images of soft tissues, MRI is the imaging modality of choice to evaluate the local extent of the primary tumor in the different anatomical compartments surrounding the tumor like muscles, fat, blood vessels, nerves, tendons, and synovial tissues.

Thanks to the ability to screen the entire patient for distant metastases without significantly increasing the radiation burden, the key role of ^{18}F-FDG-PET/CT lies largely in detecting metastases at unexpected sites, outside the standard field of view of CT and MRI, and in the exclusion of disease in equivocal results on conventional imaging (Upadhyay et al. 2020; Macpherson et al. 2018).

Regarding the detection of lymph node metastases, the power of ^{18}F-FDG-PET exists in its ability to show tumoral involvement in normal-sized nodes and to exclude disease in reactively enlarged nodes (Dwamena et al. 1999). Although lymphatic spread is not common in case of sarcoma in general, it is possible that with the growing use of ^{18}F-FDG-PET/CT, the prevalence of lymph node metastases might increase.

Despite the fact that further studies are required, preliminary clinical experiences with ^{18}F-FDG-PET/MRI seem promising. The main advantages of combining the anatomical information of MRI and the metabolic information of PET lie in joining the strength of the T staging equal to that of an MR alone, complemented by the power of N and M staging from the PET component (Partovi et al. 2014).

2.12.3 Evaluation of Response to Treatment

The purpose of treatment monitoring is to accurately distinguish responders from nonresponders with the ultimate goal to adjust therapy to the information provided: treatment can be continued in responders, whereas therapy can be adapted in case of nonresponse.

Since ^{18}F-FDG-PET can differentiate between viable cells and necrotic or fibrotic inactive tissue, it is no surprise that several studies have shown a good correlation between a significant decline in metabolic activity and response to therapy in various tumors, including sarcoma (Polverari et al. 2020; Juweid and Cheson 2006). Quantitative ^{18}F-FDG-PET outperforms the size-based criteria to distinguish responders from nonresponders to neoadjuvant therapy in high-grade soft tissue sarcomas. Using a 60% decrease in ^{18}F-FDG uptake resulted in a sensitivity of 100% and specificity of 71% for PET, whereas for RECIST, a sensitivity of 25% and specificity of 100% were seen (Evilevitch et al. 2008). Even early after the start of neoadjuvant chemotherapy in high-grade STS, histologic responders could be identified using a ≥35% reduction in ^{18}F-FDG uptake (SUVpeak) as early metabolic response threshold (sensitivity 100% and specificity 67%). Since responders have to be identified with high sensitivity to avoid withholding potentially effective treatments to patients, a high sensitivity is more important than a high specificity (Benz et al. 2009).

When using ^{18}F-FDG-PET to assess treatment response, a baseline PET scan is mandatory, since evaluation of metabolic response is based on the change in ^{18}F-FDG uptake in the tumor compared to the pretreatment study. Moreover, as mentioned before, some tumors show only slight ^{18}F-FDG uptake. In the latter case, ^{18}F-FDG-PET is not suitable for response assessment, nor follow-up.

2.12.4 Detection of Recurrence

If the intent is surgical control, early detection and treatment of local recurrence are mandatory, even if this does not necessarily influence the final outcome of the patient. Due to its high contrast resolution, MRI remains the technique of choice in case of suspected local recurrence in the extremities, although radiotherapy- and chemotherapy-induced changes can complicate the evaluation of the affected region. Yet, using an organized systematic approach and certain algorithms, these challenges can be reduced (Garner et al. 2009; Vanel et al. 1998).

First reports on the use of ^{18}F-PET/CT for detection of local recurrence of STS seem promising (Dancheva et al. 2016), especially when combining the metabolic information of ^{18}F-FDG-PET and the soft tissue contrast of MRI in an integrated ^{18}F-FDG-PET/MRI. In a study of Erfanian and coworkers, the diagnostic accuracy of PET/MRI and MRI alone was compared for the detection of local recurrences of soft tissue sarcomas (STSs) after initial surgical resection. ^{18}F-FDG-PET/MRI appeared to be an excellent imaging technique with a higher sensitivity and negative predictive value as well as a higher diagnostic confidence for the detection of recurrent STS after resection compared to MRI alone (Erfanian et al. 2017).

2.12.5 Prognostic Value

Maximum ^{18}F-FDG uptake (SUV) correlates well with pathological grade, cellularity, mitotic activity, MIB labeling index, and p53 overexpression, all of these factors known to have prognostic value (Kubota et al. 1992). Studies demonstrated that high ^{18}F-FDG uptake in sarcoma on the baseline PET/CT is associated with a significant shorter disease-free survival (DFS) ($p < 0.001$) and overall survival (OS) ($p < 0.003$) (Eary et al. 2002). Not only pretreatment SUVmax but also metabolic tumor volume (MTV) and total lesion glycolysis (TLG) were found to be prognostic factors of overall survival (OS) (Reyes Marlés et al. 2021).

3 PET/MRI

An exciting development in the nuclear medicine field is the transition of PET/MRI hybrid systems from preclinical and clinical research to clinical practice. The PET component allows the detection of metabolic alterations with high sensitivity, whereas the MRI component offers high-resolution structural information and high soft tissue contrast. An integrated PET/MRI combines these strengths in "one-stop shop" (Mannheim et al. 2018). So far, the use of PET/MRI in the clinical setting is overall accepted for those locations where MRI is clearly superior to CT, e.g., brain and certain pelvic cancers. The clinical use for other types of cancers is not yet widespread. However, since this field is still highly dynamic with an ongoing search for more advanced data analysis techniques and new tracers, a shift from PET/CT to PET/MRI might not be a faraway future not only in oncology and neurology, but also in infection and inflammatory diseases (Broski et al. 2018; Sepehrizadeh et al. 2021).

4 Conclusion

^{18}F-FDG-PET can help to distinguish intermediate/high-grade lesions from low-grade/benign lesions. However, adequate discrimination between low-grade tumors and benign soft tissue lesions by ^{18}F-FDG-PET is difficult due to the fact that an increased FDG uptake can also be seen in some inflammatory conditions, as well as infectious foci. Therefore, we must always take into account the entire medical history of the patient.

In the diagnostic workup of a malignant lesion in general, combining the anatomical information of the CT or MR and the metabolic information of ^{18}F-FDG-PET in the last-generation hybrid imaging machines improves diagnostic accuracy, provides surgery and radiation therapy planning, and can guide biopsy by merging the anatomic and metabolic information in one single procedure. ^{18}F-FDG-PET/CT allows detection of metastases at unexpected sites, outside the standard field of view of CT and MRI, and exclusion of disease in equivocal results on conventional imaging.

^{18}F-FDG-PET also seems promising for treatment monitoring. A good correlation was found between an early and significant decline in metabolic activity and response to therapy in various tumors. Consequently, PET can be used to identify those patients at high risk with regard to progression and survival in whom a closer follow-up might be desirable.

Finally, ^{18}F-FDG-PET/CT is a useful tool for the detection of local recurrences and metastases after therapy.

5 Key Points

- ^{18}F-FDG-PET/CT can guide biopsy toward the most aggressive zone by identifying the most metabolically active portion of a tumor mass.
- In the diagnostic workup of a malignancy, the strength of ^{18}F-FDG-PET/CT lies in its ability to detect metastases outside the standard field of view of CT and MRI and to rule out disease in equivocal results on conventional imaging.
- With regard to treatment monitoring, a good correlation is found between an early and significant decline in metabolic activity visualized on ^{18}F-FDG-PET and response to therapy in various tumors.
- Finally, ^{18}F-FDG-PET/CT is a useful tool for the detection of local recurrences and metastases after therapy.

References

Altini C, Lavelli V, Niccoli-Asabella A et al (2020) Comparison of the diagnostic value of MRI and whole body 18F-FDG PET/CT in diagnosis of spondylodiscitis. J Clin Med 9(5):1581

Barrington SF, Qian W, Somer EJ et al (2010) Concordance between four European centres of PET reporting criteria designed for use in multicentre trials in Hodgkin lymphoma. Eur J Nucl Med Mol Imaging 37(10):1824–1833

Barz M, Aftahy K, Janssen I et al (2021) Spinal manifestation of malignant primary (PLB) and secondary bone lymphoma (SLB). Curr Oncol 28(5):3891–3899

Benz MR, Czernin J, Allen-Auerbach MS et al (2009) FDG-PET/CT imaging predicts histopathologic treatment responses after the initial cycle of neoadjuvant chemotherapy in high-grade soft-tissue sarcomas. Clin Cancer Res 15(8):2856–2863

Broski SM, Goenka AH, Kemp BJ et al (2018) Clinical PET/MRI: 2018 update. Am J Roentgenol 211(2):295–313

Caers J, Paiva B, Zamagni E et al (2018) Diagnosis, treatment, and response assessment in solitary plasmacytoma: updated recommendations from a European Expert Panel. J Hematol Oncol 11(1):10

Cashen AF, Dehdashti F, Luo J et al (2011) 18F-FDG PET/CT for early response assessment in diffuse large B-cell lymphoma: poor predictive value of international harmonization project interpretation. J Nucl Med 52:386–392

Cerci JJ, Pracchia LF, Linardi CC et al (2010) 18F-FDG PET after 2 cycles of ABVD predicts event-free survival in early and advanced Hodgkin lymphoma. J Nucl Med 51:1337–1343

Chen B, Feng H, Xie J et al (2020) Differentiation of soft tissue and bone sarcomas from benign lesions utilizing 18 F-FDG PET/CT-derived parameters. BMC Med Imaging 20(1):85

Cheson BD, Fisher RI, Barrington SF et al (2014) Recommendations for initial evaluation, staging, and response assessment of Hodgkin and non-Hodgkin lymphoma: the Lugano classification. J Clin Oncol 32(27):3059–3068

Cook GJ, Maisey MN, Fogelman I (1997) Fluorine-18-FDG PET in Paget's disease of bone. J Nucl Med 38(9):1495–1497

Cui F, Su M, Zhang H et al (2018) Humeral metastasis of sacrococcygeal chordoma detected by fluorine-18 fluorodeoxyglucose positron emission tomography-computed tomography: a case report. Radiol Case Rep 13(2):449–452

Dancheva Z, Bochev P, Chaushev B et al (2016) Dual-time point 18FDG-PET/CT imaging may be useful in assessing local recurrent disease in high grade bone and soft tissue sarcoma. Nucl Med Rev Cent East Eur 19(1):22–27

Dimitrakopoulou-Strauss A, Strauss Ludwig G, Heichel T et al (2002) The role of quantitative (18)F-FDG PET studies for the differentiation of malignant and benign bone lesions. J Nucl Med 43(4):510–518

Domanski HA, Akerman M, Carlén B et al (2005) Core-needle biopsy performed by the cytopathologist: a technique to complement fine-needle aspiration of soft tissue and bone lesions. Cancer 105(4):229–239

Dondi F, Domenico Albano D, Giorgio Treglia G et al (2022) Paget disease as common pitfall on PET with different radiopharmaceuticals in oncology: not all that glitters is gold! J Clin Med 11(18):5372

Dwamena BA, Sonnad SS, Angobaldo JO et al (1999) Metastases from non-small cell lung cancer: mediastinal staging in the 1990s—meta-analytic comparison of PET and CT. Radiology 213:530–536

Eary JF, O'Sullivan F, Powitan Y et al (2002) Sarcoma tumor FDG uptake measured by PET and patient outcome: a retrospective analysis. Eur J Nucl Med Mol Imaging 29:1149–1154

Elhelf IAS, Maheshwarappa RP, Hodgson J et al (2019) Giant vertebral hemangioma masquerading as aggressive tumor: Tc-99m tagged RBC scan can help to solve the diagnostic conundrum! Radiol Case Rep 14(11):1360–1363

Erfanian Y, Grueneisen J, Kirchner J et al (2017) Integrated 18F–FDG PET/MRI compared to MRI alone for identification of local recurrences of soft tissue sarcomas: a comparison trial. Eur J Nucl Med Mol Imaging 44:1823–1831

Evilevitch V, Weber WA, Tap WD et al (2008) Reduction of glucose metabolic activity is more accurate than change in size at predicting histopathologic response to neoadjuvant therapy in high-grade soft-tissue sarcomas. Clin Cancer Res 14:715–720

Ferner RE, Lucas JD, O'Doherty MJ et al (2000) Evaluation of (18)fluorodeoxyglucose positron emission tomography ((18)FDG PET) in the detection of malignant peripheral nerve sheath tumours arising from within plexiform neurofibromas in neurofibromatosis 1. J Neurol Neurosurg Psychiatry 68:353–357

Ferrell J, Sharp S, Kumar A et al (2021) Discrepancies between F-18-FDG PET/CT findings and conventional imaging in Langerhans cell histiocytosis. Pediatr Blood Cancer 68(4):e28891

Garner HW, Kransdorf MJ, Bancroft LW et al (2009) Benign and malignant soft-tissue tumors: posttreatment MR imaging. Radiographics 29:119–134

Huynh KN, Nguyen BD (2021) Histiocytosis and neoplasms of macrophage-dendritic cell lineages: multimodality imaging with emphasis on PET/CT. Radiographics 41(2):576–594

Installé J, Nzeusseu A, Bol A et al (2005) (18)F-fluoride PET for monitoring therapeutic response in Paget's disease of bone. J Nucl Med 46(10):1650–1658

Ioannidis JP, Lau J (2003) 18F-FDG PET for the diagnosis and grading of soft-tissue sarcoma: a meta-analysis. J Nucl Med 44:717–724

Ishikura Y, Yoshida R, Yoshizako T et al (2021) Osteoid osteoma of the rib with strong F-18 fluorodeoxyglucose uptake mimicking osteoblastoma: a case report with literature review. Acta Radiol Open 10(6):20584601211022497

Jessop S, Crudgington D, London K et al (2020) FDG PET-CT in pediatric Langerhans cell histiocytosis. Pediatr Blood Cancer 67(1):e28034

Jones T (1996) The imaging science of positron emission tomography. Eur J Nucl Med 23:807–813

Juweid MA, Cheson BD (2006) Positron-emission tomography and assessment of cancer therapy. N Engl J Med 354:496–507

Juweid ME, Wiseman GA, Vose JM et al (2005) Response assessment of aggressive non-Hodgkin's lymphoma by integrated International Workshop Criteria (IWC) and fluorine-18-fluorodeoxyglucose positron emission tomography. J Clin Oncol 23:4652–4661

Juweid ME, Stroobants S, Hoekstra OS et al (2007) Use of positron emission tomography for response assessment of lymphoma: consensus of the Imaging Subcommittee of International Harmonization Project in Lymphoma. J Clin Oncol 25(5):571–578

Ko SW, Park JG (2013) Cavernous hemangioma of the ilium mimicking aggressive malignant bone tumor with increased activity on (18)F-FDG PET/CT. Korean J Radiol 14(2):294–298

Kouijzer IJE, Scheper H, de Rooy JWJ et al (2018) The diagnostic value of 18F-FDG-PET/CT and MRI in suspected vertebral osteomyelitis - a prospective study. Eur J Nucl Med Mol Imaging 45(5):798–805

Kreshak J, Larousserie F, Picci P et al (2014) Difficulty distinguishing benign notochordal cell tumor from chordoma further suggests a link between them. Cancer Imaging 14(1):4

Kubota R, Yamada S, Kubota K et al (1992) Intratumoural distribution of fluorine-18-fluorodeoxyglucose in vivo: high accumulation in macrophages and granulation tissues studied by microautoradiography. J Nucl Med 33:1972–1980

Lee WW, So Y, Kang SY, So MK et al (2017) F-18 fluorodeoxyglucose positron emission tomography for differential diagnosis and prognosis prediction of vascular tumors. Oncol Lett 14(1):665–672

Leitch CE, Goenka AH, Howe BM et al (2017) Imaging features of Paget's disease on 11C choline PET/CT. Am J Nucl Med Mol Imaging 7(3):105–110

Lim CH, Park YH, Lee SY et al (2007) F-18 FDG uptake in the nidus of an osteoid osteoma. Clin Nucl Med 32(8):628–630

Lodge MA, Lucas JD, Marsden PK et al (1999) A PET study of 18FDG uptake in soft tissue masses. Eur J Nucl Med 26:22–30

Loi F, Córdova LA, Pajarinen J et al (2016) Inflammation, fracture and bone repair. Bone 86:119–130

Loktev A, Lindner T, Mier W et al (2018) A tumor-imaging method targeting cancer-associated fibroblasts. J Nucl Med 59(9):1423–1429

Lucas JD, O'Doherty MJ, Cronin BF et al (1999) Prospective evaluation of soft tissue masses and sarcomas using fluorodeoxyglucose positron emission tomography. Br J Surg 86:550–556

Macpherson RE, Pratap S, Tyrrell H et al (2018) Retrospective audit of 957 consecutive 18F-FDG PET-CT scans compared to CT and MRI in 493 patients with different histological subtypes of bone and soft tissue sarcoma. Clin Sarcoma Res 8:9

Mannheim JG, Schmid AM, Schwenck J, Katiyar P et al (2018) PET/MRI hybrid systems. Semin Nucl Med 48(4):332–347

Mayerhoefer ME, Breitenseher M, Amann G et al (2008) Are signal intensity and homogeneity useful parameters for distinguishing between benign and malignant soft tissue masses on MR images?: objective evaluation by means of texture analysis. Magn Reson Imaging 26:91316–91322

Mueller WP, Melzer HI, Schmid I et al (2013) The diagnostic value of 18F-FDG PET and MRI in paediatric histiocytosis. Eur J Nucl Med Mol Imaging 40(3):356–363

Muheremu A, Ma Y, Huang Z et al (2017) Diagnosing giant cell tumor of the bone using positron emission tomography/computed tomography: a retrospective study of 20 patients from a single center. Oncol Lett 14(2):1985–1988

Müller A, Dreyling M, Roeder F et al (2020) Primary bone lymphoma: clinical presentation and therapeutic considerations. J Bone Oncol 25:100326

Nishiguchi T, Mochizuki K, Tsujio T et al (2010) Lumbar vertebral chordoma arising from an intraosseous benign notochordal cell tumour: radiological findings and histopathological description with a good clinical outcome. Br J Radiol 83(987):e49–e53

Olson JT, Wenger DE, Rose PS et al (2021) Chordoma: 18F-FDG PET/CT and MRI imaging features. Skeletal Radiol 50(8):1657–1666

Palmerini E, Picci P, Reichardt P et al (2019) Malignancy in giant cell tumor of bone: a review of the literature. Technol Cancer Res Treat 18:1533033819840000

Parghane RV, Basu S (2017) Dual-time point 18F-FDG-PET and PET/CT for differentiating benign from malignant musculoskeletal lesions: opportunities and limitations. Semin Nucl Med 47(4):373–391

Park SA, Kim HS (2008) F-18 FDG PET/CT evaluation of sacrococcygeal chordoma. Clin Nucl Med 33(12):906–908

Partovi S, Kohan AA, Zipp L et al (2014) Hybrid PET/MR imaging in two sarcoma patients - clinical benefits and implications for future trials. Int J Clin Exp Med 7(3):640–648

Phillips M, Allen C, Gerson P et al (2009) Comparison of FDG-PET scans to conventional radiography and bone scans in management of Langerhans cell histiocytosis. Pediatr Blood Cancer 52(1):97–101

Pijl JP, Kwee TC, Legger GE et al (2020) Role of FDG-PET/CT in children with fever of unknown origin. Eur J Nucl Med Mol Imaging 47(6):1596–1604

Polverari G, Ceci F, Passera R et al (2020) [18F]FDG PET/CT for evaluating early response to neoadjuvant chemotherapy in pediatric patients with sarcoma: a prospective single-center trial. EJNMMI Res 10(1):122

Pozzessere C, Cicone F, Barberio P et al (2022) Cross-sectional evaluation of FGD-avid polyostotic fibrous dysplasia: MRI, CT and PET/MRI findings. Eur J Hybrid Imaging 6(1):19

Rakheja R, Makis W, Skamene S et al (2012) Correlating metabolic activity on 18F-FDG PET/CT with histopathologic characteristics of osseous and soft-tissue sarcomas: a retrospective review of 136 patients. AJR Am J Roentgenol 198(6):1409–1416

Ran P, Dong A, Wang Y et al (2018) Increased FDG uptake in a giant bone island mimicking malignancy. Clin Nucl Med 43(6):e209–e211

Reyes Marlés RH, Navarro Fernández JL, Puertas García-Sandoval JP et al (2021) Clinical value of baseline

18F-FDG PET/CT in soft tissue sarcomas. Eur J Hybrid Imaging 5(1):16

Sang P, Park U, Raynor WY et al (2021) 18F-sodium fluoride PET as a diagnostic modality for metabolic, autoimmune, and osteogenic bone disorders: cellular mechanisms and clinical applications. Int J Mol Sci 22(12):6504

Schulte M, Brecht-Krauss D, Heymer B et al (2000) Grading of tumors and tumorlike lesions of bone: evaluation by FDG PET. J Nucl Med 41(10):1695–1701

Sepehrizadeh T, Jong I, DeVeer M et al (2021) PET/MRI in paediatric disease. Eur J Radiol 144:109987

Solav SV, Savale SV, Patil AM (2019) False-positive FDG PET CT scan in vertebral hemangioma. Asia Ocean J Nucl Med Biol 7(1):95–98

Song L, Han S, Jiang L et al (2020) F18-fluorodeoxyglucose positron emission tomography/computed tomography in the evaluation of vertebral vascular tumors. Clin Imaging 65:24–32

Ulano A, Bredella MA, Burke P et al (2016) Distinguishing untreated osteoblastic metastases from enostoses using CT attenuation measurements. AJR Am J Roentgenol 207(2):362–368

Upadhyay A, Rastogi S, Arunraj ST et al (2020) An unusual case of synovial sarcoma with breast metastasis: findings on positron emission tomography-computed tomography. Indian J Nucl Med 35(4):345–347

van Langevelde K, McCarthy CL (2020) Radiological findings of denosumab treatment for giant cell tumours of bone. Skeletal Radiol 49(9):1345–1358

Vanel D, Shapeero LG, Tardivon A et al (1998) Dynamic contrast-enhanced MRI with subtraction of aggressive soft tissue tumors after resection. Skeletal Radiol 27:505–510

Warburg O, Posener K, Negelein E (1931) The metabolism of the carcinoma cell. In: Warburg O (ed) The metabolism of tumors. Richard R. Smith, Inc, New York, pp 29–169

Yamada S, Kubota K, Kubota R et al (1995) High accumulation of fluorine-18-fluorodeoxyglucose in turpentine-induced inflammatory tissue. J Nucl Med 36:1301–1306

Zhang L, Zhang X, He Q et al (2018) The role of initial 18F-FDG PET/CT in the management of patients with suspected extramedullary plasmocytoma. Cancer Imaging 18(1):19

Local and Distant Staging

Emna Labbène and Mohamed Fethi Ladeb

Contents

E. Labbène (✉) · M. F. Ladeb
Department of Radiology, M T Kassab Institute of Orthopedics, Ksar Said, Tunisia

Faculty of Medicine of Tunis, Tunis-El Manar University, Tunis, Tunisia

Abstract

Primary spinal tumors are relatively rare, representing 11% of primary musculoskeletal tumors and about 4% of all spinal tumors. Their management depends on their local and distant spread. Whenever it is feasible, *en bloc* resection with clear margins is the preferred surgical approach for malignant and aggressive benign tumors in order to achieve local control of the disease. An accurate preoperative evaluation is therefore mandatory for adequate surgical planning.

Because spinal tumors are very rare, the main oncologic staging systems applied to them are those originally developed for appendicular location. However, the spine presents some particularities that distinguish it from extremities, namely the proximity to the spinal cord and the concern for spinal stability. These differences limit the application of the same surgical concepts that are applied in appendicular tumors. A surgical staging system dedicated to the spine and considering these particularities is therefore necessary. Imaging plays a key role in assessing the staging of tumors. Therefore, the knowledge of the main staging systems and the contribution of the different imaging modalities is necessary for the radiologist to provide an accurate staging report.

Med Radiol Diagn Imaging (2023)
https://doi.org/10.1007/174_2023_440,
Published Online: 06 July 2023

1 Introduction

Primary spinal tumors are relatively rare, representing 11% of primary musculoskeletal tumors and about 4% of all spinal tumors (Dahlin and Unni 1986; Boriani et al. 1997). Their management depends on their local and distant spread. Similar to appendicular tumors, malignant and aggressive benign spinal tumors are best managed with *en bloc* resection with clear margins whenever the procedure is feasible (Musculoskeletal Tumor Society 1985; Boriani et al. 1997; Enneking et al. 2003). Imaging plays a central role in tumor staging and preoperative surgical planning. Different modalities provide complementary information and contribute to achieving an accurate staging report.

Because spinal tumors are very rare, the main oncologic staging systems applied to them are those originally developed for appendicular location (Murphey and Kransdorf 2021). However, the spine presents two major particularities that distinguish it from other locations, namely the proximity to the spinal cord and the concern for spinal stability. These differences limit the application of the same surgical concepts that are applied to extremities. A surgical staging system dedicated to the spine and taking into account these particularities is therefore necessary. Because imaging plays a key role in assessing local and distant spread of tumors and in planning the adequate surgical approach, the knowledge of the main staging systems and the contribution of different imaging modalities is necessary for the radiologist to provide an accurate report when assessing tumor extension.

2 The Main Staging Systems Applied to Spinal Tumors

A major goal for staging tumors is to determine the suitable treatment that allows local control and minimizes the risk of recurrence. Imaging plays a central role in staging tumors. Therefore, knowing and understanding the used staging systems allow the radiologist to provide an accurate assessment of tumor spread.

2.1 Enneking/MSTS Staging System

In 1980, Dr. William Enneking published a surgical staging system for musculoskeletal tumors in which he defined the biological behavior of primary bone and soft tissue tumors based on clinical, radiological, and histological features (Enneking et al. 1980).

The system incorporates three main prognostic factors: tumor grade (based on clinical, radiological, and histological correlation), local extension, and presence or absence of regional or distant metastases. It was later adopted by the musculoskeletal tumor society (MSTS) and remains until this day one of the main oncologic staging systems (Musculoskeletal Tumor Society 1985; Murphey and Kransdorf 2021) (Table 1).

Enneking also defined the different oncologic surgical margins (Table 2) and provided a guideline for the suitable surgical treatment to choose and the adequate oncologic margins to achieve

Table 1 Enneking/MSTS staging system. Adapted from the Musculoskeletal Tumor Society (1985)

Stage	Tumor grade	Local extension	Regional or distant metastases
Benign tumors			
Stage 1: inactive/latent	G0	T0	M0
Stage 2: active	G0	T0	M0
Stage 3: aggressive	G0	T1 or T2	M0 or M1
Malignant tumors			
Stage IA	G1	T1	M0
Stage IB	G1	T2	M0
Stage IIA	G2	T1	M0
Stage IIB	G2	T2	M0
Stage IIIA	G1 or G2	T1	M1
Stage IIIB	G1 or G2	T2	M1

G0: benign; G1: low-grade malignant; G2: high-grade malignant, T0: intracapsular and intracompartmental; T1: extracapsular and intracompartmental; T2: extracapsular and extracompartmental; M0: absence of metastases; M1: presence of metastases

Table 2 Types of oncologic surgical margins. Adapted from the Musculoskeletal Tumor Society (1985)

Type of surgical margins	Plane of dissection	Histological findings
Intracapsular	Within tumor	Tumor at margin
Marginal	Within the reactive zone around the tumor	Reactive tissue with or without microsatellite tumor
Wide	In normal tissue around the reactive zone but within the anatomical compartment involved by the tumor	Normal tissue with or without skip tumor
Radical	In normal tissue outside the anatomical compartment involved by the tumor (resection of the whole anatomical compartment)	Normal tissue

Table 3 Recommended surgical margins according to the Enneking tumor stage. Adapted from the Musculoskeletal Tumor Society (1985)

Enneking stage	Recommended surgical margins for local control
Benign tumors	
Stage 1 (latent)	Intracapsular
Stage 2 (active)	Marginal (or intracapsular + adjuvant treatment)
Stage 3 (aggressive)	Wide (or marginal + adjuvant treatment)
Malignant tumors	
Stage I	Wide
Stage II	Radical
Stage III	Radical or palliative

for each tumor stage to obtain a definitive local control and avoid the risk of recurrence (Enneking et al. 1980, 2003; Musculoskeletal Tumor Society 1985) (Table 3).

This system applies only to connective tissue tumors and excludes primary lesions of round cell origin (Ewing's sarcoma, myeloma, lymphoma, and leukemias) and metastatic lesions because they have a different natural history, therapeutic management, and prognosis (Enneking et al. 1980, 2003; Musculoskeletal Tumor Society 1985). The radiological features used in this system are mainly based on the Lodwick classification (Fig. 1) and assessed with radiographs and CT.

The Enneking/MSTS staging system distinguishes three grades of tumors based on their biological behavior: benign tumors (G0), low-grade malignant tumors (G1), and high-grade malignant tumors (G2) (Table 1).

For malignant tumors, this classification distinguishes low- (G1) and high-grade (G2) tumors based mainly on histology. These two categories are further divided according to their local extension (intracompartmental (A)/extracompartmental (B)) and distant spread (presence (M1) or absence (M0) of metastasis) based mainly on imaging.

Local extension is based on the concept of anatomical compartment (an anatomical space limited by a biological barrier such as cortical bone, articular capsule, or major fascial septa). For spinal location, a tumor is considered intracompartmental when it is confined to the vertebra and extracompartmental when it extends to soft tissues or into the spinal canal (Boriani et al. 1997).

According to Enneking, low-grade bone sarcoma presents as a Lodwick type 2 lesion and high-grade tumors as a Lodwick type 3 lesion. Nevertheless, data from literature show that low-grade tumors can present as a Lodwick type 1B or 1C lesions (sometimes 1A) and mimic benign tumors, while high-grade tumors can have the pattern of a Lodwick type 1C, 2, or 3 lesion (Sans and Perroncel 2014).

Benign tumors (G0) are divided into three categories based on their activity: inactive benign lesions (stage 1), active benign lesions (stage 2), and aggressive benign lesions (stage 3). The distinction is mainly based on the radiological margins of the tumor. In stage 1, the tumor appears as a Lodwick type 1A lesion and remains confined to the anatomical compartment of origin. In stage 2, the tumor appears generally as a Lodwick type 1B (sometimes 1A) lesion, deforms the compart-

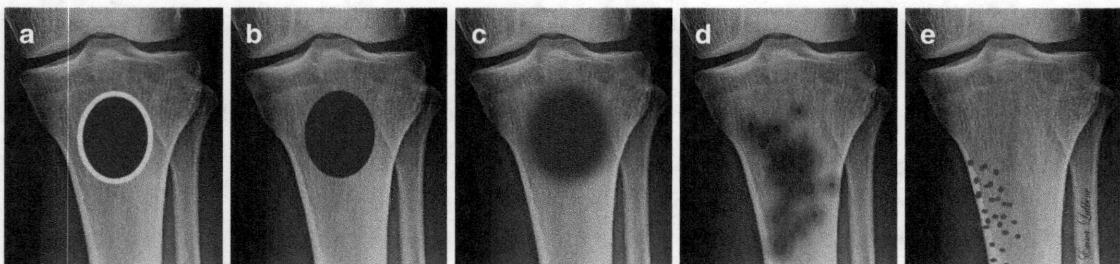

Fig. 1 Lodwick classification. (**a**) Type 1A: geographic lesion with well-defined margin surrounded by a sclerotic rim. (**b**) Type 1B: geographic lesion with well-defined and no sclerotic rim. (**c**) Type 1C: geographic lesion with ill-defined margin. (**d**) Type 2: Moth-eaten pattern. (**e**) Type 3: Permeative pattern

ment boundaries, and appears as an "expansile" lesion but remains intracompartmental. In stage 3, the tumor usually appears as a Lodwick type 1C with possible cortical breach and extension to soft tissues, and thus it can be either intracompartmental or extracompartmental. According to Enneking, the appropriate type of surgical margins that result in a definitive local control depends on the activity of benign tumors (Enneking et al. 2003) (Table 3). Different studies confirmed the effectiveness of Enneking guidelines both for appendicular and spinal tumors by showing a higher level of local recurrence when the type of surgical margins did not match the Enneking recommendations (Harrop et al. 2009; Boriani et al. 2012).

For distant staging (M0/M1), the Enneking/MSTS system includes regional lymph node metastases and distant metastases in one category. This is based on the fact that unlike most carcinoma, bone sarcoma with regional lymph node metastases has the same prognosis as those with distant spread (Musculoskeletal Tumor Society 1985).

The Enneking/MSTS staging system was originally developed for the management of appendicular musculoskeletal tumors but was later applied to spinal locations. Nevertheless, this system does not consider the particularities of the vertebral column that can limit the feasibility of the recommended surgical margins such as the proximity of the spinal cord or the impossibility to remove completely the epidural space (considered as an anatomical compartment) to obtain radical margins. Therefore, some authors proposed some modifications of Enneking recommendations to adapt to the spine (Chan et al. 2009) (Table 4).

Table 4 Modified recommendations for surgical margins according to the Enneking tumor stage. Adapted from Chan et al. (2009)

Enneking stage	Recommended surgical margins for local control
Benign tumors	
Stage 1 (latent)	No surgery unless spinal instability or neurological structure compression
Stage 2 (active)	Intralesional excision ± adjuvant treatment
Stage 3 (aggressive)	Marginal *en bloc* resection
Malignant tumors	
Stage I	Wide *en bloc* resection
Stage II	Wide *en bloc* resection + adjuvant treatment
Stage III	Palliative

2.2 AJCC Staging System (TNM Classification)

The AJCC (American Joint Committee on Cancer) staging system for bone sarcoma is an oncologic staging based on the TNM classification and histologic grading of tumors. This system is constantly evolving with the last update (eighth edition) published in 2017 (Amin et al. 2017).

This system includes different malignant tumors arising from bone but excludes primary marrow lesions (multiple myeloma and lymphoma). Until the seventh edition, a common TNM classification was used for all sites of bone sarcoma. A notable change in the eighth edition was the distinction of a separate T category both for the spine and for the pelvis (Tables 5 and 6). This was because surgical approaches and the possibility to achieve resection with free margins are different than those in extremities. However, the N (nodes), M (metastases), and G (histologic grade) categories remain the same for all sites (Table 7), and there are no prognostic stage grouping for spine and pelvis yet.

In this eighth edition of TNM classification, the sacrum is included in pelvic staging and not in spine staging.

For spinal tumors (excluding sacrum), the vertebra is divided into five segments (Fig. 2): two segments (right and left) for the vertebral body, a segment for each pedicle and ipsilateral transverse process, and finally a segment for the posterior elements. The T category is then defined by the number of segments involved by the tumor or by spinal canal and/or great vessel involvement (Table 5 and Fig. 3). The size of tumor is not considered in the T category for spinal tumors.

Sacral tumors are classified with pelvic tumors. The pelvis is divided into four segments (Fig. 4): 1) sacrum, 2) iliac wing, 3) acetabulum and periacetabulum and finally 4) pubic rami, symphysis and ischium. The T category is defined by the number of involved segments, size of tumor, and extra-osseous extension (Table 6).

Table 5 AJCC TNM definition of T category for spinal tumors (eighth edition). Adapted from Amin et al. (2017)

T category	Description
TX	Primary tumor cannot be assessed
T0	No evidence of primary tumor
T1	Primary tumor confined to one or two adjacent vertebral segments
T2	Primary tumor confined to three adjacent vertebral segments
T3	Primary tumor involving four or more adjacent vertebral segments or involving nonadjacent vertebral segments
T4	Extension into spinal canal or great vessels
T4a	Extension into the spinal canal
T4b	Gross vascular invasion or tumor thrombus in great vessels

Table 6 AJCC TNM definition of T category for pelvic tumors (eighth edition). Adapted from Amin et al. (2017)

T category	Description
TX	Primary tumor cannot be assessed
T0	No evidence of primary tumor
T1	Primary tumor confined to one segment without extraosseous extension
T1a	Greatest dimension ≤8 cm
T1b	Greatest dimension >8 cm
T2	Primary tumor confined to one segment with extra-osseous extension or two segments without extra-osseous extension
T2a	Greatest dimension ≤8 cm
T2b	Greatest dimension >8 cm
T3	Primary tumor involving two segments with extra-osseous extension
T3a	Greatest dimension ≤8 cm
T3b	Greatest dimension >8 cm
T4	Primary tumor involving three segments or crossing the sacroiliac joint
T4a	Sacroiliac joint involvement and extension medial to sacral neuroforamen
T4b	Encasement of external iliac vessels or presence of gross tumor thrombus in great pelvic vessels

Table 7 AJCC TNM definitions of N (lymph node), M (distant metastasis), and G (histologic grade) categories for bone tumors (eighth edition). Adapted from Amin et al. (2017)

Category	Description
N category	
Nx	Regional lymph node cannot be assessed
N0	Absence of regional lymph node metastasis
N1	Presence of regional lymph node metastasis
M category	
M0	Absence of distant metastasis
M1a	Pulmonary metastasis
M1b	Other distant extrapulmonary metastasis
G category	
Gx	Grade cannot be assessed
G1	Well differentiated, low grade
G2	Moderately differentiated, high grade
G3	Poorly differentiated, high grade

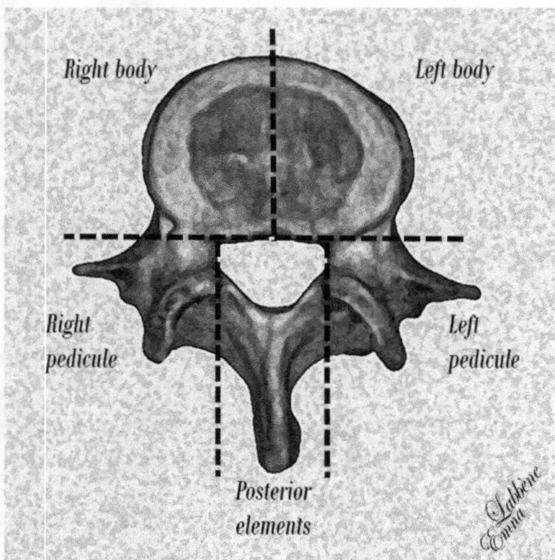

Fig. 2 Vertebral division in the eighth edition of the AJCC cancer staging. The vertebra is divided into five segments: the right and left parts of the vertebral body, the right and left pedicles and transverse processes, and the posterior elements

For distant metastatic sites, the AJCC classification separates lung metastasis from other sites (extrapulmonary location) because of its better prognosis (Zhang et al. 2021). However, it does not take into account the solitary or multiple character of lung metastases although the latter has a poorer prognosis (Amin et al. 2017; Guedes et al. 2021).

2.3 The Weinstein-Boriani-Biagini Staging System (WBB Staging System)

Similar to the appendicular location, spinal malignant tumors and Enneking stage 3 benign tumors are best managed with *en bloc* resection with negative margins (Chan et al. 2009). *En bloc* resection means that the tumor is retrieved in one piece. Giving the proximity of the spinal cord, this type of resection is more difficult to achieve compared to the extremities.

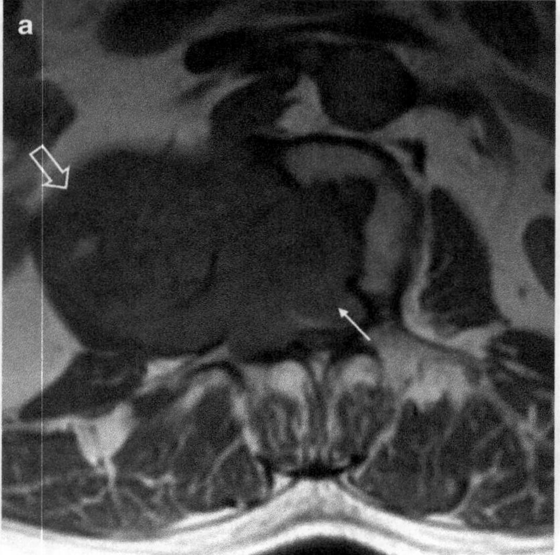

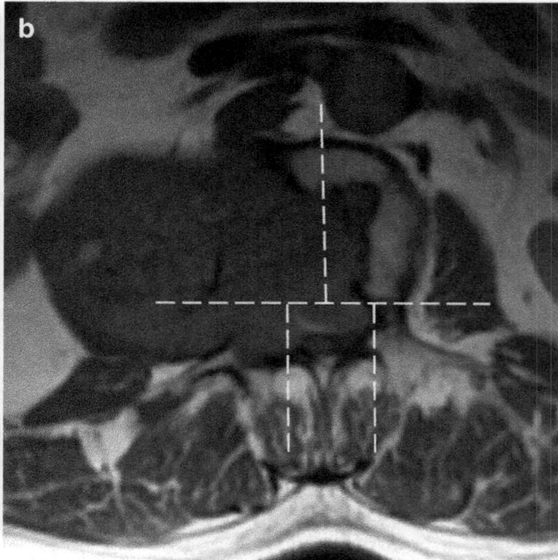

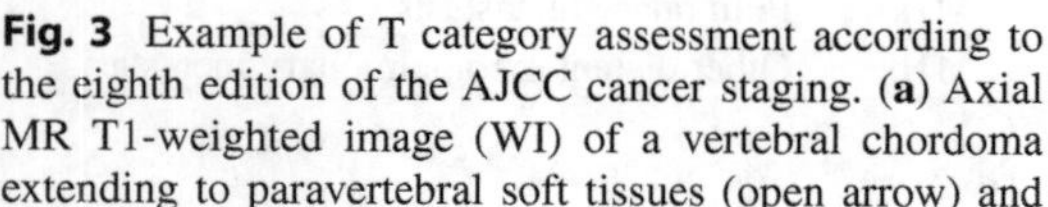

Fig. 3 Example of T category assessment according to the eighth edition of the AJCC cancer staging. (**a**) Axial MR T1-weighted image (WI) of a vertebral chordoma extending to paravertebral soft tissues (open arrow) and into the spinal canal (arrow). (**b**) According to the AJCC staging system, the tumor involves three adjacent segments (right and left vertebral body, right pedicle) with extension into the spinal canal. It is considered T4a

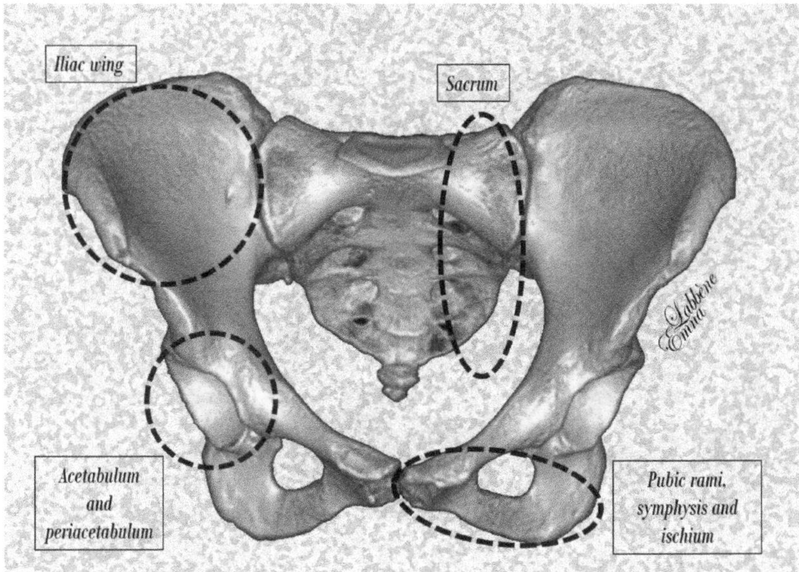

Fig. 4 Pelvic segments according to the eighth edition of the AJCC cancer staging. The pelvis is divided into four segments: 1) iliac wing, 2) sacrum, 3) acetabular and periacetabular region, 4) pubic rami, symphysis, and ischium

In 1997, Weinstein, Boriani, and Biagini published a surgical staging system that allows to evaluate the feasibility of *en bloc* resection of spinal tumors and the surgical approach to adopt when it is feasible (Boriani et al. 1997; Chan et al. 2009).

This system is based on a concept that allows the surgeon to achieve a suitable oncological resection of tumors while sparing the spinal cord.

The WBB staging system is based on imaging and consists of a combination of two division systems on the transversal plane (Fig. 5). The first division consists of dividing the vertebra into 12 radial zones with the intersection of all zones located in the center of the spinal canal. The zones are noted from 1 to 12 with the left half of the vertebra corresponding to the 1–6 zones and the right half corresponding to the 7–12 zones. The right and left pedicles are located, respectively, in zones 9 and 4. The second division consists of distinguishing five concentric layers (layers A–D) extending form paravertebral soft tissues to the intradural space. A sixth layer (layer F) is individualized in the cervical spine and corresponds to the transverse foramen with the vertebral artery (Gasbarrini et al. 2009). The limit between layers B (superficial intra-osseous) and C (deep intra-osseous) is not clearly defined in this system.

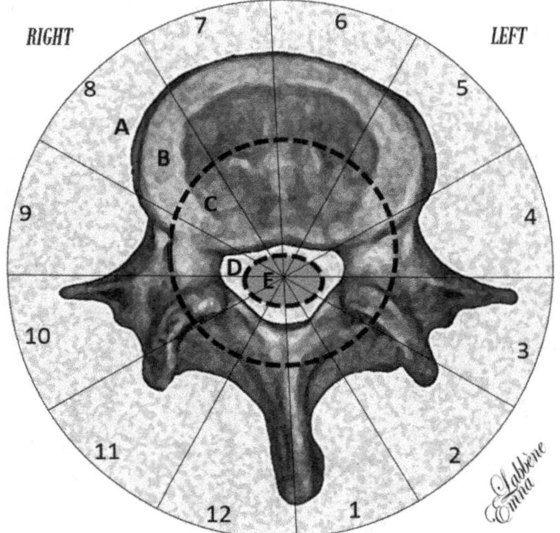

Fig. 5 The vertebral division according to the WBB staging system. The vertebra is divided into 12 radiating zones from the left side of the spinous process (zone 1) to the right side of the spinous process (zone 12) with the left and right pedicles included, respectively, in zones 4 and 9. A second division consisting of five concentric layers distinguishes extra-osseous paravertebral soft tissues (layer A), superficial intra-osseous layer (layer B), deep intra-osseous layer (layer C), extra-osseous extradural space (layer D), and extra-osseous intradural space (layer E)

The location of the tumor is thus specified in terms of zones and layers (Figs. 6 and 7).

The zones involved by the tumor are indicated in one direction from 1 to 12: for example, a

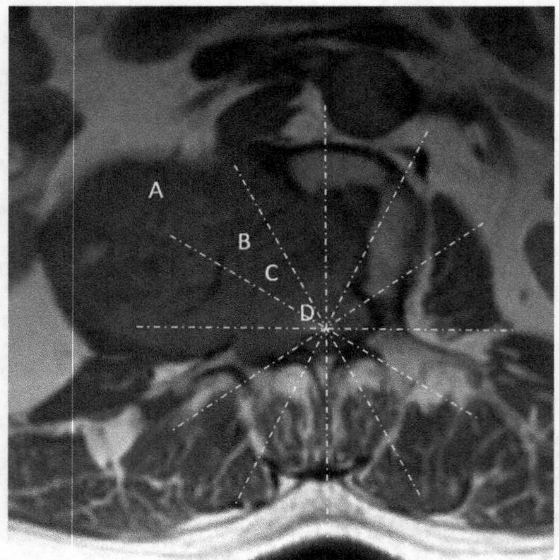

Fig. 6 Example of a spinal tumor staging according to the WBB system (same patient as in Fig. 3). A chordoma involving the vertebra from zone 5 to zone 10. The tumor involves the superficial (layer B) and the deep (layer C) parts of the vertebra and extends to the paravertebral soft tissues (layer A) and into the spinal canal to the epidural space (layer D). WBB classification: zones 5–10, layers A–D

tumor that occupies the zones 3–10 means that the tumor involves the zones 3, 4, 5, 6, 7, 8, 9, and 10 while a tumor that occupies the zones 10–3 means that it involves the zones 10, 11, 12, 1, 2, and 3 (Boriani et al. 1997, 2000).

According to the location of the tumor based on this system, the adequate type of *en bloc* resection (vertebrectomy, sagittal resection, or posterior arch resection) is determined (Table 8).

The WBB staging system is a surgical staging that can be applied to all types of spinal tumors and not only sarcoma.

Table 8 Recommended surgical approach according to the location of the spinal tumor based on the WBB staging system. Adapted from Boriani et al. (1997)

WBB staging (zones involved by the tumor)	Recommended surgical approach (*en bloc* resection)
4–8 or 5–9	Vertebrectomy
2–5 or 7–11	Sagittal resection
10–3	Resection of the posterior arch

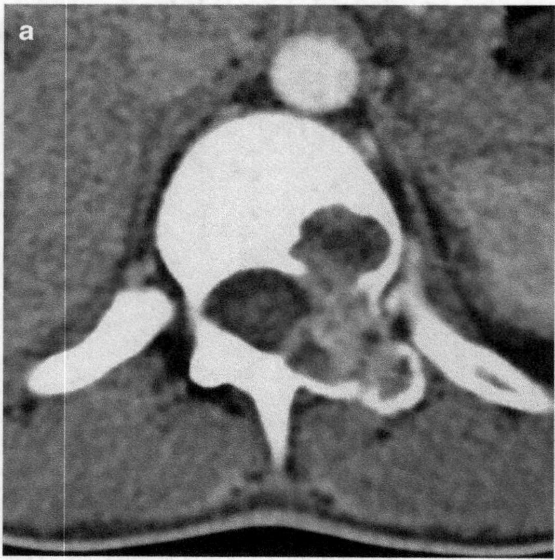

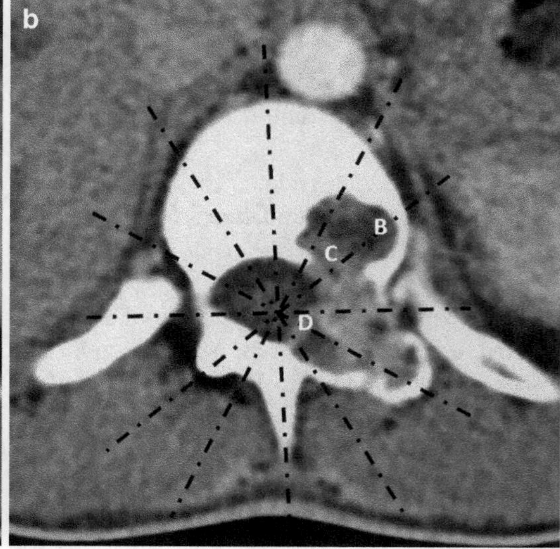

Fig. 7 Example of a spinal tumor staging according to the WBB system. Vertebral aneurysmal bone cyst extending from zone 1 to zone 6 and involving the superficial (layer B) and the deep (layer C) parts of the vertebra and the epidural space (layer D). WBB classification: zones 1–6, layers B–D

3 Imaging of Spinal Tumor Local Extension and Distant Spread

3.1 Spinal Tumor Local Extension

Imaging is the keystone in assessing the local extension of spinal tumors. A detailed description of tumor spread and relationship with adjacent structures is mandatory for the surgeon to choose the appropriate, free of tumor, resection plan whenever it is feasible.

3.1.1 Conventional Radiography, Computed Tomography, and Angiography

Conventional radiography (CR) is usually the first-line modality used to assess bone pain and other clinical symptoms. It allows assessing tumor aggressiveness based on the Lodwick classification, the pattern of periosteal reaction, and the extent to soft tissues. However, this is generally true for appendicular tumors. Spinal tumors are more difficult to analyze due to the anatomical complexity of the vertebral column and further evaluation with CT and/or MRI is often necessary.

Although MRI is superior to CT to evaluate intra-osseous extension of tumors (O'Flanagan et al. 1991), the assessment of bony margins, Lodwick type, and pattern of periosteal reaction is based on CR, with CT being the modality of choice for spine. These features allow the classification of benign tumors according to their biological activity based on the Enneking system, which provides a guideline for the management of these tumors (no treatment for latent tumors, curettage for active tumors, and resection for aggressive tumors) (Boriani et al. 1995, 2012; Enneking et al. 2003; Chan et al. 2009) (Table 4).

CT can also assess extracompartmental extension of the tumor into the spinal canal and paravertebral soft tissues although MRI provides a better evaluation.

Within cervical spine, scarifying the vertebral artery with *en bloc* resection may require preoperative CT angiography to assess vascular anatomical variations and risks of neurological ischemia (Westbroek et al. 2020; Smith et al. 2022).

Spinal angiography remains the gold standard for studying the vascularization of the lesion and is realized whenever embolization is considered for hypervascular tumors (Gailloud 2019; Facchini et al. 2021).

3.1.2 MRI

Based on data from appendicular bone and soft tissue sarcoma, MRI is the modality of choice for defining tumor local extension (Pennington et al. 2019). It should be performed before the biopsy because signal abnormalities along the biopsy tract can compromise the accuracy of MRI interpretation (Amin et al. 2017). Although not specified in the guidelines, assessing the whole spine with MRI is recommended.

Assessing local extension consists of evaluating intra-osseous and extra-osseous spread of the tumor. Extra-osseous spread includes paravertebral soft tissue extension (including the major vascular structures) and extension in the spinal canal (including spinal cord and nerve roots).

Non-contrast T1-weighted images (WI) are most accurate to assess intra-osseous tumor margins and guide the plan of surgical resection as it provides an excellent contrast between the low to intermediate signal of the tumor and the high signal of the surrounding fatty bone marrow (Pennington et al. 2019). Nevertheless, the presence of abundant red marrow in the spine of young patients can limit the accuracy of this sequence. The use of chemical shift imaging and contrast-enhanced sequences can be useful in these cases (Shiga et al. 2013; Del Grande et al. 2014; van Vucht et al. 2019). Along with intra-osseous extension in the transversal plane, the longitudinal spread of the tumor to adjacent disks and vertebrae is also important to report (Smith et al. 2022) (Fig. 8).

When the tumor has an extracompartmental extension into paravertebral soft tissues, assessing the relationship of the tumor with the major vascular structures (aorta, inferior vena cava, and iliac vessels) is essential because it influences the feasibility of tumor resection with free margins. The neurovascular structures are normally sur-

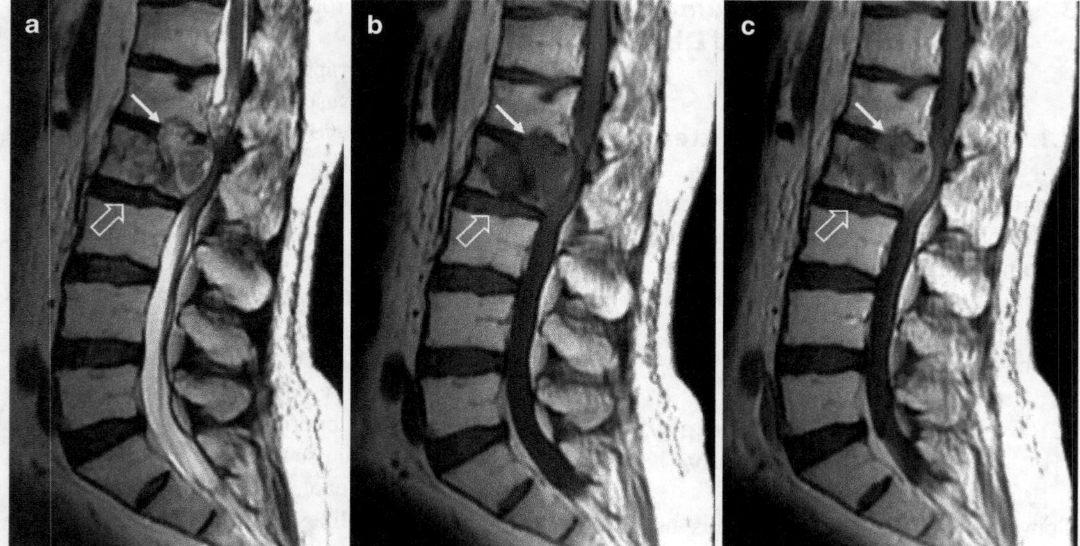

Fig. 8 Chordoma of L2 vertebra. Sagittal MR T2-WI (**a**), T1-WI (**b**), and enhanced T1-WI (**c**) images show extension of the tumor to the superior adjacent disk and the end plate of L1 (arrow). The inferior adjacent disk has a normal signal and seems to be free of tumor (open arrow). *En bloc* resection with a plane of resection through the superior disk (discectomy) would result in contaminated margins (intracapsular margins)

rounded by fat tissue. Preservation of a fat plane between the tumor and vascular structures is a reliable sign indicating absence of vascular involvement, while a circumferential encasement or tumor thrombus is a sign of vascular involvement. However, between these two situations (contact with loss of fat plane, partial encasement), there are no clearly defined criteria (van Trommel et al. 1997; Holzapfel et al. 2015; Saifuddin et al. 2019) (Fig. 9). Some authors consider encasement of 180° or more of the circumference of neurovascular structures a good sign indicating involvement (Holzapfel et al. 2015). Neurovascular bundle involvement should be described both in the transverse and in the longitudinal planes (Fig. 9).

When there is extension into the spinal canal, evaluation of spinal cord compression and signal abnormalities is better achieved with T2-weighted images.

For sacral tumors, extension through the sacroiliac joint is among the important elements to mention. While the cartilage in the synovial portion constitutes a barrier to the tumor extension, the crossing of the joint occurs preferentially through the ligamentous portion. Therefore, it is important to pay attention to this part of the sacroiliac joint when assessing tumors located adjacent to this articulation (Fig. 10).

The size of the tumor should also be reported although it is not taken into account in the different staging systems used for spinal tumors.

Dynamic contrast-enhanced MRI can be used to evaluate tumor vascularity, to target the most appropriate site for biopsy, and to guide the decision for preoperative embolization (Meng et al. 2016).

3.2 Spinal Tumor Distant Spread

Similar to appendicular musculoskeletal tumors, the main distant metastatic sites of primary malignant bone tumors are lung and bone. Imaging evaluation of distant staging is mainly based on assessing these sites (Amin et al. 2017; Billingsley et al. 1999; Nakamura et al. 2011; Zhang et al. 2021; Stanborough et al. 2022).

Pulmonary metastases have a better prognosis than extrapulmonary metastases (Ward et al.

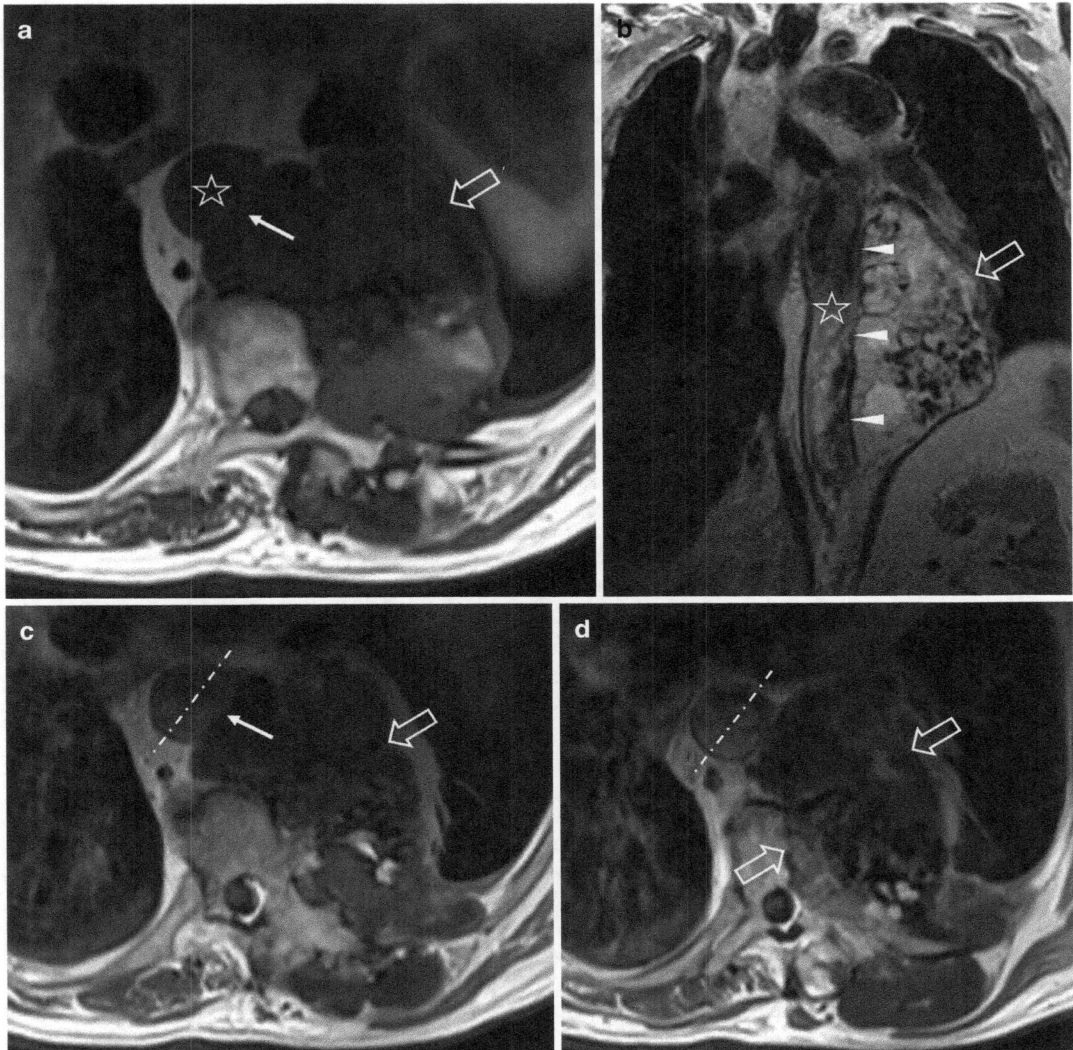

Fig. 9 Vertebral chondrosarcoma extending to the paravertebral soft tissues and coming close to the aorta. Axial MR T1-WI (**a**), coronal T2-WI (**b**), and axial enhanced T1-WI (**c** and **d**) show a vertebral chondrosarcoma (open arrow) extending to paravertebral soft tissues. The tumor extends adjacent to the descending thoracic aorta (star) with loss of fat plane (white arrow) and encasement <180° of the circumference of the artery (broken line). The extent of the encasement on the longitudinal plane is well assessed on the coronal image (**b**) (arrowheads)

1994; Cotterill et al. 2000). Regional lymph node metastases are extremely rare (Amin et al. 2017).

Some aggressive benign tumors such as giant cell tumor can rarely metastasize to the lung.

3.2.1 Pulmonary Metastases

With the improvement of imaging modalities, chest CT has replaced chest plain radiograph for the detection of lung metastases, offering higher sensibility and specificity (Stanborough et al. 2022).

Nonenhanced chest CT is the modality of choice (Fig. 11). There is no relevant literature regarding the superiority of contrast-enhanced CT scans in detecting pulmonary nodules (Stanborough et al. 2022). PET/CT is also less sensitive than chest CT partly because of the inferior resolution of PET/CT technique that does not

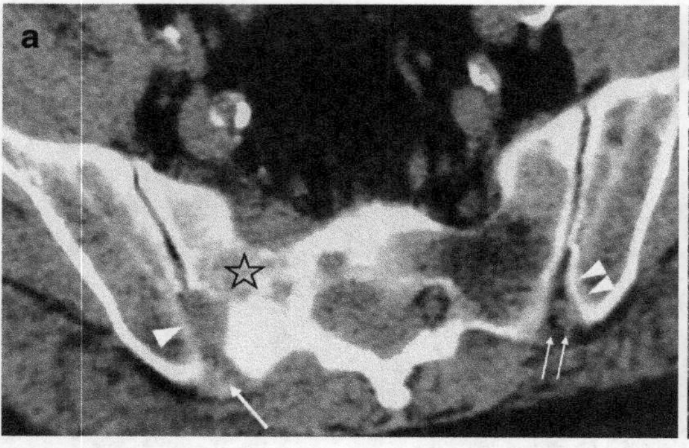

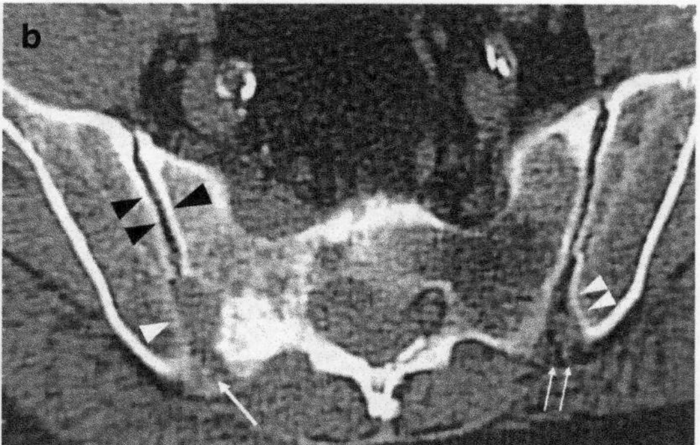

Fig. 10 Sacral location of lymphoma with extension to the right iliac bone throughout the ligamentous portion of the sacroiliac joint. Axial CT images with soft tissue (**a**) and bone (**b**) windows showing a sacral lesion (star) extending to ligamentous portion of the right sacroiliac joint shown by the soft tissue density of this area (white arrow). Note the normal aspect of the ligamentous portion of the left sacroiliac joint with areas of fat density (double white arrows). Cortical lysis (white arrowhead) reveals extension to the iliac bone. Note the normal cortical aspect of the contralateral iliac bone (double white arrowheads). The synovial portion of the right sacroiliac joint is not involved by the tumor (black arrowheads)

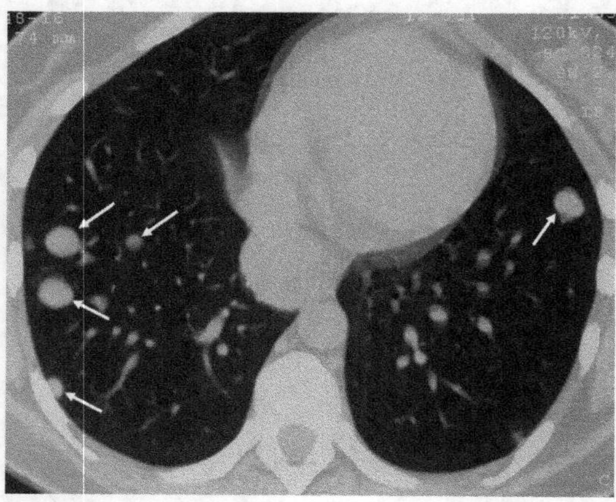

Fig. 11 Axial CT image showing pulmonary metastases (arrows) from a vertebral giant cell tumor

allow the detection and characterization of small nodules (<5–6 mm) (London et al. 2012; Chiesa et al. 2021). Although some studies showed that PET/CT had a higher specificity (London et al. 2012; Cistaro et al. 2012), it has little benefit over chest CT (Stanborough et al. 2022).

3.2.2 Extrapulmonary Metastases

Detection of bone metastases was, for a long time, based on bone scan. However, with the development of imaging techniques, other modalities have emerged. PET/CT proved to be superior to bone scan in detecting bone metastases both in general oncology and bone sarcoma (Chang et al. 2016; Hurley et al. 2016). It has also the advantage to detect nonskeletal metastases such as lymph nodes (Völker et al. 2007). Whole-body MRI is another option to assess extrapulmonary locations. Similar to PET/CT, it is superior to bone scan in detecting skeletal metastases (Kalus and Saifuddin 2019; Sun et al. 2020). Whole-body MRI is also superior to PET/CT in characterizing bone lesions and distinguishing metastases from other benign bone marrow abnormalities (Stanborough et al. 2022). Nevertheless, there is no consensus on which modality should be preferred (Sun et al. 2020).

4 Assessing Spinal Instability

Although assessing spinal instability is not part of oncological tumor staging, it is important to consider it in surgical treatment. There is no clear criterion-based definition of spinal instability in neoplastic disease, and many radiological and non-radiological features have been described in literature such as those in the SINS score (Tomita et al. 2001; Fisher et al. 2010) (Table 9). Imaging plays a key role in evaluating spinal stability. While some radiological features such as vertebral collapse can be assessed by MRI, other signs such as the bone tumor pattern (sclerotic, lytic, or

Table 9 Spine Instability Neoplastic Score (SINS). Adapted from Fisher et al. (2010)

SINS features	Score
Location	
Junctional (occiput-C2, C7–T2, T11–L1, L5–S1)	3
Mobile spine (C3–C6, L2–L4)	2
Dorsal spine from T3 to T10	1
Sacrum from S2 to S5	0
Clinical features: Pain relief with rest and/or pain triggered by movement/standing position	
Yes	3
No (occasional pain but not mechanical)	1
No pain at all	0
Imaging features	
Bone lesion appearance	
Lytic	2
Mixed	1
Sclerotic	0
Vertebral body collapse	
>50% vertebral collapse	3
<50% vertebral collapse	2
Involvement of more than 50% of vertebral body but without collapse	1
None of the above	0
Posterior elements' involvement (fracture or tumor extension to the facet, pedicle, or costovertebral joint)	
Bilateral	3
Unilateral	1
No involvement	0
Spinal alignment	
Presence of subluxation/translation	4
De novo deformity (kyphosis/scoliosis)	2
Normal alignment	0

Scores of 0–6 = stability; 7–12 = undetermined instability; 13–18 = instability

mixed), the extent of vertebral bony destruction, and the presence of posterior element fracture are better delineated by CT. Dynamic radiographs can also be useful to assess spine alignment (Fisher et al. 2010; Caracciolo and Letson 2016).

5 Conclusion

Spinal primary tumors are rare, and the main staging systems and recommended imaging techniques applied to the spine are based on data from appendicular neoplasms. Nevertheless, some particularities distinguish the spine from other locations and need to be considered for an appropriate management. Imaging plays a pivotal role in staging these tumors and planning the adequate treatment.

6 Key Points

- The Enneking/MSTS, the AJCC, and the WBB staging systems are the main used systems for spinal primary tumors.
- The role of conventional radiography in staging bone tumors is less important on the level of the spine compared to extremities due to the complex anatomy of the vertebral column.
- MRI is the modality of choice for local staging of spinal bone tumors.
- CT is the modality of choice for assessing lung metastases.
- PET/CT, whole-body MRI, or bone scan can be used to assess extrapulmonary metastases.

References

Amin MB, Greene FL, Edge SB et al (2017) AJCC Cancer Staging Manual, 8th edn. Springer

Billingsley KG, Lewis JJ, Leung DH et al (1999) Multifactorial analysis of the survival of patients with distant metastasis arising from primary extremity sarcoma. Cancer 85:389–395

Boriani S, Biagini R, De Iure F et al (1995) Primary bone tumors of the spine: a survey of the evaluation and treatment at the Istituto Ortopedico Rizzoli. Orthopedics 18:993–1000

Boriani S, Weinstein JN, Biagini R (1997) Primary bone tumors of the spine. Terminology and surgical staging. Spine (Phila Pa 1976) 22:1036–1044

Boriani S, De Iure F, Bandiera S et al (2000) Chondrosarcoma of the mobile spine: report on 22 cases. Spine (Phila Pa 1976) 25:804–812

Boriani S, Bandiera S, Casadei R et al (2012) Giant cell tumor of the mobile spine: a review of 49 cases. Spine (Phila Pa 1976) 37:37–45

Caracciolo JT, Letson GD (2016) Radiologic approach to bone and soft tissue sarcomas. Surg Clin North Am 96:963–976

Chan P, Boriani S, Fourney DR et al (2009) An assessment of the reliability of the Enneking and Weinstein-Boriani-Biagini classifications for staging of primary spinal tumors by the Spine Oncology Study Group. Spine (Phila Pa 1976) 34:384–391

Chang CY, Gill CM, Joseph Simeone F et al (2016) Comparison of the diagnostic accuracy of 99m-Tc-MDP bone scintigraphy and 18F-FDG PET/CT for the detection of skeletal metastases. Acta Radiol 57:58–65

Chiesa AM, Spinnato P, Miceli M, Facchini G (2021) Radiologic assessment of osteosarcoma lung metastases: state of the art and recent advances. Cell 10:553

Cistaro A, Lopci E, Gastaldo L et al (2012) The role of 18F-FDG PET/CT in the metabolic characterization of lung nodules in pediatric patients with bone sarcoma. Pediatr Blood Cancer 59:1206–1210

Cotterill SJ, Ahrens S, Paulussen M et al (2000) Prognostic factors in Ewing's tumor of bone: analysis of 975 patients from the European Intergroup Cooperative Ewing's Sarcoma Study Group. J Clin Oncol 18:3108–3114

Dahlin DC, Unni KK (1986) Bone tumors: general aspects and data on 8,547 cases, 4th edn. Charles C Thomas Pub, Springfield, IL

Del Grande F, Tatizawa-Shiga N, Jalali Farahani S et al (2014) Chemical shift imaging: preliminary experience as an alternative sequence for defining the extent of a bone tumor. Quant Imaging Med Surg 4:173–180

Enneking WF, Spanier SS, Goodman MA (1980) A system for the surgical staging of musculoskeletal sarcoma. Clin Orthop Relat Res 153:106–120

Enneking WF, Spanier SS, Goodman MA (2003) A system for the surgical staging of musculoskeletal sarcoma. 1980. Clin Orthop Relat Res (415):4–18

Facchini G, Parmeggiani A, Peta G et al (2021) The role of percutaneous transarterial embolization in the management of spinal bone tumors: a literature review. Eur Spine J 30:2839–2851

Fisher CG, DiPaola CP, Ryken TC et al (2010) A novel classification system for spinal instability in neoplastic disease: an evidence-based approach and expert consensus from the Spine Oncology Study Group. Spine (Phila Pa 1976) 35:1221–1229

Gailloud P (2019) Introduction to diagnostic and therapeutic spinal angiography. Neuroimaging Clin N Am 29:595–614

Gasbarrini A, Cappuccio M, Donthineni R et al (2009) Management of benign tumors of the mobile spine. Orthop Clin North Am 40:9–19

Guedes A, Oliveira MBDR, Costa FM, de Melo AS (2021) Updating on bone and soft tissue sarcomas staging. Rev Bras Ortop 56:411–418

Harrop JS, Schmidt MH, Boriani S, Shaffrey CI (2009) Aggressive "benign" primary spine neoplasms: osteoblastoma, aneurysmal bone cyst, and giant cell tumor. Spine (Phila Pa 1976) 34:S39–S47

Holzapfel K, Regler J, Baum T et al (2015) Local staging of soft-tissue sarcoma: emphasis on assessment of neurovascular encasement-value of MR imaging in 174 confirmed cases. Radiology 275:501–509

Hurley C, McCarville MB, Shulkin BL et al (2016) Comparison of (18) F-FDG-PET-CT and bone scintigraphy for evaluation of osseous metastases in newly diagnosed and recurrent osteosarcoma. Pediatr Blood Cancer 63:1381–1386

Kalus S, Saifuddin A (2019) Whole-body MRI vs bone scintigraphy in the staging of Ewing sarcoma of bone: a 12-year single-institution review. Eur Radiol 29:5700–5708

London K, Stege C, Cross S et al (2012) 18F-FDG PET/CT compared to conventional imaging modalities in pediatric primary bone tumors. Pediatr Radiol 42:418–430

Meng XX, Zhang YQ, Liao HQ et al (2016) Dynamic contrast-enhanced MRI for the assessment of spinal tumor vascularity: correlation with angiography. Eur Spine J 25:3952–3961

Murphey MD, Kransdorf MJ (2021) Staging and classification of primary musculoskeletal bone and soft-tissue tumors according to the 2020 WHO update, from the AJR special series on cancer staging. AJR Am J Roentgenol 217:1038–1052

Musculoskeletal Tumor Society (1985) Staging of musculoskeletal neoplasms. Skeletal Radiol 13:183–194

Nakamura T, Matsumine A, Matsubara T et al (2011) Retrospective analysis of metastatic sarcoma patients. Oncol Lett 2:315–318

O'Flanagan SJ, Stack JP, McGee HM et al (1991) Imaging of intramedullary tumour spread in osteosarcoma. A comparison of techniques. J Bone Joint Surg Br 73:998–1001

Pennington Z, Ahmed AK, Cottrill E et al (2019) Systematic review on the utility of magnetic resonance imaging for operative management and follow-up for primary sarcoma-lessons from extremity sarcomas. Ann Transl Med 7:225

Saifuddin A, Sharif B, Gerrand C, Whelan J (2019) The current status of MRI in the pre-operative assessment of intramedullary conventional appendicular osteosarcoma. Skeletal Radiol 48:503–516

Sans N, Perroncel G (2014) Imagerie des tumeurs osseuses. Sauramps Médical, Montpellier

Shiga NT, Del Grande F, Lardo O, Fayad LM (2013) Imaging of primary bone tumors: determination of tumor extent by non-contrast sequences. Pediatr Radiol 43:1017–1023

Smith E, Hegde G, Czyz M et al (2022) A radiologists' guide to en bloc resection of primary tumors in the spine: what does the surgeon want to know? Indian J Radiol Imaging 32:205–212

Stanborough R, Demertzis JL, Wessell DE et al (2022) ACR Appropriateness Criteria® malignant or aggressive primary musculoskeletal tumor-staging and surveillance: 2022 update. J Am Coll Radiol 19:S374–S389

Sun G, Zhang Y-X, Liu F, Tu N (2020) Whole-body magnetic resonance imaging is superior to skeletal scintigraphy for the detection of bone metastatic tumors: a meta-analysis. Eur Rev Med Pharmacol Sci 24:7240–7252

Tomita K, Kawahara N, Kobayashi T et al (2001) Surgical strategy for spinal metastases. Spine (Phila Pa 1976) 26:298–306

Van Trommel MF, Kroon HM, Bloem JL et al (1997) MR imaging based strategies in limb salvage surgery for osteosarcoma of the distal femur. Skeletal Radiol 26:636–641

Van Vucht N, Santiago R, Lottmann B et al (2019) The Dixon technique for MRI of the bone marrow. Skeletal Radiol 48:1861–1874

Völker T, Denecke T, Steffen I et al (2007) Positron emission tomography for staging of pediatric sarcoma patients: results of a prospective multicenter trial. J Clin Oncol 25:5435–5441

Ward WG, Mikaelian K, Dorey F et al (1994) Pulmonary metastases of stage IIB extremity osteosarcoma and subsequent pulmonary metastases. J Clin Oncol 12:1849–1858

Westbroek EM, Pennington Z, Ehresman J et al (2020) Vertebral artery sacrifice versus skeletonization in the setting of cervical spine tumor resection: case series. World Neurosurg 139:601–607

Zhang L, Xiong L, Wu L-M et al (2021) The patterns of distant metastasis and prognostic factors in patients with primary metastatic Ewing sarcoma of the bone. J Bone Oncol 30:100385

Imaging-Guided Biopsy

Yet Yen Yan, Hong Chou, and Wilfred C. G. Peh

Contents

Abstract

Since Coley first described the method of percutaneous biopsy for the diagnosis of skeletal lesions in 1931, imaging-guided bone biopsy has advanced significantly. Unlike spinal metastases, primary tumors localized to a single location may offer the potential for curative resection. However, a spinal biopsy that is not performed correctly can compromise a patient's survival. The high accuracy, lower costs, reduced complication rate and morbidity, and decreased risk of tumor seeding as opposed to open surgical biopsy have supported imaging-guided biopsy as the preferred mode of biopsy. This chapter aims to provide an overview of the various imaging-guided biopsy techniques and their technical considerations.

Abbreviations

CT Computed tomography
MRI Magnetic resonance imaging
US Ultrasound

Y. Y. Yan (✉)
Department of Radiology, Changi General Hospital, Singapore, Republic of Singapore
e-mail: yanyetyen@gmail.com

H. Chou · W. C. G. Peh
Department of Diagnostic Radiology, Khoo Teck Puat Hospital, Singapore, Republic of Singapore
e-mail: chou.hong@ktph.com.sg; Wilfred.peh@gmail.com.sg

Med Radiol Diagn Imaging (2023)
https://doi.org/10.1007/174_2023_429, © The Author(s), under exclusive license to Springer Nature Switzerland AG
Published Online: 25 April 2023

1 General Considerations

An optimal biopsy is crucial in the management of primary bone tumors, which accounts for 4% of all spinal tumors (Boriani et al. 1995). Spinal biopsies are preferably obtained by percutaneous biopsy as open biopsies are more invasive, require the use of operating room facilities and general anesthesia, are more costly, and are associated with increased morbidity and risk of complications, longer hospital stays, and a higher risk of tumor seeding (Rehm et al. 2016). Percutaneous biopsy, on the contrary, is usually performed in an outpatient setting, rarely requires general anesthesia as it is mostly performed under local anesthesia and/or sedation, cheaper, and is minimally invasive with a low risk of infection and wound-related complications. The low complication rates for percutaneous biopsy vary between 1% and 3% and are lower than that of open biopsy which is approximately 16% (Harris et al. 2021). Major complications for percutaneous biopsy are rare and include hemorrhage, infection, neurological compromise, pneumothorax, tumor seeding, device failure, and potential for sinus tract/fistula formation secondary to infection (both primary and secondary) (Peh 2006). Limitations of percutaneous biopsy include a small risk of having a non-diagnostic sample and a lower accuracy in assessing the exact pathology and grade of spinal tumor.

2 Indications and Contraindications

Typical indications for biopsy in the setting of a primary spinal tumor consist of the following: histological assessment of vertebral lesions, receptor/immunohistochemical analysis in known neoplasms, and evaluation of the cause of potential pathological vertebral fractures. Surgical planning, chemotherapy, and radiotherapy can only commence once the histological diagnosis of a spinal tumor has been obtained. Furthermore, pretreatment biopsy is frequently requested when the lesion involves a critical structure or when neoadjuvant chemotherapy is considered (Hueman et al. 2008).

Contraindications of percutaneous biopsy include bleeding diathesis, thrombocytopenia (platelet count <50,000/mm^3), suspected hypervascular lesion with potential for hemorrhage and subsequent spinal cord/nerve compression, suspected spinal echinococcosis, infection involving the proposed biopsy trajectory, and uncooperative patient. Cessation of anticoagulants prior to the biopsy should be in accordance with the Society of Interventional Radiology consensus guidelines, in addition to ensuring normal international normalized ratio (INR), prothrombin time, and platelet counts (Patel et al. 2019). Prophylactic antibiotics are usually not necessary. The only absolute contraindication to performing a vertebral biopsy is when a lesion can be confidently diagnosed on imaging and in which no extra information can be yielded from the biopsy to alter patient management, such as a benign lesion with classical imaging features. Examples include benign vertebral compression fracture, vertebral hemangioma, osteoid osteoma, fibrous dysplasia, enostosis, and focal nodular marrow hyperplasia. In addition, when the diagnosis of multiple myeloma is obvious with concordant biologic parameters and bone marrow cytology/histology, a vertebral biopsy is not necessary.

3 Technique

3.1 Imaging Review and Lesion Characteristics

A major factor for a failed biopsy is inability to target the lesion (Rehm et al. 2016). Comprehensive pre-biopsy planning is pivotal when attempting technically challenging biopsies. All relevant imaging should be reviewed. MRI and CT should be examined for targetable enhancing portions of the lesion, and [Fluorine-18]-fluoro-2-deoxy-D-gluose (^{18}F-FDG) positron-emission tomography (PET)-CT should be assessed for the presence of hypermetabolic areas, which correspond with viable or hypercellular tissue (Wu et al. 2019). If there is concern for possible vascular injury during the biopsy, performing vascular imaging such as CT angiogram should be considered.

In the setting of primary spinal tumor presenting with multiple spinal metastases, the safest, largest, and most accessible/superficial lesion should be targeted, keeping in view the need to balance procedural risk against diagnostic yield. When encountering a mixed sclerotic–lytic lesion, the lytic component should be targeted. The necrotic and cystic areas of the lesion do not yield sufficient cells for satisfactory evaluation compared with the solid components. The entry point and angle of approach for each biopsy tract should be coordinated with the definitive surgical plan. Hence, the biopsy tract entry site and trajectory should be aligned with the plane of incision for excisional surgery, with a view of resection of the biopsy tract in curative resection. Hence, it is beneficial for every biopsy tract to be reviewed with the oncologic spine surgeon involved in the definitive surgical management. The general principles for appropriate needle paths are those which avoid critical neurovascular structures, respect the boundaries of uncontaminated tissue planes, and never pass through the pleural cavity, abdominal cavity, or the spinal canal if it has not yet been invaded (Missenard et al. 2020).

As most en bloc vertebrectomies are performed with the patient prone and involves a midline longitudinal incision, a direct posterior midline approach is the most common needle trajectory. Slight varying degrees of obliquity and para-midline entry may be acceptable to the surgeon (Figs. 1, 2, and 3). The needle tract is usually indicated by the proceduralist, often with agents such as methylene blue, to assist with identification of the biopsy tract at the time of subsequent resection. Alternatively, depending on the surgeon's comfort, aligning the visible skin incision or suture with the needle entry site of the target lesion is also a feasible option. In situations when curative resection is not considered and resection of the biopsy tract is not required, such as in the presence of metastases, a biopsy route alternative to the mentioned posterior midline or paramedian approach may be considered.

Pre-biopsy imaging should also be evaluated for any areas of active infection around the proposed biopsy site, especially if the target lesion is not infected, to avoid unintentional seeding (Peh 2006). In the event the biopsy is negative or non-interpretable (10–20% of cases), a repeat percutaneous biopsy must be discussed, potentially using a different target from the initial biopsy, particularly if technical difficulties were encountered during the first biopsy (Missenard et al. 2020). A surgical biopsy should only be considered as a last recourse, as it is much more invasive in the spine compared to the limbs.

3.2 Needle Types and Sizes

Biopsy needles can be classified into three types: fine aspiration needles, cutting needles, and trephine needles. Needle sizes range from 22 G or smaller for fine needle aspiration to 11 G for trephine biopsy. The selected needle types are determined by the nature of the lesion to be biopsied and the operator's preference. The needles selected should have enough length to reach the lesion and obtain sufficient samples. Smaller needles decrease patient discomfort, have a smaller risk of injury to adjacent structures, and cause less bleeding, as compared to larger needles. Smaller needles are best suited for fluid aspiration and for cytology of soft tissue lesions. Cutting needles can obtain larger cores of tissue from bone and soft tissue.

Fine needles (20–22 G) are utilized for cytology and fluid aspiration and have a lower risk of bleeding and tract seeding. Fine needles are limited by their inability to penetrate intact bone, tendency to bend when targeting deep lesions, and limited quantity of cells obtained from each sample, which may be under-representative of the entire lesion. The utility of fine needle aspiration biopsy in the diagnosis of primary malignant tumors is limited and controversial (Wu et al. 2008), although it has been reported to yield a tissue diagnosis in 70–80% of procedures (Carson et al. 1994; Phadke et al. 2001).

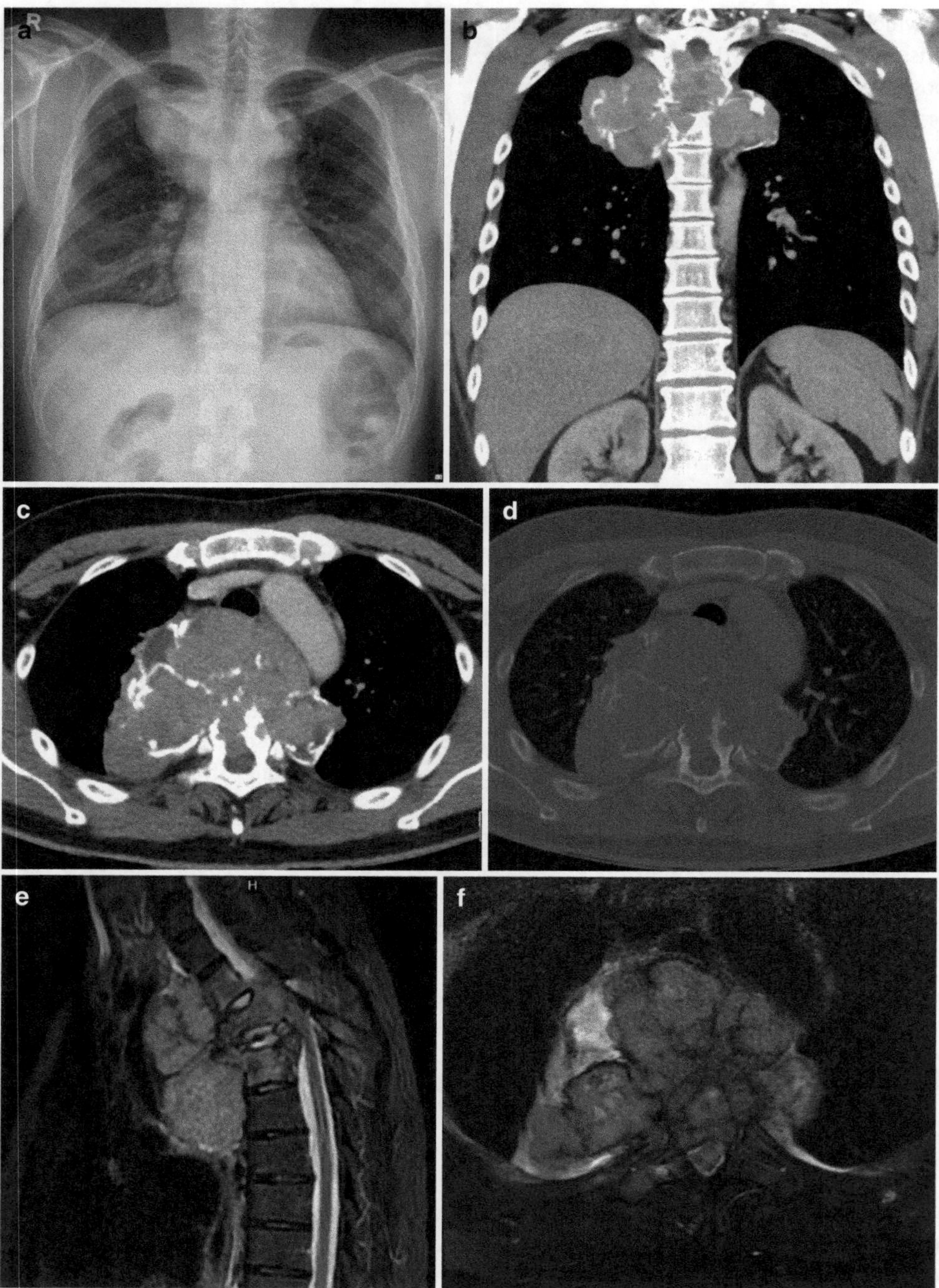

Fig. 1 A 36-year-old man who presented with bilateral lower limb weakness and numbness. (**a**) Frontal chest radiograph shows a lobulated upper mediastinal mass. (**b**) Coronal CT image shows a posterior mediastinal mass with destruction of the adjacent T3 and T4 vertebral bodies. Axial CT images obtained in (**c**) soft tissue and (**d**) bone settings show an expansile lesion arising from and destroying the vertebral body. A large soft tissue component is seen with irregular bands of internal calcifications. (**e**) Sagittal fat-suppressed T2-W and (**f**) axial contrast-enhanced fat-suppressed T1-W MR images show dural extension and cord compression. Axial CT images obtained in bone setting show the (**g**) planning image, (**h**) needle position above the adjacent rib minimizing risk of neurovascular injury, and (**i**) sampling of soft tissue component of vertebral mass with a 20 G × 15 cm × 20 T Quickcore biopsy needle. A right posterior para-midline approach was utilized. Histopathology revealed an unusual case of giant cell tumor of the vertebral body

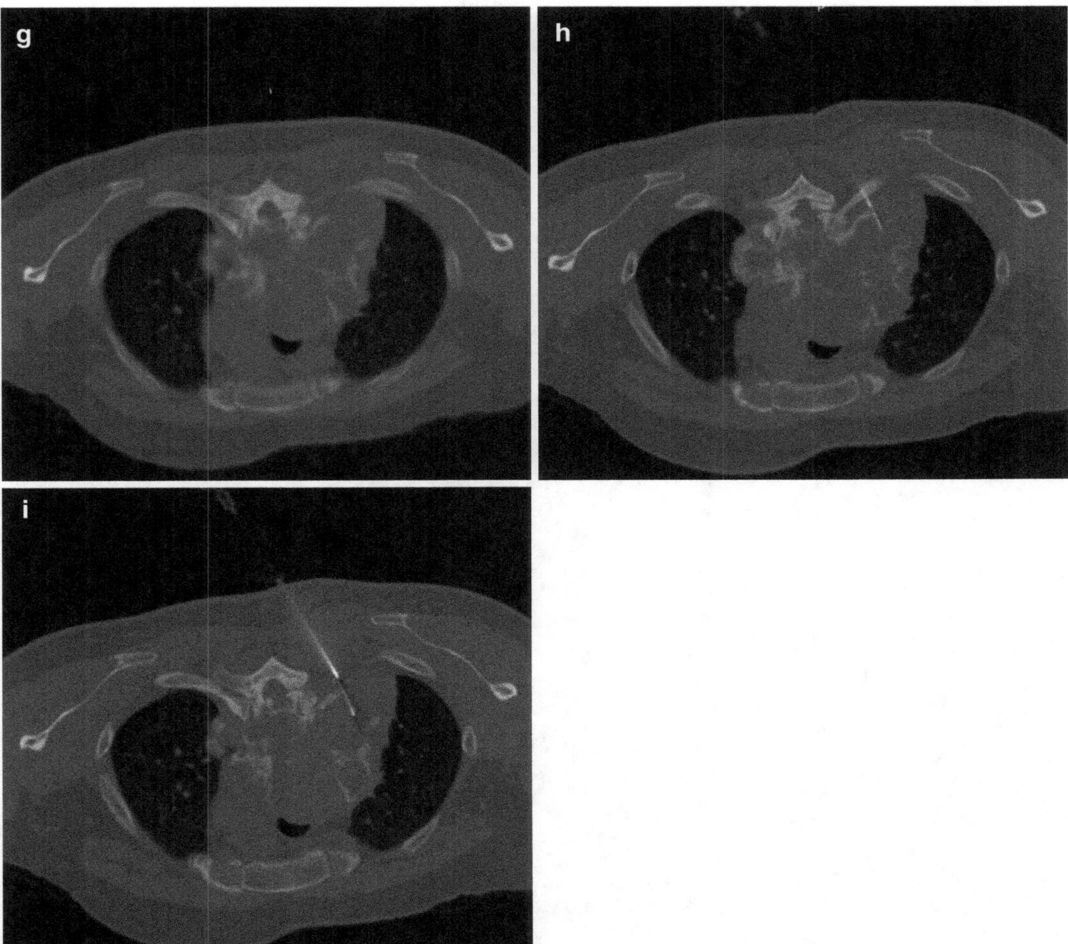

Fig. 1 (continued)

However, the perceived accuracy of fine needle aspiration biopsy is often positively confounded by a large number of benign lesions in the study population in some of these studies, as these benign tumors are easier to diagnose (Gogna et al. 2008). Fine needle aspiration biopsy can be repeated to ensure sufficient tissue for diagnosis whenever indicated. It is common for the biopsy results to be interpreted as normal bone marrow in vertebral lesions such as typical or atypical hemangiomas (Clarke et al. 2014). The utility of fine needle aspiration biopsy is therefore heavily reliant on the interpreting pathologist's experience and skill.

Important factors for a non-diagnostic biopsy include insufficient sample size and crush artifact. Larger volumes of tissue are also frequently requested, given the increasing number of tests being performed on specimens, such as flow cytometry, immunohistochemistry, and chromosomal analysis (Nourbakhsh and Hanson 2021). Larger bore needles are able to address these concerns and are more likely to provide adequate material and decrease crush artifact (Rehm et al. 2016), although at the expense of increased patient discomfort and increased complications such as bleeding. Unlike fine needle aspirate, a core biopsy preserves tissue architecture, aiding

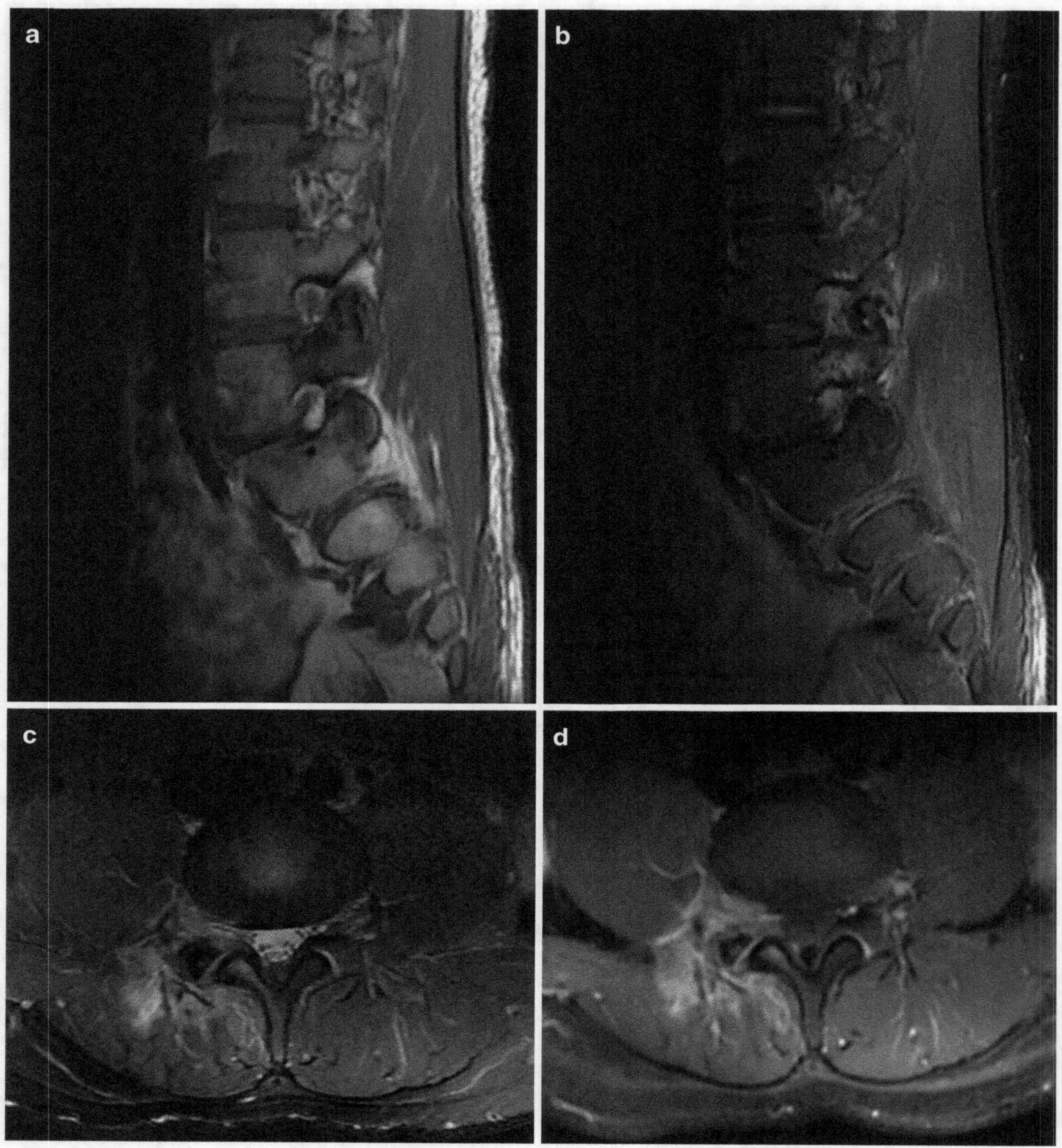

Fig. 2 A 24-year-old man who presented with low back pain with right sciatica. Sagittal (**a**) T1-W and (**b**) fat-suppressed T2-W, and axial fat-suppressed (**c**) T2-W and (**d**) contrast-enhanced fat-suppressed T1-W MR images show a T1- and T2-hypointense lesion in the right superior articular process of L5 vertebra with florid surrounding soft tissue edema and enhancement. (**e**) Axial (**f**) sagittal and (**g**) coronal CT images show a sclerotic nidus and surrounding new bone formation. (**h**) SPECT-CT images show intense activity of the same lesion. (**i**) CT-guided biopsy was performed using 14.5 G Ostycut bone biopsy needle, retrieving a 1.5 cm solid bone core via a right posterior para-midline route. (**j**) Axial and (**k**) sagittal CT images show position of radiofrequency ablation needle (1 cm, non-cooled active tip) during CT-guided ablation. (**l**) Axial and (**m**) sagittal CT images show position of 22 G spinal needle placed in the right L4–5 neural foramen for administration of nerve root block as well as neuroprotection using slow infusion of cooled Dextrose 5% solution. Patient made a good recovery with resolution of symptoms. The final diagnosis of osteoblastoma was confirmed on histopathology

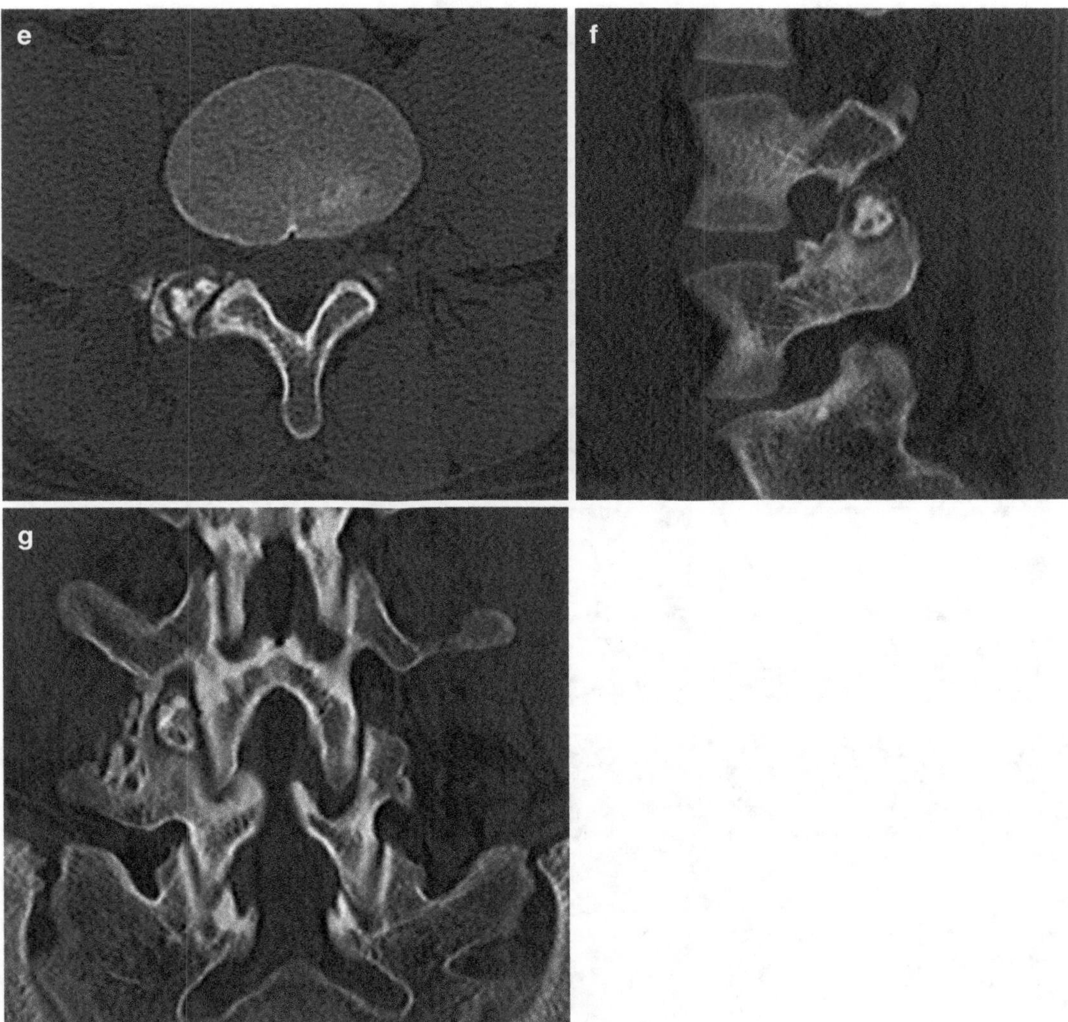

Fig. 2 (continued)

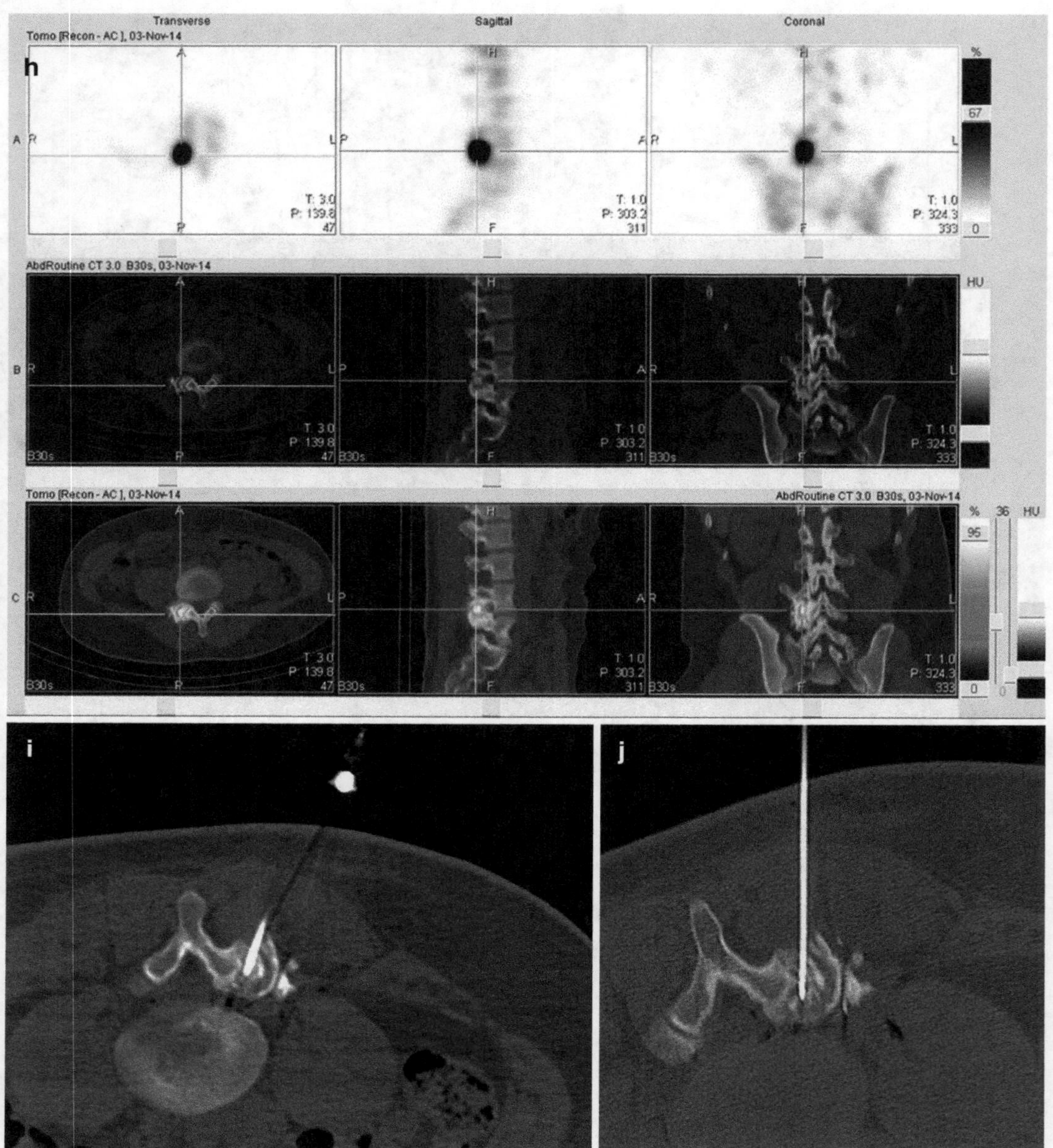

Fig. 2 (continued)

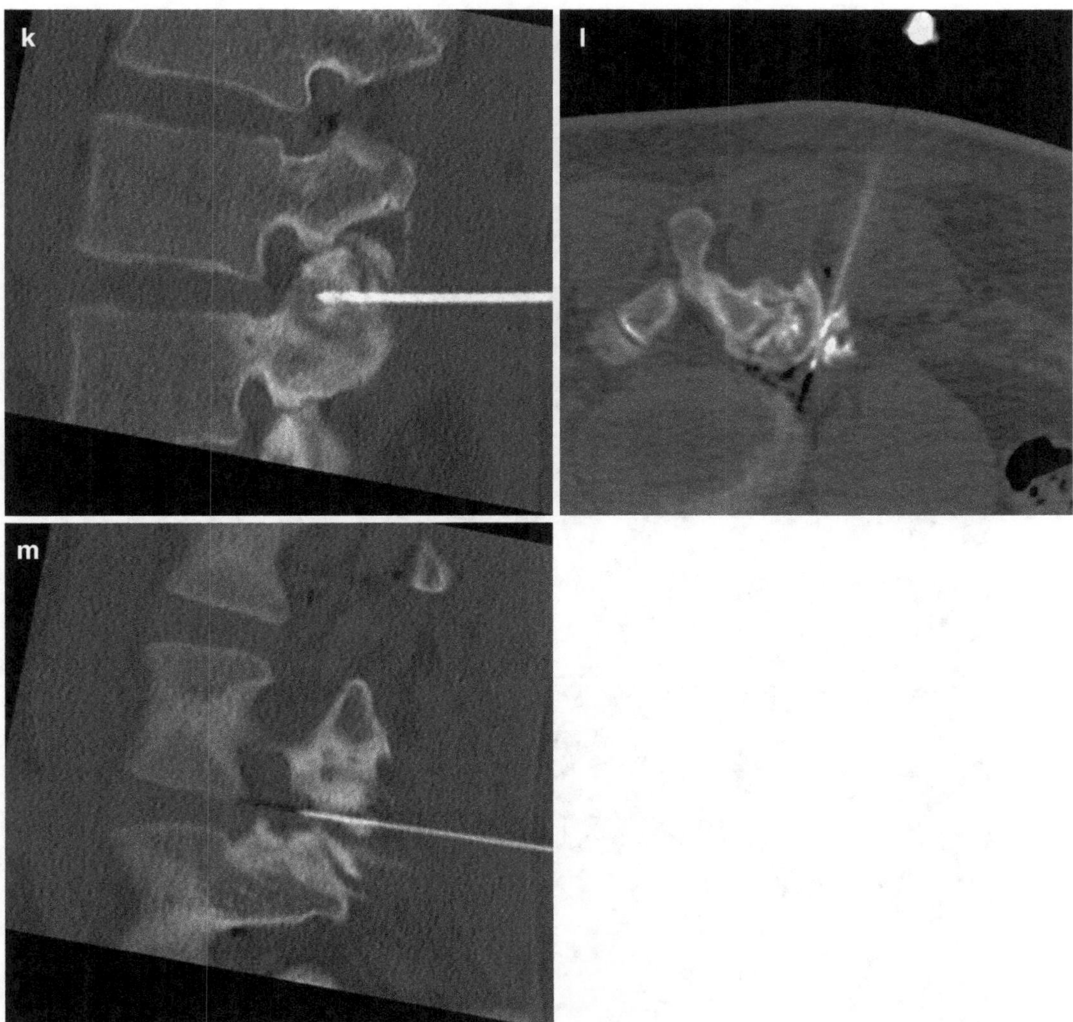

Fig. 2 (continued)

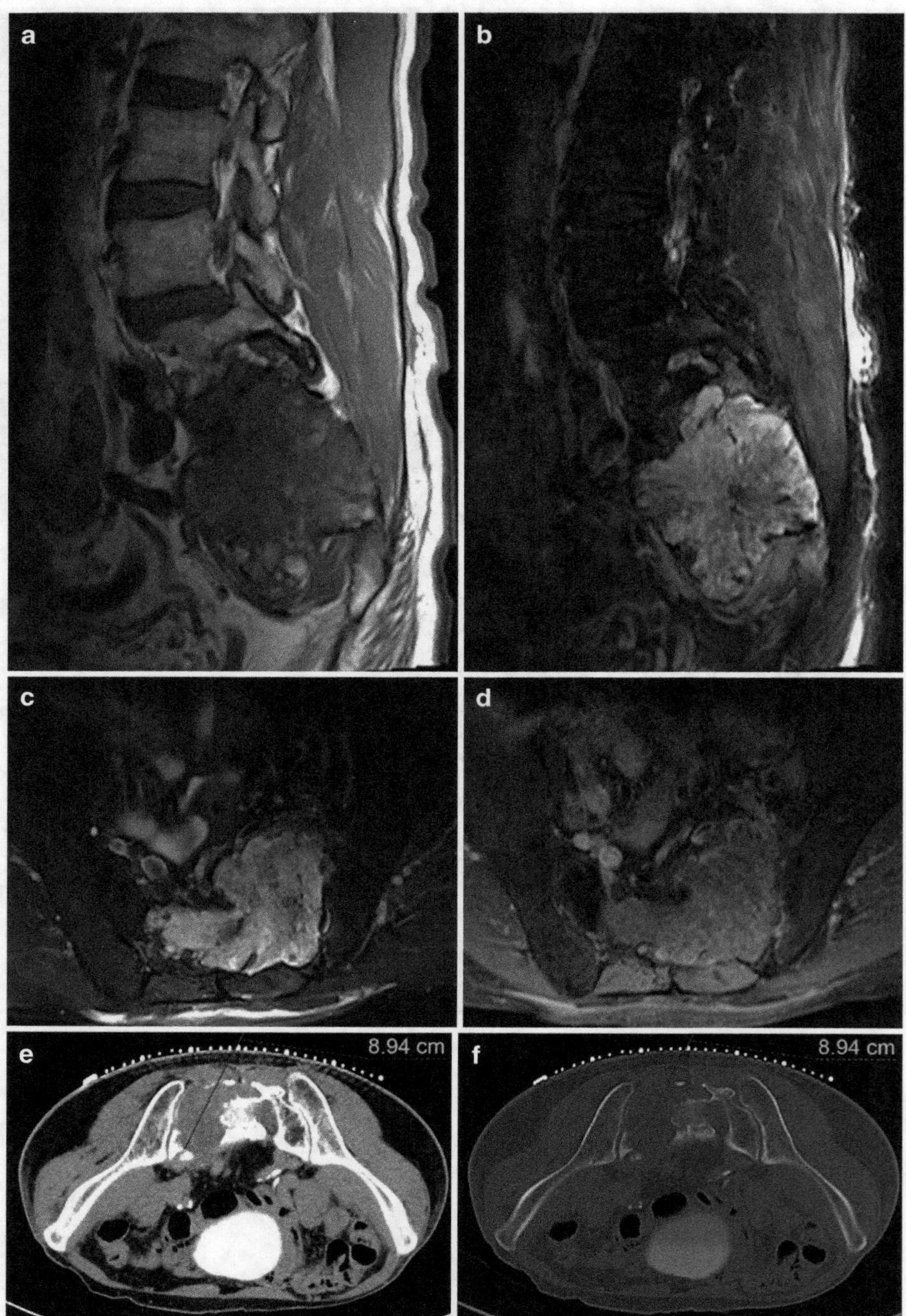

Fig. 3 A 68-year-old man who presented with low back pain radiating to the left leg. Sagittal (**a**) T1-W and (**b**) fat-suppressed T2-W, and axial fat-suppressed (**c**) T2-W and (**d**) contrast-enhanced fat-suppressed T1-W MR images show a large enhancing T2-hyperintense mass centered in the left hemisacrum with involvement of the sacral foramina and consequent nerve root impingement. Axial planning images for CT-guided biopsy obtained in (**e**) soft tissue and (**f**) bone settings with surface marking grid in place and intended biopsy tract marked. Note midline position of the skin puncture site. CT images obtained in (**g**) soft tissue and (**h**) bone settings show position of 18 G × 9 cm Quickcore biopsy needle inserted through a 16 G × 5.5 cm coaxial needle (not shown) via a direct posterior approach with slight needle path obliquity through a cortical breach. Multiple cores of fragmented soft tissue were obtained for histopathology which confirmed the diagnosis of chordoma

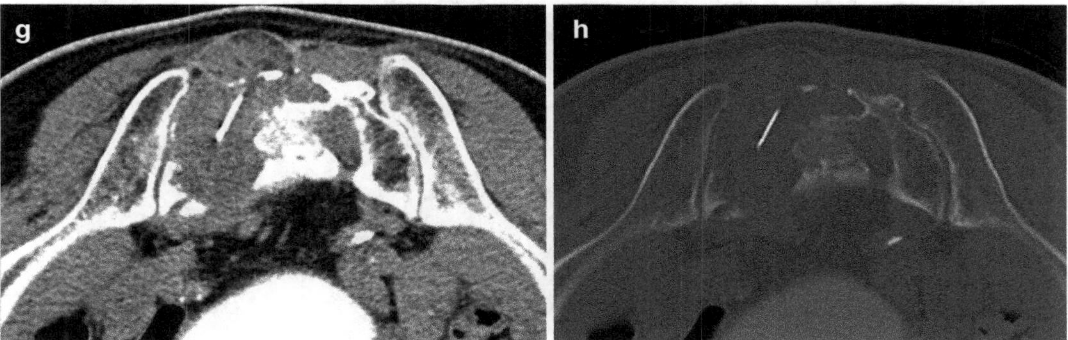

Fig. 3 (continued)

in the diagnosis. Larger needles can be drilled into bone, permitting coaxial insertion of smaller needles. The coaxial method also allows multiple passes through a single skin puncture and single bone entry site, reducing risk of injury to adjacent structures, increasing patient comfort, and decreasing tract seeding. Percutaneous biopsy can be directly performed using an aspiration or cutting needle whenever the vertebral lesion displays cortical breach. In the presence of an intact cortex, cortex must be breached using a trephine needle, which has a cutting tip to allow penetration of bone or drill-based systems. Comprehensive hemostasis must be achieved as an expanding hematoma may contaminate adjacent fascial planes (Williams et al. 2012). The risk of procedural bleeding can be minimized through the administration of autologous clots, Gelfoam pledgets or slurry along the coaxial needle tract by inserting the stylet into the access cannula between passes and/or after the biopsy (Yaffe et al. 2003).

In our institutions' practice, the minimum core biopsy needle caliber used for both soft tissue and bone is 18 G. When obtaining biopsies of soft tissue components via a cutting needle, the Quickcore (IZI Medical, Maryland; the authors declare that they have no conflict of interest) (Fig. 1, 3, and 4), which comprises of a 18 G (9 cm, 15 cm, or 20 cm) biopsy needle or SuperCore Semi-Automatic biopsy set (Argon Medical, Texas; the authors declare that they have no conflict of interest), which consists of a 14 G biopsy needle (6 cm, 9 cm, 15 cm, or 20 cm) is used. Using a much larger caliber needle such as a 14 G core biopsy needle reduces the need for multiple passes, with the volume acquired from two 2 cm cores often being sufficient. With a decreased number of passes made, the risk of complications or biopsy tract seeding is minimized, in tandem with a reduction in procedural time.

Vertebral bone biopsy kits use a coaxial system with larger gauge needles than those used for soft tissues and employ the use of a trephine needle with a cutting tip or drill system to enter the bone. In the authors' experience, 11 G or 13 G (10 cm or 15 cm) Confidence access needles (DePuy Spine, Leeds, UK; the authors declare that they have no conflict of interest), 10 G or 11 G (6 cm, 10 cm, or 15 cm) Arrow OnControl powered bone access needles (Teleflex, Pennsylvania; the authors declare that they have no conflict of interest) (Fig. 5), or 14.5 G or 15 G (5 cm, 7.5 cm or 10 cm) Ostycut access needles (Ostycut, Bard, Karlsruhe, Germany; the authors declare that they have no conflict of interest) (Fig. 2) are utilized. The Arrow OnControl powered bone access system is a coaxial drill-assisted bone biopsy set that reduces procedural time, without any increased risk of crush artifact (Wallace et al. 2016). The diagnostic rate in sclerotic bone lesion may also improve slightly with a battery-powered drill system, as opposed to a manual device (Suh and Yun 2019). The OnControl system is also packaged with 12 G or 13 G biopsy needles (10 cm, 14 cm, or 19 cm), though a cutting needle such

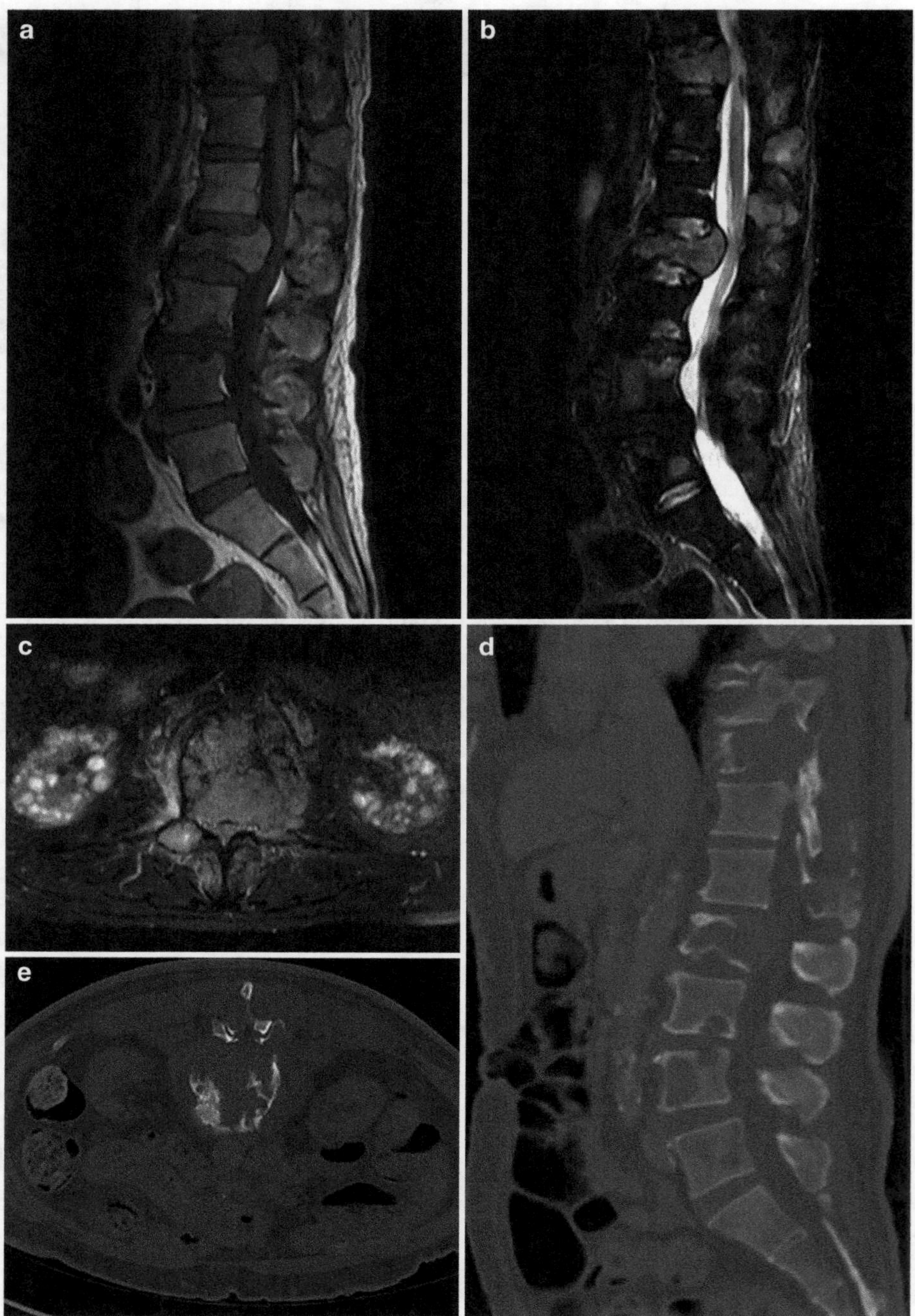

Fig. 4 A 66-year-old man with history of end-stage renal failure and incidental multiple lytic lesions who presented with a L2 pathological fracture. Sagittal (**a**) T1-W and (**b**) fat-suppressed T2-W MR images show multiple T2-hyperintense vertebral lesions involving the vertebral bodies and posterior elements. Pathological fractures at T11 and L2 levels cause significant spinal stenosis. (**c**) Axial fat-suppressed T2-W MR image at L2 level shows an expanded vertebral body lesion with cauda equina compression along with features of chronic renal failure. (**d**) Sagittal CT image shows multiple lytic bony lesions in the lower thoracic and lumbar spine. Axial CT images show the (**e**) planning stage, and insertion of the (**f**) 14 G × 5.5 cm coaxial needle and (**g**) 16 G × 9 cm (20 mm throw) Quickcore soft tissue biopsy needle via a left posterolateral route through a cortical breach. Histopathology confirmed the diagnosis of multiple myeloma

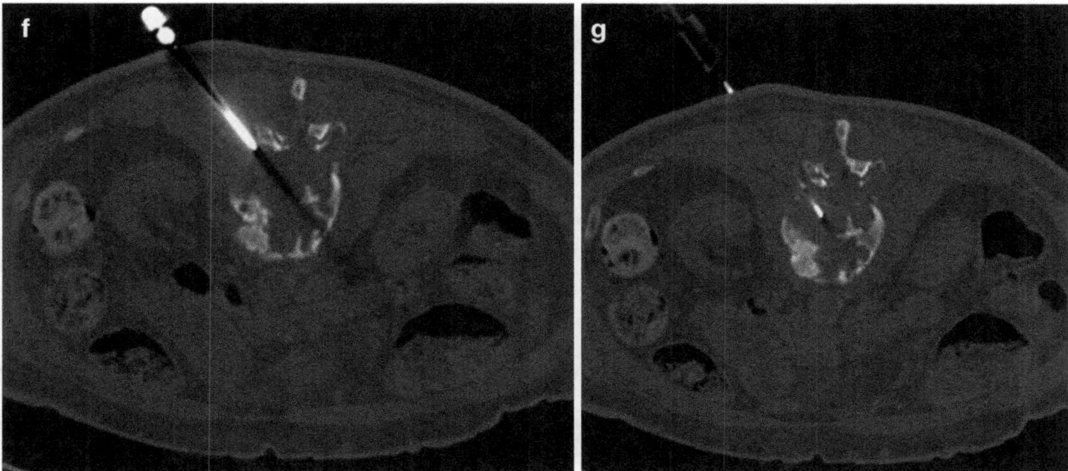

Fig. 4 (continued)

as the Quickcore or SuperCore needles can be passed through the OnControl or Confidence access needles to increase the diagnostic yield in lytic vertebral tumors. The availability of on-site intraoperative cytology ensures adequacy of the biopsy specimen, has been shown to have a cytological diagnosis that correlated with final histology in 95.7% of cases, and adds only 7–10 min to the overall procedural time (Naresh-Babu et al. 2014).

3.3 Positioning

It is important to ensure that the patient is comfortable and able to lie still and remain cooperative for a prolonged time period, particularly if the procedure is performed under local anesthesia or conscious sedation. The majority of thoracolumbar and sacral spinal biopsies are performed in the prone position, while cervical spine biopsies may be performed in either the prone or supine position, depending on the level and exact site to be biopsied (Peh 2006).

The choice of anesthesia is dependent on various factors. These include patient-related factors such as medical comorbidities and the patient's ability to cooperate and lie still, technical factors such as biopsy approaches that can potentially lead to excessive anxiety or pain, biopsy of sclerotic lesions which might lead to difficulty in obtaining samples, or biopsy of deep-seated vertebral lesions. Pediatric patients may require referral for general anesthesia.

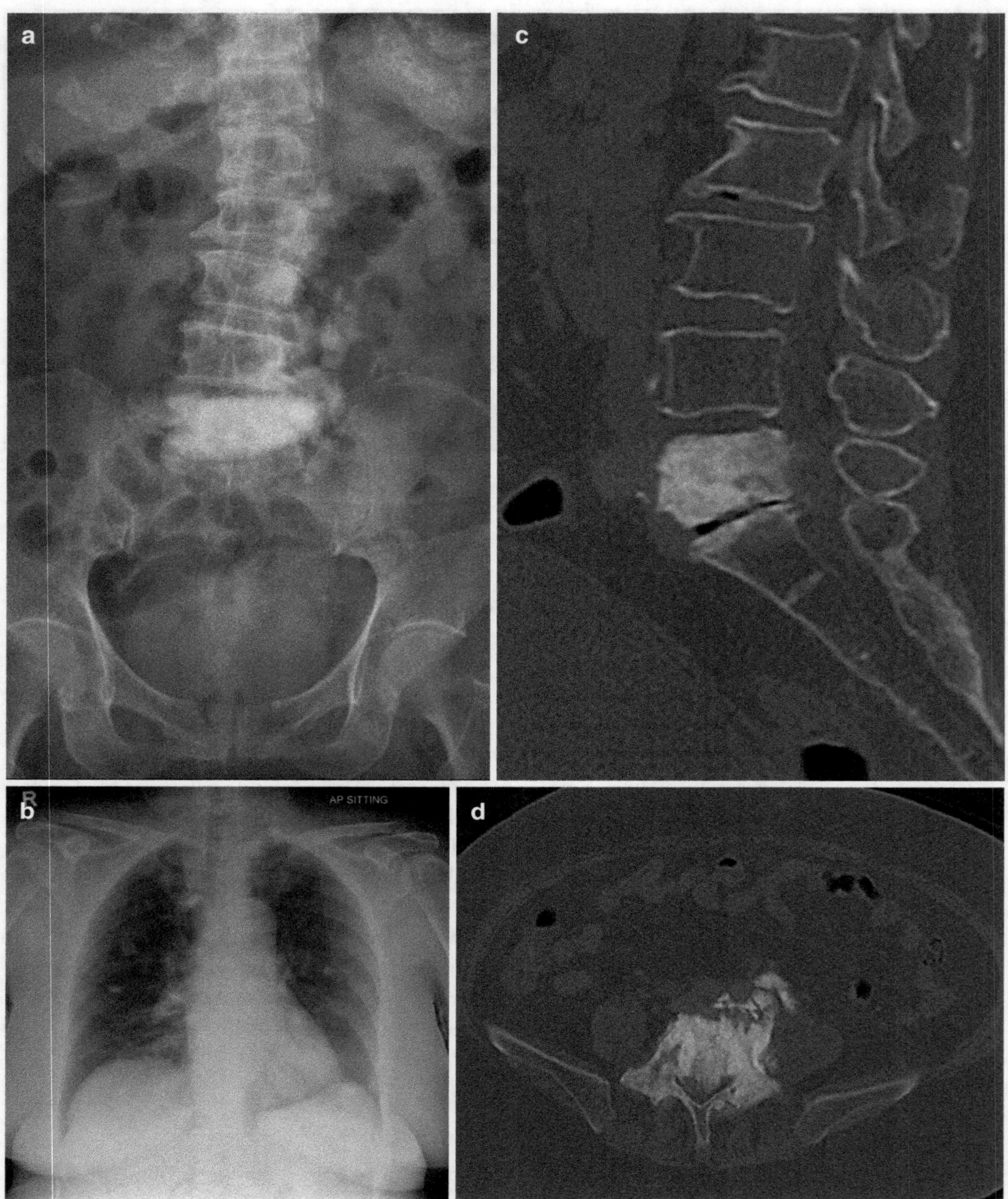

Fig. 5 A 75-year-old woman with history of cervical cancer who presented with low back and bilateral hip pain after a fall. (**a**) Frontal radiograph of the lumbar spine shows a sclerotic lesion in L5 vertebral body as well as nodular left paravertebral ossifications. (**b**) Frontal chest radiograph shows several calcified nodules in both lungs. (**c**) Sagittal and (**d**) axial CT images obtained in bone setting show sclerotic bony lesion involving both the body and posterior elements of L5 vertebra, which encroaches into the spinal canal. Associated calcified left para-aortic lymph nodes are evident. (**e–h**) Axial CT images from the CT-guided biopsy using an Arrow OnControl powered drill-assisted bone biopsy set via a left transpedicular approach. Two solid cores of bone were obtained using 13 G × 10 cm bone biopsy needle through an 11 G coaxial needle. Histological analysis revealed the diagnosis of osteosarcoma

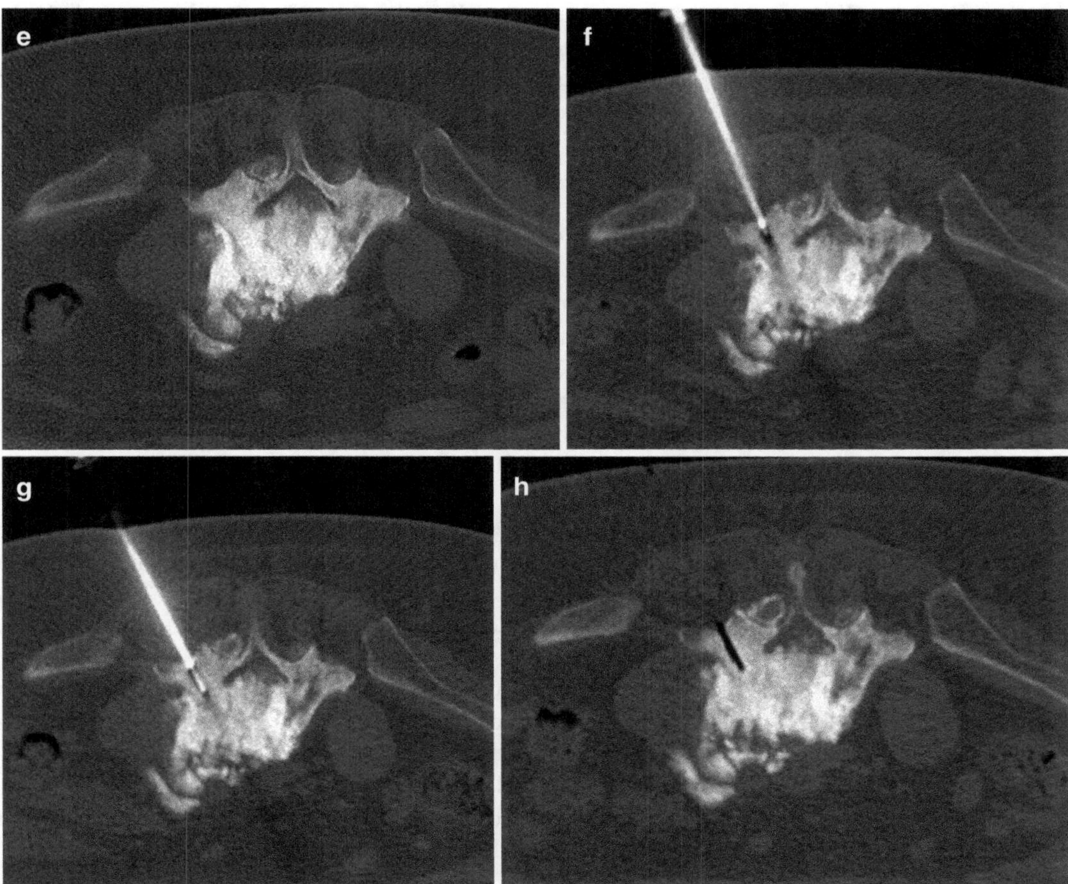

Fig. 5 (continued)

4 Imaging Types

When considering the imaging modality used to guide a spinal biopsy, the lesion should ideally be conspicuous on the chosen modality, and prior imaging should have already been done with the selected modality. Information gleaned from different modalities should be combined to achieve optimal targeting (e.g., hypermetabolic, solid, and non-sclerotic portions). No significant difference has been found between fluoroscopic and CT-guided spinal biopsy in terms of diagnostic accuracy and procedural pain (Lee et al. 2020). Continuous or intermittent imaging monitoring should be performed initially to ensure that the needle tip is in a safe position during its insertion and subsequently to confirm its placement within the lesion (Chelli Bouaziz et al. 2021).

In our institutions, fluoroscopy coupled with cone-beam CT-guided biopsy and CT-guided biopsy are the main imaging modalities used. Fluoroscopy is more accessible, inexpensive and results in a lower radiation dose compared with CT for the same imaging period (Lee et al. 2020). Biplanar fluoroscopy allows real-time guidance in needle advancement and the ability to approach a lesion from technically challenging angles of entry. Cone-beam CT can also be carried out during fluoroscopy for both planning purposes and guidance through complex anatomy, though with additional radiation dose to the patient (Filippiadis et al. 2021). In addition, patient movement does not degrade image quality as severely, compared to CT or MRI (Gogna et al. 2008). Furthermore, there is no image degradation by metallic streak artifacts in the presence of metallic implants as opposed to CT.

The accuracy of fluoroscopic-guided spinal biopsy ranges between 80% and 90% (Mireles-Cano et al. 2021; Pierot and Boulin 1999). Furthermore, the availability of real-time three-dimensional fluoroscopic needle guidance systems has further assisted fluoroscopic biopsy and is particularly useful in difficult biopsies or targeting of desired portions of a lesion. These fluoroscopic needle guidance systems allow the planning of the needle path in three planes through a pre-procedural cone-beam CT, enabling increased success of targeting the desired portions of the lesion, and avoidance of critical structures such as neurovascular structures. The error margin for this is reported at less than 5 mm (Saththianathan et al. 2022).

Limitations of fluoroscopy include poor visualization of small intramedullary lesions and neural arch lesions, as well as soft tissue component of osseous spinal tumors. Limitations of fluoroscopic needle guidance systems include the system's inherent susceptibility to patient motion artifact, which can trigger a mis-registration between real-time fluoroscopy and the initial planning cone-beam CT acquisition. Measures to circumvent these shortfalls include the use of general anesthesia to minimize patient motion or repeat cone-beam CT for updated needle guidance planning (Leschka et al. 2012).

CT-guided biopsy provides excellent spatial resolution with accuracy rates reported over 90% (Rimondi et al. 2008), with the accuracy rate reduced to 81% in CT-occult lesions (Lis et al. 2004). Intermittent CT fluoroscopy, using a quick check method, where only a few consecutive slices are imaged at a time and the needle is advanced after studying these images, permits a quick evaluation of needle advancement and progress. Although there have been concerns of increased radiation dose with CT-guided biopsy (Silverman et al. 1999), this can be minimized through the use of low-dose scanning techniques and alterations in the scanning protocols.

Limitations of CT-guided biopsy include the inability to utilize a wide range of angles of approach as compared to fluoroscopy. Furthermore, in view of the complex curved spinal anatomy, a true-axial plane needle path might not allow access to the target lesion and while this limitation can potentially be overcome with a gantry tilt, there remain circumstances where complicated out-of-plane imaging and alternate approaches will still have to be employed. Some authors recommend CT-guided biopsy for lesions closely related to the dura, spinal cord, nerve roots, or vascular structures, as well as lesions not well visualized on fluoroscopy (Saththianathan et al. 2022).

MRI-guided biopsy offers excellent spatial and temporal resolution, enabling real-time three-dimensional guidance without the use of ionizing radiation and accuracy rates of 94%. Localization and entry point planning are assisted by multiplanar guidance (Liu et al. 2015). MRI image overlay navigation allows concurrent visualization of both the MR images and target results (Saththianathan et al. 2022). However, a longer procedural time (Yang et al. 2018), high costs, requirement for MR-compatible non-ferromagnetic equipment, and difficulty in procuring MR imaging scan room time limit MRI's role in biopsy.

^{18}F-FDG PET-CT-guided bone biopsy has excellent diagnostic accuracy, reported at over 95%. However, such systems are expensive, not widely available and cause increased radiation dose to both patient and proceduralist (Wu et al. 2019). A careful review of prior ^{18}F-FDG PET-CT studies and correlation with the planning CT can provide similar advantages without the additional radiation dose from the radioisotope. US imaging allows real-time imaging guidance, flexible patient positioning, and identification of blood flow, without the hazards of ionizing radiation. However, US has a limited role in percutaneous biopsy unless there is superficial extra-osseous soft tissue extension of the vertebral lesion or it is used as a supplement to guide needles past crucial neurovascular structures, such as in the neck.

5 Location-Specific Considerations

5.1 Cervical

The cervical spine is the most challenging spinal segment to biopsy, with the lowest accuracy rate (70%) compared to the rest of the spine (accuracy rate > 90%) (Rimondi et al. 2008). This technical difficulty is attributed by the smaller size of the cervical vertebra, and the proximity of the surrounding critical neurovascular structures and the aerodigestive tract (Brugieres et al. 1990). CT is predominantly used, with or without supplementary assistance from US imaging to guide the needle through the soft tissues prior to entering the vertebra (Peh 2006). A pre-procedural CT angiogram can be performed to evaluate the vascular anatomy and detect variant or anomalous vessels that might complicate the biopsy. Coordination with the oncologic spine surgeon to determine the safest biopsy route that aligns with the surgical approach is recommended.

In the cervical spine, both anterior and posterior approaches may be used. With the patient prone, a posterolateral or direct posterior approach can be employed, with the direct posterior approach being the most commonly employed as this coincides with the surgical approach. The posterolateral approach may be appropriate in selected cases, although it may limit potential surgical options and a longer needle biopsy path is usually required compared to other approaches (Brugieres et al. 1990). A thorough review of the vertebral artery course is required for the posterior and posterolateral approaches. A transpedicular approach is frequently difficult due to the shorter and smaller caliber of cervical pedicle.

An anterolateral approach can be utilized in situations when an anterior surgical approach is considered, and has been described for the C3–C7 vertebral bodies. An anterolateral approach is performed with the patient supine, with the entry point anterior to the sternocleidomastoid and the biopsy route coursing lateral to the carotid and jugular vessels and medial to the aerodigestive tract. Approach from the right side is preferred when using the anterolateral approach to avoid injury to the esophagus, especially from C5 to C7 (Brugieres et al. 1990; Nourbakhsh and Hanson 2021). When performing biopsy of the lower cervical spine, additional risks of thyroid injury and pneumothorax should be conveyed to the patient (Brugieres et al. 1990). The proceduralist's fingers are used to displace the carotid and jugular vessels laterally, guarding them while the needle is advanced (Peh 2006).

The C1 and C2 vertebra can be approached transorally, involving the use of an ENT mouth retractor and general anesthesia (Peh 2006). It is vital to exclude a retropharyngeal course of the internal carotid artery prior to attempting a transoral approach. A lateral approach should not be employed as it is virtually a non-resectable approach (Singh et al. 2020).

5.2 Thoracolumbar

Thoracolumbar spinal lesions are usually biopsied with the patient prone. An approach with patient in a decubitus position is rarely used and is typically avoided. When approaching a thoracic spinal lesion, related complications include injury to the major vessels, pleura, lung parenchyma, esophagus, and posterior mediastinal structures (Tehranzadeh et al. 2007). Depending on the operator's preference, thoracolumbar spinal biopsies can be performed under fluoroscopy or CT guidance.

The biopsy approach for a thoracic spinal lesion is determined by future management of the lesion. If curative resection is a possibility, a transpedicular approach is utilized. If not, an extrapedicular costotransverse approach may be used, especially for lesions sited centrally in the vertebral body (Saifuddin et al. 2021; Saththianathan et al. 2022). When approaching a lumbar spinal lesion, a transpedicular route is employed if curative resection is a possibility (Fig. 5), while posterolateral and lateral approaches are usually non-resectable (Saththianathan et al. 2022) (Fig. 4). In a transpedicular approach, the patient is kept prone. This technique employs a short needle tract and takes advantage of the groove between the mamillary process and transverse process to guide the needle into the pedicle. It is essential to align the vertebral endplates of the target vertebra at the beginning of the procedure on fluoroscopy or through a gantry tilt on CT. This step should be performed prior to any further angulation that may be required fluoroscopically.

When using fluoroscopy, the medial and inferior borders of the pedicle must be identified throughout the procedure. Breach of the pedicle, particularly in these directions, increases the risks associated with the procedure. Needle entry into the pedicle depends on which part of the vertebra needs to be accessed. Additionally, the relative anterior–posterior orientation of the thoracic pedicles limits the accessibility of the posteromedian aspect of the vertebral body. Bipedicular access can increase yield. When the pedicle margin conspicuity is diminished on fluoroscopy due to a lytic pedicular lesion, it is possible to rely on the neighboring pedicles above and below the target vertebra to guide needle placement on the posteroanterior view under fluoroscopy. In pedicular tumor infiltration and pathological vertebral body collapse, a pedicular biopsy could be considered with a more inferior placement of the needle (Singh et al. 2020; Saifuddin et al. 2021).

5.3 Sacrum

The sacrum is usually biopsied with the patient in a prone position. A direct posterior approach is preferred (Oñate Miranda and Moser 2018) (Fig. 3). A trans-foraminal technique can be utilized via CT guidance if there is clear visualization of the sacral foramina and nerve roots. In the event a trans-foraminal approach is selected, a concomitant nerve root block can be administered to decrease any risk of adjacent nerve root irritation. Although more laterally angulated biopsy routes or a trans-iliosacral path may be technically more easily performed, such approaches are non-resectable and should not be attempted. Bowel injury can be a significant risk, especially when targeting sacral lesions with extra-osseous presacral extension.

6 Handling of Specimens

Every obtainable material, tissue or fluid and including blood clots, should be dispatched for cytology, culture, and histopathological examination whenever applicable. The histological examination of the osseous blood increases the accuracy of the biopsy and should be treated like a tissue specimen (Nourbakhsh and Hanson 2021). In view of the different methods of specimen handling and fixation, a pre-procedure consultation between the radiologist and pathologist to ensure acquisition of sufficient number of specimens and proper tests to be ordered is recommended. Generally, if ancillary studies are anticipated, then a minimum of three cores may be required (Mangham and Athanasou 2011). Some authors recommend 2–3 bone cores and if possible, a medullary aspirate for sclerotic lesions; an aspiration biopsy to obtain 10–20 mL of lesional tissue for lytic lesions; and a minimum of 3 soft tissue cores using a cutting needle for lesions with a large (>1–1.5 cm depth) extra-osseous component (Saifuddin et al. 2021).

All the specimens should be carefully labeled and dispatched promptly by a responsible person. The proceduralist should be familiar with smear preparation on glass slides and the various types of containers to be used for histopathological specimens (Peh 2006). Clinical information should be stated on the request form because further testing may be required. The fine needle aspirate specimens can be injected onto glass slides and smeared using a second glass slide. Some slides are air-dried and stained with Diff-Quick (Fisher Scientific Biomedical Sciences Incorporated, Swedesboro, New Jersey) for immediate cytological assessment (to check for an adequate sample). Other slides are fixed immediately with 95% ethanol for later staining using the Papanicolaou method. For suspected lymphoma, flushing some aspirate into Hank's solution for flow cytometric immunophenotyping can be considered (Domanski et al. 2005). Fine needle material can be applied to rapid staining and preliminary assessment techniques.

Core biopsy specimens can be placed on wet gauze and sent to the pathology department immediately. If the core is 5 mm or more in thickness, it should be divided. Most bone tumor specimens are further processed by decalcification with strong or weak acid solutions. Samples of the biopsy specimen that are not heavily mineralized should be selected to reduce the duration required for decalcification. Receiving specimens fresh (unfixed) in the laboratory allows additional tissue processing and application of a number of specialized investigations where appropriate. These include providing material for frozen section diagnosis, the use of specific fixatives for histochemistry, and snap freezing of tissue for molecular genetic studies (Rubin et al. 2010). Fresh tissue can also be sent for microbiological culture or cytogenetic studies.

Alternatively, specimens may be placed in 10% neutral buffered formalin if ancillary tests are not anticipated or when there is likely to be a delay in the processing of the specimen. Fixation of specimens in absolute alcohol is useful for identifying glycogen in Ewing's sarcoma cells (Mangham and Athanasou 2011). It is important that specimens are not placed in a freezer as this may result in formation of ice crystal artifacts. If infection remains a differential diagnosis, additional material should be sent in a sterile container and/or placed directly into culture material. Imprints of the core specimen may be obtained by touching the tissue core onto a glass slide before dislodging it into the specimen container. The imprint cytology enables a quick review for adequacy and may even provide a provisional diagnosis (Domanski et al. 2005).

7 Post-procedure Care

The patient should be monitored in the recovery area after the biopsy for 2–4 h for any alteration of vital signs and puncture site hematoma. As a general guide, vital signs should be recorded every 15 min for the first hour, 30 min for the following 2 h, and hourly thereafter. If clinically warranted, the monitoring can be extended to overnight observation. A chest radiograph should be performed after a thoracic spine biopsy to exclude a pneumothorax, although this may not be necessary if the biopsy had been performed under CT guidance. In high-risk patients, cardiopulmonary monitoring and post-procedural pain management are recommended (Nourbakhsh and Hanson 2021).

Upon discharge, the patient is given a patient information sheet detailing potential late complications and instructions on how to proceed and whom to contact if signs or symptoms occur. Sufficient, preferable long-acting pain medications should be prescribed for at least 2 days post-procedure. It is important to ensure that a follow-up appointment had been scheduled with the referring clinician to discuss the biopsy findings. The patient should be discouraged from driving on the procedure day, especially if sedation had been administered. The biopsy results should ideally be discussed together by the interventional radiologist, surgeon, and pathologist.

8 Conclusion

Imaging-guided biopsy is crucial in the management of primary bone tumors. Familiarization with the advantages and disadvantages of the different imaging modalities, biopsy methods, needle types as well as awareness of how the different anatomical locations can influence the biopsy approach, enables the radiologist in becoming an essential member of the management team.

9 Key Messages

1. Every biopsy tract should be reviewed with the oncologic spine surgeon involved in the definitive surgical management.
2. In the event curative resection is not considered and resection of the biopsy tract is not required, such as in the presence of metastases, a biopsy route alternative to a posterior midline or paramedian approach may be considered.
3. When a percutaneous biopsy is negative or non-interpretable, a repeat percutaneous biopsy must be considered, potentially targeting a different area from the initial biopsy,

particularly if technical difficulties were encountered during the first biopsy.

4. Every obtainable material, tissue or fluid and including blood clots, should be dispatched for cytology, culture and histopathological examination whenever applicable.

References

Boriani S, Biagini R, de Iure F et al (1995) Primary bone tumors of the spine: a survey of the evaluation and treatment at the Istituto Ortopedico Rizzoli. Orthopedics 18:993–999

Brugieres P, Gaston A, Heran F et al (1990) Percutaneous biopsies of the thoracic spine under CT guidance: transcostovertebral approach. J Comput Assist Tomogr 14:446–448

Carson HJ, Castelli MJ, Reyes CV et al (1994) Fine-needle aspiration biopsy of vertebral body lesions: cytologic, pathologic, and clinical correlations of 57 cases. Diagn Cytopathol 11:348–351

Chelli Bouaziz M, Ladeb MF, Rammeh S et al (2021) Percutaneous biopsy of spinal infection. In: Ladeb MF, Peh WCG (eds) Imaging of spinal infection. Springer Nature, Switzerland AG, pp 89–104

Clarke MJ, Mendel E, Vrionis FD (2014) Primary spine tumors: diagnosis and treatment. Cancer Control 21:114–123

Domanski HA, Akerman M, Carlén B et al (2005) Core-needle biopsy performed by the cytopathologist: a technique to complement fine-needle aspiration of soft tissue and bone lesions. Cancer 105:229–239

Filippiadis D, Moschovaki-Zeiger O, Kelekis A (2021) Percutaneous bone and soft tissue biopsies: an illustrative approach. Tech Vasc Interv Radiol 24:100772

Gogna A, Peh WCG, Munk PL (2008) Image-guided musculoskeletal biopsy. Radiol Clin North Am 46:455–473

Harris L, Rajashekar D, Sharma P et al (2021) Performance of computed tomography-guided spine biopsy for the diagnosis of malignancy and infection. Oper Neurosurg (Hagerstown) 21:126–130

Hueman MT, Thornton K, Herman JM et al (2008) Management of extremity soft tissue sarcomas. Surg Clin North Am 88:539–557

Lee SA, Chiu CK, Chan CYW et al (2020) The clinical utility of fluoroscopic versus CT guided percutaneous transpedicular core needle biopsy for spinal infections and tumours: a randomized trial. Spine J 20:1114–1124

Leschka SC, Babic D, El Shikh S et al (2012) C-arm cone beam computed tomography needle path overlay for image-guided procedures of the spine and pelvis. Neuroradiology 54:215–223

Lis E, Bilsky MH, Pisinski L et al (2004) Percutaneous CT-guided biopsy of osseous lesion of the spine in patients with known or suspected malignancy. AJNR Am J Neuroradiol 25:1583–1588

Liu M, Sequeiros RB, Xu Y et al (2015) MRI-guided percutaneous transpedicular biopsy of thoracic and lumbar spine using a 0.23t scanner with optical instrument tracking. J Magn Reson Imaging 42:1740–1746

Mangham DC, Athanasou NA (2011) Guidelines for histopathological specimen examination and diagnostic reporting of primary bone tumours. Clin Sarcoma Res 1:6

Mireles-Cano JN, Gonzalez AM, García-González OG, Pérez RM (2021) Effectiveness of fluoroscopy-guided percutaneous vertebral biopsy. Rev Bras Ortop (Sao Paulo) 56:453–458

Missenard G, Bouthors C, Fadel E et al (2020) Surgical strategies for primary malignant tumors of the thoracic and lumbar spine. Orthop Traumatol Surg Res 106:S53–S62

Naresh-Babu J, Neelima G, Reshma-Begum SK (2014) Increasing the specimen adequacy of transpedicular vertebral body biopsies. Role of intraoperative scrape cytology. Spine J 14:2320–2325

Nourbakhsh A, Hanson ZC (2021) Percutaneous spine biopsy: a review of the current literature. J Am Acad Orthop Surg 29:e681–e692

Oñate Miranda M, Moser TP (2018) A practical guide for planning pelvic bone percutaneous interventions (biopsy, tumour ablation and cementoplasty). Insights Imaging 9:275–285

Patel IJ, Rahim S, Davidson JC et al (2019) Society of Interventional Radiology consensus guidelines for the periprocedural management of thrombotic and bleeding risk in patients undergoing percutaneous image-guided interventions - Part II: Recommendations: endorsed by the Canadian Association for Interventional Radiology and the Cardiovascular and Interventional Radiological Society of Europe. J Vasc Interv Radiol 30:1168–1184.e1

Peh WCG (2006) CT-guided percutaneous biopsy of spinal lesions. Biomed Imaging Interv J 2:e25

Phadke DM, Lucas DR, Madan S et al (2001) Fine-needle aspiration biopsy of vertebral and intervertebral disc lesions: specimen adequacy, diagnostic utility, and pitfalls. Arch Pathol Lab Med 125:1463–1468

Pierot L, Boulin A (1999) Percutaneous biopsy of the thoracic and lumbar spine: transpedicular approach under fluoroscopic guidance. AJNR Am J Neuroradiol 20:23–25

Rehm J, Veith S, Akbar M et al (2016) CT-guided percutaneous spine biopsy in suspected infection or malignancy: a study of 214 patients. Rofo 188:1156–1162

Rimondi E, Staals EL, Errani C et al (2008) Percutaneous CT-guided biopsy of the spine: results of 430 biopsies. Eur Spine J 17:975–981

Rubin BP, Antonescu CR, Gannon FH et al (2010) Members of the Cancer Committee, College of American Pathologists. Protocol for the examination of specimens from patients with tumors of bone. Arch Pathol Lab Med 134:e1–e7

Saifuddin A, Palloni V, du Preez H et al (2021) Review article: The current status of CT-guided needle biopsy of the spine. Skeletal Radiol 50:281–299

Saththianathan M, Mallinson PI, Munk PL et al (2022) Percutaneous spine biopsy: reaching those hard-to-reach places. Skeletal Radiol. https://doi.org/10.1007/s00256-022-04120-7

Silverman SG, Tuncali K, Adams DF et al (1999) CT fluoroscopy-guided abdominal interventions: techniques, results, and radiation exposure. Radiology 212:673–681

Singh DK, Kumar N, Nayak BK et al (2020) Approach-based techniques of CT-guided percutaneous vertebral biopsy. Diagn Interv Radiol 26:143–146

Suh CH, Yun SJ (2019) Diagnostic outcome of image-guided percutaneous core needle biopsy of sclerotic bone lesions: a meta-analysis. AJR Am J Roentgenol 212:625–631

Tehranzadeh J, Tao C, Browning CA (2007) Percutaneous needle biopsy of the spine. Acta Radiol 48:860–868

Wallace AN, Pacheco RA, Vyhmeister R et al (2016) Fluoroscopy-guided intervertebral disc biopsy with a coaxial drill system. Skeletal Radiol 45:273–278

Williams R, Foote M, Deverall H (2012) Strategy in the surgical treatment of primary spinal tumors. Global Spine J 2:249–266

Wu JS, Goldsmith JD, Horwich PJ et al (2008) Bone and soft-tissue lesions: what factors affect diagnostic yield of image-guided core-needle biopsy? Radiology 248:962–970

Wu MH, Xiao LF, Liu HW et al (2019) PET/CT-guided versus CT-guided percutaneous core biopsies in the diagnosis of bone tumors and tumor-like lesions: which is the better choice? Cancer Imaging 19:69

Yaffe D, Greenberg G, Leitner J et al (2003) CT-guided percutaneous biopsy of thoracic and lumbar spine: a new coaxial technique. AJNR Am J Neuroradiol 24:2111–2113

Yang SY, Oh E, Kwon JW et al (2018) Percutaneous image-guided spinal lesion biopsies: factors affecting higher diagnostic yield. AJR Am J Roentgenol 211:1068–1074

Part III

Imaging of Primary Bone Tumors of the Spine and Its Mimics

Vertebral Hemangioma and Angiomatous Neoplasms

Olivier Leroij and Filip Vanhoenacker

Contents

O. Leroij (✉)
Department of Radiology, AZ Sint-Maarten Mechelen, Mechelen, Belgium

University Hospital Antwerp, Antwerp, Belgium

University Antwerp, Antwerp, Belgium

F. Vanhoenacker
Department of Radiology, AZ Sint-Maarten Mechelen, Mechelen, Belgium

University Hospital Antwerp, Antwerp, Belgium

University Antwerp, Ghent and Leuven, Belgium
e-mail: filip.vanhoenacker@telenet.be

Abstract

Vertebral hemangiomas and angiomatous neoplasms consist of a group of vascular tumors that arise from the abnormal proliferation of blood vessels within the bone.

Vertebral hemangiomas are common, benign vascular tumors and are often discovered incidentally during routine imaging studies. These tumors are typically slow-growing and asymptomatic. Conventional radiography (CR) and computed tomography (CT) typically show a well-demarcated mass-like lesion of reduced bone density with thickened trabeculae. CR is not sensitive in the detection of these lesions. Thickened trabeculae are best seen on CT. On magnetic resonance imaging (MRI), the thickened trabeculae appear as low signal foci. Typical vertebral hemangiomas are of high signal intensity (SI) on T1- and T2-weighted images (WI). Atypical vertebral hemangiomas have a lower fat content and are of low SI on T1-WI and of high SI on T2-WI. Aggressive vertebral hemangiomas display aggressive behavior on imaging causing pain and neurological deficit. In general, aggressive vertebral hemangiomas are of low SI on T1-WI and of high SI on T2-WI.

Epithelioid hemangioma is a rare mesenchymal tumor of vascular origin. CT shows well-defined, septate, lytic lesions with cortical destruction and bony expansion. On MRI, lesions are hypointense or iso-intense to muscle on T1-WI, and hyperintense on T2-WI.

Med Radiol Diagn Imaging (2024)
https://doi.org/10.1007/174_2023_468,
Published Online: 17 January 2024

Epithelioid hemangioendothelioma is an intermediate-grade malignant vascular neoplasm. It presents as a mild expansile osteolysis, with ill-defined boundaries and a surrounding soft-tissue mass and uncommonly a sclerotic rim.

Angiosarcoma is a rare, aggressive, vascular malignancy with only rare cases reported in the spine. Angiosarcoma and epithelioid hemangioendothelioma show similar features radiologically.

1 Vertebral Hemangioma

1.1 Definition

Vertebral hemangiomas (VHs) are benign tumors of malformed blood vessels. They are not considered to be true vascular neoplasms, but rather congenital vascular malformations. Therefore, they cannot be classified as tumors, but rather as hamartomas (Slon et al. 2015; Nigro and Donnarumma 2017; Rodallec et al. 2008). Depending on the predominant vessel, they are classified into four histological types: capillary, cavernous, venous, and arteriovenous malformations. The cavernous type seems to be the most prevalent in the spine (Nigro and Donnarumma 2017). Differences in clinical history and radiological features exist among these histological types (Pastushyn et al. 1998).

1.2 Epidemiology

VHs are very common lesions; the prevalence ranges from 11% to 26% and is probably still underestimated. Patients can present with single or occasionally multiple VHs. There is a slight female predilection. VHs can be observed at any age, but older individuals (over 50 years old) are more commonly affected (Slon et al. 2015). The most common location is the vertebral body, with occasional extension to the posterior arch, with preferential involvement of the thoracic and lumbar spine (Gaudino et al. 2015).

1.3 Clinical Features

VHs are most frequently asymptomatic, quiescent lesions discovered incidentally on routine imaging. Rarely, they can become symptomatic (aka symptomatic VHs) and cause pain. If accompanied by neurological symptoms due to compression of the spinal cord or nerve roots resulting in myelopathy and/or radiculopathy, they are called "compressive VHs." Compression is caused by bone expansion, extension into the spinal canal, disturbance of blood flow, or epidural hemorrhage (Fox and Onofrio 1993; Gaudino et al. 2015). A unique form of onset occurs during pregnancy with rapid onset of symptoms in a previously asymptomatic VH (Nigro and Donnarumma 2017).

1.4 Histopathology

VHs are vascular malformations composed of capillary-sized to cavernous blood vessels. Macroscopically, the tissue appears as a well-delineated homogeneous or heterogeneous dark red mass with multiple interspersed discernible dots of a different reddish color (Baudrez et al. 2001). There are two main microscopic types, which frequently coexist.

Cavernous VHs are composed of large, dilated blood vessels closely clustered together. They are not separated by normal bone tissue.

Capillary VHs are formed by thin-walled vessels of various sizes separated by normal bone tissue or stroma tissue (Pastushyn et al. 1998). As a general characteristic, they are situated within a stroma composed of adipocytes and interstitial edema. The vessels permeate the bone marrow and surround preexisting trabeculae (Gaudino et al. 2015).

1.5 Imaging Features

On imaging, we can distinguish three different types of vertebral hemangiomas.

1.5.1 Typical Vertebral Hemangioma

These hemangiomas are rich in fat content and display typical imaging features, resulting from the fatty composition of the lesion, osseous rarefaction, and thickening of the trabeculae, caused by bone resorption from the crowding vessels (Persaud 2008).

- Conventional Radiography (CR)

  CR shows an area of reduced bone density with intralesional thickened vertical trabeculae. This may result in a "*corduroy cloth*" or "*jail bar*" appearance (Gaudino et al. 2015). One-third of the vertebral body must be involved for these characteristic findings to be apparent on CR. The vertical trabecular pattern is most clear on the lateral view (Fig. 1). The disk spaces are intact, and the vertebral cortex is preserved (Fox and Onofrio 1993). The presence of a vertebral fracture is rather a coincidental finding than a true complication of a VH. The hypothesis that VHs can lead to compression fractures due to weakening of the vertebral body is not accepted (Baudrez et al. 2001).

- Computed Tomography (CT)

  On unenhanced CT images, VHs typically appear as hypodense lesions with interspersed thickened trabeculae.

  In bone window, which is best suited for osseous evaluation, axial slices reveal small punctate areas of higher attenuation that correspond to thickened trabeculae. This results in a characteristic appearance that is commonly referred to as the "*polka-dot*" sign (Kim et al. 2017), due to its resemblance to a spotted or polka-dot pattern. On sagittal and coronal images, the thickened trabeculae are oriented vertically, creating the pattern known as the "*corduroy cloth*" sign (Fig. 2). Importantly, the bony cortex always appears intact without any evidence of extra-osseous extension.

  In soft tissue window, these thickened trabeculae can also be visualized, but this window is more suited for evaluation of attenuation of a hemangioma. The lesion can have fatty tissue or soft tissue attenuation or both (Laredo et al. 1990).

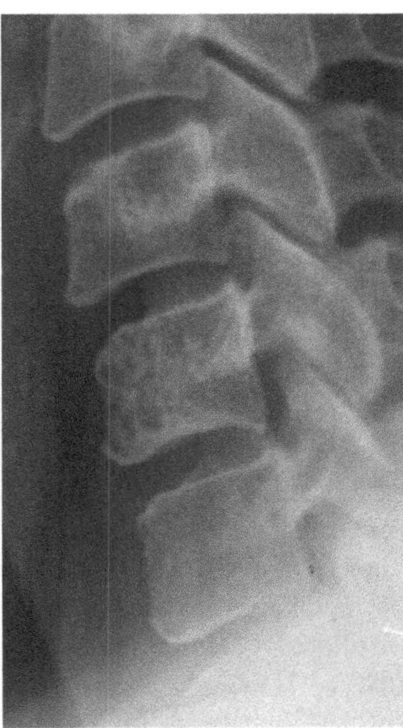

Fig. 1 Typical vertebral hemangioma. Sagittal CR showing a translucent lesion in the cervical vertebra. Irregular vertical struts can be seen within lesion

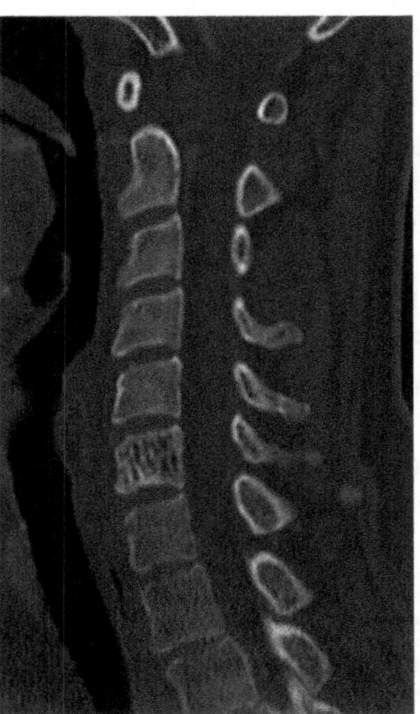

Fig. 2 Typical vertebral hemangioma. Sagittal CT image of the same patient as in Fig. 1. The thickened vertical trabeculae are better appreciated resulting in the "corduroy cloth" sign or "jail bar" appearance

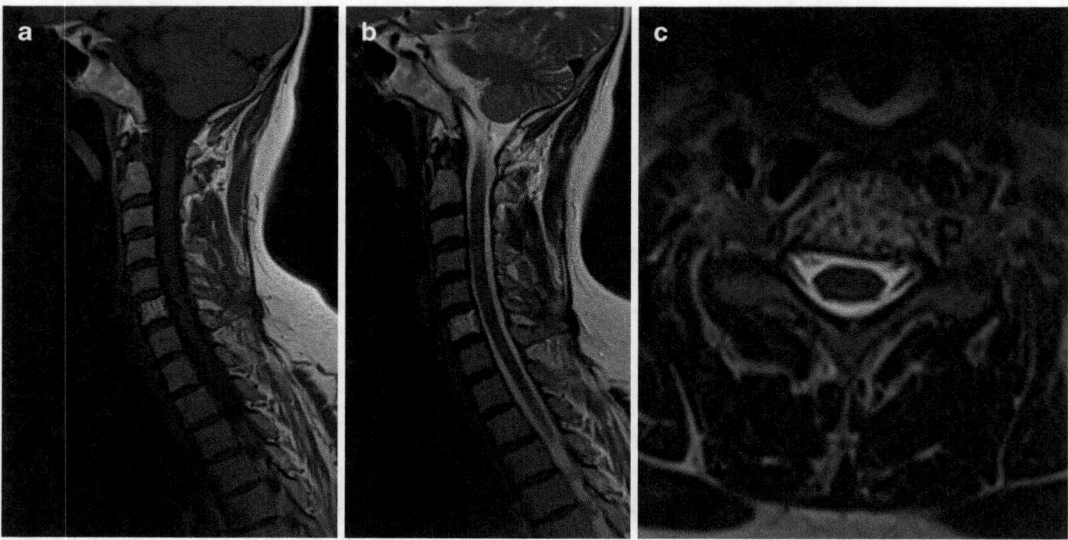

Fig. 3 Typical vertebral hemangioma. (**a**) Sagittal T1-WI of the cervical spine showing a hyperintense vertebral lesion with vertically oriented hypointense struts representing thickened trabeculae. (**b**) On sagittal T2-WI, the vertebral lesion is hyperintense. (**c**) Axial T2-WI showing an overall hyperintense signal of the vertebral body with intralesional hypointense dots. The low-signal-intensity dots represent the thickened trabeculae causing a "polka-dot" appearance

- Magnetic Resonance Imaging (MRI)

  The histological composition reflects the signal intensity on T1- and T2-WI, which is related to the relative number of adipocytes, vessels, and interstitial edema.

  The lesion is well defined, and the thickened trabeculae can be seen as low-signal-intensity dots on axial images or vertical struts on sagittal images on both T1- and T2-WI (Rodallec et al. 2008; Fox and Onofrio 1993). Overall, the lesion appears hyperintense on T1-WI due to its high fat content (Fig. 3). The Dixon method can be used as a fat suppression technique and is suitable for large field-of-view applications such as spinal imaging. The Dixon method is able to replace the information provided by the T1-WI sequence on bone marrow fat content. The fat content of VHs will show a higher SI on fat-only (FO) images compared to T1-WI. Areas of decreased fat content show lower SI compared to normal marrow (Omoumi 2022).

  It appears even more hyperintense on T2-WI, as compared to T1-WI, due to vascular tissue and a high water content (Baudrez et al. 2001; Gaudino et al. 2015; Ross et al. 1987).

  On fluid-sensitive sequences, the hyperintense signal is even more pronounced. Enhancement is variable on T1-WI after intravenous gadolinium contrast administration.

1.5.1.1 Nuclear Medicine

- Scintigraphy

  Planar bone scintigraphy with technetium-99m (99mTc)-labeled diphosphonates may demonstrate no uptake, increased uptake, or decreased uptake. Most VHs show a normal uptake; this means an equal uptake relative to the background vertebral uptake meaning that the lesion is not visible. The reason for the variable uptake is not known (Abdel Razek and Castillo 2010; Han et al. 1995).
- SPECT/CT

  SPECT/CT can be useful for a better delineation of the lesion compared to bone scintigraphy. Most VHs show normal uptake of 99mTc, and larger VHs show increased or decreased uptake (Han et al. 1995).

- PET/CT

  VHs can show as a "hot" or a "cold" lesion on fluorodeoxyglucose (FDG) PET/CT (Basu and Nair 2006).

Somatostatin receptor scintigraphy with ^{68}Ga DOTATATE, which is an established modality for imaging of well-differentiated neuroendocrine tumors, can also show uptake of ^{68}Ga DOTATATE in VHs and thus should be kept in mind as a benign differential diagnosis (Brogsitter et al. 2014).

1.5.2 Atypical Vertebral Hemangioma

These hemangiomas have less fatty and greater vascular content resulting in different signal intensities on MRI and therefore differing from the typical VHs.

On CR, however, they exhibit similar features as typical VHs.

On CT, the lesion may exhibit higher Hounsfield units, which can indicate lower fat content (Fig. 4). Sclerosis may be seen as well.

The signal intensity is low on T1-WI, as opposed to a high signal for a typical VHs.

Usually, the lower signal is homogeneous, but heterogeneous signal with low SI and high SI areas may be seen as well (Fig. 5).

The signal intensity is high on T2-WI due to the vascular contents.

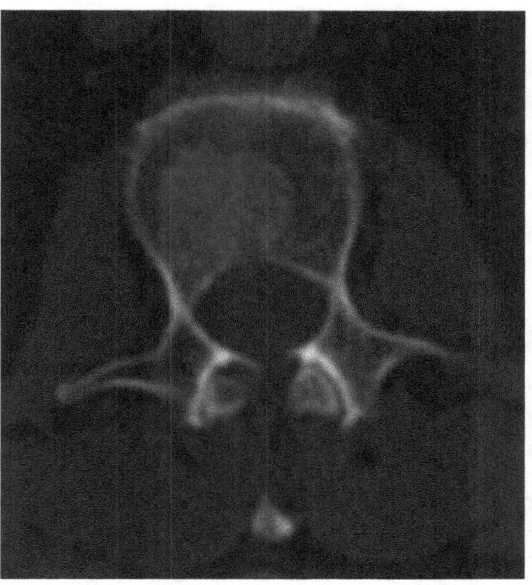

Fig. 4 Atypical sclerotic vertebral hemangioma. Axial CT showing a sharply demarcated focal area of sclerosis in the vertebral body. In this case, the thickened trabeculae are not visible

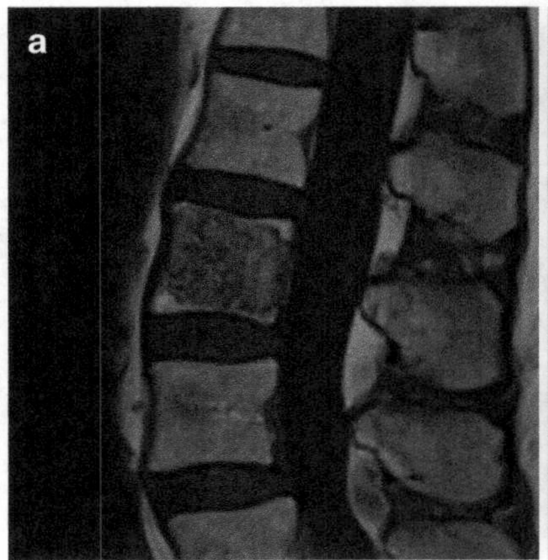

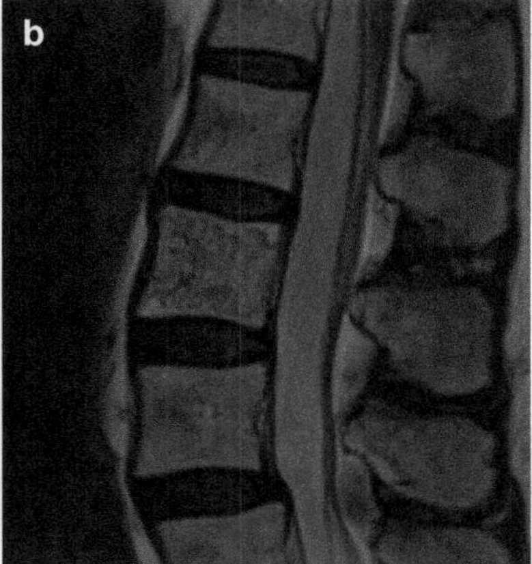

Fig. 5 Atypical vertebral hemangioma. (**a**) Sagittal T1-WI of the vertebral spine showing a well-delineated heterogenous predominantly hypointense lesion representing a vertebral hemangioma with a lower fat content. (**b**) On sagittal T2-WI, the lesion has a slightly heterogeneous signal, but overall slightly hyperintense compared to the other vertebra

The characteristic thickened trabeculae can be more difficult to appreciate on the different modalities, but this should always be sought meticulously as this is a major clue to the diagnosis of a vertebral hemangioma (Laredo et al. 1990; Hoyle et al. 2020; Gaudino et al. 2015).

In this regard, CT can be problem-solving by demonstrating these thickened trabeculae if MRI is not straightforward.

Atypical hemangiomas behave clinically similar to typical hemangioma; therefore, the term "lipid-poor" hemangioma is preferable to atypical because the term "atypical" has been associated with aggressive biological behavior (Hoyle et al. 2020).

1.5.3 Aggressive Vertebral Hemangioma

VHs can rarely display aggressive behavior on imaging and histopathology. This may result in neurological deficit, because of mass effect on the nerve roots and the spinal cord (Gaudino et al. 2015; Rodallec et al. 2008).

Neurological deficit may be caused by bony compression resulting from hypertrophy or "ballooning" of the posterior cortex of the vertebral body, enlargement of the laminae or the facets causing narrowing of the epidural and/or neuroforaminal space. Intraspinal or paravertebral bone formation can also cause bone compression, which is not uncommon and has important clinical significance. Deficit may also be caused directly by soft tissue compression of the VH on the spinal cord and nerves in the epidural and foraminal space. A combination of all the above effects can also cause neurological deficit (Jiang et al. 2014; Vilanova et al. 2004; Mohan et al. 1980). Spinal cord ischemia resulting from hemodynamic effects such as arterial "steal" and venous hypertension has also been described as a potential pathological mechanism (Urrutia et al. 2011).

CR may be unremarkable or show nonspecific findings, such as osteoporosis, poor delineation or expansion of cortex, vertebral collapse, or pedicle erosion associated with lytic areas of varying sizes.

CT is optimal for the visualization of osseous involvement. Bone window can reveal the bony compression as well as the ossification in the intraspinal or paraspinal regions and show osteolytic regions. CT is better to demonstrate thickened trabeculae. Soft tissue expansion can also be appreciated in the soft tissue window (Fig. 6) (Zhang et al. 2021; Gaudino et al. 2015). CT after intravenous contrast administration can be useful in evaluating the vascular nature of the lesion (Yu et al. 1984).

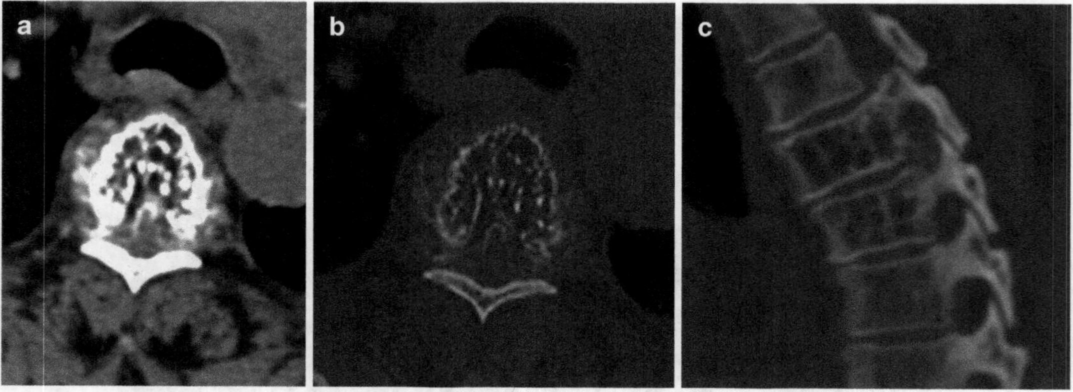

Fig. 6 Aggressive vertebral hemangioma. (**a**) Axial CT in soft tissue window showing an expansile vertebral lesion with poorly demarcated paravertebral soft tissue extension. The intralesional foci of low attenuation are in keeping with fat. (**b**) Axial CT in bone window showing subtle destruction of the cortical delineation of the vertebral body and narrowing of the spinal canal. Thickened trabeculae are the clue to the correct diagnosis of a vertebral hemangioma. (**c**) Sagittal CT in bone window showing a hypodense lesion with a discrete "jail bar" appearance and extension in the right neuroforamen

Aggressive VHs are difficult to diagnose on MRI. Aggressive VHs contain less fat than typical VHs, and therefore the signal intensity is hypointense on T1-WI. Intra-osseous signal intensity voids, corresponding to thickened trabeculae, may not be easily recognized on MRI. However, such voids represent the most useful MR imaging sign to characterize a VH, even in hypointense lesions on T1-WI, and are best recognized on axial images. A decreased fat content, leading to the atypical low T1-WI and high T2-WI MRI appearance, may suggest an active lesion and has a higher risk of having aggressive features (Nabavizadeh et al. 2016). However, there are studies that show no strong evidence that an atypical MRI appearance of a hemangioma predicts aggressive behavior (Hoyle et al. 2020). This hypothesis is therefore unreliable. Aggressive VHs with a high T1- and T2-WI signal, the MRI features of a typical VH, also do exist.

Most authors recognize that mottled high signal intensity on T1-WI is highly suggestive for aggressive VH (Cross et al. 2000). A minority can appear iso-intense to normal bone marrow on T2-WI, reflecting the relatively lower lipid and vascular content. Occasionally, symptomatic VHs are of hypointense or heterogeneous signal on T2-WI. This is related to several factors such as bone sclerosis, intralesional hemorrhage, or compression fracture (Zhang et al. 2021). A sharp margin with normal marrow and enlarged paraspinal vessels is only present in a minority of lesions (Gaudino et al. 2015; Cross et al. 2000; Puvaneswary et al. 2003).

CT-guided biopsy is useful for the final diagnosis and to differentiate with malignant tumors of the osseous spine. Biopsy should be recommended for aggressive VHs with atypical features (Wang et al. 2019).

Angiography can also be a useful diagnostic tool when an aggressive VH is suspected (Alexander et al. 2010). The angiographic appearance of aggressive vertebral hemangiomas is usually characteristic, with dilatation of arterioles, multiple blood pools in the capillary phase, and intense opacification extending beyond the normal vertebral territory (Friedman 1996; Healy et al. 1983).

1.6 Treatment

In general, treatment is only indicated for aggressive VHs to prevent neurological compression. It consists of radiotherapy, surgery, embolization, or vertebroplasty (Nigro and Donnarumma 2017). Treatment or follow-up for the typical and atypical VH is not necessary.

Observation for asymptomatic aggressive lesions is appropriate. For VHs presenting with pain, vertebroplasty is the treatment of choice. VHs with neurologic deficit or pain unresponsive to vertebroplasty, decompressive surgery, and stabilization are indicated (Dang et al. 2012). Recurrent VHs (Teferi et al. 2020) or painful VHs (Aksoy et al. 2022) can be treated with radiation therapy. Radiation can even be a first-line therapy for symptomatic VHs (Asthana et al. 1990).

Preoperative embolization of the lesion, if possible, for example during angiography, should be performed to avoid major bleeding during surgery (Jayakumar et al. 1997). Sclerotherapy by direct ethanol injection for treatment of aggressive VHs has promising results (Alexander et al. 2010). The best treatment of aggressive VH in pregnancy remains controversial, but the suggestion is to be as radical as possible with a prompt and wide decompression (Santagada et al. 2020; Hu et al. 2018; Dobran et al. 2018).

1.7 Differential Diagnosis

There is a big overlap between the imaging features of atypical as well as aggressive VHs and metastatic disease.

Metastases are the most common vertebral tumors and can be either osteolytic, osteoblastic, or both. Osteolytic metastases are more frequent than osteoblastic metastases, and osteolytic lesions may be of hypointense signal on T1-WI, a feature similar to atypical VHs. Aggressive VHs may display soft tissue extension mimicking metastasis (Rodallec et al. 2008; Gaudino et al. 2015).

CT is the most useful imaging tool in distinguishing the thickened trabeculae characteristic of VH, thus differentiating the two entities. If thickened trabeculae are not recognized, other imaging signs, as discussed below, should be sought.

The shape of time-intensity curves after dynamic contrast-enhanced MR imaging helps in differentiating between atypical VHs and metastases. The time-intensity curve of metastases shows a steeper slope with a higher peak and a faster washout. On the contrary, atypical VH shows minimal and delayed signal intensity without a steep slope and with slow washout (Morales et al. 2018). It is said that an atypical VH has a higher level of fat content compared to metastasis and can show a higher T1-WI signal. The ratio of signal intensity loss between T1-WI and fat-suppressed T1-WI is higher with atypical VH, compared to metastases (Shi et al. 2017). Diffusion-weighted images can also be used to differentiate atypical VH and metastases. The mean ADC value for atypical hemangiomas is 1884 ± 74 ($\times 10^{-6}$ mm^2/s), and the mean for metastatic lesions is 1008 ± 81 ($\times 10^{-6}$ mm^2/s) (Hajalioghli et al. 2020). Finally, all radiological modalities in addition to histopathological examination are often required for the correct diagnosis.

Fatty marrow islands (see also chapter "Lipogenic Tumors") are well-defined focal fat islands within the bone marrow of the spine or other parts of the axial skeleton. Fatty marrow islands are a developmental variation of the bone marrow conversion process. These islands are of high signal on T1-WI and vanish on fat-suppressed images. Fatty marrow islands are isointense to normal bone marrow on TIR sequences, whereas typical VHs are of high SI on TIR sequences (Nouh and Eid 2015).

Plasmacytoma (see also chapter "Plasmacytoma") represents a focal proliferation of malignant plasma cells without diffuse bone marrow involvement, and it is thought to be a precursor to multiple myeloma. Solitary plasmacytoma is an uncommon tumor in patients with plasma cell neoplasms. The majority of patients are over 60 years old and often manifest with a single collapsed vertebra (Gaudino et al. 2015). The vertebral body is the most common site of involvement. The radiological appearance is that of a purely lytic process replacing cancellous bone, which may result in a "mini brain" appearance on axial CT and MR imaging due to thickened cortical struts, resembling the sulci in the brain (Rodallec et al. 2008). Although previously reported as pathognomonic for plasmacytoma, this classical mini brain sign has also been reported in a case of a VH, so caution is warranted (Zhang et al. 2020). In one-third of cases, there is a multicystic "soap bubble" appearance. MRI often demonstrates a nonspecific pattern of decreased T1 and increased T2 signal, which makes the differential diagnosis very challenging. Age is probably a more helpful differentiating feature, because the majority (70%) of patients with plasmacytoma are over 60 years old, as stated earlier (Zbojniewicz et al. 2010).

Focal involvement of *multiple myeloma*, another differential diagnosis, may mimic atypical VHs. Changes between pre- and posttreatment MR images for multiple myeloma, in terms of dimension and signal intensity, can help to differentiate these two entities. A response of the lesion after treatment for multiple myeloma favors the diagnosis of multiple myeloma. The combination of a focal bone lesion with signs of osteoporosis or a pattern of diffuse bone marrow infiltration can suggest the diagnosis of multiple myeloma (Gaudino et al. 2015; Walker et al. 2007).

Primary spinal bone lymphoma (see also chapter "Lymphoma") is an extremely rare condition, which usually manifests as a combination of paraspinal, vertebral, and epidural involvement. Aggressive VHs and lymphoma lesions are usually lytic, showing an infiltrating pattern of growth. The epidural component of a vertebral lymphoma appears less hyperintense due to its high cellularity compared with the hypervascular component of VHs on fluid-sensitive MR images (Gaudino et al. 2015).

Chordomas (see also chapter "Notochordal Tumors") are the second most common primary malignant neoplasms of the spine. Chordomas arise from the remnants of the primitive notochord. The tumor shows gelatinous mucoid substance, hemorrhage, and necrotic areas and may contain osseous sequestra. Chordomas are most commonly located at the sacrococcygeal region and the clivus (Abdel Razek and Castillo 2010). Chordomas appear as a destructive, often expansile lesion centered in the midline. The lesion has a low attenuation on CT scans. Intratumoral areas of high attenuation on CT, representing osseous sequestra or destroyed bone rather than calcifications, can be present. Chordomas enhance heterogeneously after contrast administration.

Chordomas show low signal intensity on T1-WI, high signal on T2-WI, and heterogeneous contrast enhancement on MR imaging.

These features somewhat overlap with the radiological appearance of aggressive VHs, but the involvement of several vertebral segments, sparing of the posterior elements, osseous sequestra, and intratumoral hemorrhage are atypical features in aggressive VHs (Gaudino et al. 2015).

Paget's disease (see also chapter "Paget of the Spine") is a chronic metabolically active bone disease, characterized by a disturbance in bone modeling and remodeling due to an increase in osteoblastic and osteoclastic activity. The spine is the second most affected site. Paget's disease can involve either a single level or more than one level. The lumbar spine and more commonly the L4 and L5 levels are the most frequently involved sites. The earliest phase seen radiologically in the vertebra is the mixed phase. The apparently "early" radiographic appearance of vertebral body involvement in Paget's disease is thickening and hypertrophy of the trabecular bone, parallel to the end plates, which can appear similar to a thickened cortex and the trabecular thickening in VHs. The marrow signal changes in established Paget's disease vary with the stage of the disease. Low signal on T1-WI and mild high signal on T2-WI in the mixed hypervascular phase are seen, mimicking atypical VHs. The sclerotic phase of Paget's disease results in low signal on both T1- and T2-WI in the vertebra due to increased trabecular thickness, sclerosis, and marrow fibrosis. There is fatty transformation in the later stages when there is high signal on both T1- and T2-WI, similar to the signal intensities in typical VHs. Bone expansion is a common denominator in Paget's disease and an important differentiating feature (Dell'Atti et al. 2007).

2 Other Angiomatous Neoplasms

2.1 Epithelioid Hemangioma

Epithelioid hemangioma (EH) is a rare mesenchymal tumor of vascular origin. EH usually occurs as a reddish-brown mass forming in the skin of the head, neck, or extremities and is mostly found in young and middle-aged adults. EH was first recognized as a distinct entity in 1983 and has been called angiolymphoid hyperplasia with eosinophilia, inflammatory angiomatous nodule, and histiocytoid hemangioma. The new World Health Organization classification (2020) now recognizes EH as a separate entity that can be polyostotic. It is classified as locally aggressive, rarely presenting with lymphatic metastasis (Ahlawat and Fayad 2020). Previous reports indicate that EH in the spine arises mostly from the vertebral body and less commonly from the transverse processes. When EH occurs in osseous tissues, it is found most frequently in the long tubular bones of the proximal and distal extremities (Nielsen et al. 2009), followed by the short tubular bones of the distal lower extremities and flat bones. The prevalence of EH of the spine is 6–16%. EH presents most commonly with back pain and without neurological symptoms, and primary EH of the spine with neurological deficits appears to be extremely rare. Whether en bloc or piecemeal resection is optimal for treating spinal EH is controversial. Although the malignant potential of EH of the spine makes total resection desirable, radical resection might result in massive bleeding or neurological deterioration (Okada et al. 2019).

2.1.1 Imaging Features

On radiographs, the bone lesions often appear lytic, septate, and expansile. A lesion can show a smooth, thick periosteal reaction. CT shows well-defined, septate, lytic lesions with cortical destruction and bony expansion. The lesions are well defined on MRI, being hypointense or isointense to muscle on T1-WI and hyperintense on T2-WI (Errani et al. 2012).

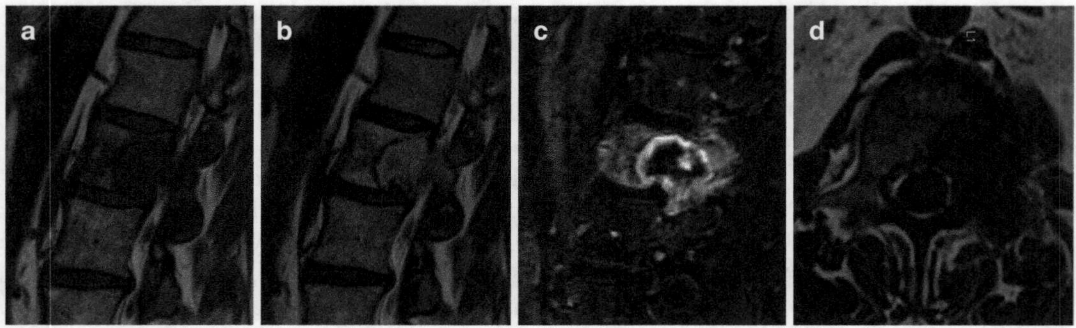

Fig. 7 Epithelioid hemangioendothelioma. (**a**) Sagittal T1-WI shows an aggressive hypointense ill-defined lesion with invasion of the lower end plate and the intervertebral disk. (**b**) On sagittal T2-WI, the lesion is mainly hyperintense with a peripheral sclerotic rim of low signal anteriorly. (**c**) Sagittal T1-WI with fat suppression after gadolinium contrast. Note vivid peripheral contrast enhancement with a nonenhancing center. Note the moderate contrast enhancement of the perilesional bone marrow and the soft tissue. (**d**) Axial T1-WI shows the hypointense lesion with invasion of the left pedicle and cortical destruction with extension into the paravertebral soft tissue on the left side

2.2 Epithelioid Hemangioendothelioma

Epithelioid hemangioendothelioma (EHE) is a true vascular neoplasm that can occur at any age but is most frequently seen during the second and third decades. It is defined as an intermediate-grade malignant vascular neoplasm that is less aggressive than angiosarcoma. EHE is typically painful and, when involving bone, most frequently involves the calvarium, axial skeleton, and lower limbs. Multifocal disease is seen in over 50% of cases, and given the potential for visceral involvement, CT examination of the chest, abdomen, and pelvis should be considered when the diagnosis is made. MRI is recommended for the extension of the soft tissues. The place of bone scintigraphy or PET/CT is not clearly established (Cousin et al. 2019).

Pathologically, the tumor consists of solid nests and anastomosing cords of round, polygonal, or spindle-shaped cells with eosinophilic cytoplasm. Intracytoplasmic vacuolization is a characteristic feature indicative of primitive vascular channels (Rosenberg and Agulnik 2018; Okada et al. 2019).

2.2.1 Imaging Features

In general, EHE manifests as a mild expansile osteolysis, with ill-defined boundaries and a surrounding soft tissue mass and uncommonly a sclerotic rim. It is prone to pathological compression fractures, which appear as a high signal on T2-WI. EHE is iso-intense on T1-WI and hyperintense on T2-WI with marked enhancement after contrast administration due to the vascular elements of the tumor (Fig. 7). EHE remains difficult to diagnose; some of the imaging features lack specificity, overlapping with other tumors (Chen et al. 2022).

2.3 Angiosarcoma

Angiosarcoma (AS) is a rare, aggressive, vascular malignancy with high local recurrence rate and distant metastasis, accounting for 2% of all sarcomas. Pathologically, these tumors may contain either hemangiomatous or lymphangiomatous cellular elements, which are often difficult or impossible to distinguish histologically, particularly with higher degrees of anaplasia. Identification of vascular channels allows to suggest the diagnosis. They occur predominantly in the soft tissue of the head and neck, followed by the extremities and the breast. Primary AS of bone has been described but makes up only 1% of ASs and has a predilection for the long tubular bones. Among osseous AS, only a handful of cases were reported in the spine. It occurs more frequently in males than females with a peak incidence in the sixth decade (Pülhorn et al. 2017).

Imaging signs on CR are not pathognomonic and are similar to the general features of malignant tumors, such as bone destruction, ill-defined margins, and involvement of surrounding soft tissue. Preoperatively, CT is necessary to define the extent of bony destruction, while MRI helps to assess the involvement of neural structures and relationship to other surrounding soft tissues (Murphey et al. 1995).

3 Conclusion

A typical hemangioma is a common incidental finding on imaging of the spine and is mostly easily characterized. The diagnosis of atypical and aggressive hemangiomas and other angiomatous tumors may be challenging. Indeterminate lesions should be referred for biopsy and interdisciplinary discussion in a tumor center.

4 Key Points

- The diagnosis of a typical vertebral hemangioma is relatively straightforward and has no clinical implications. The lesion is considered as a do not touch lesion, and no further treatment is needed.
- CT is more sensitive for detection compared to CR.
- The signal intensities on MRI vary along with the tissue composition of the lesion: T1 hyperintense signal correlates with fat content, whereas T2 hyperintense signal correlates with vascular tissue/edema.
- Atypical hemangiomas should be suspected when a lesion is T1 hypointense and T2 hyperintense.
- Aggressive hemangioma may be challenging to differentiate from metastasis.
- CT can be a problem solver by demonstrating the thickened trabeculae if MRI is inconclusive.
- Other vascular tumors of the osseous spine are rare and difficult to characterize on imaging. Histopathological examination is usually required for definitive diagnosis.

References

Abdel Razek AA, Castillo M (2010) Imaging appearance of primary bony tumors and pseudo-tumors of the spine. J Neuroradiol 37(1):37–50. https://doi.org/10.1016/j.neurad.2009.08.006

Ahlawat S, Fayad LM (2020) Revisiting the WHO classification system of bone tumours: emphasis on advanced magnetic resonance imaging sequences. Part 2. Pol J Radiol 85:e409–e419. https://doi.org/10.5114/pjr.2020.98686

Aksoy RA, Aksu MG, Korcum AF, Genc M (2022) Radiotherapy for vertebral hemangioma: the single-center experience of 80 patients. Strahlenther Onkol 198(7):648–653. https://doi.org/10.1007/s00066-022-01915-4

Alexander J, Meir A, Vrodos N, Yau YH (2010) Vertebral hemangioma: an important differential in the evaluation of locally aggressive spinal lesions. Spine (Phila Pa 1976) 35(18):E917–E920. https://doi.org/10.1097/brs.0b013e3181ddfb24

Asthana AK, Tandon SC, Pant GC, Srivastava A, Pradhan S (1990) Radiation therapy for symptomatic vertebral haemangioma. Clin Oncol (R Coll Radiol) 2(3):159–162. https://doi.org/10.1016/s0936-6555(05)80151-7

Basu S, Nair N (2006) "Cold" vertebrae on F-18 FDG PET: causes and characteristics. Clin Nucl Med 31(8):445–450. https://doi.org/10.1097/01.rlu.0000227011.21544.19

Baudrez V, Galant C, Vande Berg BC (2001) Benign vertebral hemangioma: MR-histological correlation. Skeletal Radiol 30(8):442–446. https://doi.org/10.1007/s002560100390

Brogsitter C, Hofmockel T, Kotzerke J (2014) (68)Ga DOTATATE uptake in vertebral hemangioma. Clin Nucl Med 39(5):462–463. https://doi.org/10.1097/rlu.0000000000000282

Chen Y, Xing X, Zhang E, Zhang J, Yuan H, Lang N (2022) Epithelioid hemangioendothelioma of the spine: an analysis of imaging findings. Insights Imaging 13(1):56. https://doi.org/10.1186/s13244-022-01197-5

Cousin S, Le Loarer F, Crombé A, Karanian M, Minard-Colin V, Penel N (2019) Epithelioid hemangioendothelioma. Bull Cancer 106(1):73–83. https://doi.org/10.1016/j.bulcan.2018.11.004

Cross JJ, Antoun NM, Laing RJ, Xuereb J (2000) Imaging of compressive vertebral haemangiomas. Eur Radiol 10(6):997–1002. https://doi.org/10.1007/s003300051051

Dang L, Liu C, Yang SM, Jiang L, Liu ZJ, Liu XG, Yuan HS, Wei F, Yu M (2012) Aggressive vertebral hemangioma of the thoracic spine without typical radiological appearance. Eur Spine J 21(10):1994–1999. https://doi.org/10.1007/s00586-012-2349-1

Dell'Atti C, Cassar-Pullicino VN, Lalam RK, Tins BJ, Tyrrell PN (2007) The spine in Paget's disease. Skeletal Radiol 36(7):609–626. https://doi.org/10.1007/s00256-006-0270-6

Dobran M, Mancini F, Nasi D, Gladi M, Sisti S, Scerrati M (2018) Surgical treatment of aggressive vertebral hemangioma causing progressive paraparesis. Ann Med Surg (Lond) 25:17–20. https://doi.org/10.1016/j.amsu.2017.12.001

Errani C, Zhang L, Panicek DM, Healey JH, Antonescu CR (2012) Epithelioid hemangioma of bone and soft tissue: a reappraisal of a controversial entity. Clin Orthop Relat Res 470(5):1498–1506. https://doi.org/10.1007/s11999-011-2070-0

Fox MW, Onofrio BM (1993) The natural history and management of symptomatic and asymptomatic vertebral hemangiomas. J Neurosurg 78(1):36–45. https://doi.org/10.3171/jns.1993.78.1.0036

Friedman DP (1996) Symptomatic vertebral hemangiomas: MR findings. AJR Am J Roentgenol 167(2):359–364. https://doi.org/10.2214/ajr.167.2.8686604

Gaudino S, Martucci M, Colantonio R, Lozupone E, Visconti E, Leone A, Colosimo C (2015) A systematic approach to vertebral hemangioma. Skeletal Radiol 44(1):25–36. https://doi.org/10.1007/s00256-014-2035-y

Hajalioghli P, Daghighi MH, Ghaffari J, Mirza-Aghazadeh-Attari M, Khamanian J, Ghaderi P, Yazdaninia I, Daghighi S, Zarrintan A (2020) Accuracy of diffusion-weighted imaging in discriminating atypical vertebral haemangiomas from malignant masses in patients with vertebral lesions: a cross-sectional study. Pol J Radiol 85:e340–e347. https://doi.org/10.5114/pjr.2020.97602

Han BK, Ryu JS, Moon DH, Shin MJ, Kim YT, Lee HK (1995) Bone SPECT imaging of vertebral hemangioma correlation with MR imaging and symptoms. Clin Nucl Med 20(10):916–921. https://doi.org/10.1097/00003072-199510000-00014

Healy M, Herz DA, Pearl L (1983) Spinal hemangiomas. Neurosurgery 13(6):689–691. https://doi.org/10.1227/00006123-198312000-00013

Hoyle JM, Layfield LJ, Crim J (2020) The lipid-poor hemangioma: an investigation into the behavior of the "atypical" hemangioma. Skeletal Radiol 49(1):93–100. https://doi.org/10.1007/s00256-019-03257-2

Hu W, Kan SL, Xu HB, Cao ZG, Zhang XL, Zhu RS (2018) Thoracic aggressive vertebral hemangioma with neurologic deficit: a retrospective cohort study. Medicine (Baltimore) 97(41):e12775. https://doi.org/10.1097/md.0000000000012775

Jayakumar PN, Vasudev MK, Srikanth SG (1997) Symptomatic vertebral haemangioma: endovascular treatment of 12 patients. Spinal Cord 35(9):624–628. https://doi.org/10.1038/sj.sc.3100438

Jiang L, Liu XG, Yuan HS, Yang SM, Li J, Wei F, Liu C, Dang L, Liu ZJ (2014) Diagnosis and treatment of vertebral hemangiomas with neurologic deficit: a report of 29 cases and literature review. Spine J 14(6):944–954. https://doi.org/10.1016/j.spinee.2013.07.450

Kim DJ, Shim E, Kim BH, Yeom SK (2017) The "polka-dot" sign. Abdom Radiol (NY) 42(8):2194–2196. https://doi.org/10.1007/s00261-017-1109-4

Laredo JD, Assouline E, Gelbert F, Wybier M, Merland JJ, Tubiana JM (1990) Vertebral hemangiomas: fat content as a sign of aggressiveness. Radiology 177(2):467–472. https://doi.org/10.1148/radiology.177.2.2217787

Mohan V, Gupta SK, Tuli SM, Sanyal B (1980) Symptomatic vertebral haemangiomas. Clin Radiol 31(5):575–579. https://doi.org/10.1016/s0009-9260(80)80055-9

Morales KA, Arevalo-Perez J, Peck KK, Holodny AI, Lis E, Karimi S (2018) Differentiating atypical hemangiomas and metastatic vertebral lesions: the role of T1-weighted dynamic contrast-enhanced MRI. AJNR Am J Neuroradiol 39(5):968–973. https://doi.org/10.3174/ajnr.A5630

Murphey MD, Fairbairn KJ, Parman LM, Baxter KG, Parsa MB, Smith WS (1995) From the archives of the AFIP. Musculoskeletal angiomatous lesions: radiologic-pathologic correlation. Radiographics 15(4):893–917. https://doi.org/10.1148/radiographics.15.4.7569134

Nabavizadeh SA, Mamourian A, Schmitt JE, Cloran F, Vossough A, Pukenas B, Loevner LA, Mohan S (2016) Utility of fat-suppressed sequences in differentiation of aggressive vs typical asymptomatic haemangioma of the spine. Br J Radiol 89(1057):20150557. https://doi.org/10.1259/bjr.20150557

Nielsen GP, Srivastava A, Kattapuram S, Deshpande V, O'Connell JX, Mangham CD, Rosenberg AE (2009) Epithelioid hemangioma of bone revisited: a study of 50 cases. Am J Surg Pathol 33(2):270–277. https://doi.org/10.1097/PAS.0b013e31817f6d51

Nigro L, Donnarumma P (2017) Vertebral hemangiomas: common lesions with still many unknown aspects. J Spine Surg 3(2):309–311. https://doi.org/10.21037/jss.2017.05.11

Nouh MR, Eid AF (2015) Magnetic resonance imaging of the spinal marrow: basic understanding of the normal marrow pattern and its variant. World J Radiol 7(12):448–458. https://doi.org/10.4329/wjr.v7.i12.448

Okada EM, Matsumoto MM, Nishida M, Iga T, Morishita M, Tezuka M, Mukai K, Kobayashi E, Watanabe K (2019) Epithelioid hemangioma of the thoracic spine: a case report and review of the literature. J Spinal Cord Med 42(6):800–805. https://doi.org/10.1080/10790268.2017.1390032

Omoumi P (2022) The Dixon method in musculoskeletal MRI: from fat-sensitive to fat-specific imaging. Skeletal Radiol 51(7):1365–1369. https://doi.org/10.1007/s00256-021-03950-1

Pastushyn AI, Slin'ko EI, Mirzoyeva GM (1998) Vertebral hemangiomas: diagnosis, management, natural history and clinicopathological correlates in 86 patients. Surg Neurol 50(6):535–547. https://doi.org/10.1016/s0090-3019(98)00007-x

Persaud T (2008) The polka-dot sign. Radiology 246(3):980–981. https://doi.org/10.1148/radiol.2463050903

Pülhorn H, Elliot T, Clark J, Gonzalvo A (2017) Case report: Angiosarcoma of the cervical spine. J Clin Neurosci 45:129–131. https://doi.org/10.1016/j.jocn.2017.07.018

Puvaneswary M, Cuganesan R, Barbarawi M, Spittaler P (2003) Vertebral haemangioma causing cord compression: MRI findings. Australas Radiol 47(2):190–193. https://doi.org/10.1046/j.0004-8461.2003.01151.x

Rodallec MH, Feydy A, Larousserie F, Anract P, Campagna R, Babinet A, Zins M, Drapé JL (2008) Diagnostic imaging of solitary tumors of the spine: what to do and say. Radiographics 28(4):1019–1041. https://doi.org/10.1148/rg.284075156

Rosenberg A, Agulnik M (2018) Epithelioid hemangioendothelioma: update on diagnosis and treatment. Curr Treat Options Oncol 19(4):19. https://doi.org/10.1007/s11864-018-0536-y

Ross JS, Masaryk TJ, Modic MT, Carter JR, Mapstone T, Dengel FH (1987) Vertebral hemangiomas: MR imaging. Radiology 165(1):165–169. https://doi.org/10.1148/radiology.165.1.3628764

Santagada DA, Perna A, Meluzio MC, Ciolli G, Proietti L, Tamburrelli FC (2020) Symptomatic vertebral hemangioma during pregnancy period: a case series and systematic literature review. Orthop Rev (Pavia) 12(Suppl 1):8685. https://doi.org/10.4081/or.2020.8685

Shi YJ, Li XT, Zhang XY, Liu YL, Tang L, Sun YS (2017) Differential diagnosis of hemangiomas from spinal osteolytic metastases using 3.0 T MRI: comparison of T1-weighted imaging, chemical-shift imaging, diffusion-weighted and contrast-enhanced imaging. Oncotarget 8(41):71095–71104. https://doi.org/10.18632/oncotarget.20533

Slon V, Stein D, Cohen H, Sella-Tunis T, May H, Hershkovitz I (2015) Vertebral hemangiomas: their demographical characteristics, location along the spine and position within the vertebral body. Eur Spine J 24(10):2189–2195. https://doi.org/10.1007/s00586-015-4022-y

Teferi N, Abukhiran I, Noeller J, Helland LC, Bathla G, Ryan EC, Nourski KV, Hitchon PW (2020) Vertebral hemangiomas: diagnosis and management. A single center experience. Clin Neurol Neurosurg 190:105745. https://doi.org/10.1016/j.clineuro.2020.105745

Urrutia J, Postigo R, Larrondo R, Martin AS (2011) Clinical and imaging findings in patients with aggressive spinal hemangioma requiring surgical treatment. J Clin Neurosci 18(2):209–212. https://doi.org/10.1016/j.jocn.2010.05.022

Vilanova JC, Barceló J, Smirniotopoulos JG, Pérez-Andrés R, Villalón M, Miró J, Martin F, Capellades J, Ros PR (2004) Hemangioma from head to toe: MR imaging with pathologic correlation. Radiographics 24(2):367–385. https://doi.org/10.1148/rg.242035079

Walker R, Barlogie B, Haessler J, Tricot G, Anaissie E, Shaughnessy JD Jr, Epstein J, van Hemert R, Erdem E, Hoering A, Crowley J, Ferris E, Hollmig K, van Rhee F, Zangari M, Pineda-Roman M, Mohiuddin A, Yaccoby S, Sawyer J, Angtuaco EJ (2007) Magnetic resonance imaging in multiple myeloma: diagnostic and clinical implications. J Clin Oncol 25(9):1121–1128. https://doi.org/10.1200/jco.2006.08.5803

Wang B, Zhang L, Yang S, Han S, Jiang L, Wei F, Yuan H, Liu X, Liu Z (2019) Atypical radiographic features of aggressive vertebral hemangiomas. J Bone Joint Surg Am 101(11):979–986. https://doi.org/10.2106/jbjs.18.00746

Yu R, Brunner DR, Rao KC (1984) Role of computed tomography in symptomatic vertebral hemangiomas. J Comput Tomogr 8(4):311–315. https://doi.org/10.1016/0149-936x(84)90081-x

Zbojniewicz AM, Hartel J, Nguyen T, Wilks K, Mace A, Hogg JP (2010) Neoplastic disease of the vertebral column: radiologic-pathologic correlation. Curr Probl Diagn Radiol 39(2):74–90. https://doi.org/10.1067/j.cpradiol.2009.07.004

Zhang D, Andrade JP, Cassis J, Soares P (2020) The "mini brain" sign in a case of vertebral hemangioma mimicking solitary plasmacytoma of the spine: refutal of a pathognomonic sign? Clin Neuroradiol 30(1):173–175. https://doi.org/10.1007/s00062-019-00788-y

Zhang L, Wang B, Han S, Yang S, Jiang L, Yuan H, Liu Z (2021) Imaging features and atypical signs of symptomatic vertebral haemangioma: a retrospective single-centre analysis of 118 patients. Br J Radiol 94(1121):20201250. https://doi.org/10.1259/bjr.20201250

Bone Island

Filip M. Vanhoenacker and Aseel Al-Musaedi

Contents

F. M. Vanhoenacker (✉)
Department of Radiology, AZ Sint-Maarten, Mechelen, Belgium

Antwerp University Hospital, Edegem, Belgium

Faculty of Medicine and Health Sciences, University of Antwerp, Ghent and Leuven, Belgium
e-mail: filip.vanhoenacker@telenet.be

A. Al-Musaedi
Department of Radiology, AZ Sint-Maarten, Mechelen, Belgium

Abstract

Bone islands (enostoses) are osteoblastic benign bony lesions. They consist of focal regions of mature bone cortex at the site of trabecular bone. Bone islands are thought to result from failure of bone resorption during endochondral ossification process or due to congenital etiology or failure of the development during childhood. The prevalence of bone islands is variable; the incidence of bone islands in the spine ranges between 1% and 15% on imaging studies. Clinically, bone islands are asymptomatic and mostly diagnosed incidentally on imaging done for other indications. This chapter focuses on the imaging features of bone islands involving the spine and their differential diagnosis with osteoblastic metastases. Meticulous analysis of the imaging features allows final characterization of bone islands in most cases. Although the lesions may be detected on conventional radiography, this examination is less sensitive for detection because of the complex anatomy of the spine. Computed tomography is better suited for detection and plays a pivotal role in the characterization of dense bone islands based on morphological (spicular margins) and quantitative parameters (Hounsfield units). On magnetic resonance imaging, dense bone islands are hypointense on all pulse sequences. As bone islands need no further intervention or treatment, it is of utmost importance to avoid unnecessary biopsy and potential harmful treatment.

Med Radiol Diagn Imaging (2023)
https://doi.org/10.1007/174_2023_448,
Published Online: 31 October 2023

1 Introduction

Since the first description of enostosis by Stieda in 1905 (Stieda 1905; Greenspan 1995), bone islands have been reported extensively in the literature.

The WHO recommends the term bone island as the correct terminology (Baumhoer et al. 2020).

Bone island is an idiopathic osteoblastic benign lesion, consisting of intramedullary foci of mature compact bone merging with the adjacent trabecular bone (Broski et al. 2022; Baumhoer et al. 2020).

Pathophysiologically, bone islands are believed to be a failure at the end stage of bone resorption during the endochondral ossification process and are of congenital or developmental origin (Diab et al. 2014). Other authors considered bone islands as an anatomic variant consisting of hamartomatous cortical bone embedded within the spongiosa (Alfahad et al. 2021). Bone islands are often incidental findings on imaging. They are mostly solitary and sporadic lesions, but they may be multiple particularly in osteopoikilosis (Baumhoer et al. 2020; Vanhoenacker et al. 2000). The clinical and practical importance of these benign lesions is that they may mimic neoplastic pathology and thus require recognition to prevent unnecessary investigations (Greenspan 1995).

This chapter focuses on bone islands involving the osseous spine.

2 Pathologic and Histologic Features

Macroscopically, a bone island arises in the medullary cavity as a solid, hard, and tan-white area blending peripherally into the surrounding cancellous trabecula (Baumhoer et al. 2020). Microscopically, they consist of bone cortex of the predominantly dense lamellar bone or as focal woven bone and contain Haversian-like canals (Greenspan et al. 1991). The surface lining of osteoblasts is quiescent and flat, whereas osteocytes are banal and small.

They range in size from 1 to 20 mm. When they become larger, they are referred to as the giant-type bone islands (White and Kandel 2000).

3 Epidemiology

Bone islands are rare in the pediatric population (Alfahad et al. 2021).

There is no sex or age preference (Greenspan et al. 1991).

Its incidence in the spine is estimated between 1% and 15% (Olvi et al. 2015).

4 Localization

Bone islands may be located in virtually any bone (Alfahad et al. 2021; Baumhoer et al. 2020). They are usually located in the axial skeleton including spine, ribs, pelvis, and long bones, particularly the femora. In the long bones, they are mostly seen in the epiphysis and metaphysis (Greenspan et al. 1991; Broski et al. 2022).

Within the spine, a bone island is typically located within the vertebral body (Figs. 1, 3, 4, and 6) and occasionally within the posterior elements (Fig. 2).

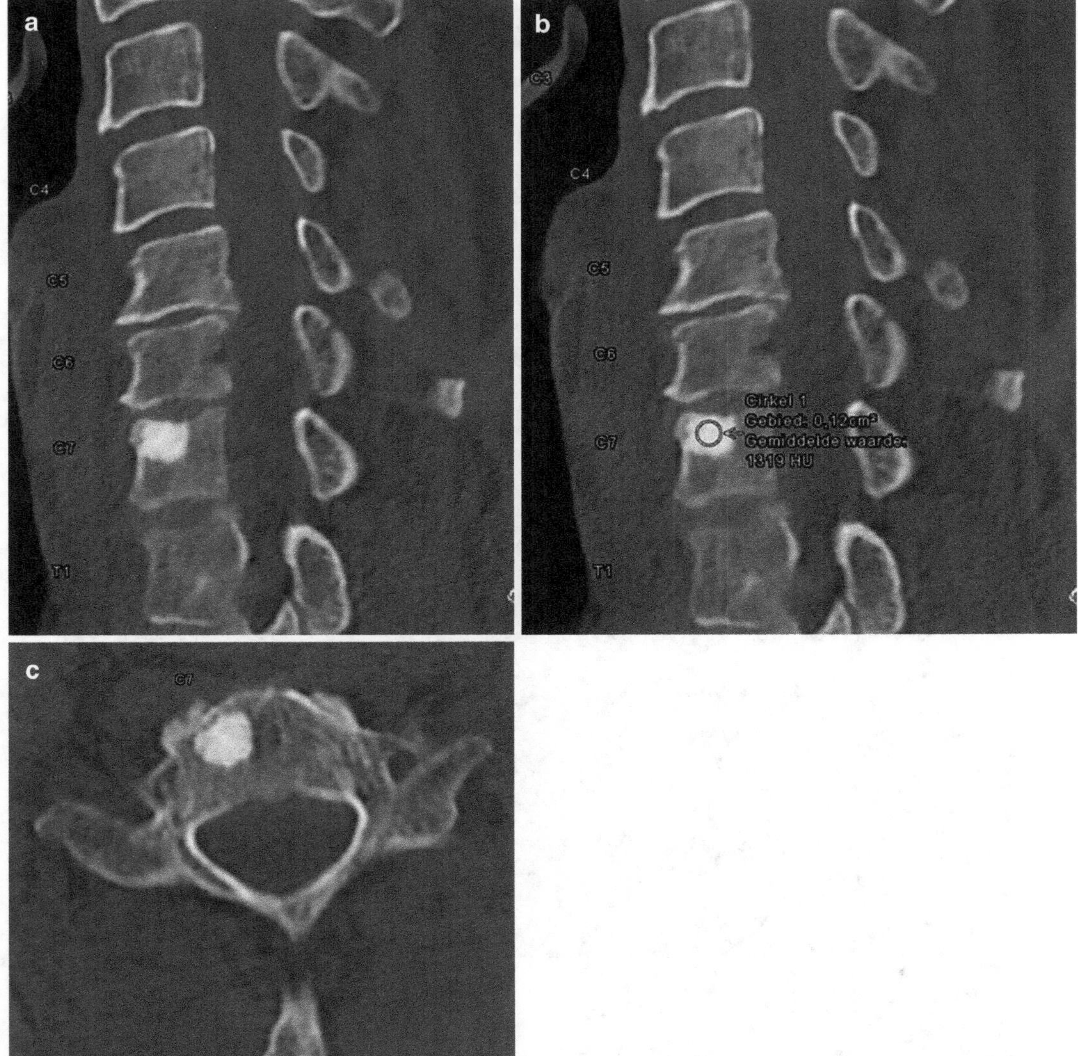

Fig. 1 Sagittal (**a**, **b**) and axial (**c**) CT shows a sclerotic intramedullary focus with spiculated margins in the vertebral body C7 with a mean attenuation of 1319 HU, in keeping with a bone island. The lesion contacts the superior end plate of C7

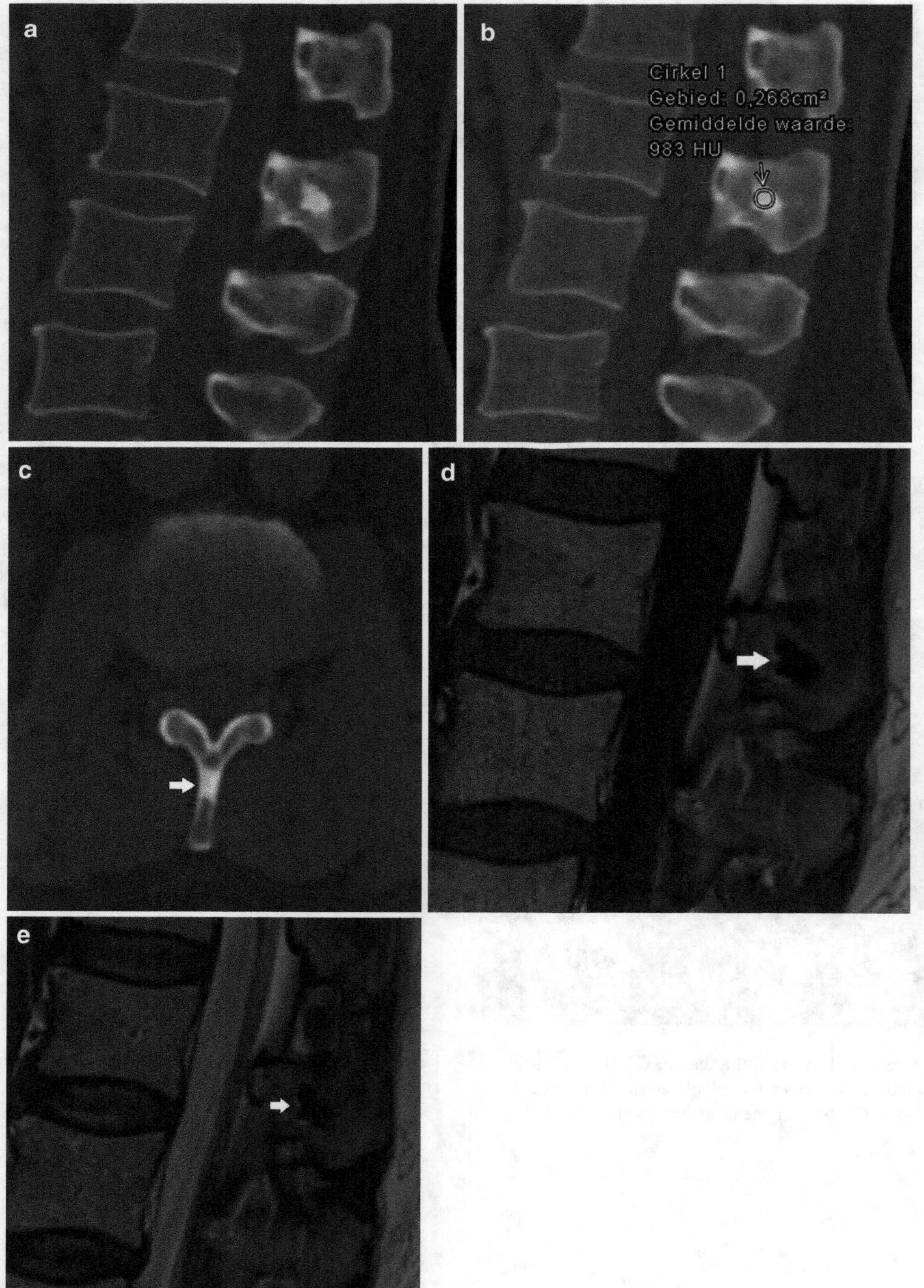

Fig. 2 Sagittal (**a**, **b**) and axial (**c**) CT shows a sclerotic intramedullary focus with spiculated margins in spinous process of a lumbar vertebra (**a**) with a mean attenuation of 983 HU (**b**). The lesion abuts the cortex of the spinous process (white arrow) (**c**). The lesion (white arrow) is hypointense to fatty bone marrow on T1-weighted images (WI) (**d**) and T2-WI (**e**)

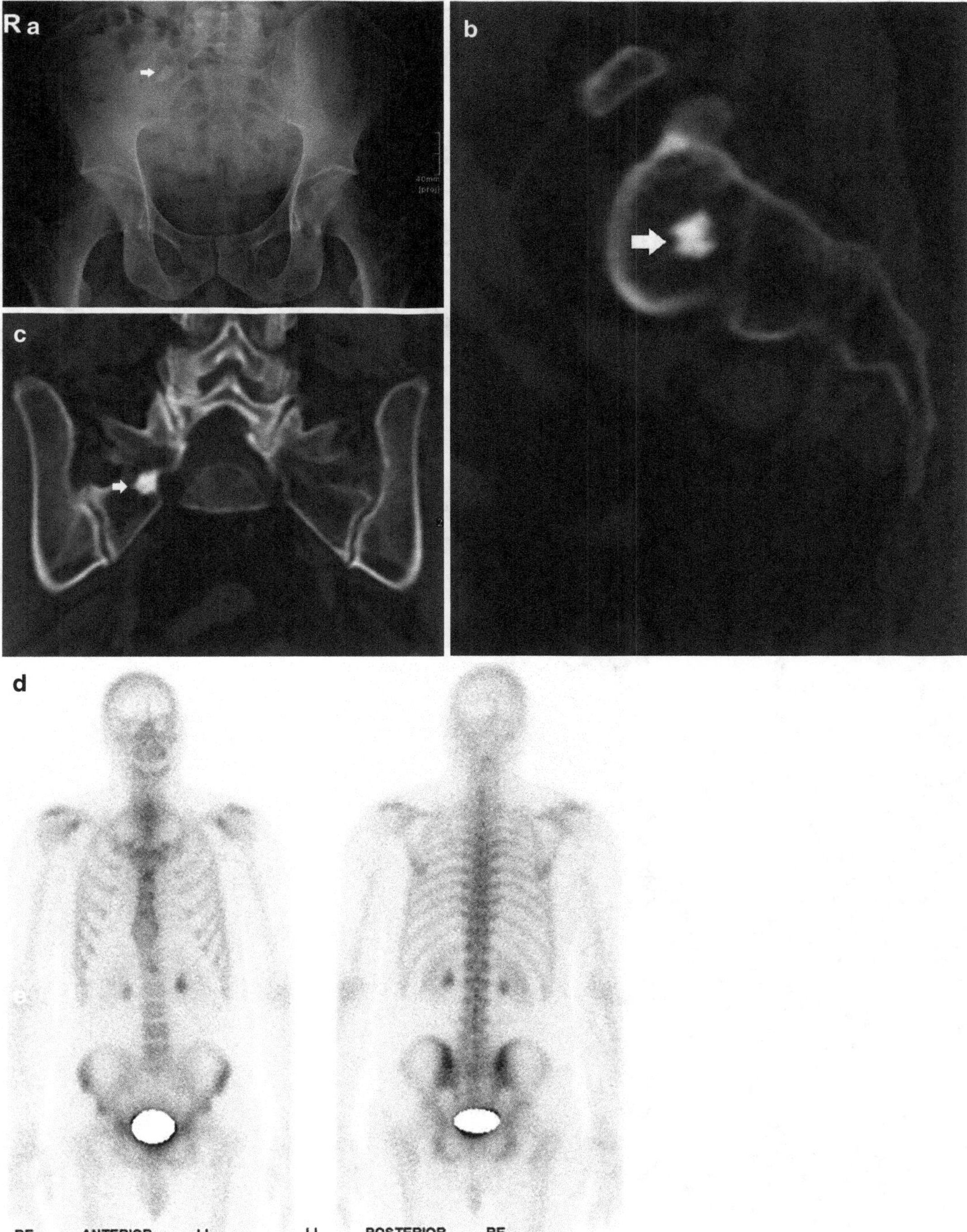

Fig. 3 Anteroposterior radiograph of the pelvis (**a**), sagittal (**b**), and coronal CT (**c**) of the sacrum shows a sclerotic focus with spiculated margins in the sacral ala (white arrow). (**d**) Bone scintigraphy shows no uptake

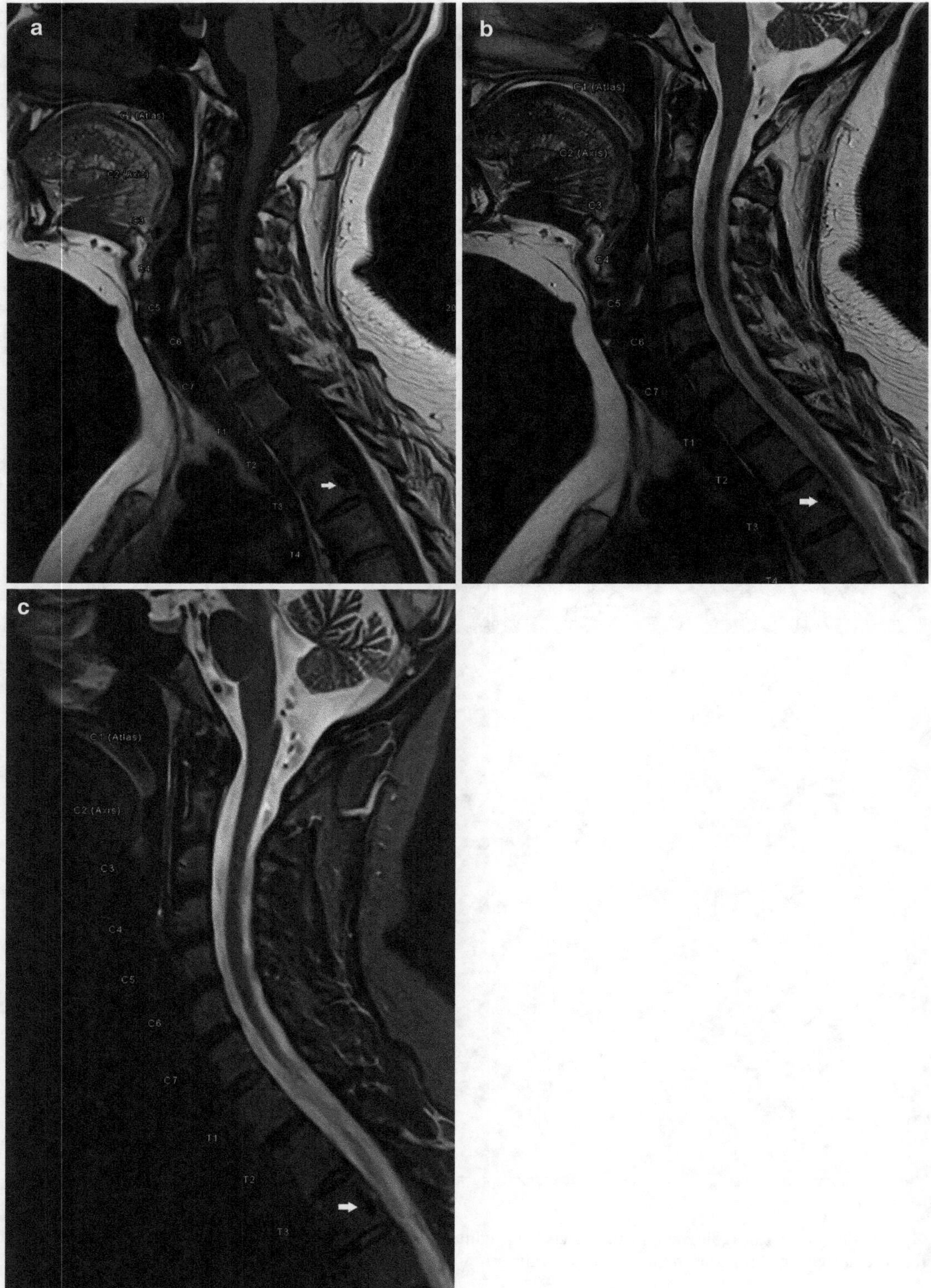

Fig. 4 Sagittal T1-WI (**a**), T2-WI (**b**), and STIR (**c**) show a hypointense lesion on all pulse sequences in the vertebral body Th3 (white arrows)

5 Clinical Presentation

Bone island is almost always an asymptomatic benign lesion and is incidentally detected on imaging (Greenspan et al. 1991). Usually, they are stable on follow-up. The size of the lesion may rarely fluctuate due to the presence of intrinsic osteoblastic or osteoclastic activities (Alfahad et al. 2021).

Multiple bone islands, with or without associated osteomas, may be part of Gardner's syndrome (Sinnott and Hodges 2020).

Some lesions are progressive and become symptomatic especially if more than 2 cm in size (giant bone islands). Small bone islands are very rarely painful (Diab et al. 2014).

6 Imaging

6.1 Conventional Radiography (CR)

Imaging often starts with CR, because this examination is inexpensive, easy to perform, and accessible.

Bone islands appear as homogeneously sclerotic dense lesions equivalent to cortical bone with a rounded, oval, or oblong shape and spiculated margins (Broski et al. 2022) (Fig. 3).

They may be single or multiple. The lesions may be either located within the trabecular bone or based on the endosteal surface of bone. Unlike osteoma, they do not involve the external cortex. Periosteal reaction is absent (Baumhoer et al. 2020).

6.2 Computed Tomography (CT)

CT is regarded as the gold standard for detection and characterization of these lesions (Broski et al. 2022). CT is more sensitive than CR to detect small bone islands in the spine, because—unlike CR—there is no superimposition of adjacent structures. Similar to CR, bone islands present as a rounded or oval-shape areas of sclerosis with an irregular and a spiculated margin (Figs. 1, 2, 3, 5, and 6). The spicules tend to blend with the trabeculae of the surrounding cancellous bone, resulting in so-called brush border margins (Murphey et al. 1996; Riahi et al. 2018). These morphological features of the island's morphology are the key imaging features in distinguishing bone islands from osseous metastases or primary bone-forming tumors on CR and CT. In addition, by measuring Hounsfield units (HU), CT provides quantitative data that allows further differentiation of a bone island from an untreated metastasis, since a bone island is denser than metastasis (Broski et al. 2022). In a large study of metastatic lung cancer, CT scan has been found to be better at differentiating bone metastasis from bone islands in 122 vertebral lesions (43

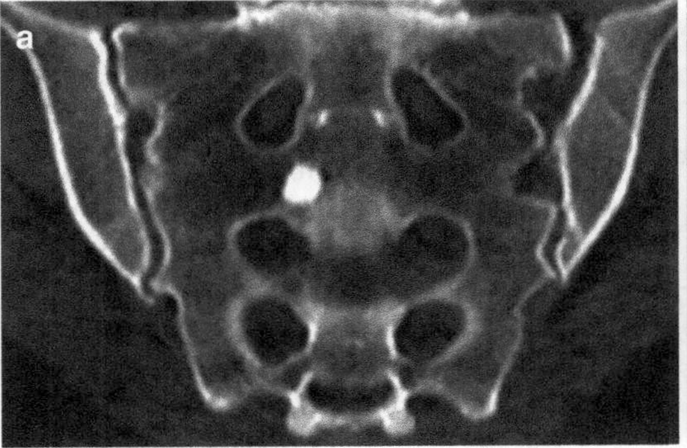

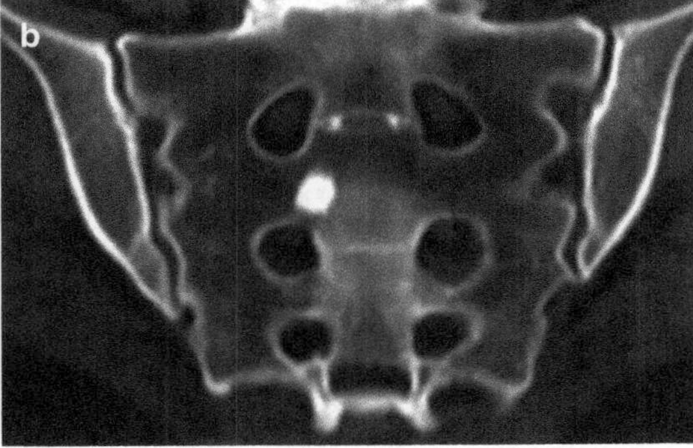

Fig. 5 Oblique coronal conventional CT (**a**) and synthetic CT (**b**) show a typical bone island in the sacrum. The morphology of the lesion can be equally evaluated on conventional as on synthetic CT. (Images courtesy of Lieve Morbée, MD, PhD, Ghent, Belgium)

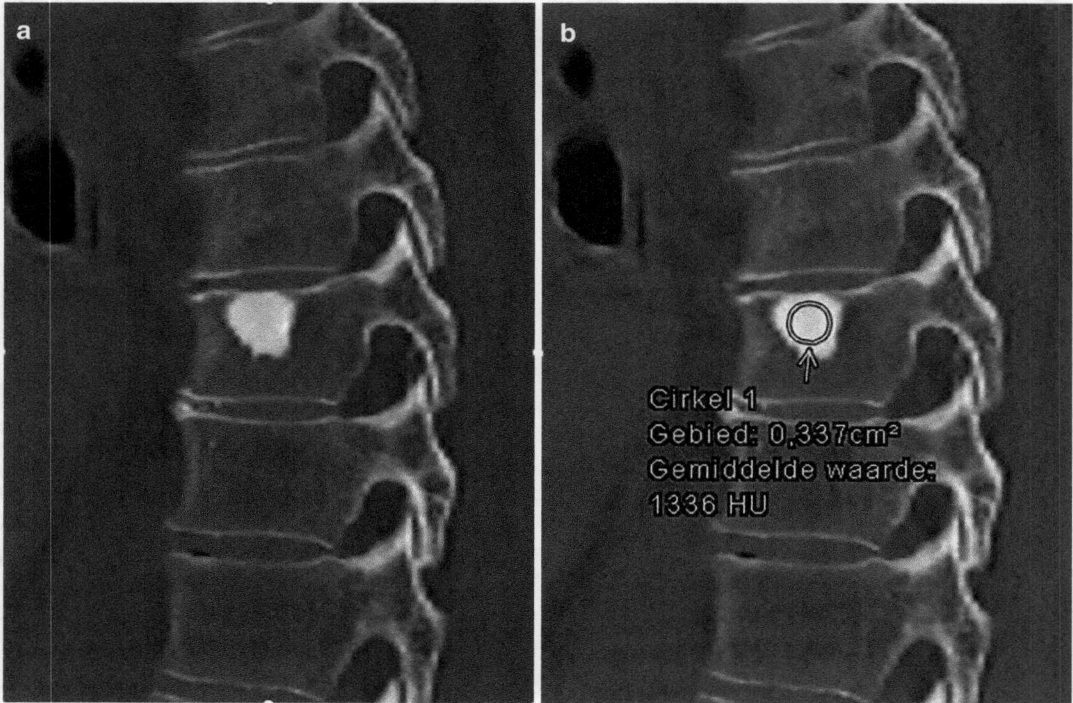

Fig. 6 Sixty-nine-year-old female with a medical history of a breast carcinoma. Sagittal (**a**, **b**) CT shows a sclerotic intramedullary focus with spiculated margins in vertebral body of a lower thoracic vertebra (**a**) with a mean attenuation of 1336 HU (**b**). Both the morphology and the attenuation of the lesion are indicative for a bone island and argue against an osteoblastic metastasis

bone islands and 79 metastatic lesions) (Dong et al. 2015). Ulano et al. showed that the mean attenuation of 885 Hounsfield units (HU) and maximum attenuation of 1060 HU provide reliable thresholds (Figs. 1, 2, and 6) under which osteoblastic metastatic lesions would be favorable (Fig. 7) (Ulano et al. 2016). The mean and maximum CT attenuations can also differentiate between bone islands and sclerotic metastases after chemotherapy, but the accuracy drops from 81.3% to 72.5% in untreated and treated metastases, respectively (Elangovan and Sebro 2018). Furthermore, these threshold levels are intended to differentiate bone island from osteoblastic metastases and should not be extrapolated to other sclerotic lesions (Azar et al. 2021).

Recently, dual-energy computed tomography (DECT) has been used to differentiate osteoblastic metastasis from bone islands. DECT can provide quantitative values of electronic density (Rho), effective atomic number (*Z*), and dual energy index (DEI), reflecting the composition of the scanned object. In a study by Xu et al., the *Z*, Rho, and DEI values for bone islands were found to be significantly higher than those for osteoblastic metastasis. In their study population, the mean *Z* had the highest accuracy with an optical cutoff value of 11.86 rendering an area under the receiving operation characteristic curve of 0.91, with 91.20% sensitivity and 82.50% specificity, performing better than CT attenuation values on conventional CT (Xu et al. 2022).

6.3 Magnetic Resonance Imaging (MRI)

On MRI, a bone island demonstrates very low signal intensities over all pulse sequences even on fluid-sensitive sequences (Figs. 2 and 4) with the

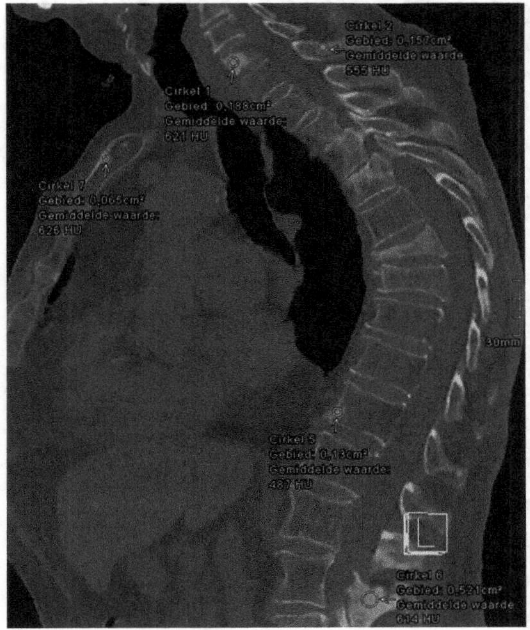

Fig. 7 Eighty-six-year-old male with a medical history of a prostate carcinoma. Sagittal reformatted CT of the chest and upper abdomen shows multiple sclerotic foci in the vertebral column and sternum diagnosis as well as mid-thoracic vertebral collapse. The mean attenuation less than 885 HU of the different osteosclerotic foci indicating osteoblastic metastases

surrounding bone marrow being normal (Baumhoer et al. 2020; White and Kandel 2000; Murphey et al. 1996; Riahi et al. 2018). MRI-based synthetic CT (SCT), also known as bone MRI, is a post-processing technology, performing a 3D MRI to CT mapping and generating "CT-like" images from the MR data. It has been shown that SCT is equally useful to characterize a bone island as conventional CT by analyzing the morphology (spicular margins) (Fig. 5) and measurement of signal intensities on SCT similar to HU on conventional CT (Morbée et al. 2022, 2023).

6.4 Nuclear Medicine

On bone scintigraphy, bone islands typically appear as cold areas (Fig. 3d), but they may exhibit uptake on bone scintigraphy occasionally (Baumhoer et al. 2020), which is histologically related to higher bone remodeling and osteoblastic activity, proliferating and active fibroblasts, and increased blood flow (Greenspan and Stadalnik 1995; Ran et al. 2018).

Generally, a bone island is not avid on fluorodeoxyglucose (FDG) PET/CT (Broski et al. 2022). Although this may be useful to differentiate bone islands from metastatic bone lesions, (FDG) PET is not recommended in the general workup (see chapter "PET/CT in Primary Tumors of the Osseous Spine").

7 Differential Diagnosis

The main differential diagnosis consists of osteoblastic metastasis, particularly in patients with known malignancy (predominantly prostate, breast).

On CR and CT, metastases typically show no radiating spicules and are less homogeneous. Mean CT attenuation is lower than 885 HU and maximum attenuation less than 1060 HU (Fig. 7) (see paragraph 6).

Another differential diagnosis consists of unilateral hypertrophy and sclerosis of the pars interarticularis resulting from a contralateral mechanical stress phenomenon in patients with unilateral spondylolysis. The location of the sclerosis in the pars interarticularis and the presence of contralateral spondylolysis are the clues to the correct diagnosis (Fig. 8).

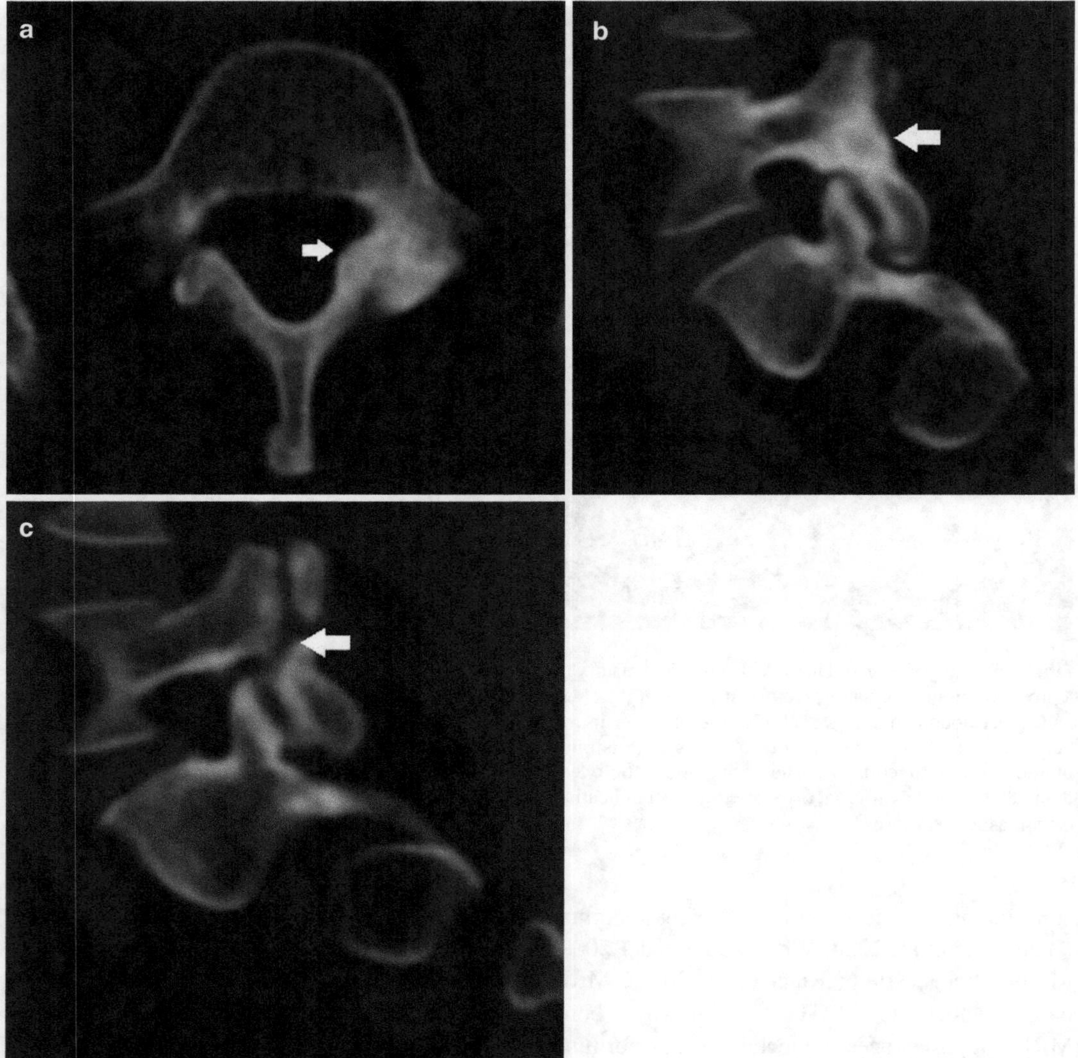

Fig. 8 Hypertrophy and sclerosis of the pars interarticularis due to increased mechanical stress caused by contralateral spondylolysis. Axial and left parasagittal reformatted CT (**a, b**) shows hypertrophy and sclerosis of the left pars interarticularis (arrows). Right parasagittal reformatted CT (**c**) shows spondylolysis at the right pars interarticularis (arrow)

8 Management and Prognosis

In case of typical presentation on imaging, the lesion can be considered as a "do-not-touch lesion" and no further treatment is required.

The prognosis is excellent as for other benign lesions.

Bone islands in adults are typically stable over time. Biopsy should be considered if the lesion increases in diameter by more than 25% during a 6-month period (White and Kandel 2000) or in atypical cases or giant bone islands in which the lesion remains undetermined.

9 Key Points

- Bone islands are almost always clinically silent and present as incidental findings on imaging studies.
- Within the spine, a bone island is typically located within the vertebral body.
- On CR and CT, bone islands are radiopaque with peripheral spicules, blending into the surrounding trabeculae (rose thorns).
- Mean CT attenuation values exceed 885 HU, and the maximum CT attenuation exceeds 1060 HU. These provide reliable thresholds and are useful in the differential diagnosis with untreated osteoblastic metastasis.
- On MRI, a bone island is hypointense on all pulse sequences.
- Bone scintigraphy is typically negative.
- Bone islands have a high rate of stability.

References

Alfahad S, Alostad M, Dunkley S et al (2021) Dense bone islands in pediatric patients: a case series study. Eur Arch Paediatr Dent 22:751–757. https://doi.org/10.1007/s40368-020-00596-w

Azar A, Garner HW, Rhodes NG et al (2021) CT attenuation values do not reliably distinguish benign sclerotic lesions from osteoblastic metastases in patients undergoing bone biopsy. AJR Am J Roentgenol 216:1022–1030. https://doi.org/10.2214/AJR.20.24029

Baumhoer D, Bredella M, Sumathi V (2020) Osteoma. In: WHO Classification of Tumours Editorial Board (ed) Soft tissue and bone tumours. WHO classification of tumours (medicine), 5th edn. IARC Publications, Lyon, France, pp 391–393

Broski SM, Littrell LA, Howe BM, Wenger DE (2022) Bone tumors: common mimickers. Radiol Clin North Am 60:239–252. https://doi.org/10.1016/J.RCL.2021.11.004

Diab MG, Glard Y, Launay F et al (2014) Small bone islands: unusual clinical symptomatology. Orthopedics 37:e79. https://doi.org/10.3928/01477447-20131219-21

Dong Y, Zheng S, Machida H et al (2015) Differential diagnosis of osteoblastic metastases from bone islands in patients with lung cancer by single-source dual-energy CT: advantages of spectral CT imaging. Eur J Radiol 84:901–907. https://doi.org/10.1016/J.EJRAD.2015.01.007

Elangovan SM, Sebro R (2018) Accuracy of CT attenuation measurement for differentiating treated osteoblastic metastases from enostoses. Am J Roentgenol 210:615–620. https://doi.org/10.2214/AJR.17.18638

Greenspan A (1995) Bone island (enostosis): current concept - a review. Skeletal Radiol 24:111–115. https://doi.org/10.1007/BF00198072

Greenspan A, Stadalnik R (1995) Bone island: scintigraphic findings and their clinical application. Can Assoc Radiol J 46:368–379

Greenspan A, Steiner G, Knutzon R (1991) Bone island (enostosis): clinical significance and radiologic and pathologic correlations. Skeletal Radiol 20:85–90. https://doi.org/10.1007/BF00193816

Morbée L, Vereecke E, Laloo F et al (2022) MR imaging of the pelvic bones: the current and cutting-edge techniques. J Belg Soc Radiol 106:123. https://doi.org/10.5334/JBSR.2874

Morbée L, Vereecke E, Laloo F et al (2023) Common incidental findings on sacroiliac joint MRI: added value of MRI-based synthetic CT. Eur J Radiol 158:110651. https://doi.org/10.1016/J.EJRAD.2022.110651

Murphey MD, Andrews CL, Flemming DJ et al (1996) From the archives of the AFIP. Primary tumors of the spine: radiologic pathologic correlation. Radiographics 16:1131–1158. https://doi.org/10.1148/RADIOGRAPHICS.16.5.8888395

Olvi L, Lembo G, Santini-Araujo E (2015) Medullary osteoma. In: Santini-Araujo E, Kalil R, Bertoni F, Park Y (eds) Tumors and tumor-like lesions of bone. Springer, London

Ran P, Dong A, Wang Y et al (2018) Increased FDG uptake in a giant bone island mimicking malignancy. Clin Nucl Med 43:e209–e211. https://doi.org/10.1097/RLU.0000000000002095

Riahi H, Mechri M, Barsaoui M et al (2018) Imaging of benign tumors of the osseous spine. J Belg Soc Radiol 102:13. https://doi.org/10.5334/JBSR.1380

Sinnott PM, Hodges S (2020) An incidental dense bone island: a review of potential medical and orthodontic implications of dense bone islands and case report. J Orthod 47:251–256. https://doi.org/10.1177/1465312520917975

Stieda (1905) Ueber umschriebene Knochenverdichtungen im Bereich der Substantia spongiosa im Rontgenbilde. Beitr Klin Chir 45:700–703

Ulano A, Bredella MA, Burke P et al (2016) Distinguishing untreated osteoblastic metastases from enostoses using CT attenuation measurements. AJR Am J Roentgenol 207:362–368. https://doi.org/10.2214/AJR.15.15559

Vanhoenacker FM, De Beuckeleer LH, Van Hul W et al (2000) Sclerosing bone dysplasias: genetic and radioclinical features. Eur Radiol 10:1423–1433. https://doi.org/10.1007/S003300000495

White LM, Kandel R (2000) Osteoid-producing tumors of bone. Semin Musculoskelet Radiol 4:25–43. https://doi.org/10.1055/S-2000-6853

Xu C, Kong L, Deng X (2022) Dual-energy computed tomography for differentiation between osteoblastic metastases and bone islands. Front Oncol 12:1–7. https://doi.org/10.3389/fonc.2022.815955

Osteoid Osteoma and Osteoblastoma

Marc-André Weber, Christoph Rehnitz, and Mouna Chelli-Bouaziz

Contents

M.-A. Weber (✉)
Institute of Diagnostic and Interventional Radiology, Pediatric Radiology and Neuroradiology, University Medical Center Rostock, Rostock, Germany
e-mail: marc-andre.weber@med.uni-rostock.de

C. Rehnitz
Clinic of Diagnostic and Interventional Radiology, University Hospital Heidelberg, Heidelberg, Germany

M. Chelli-Bouaziz
Institute Mohamed-Kassab d'Orthopédie, Tunis, Tunisia

Med Radiol Diagn Imaging (2023)
https://doi.org/10.1007/174_2023_444,
Published Online: 26 August 2023

Abstract

An osteoid osteoma is a benign bone-forming tumor, which usually presents in childhood and adolescence and typically is characterized by extensive nocturnal pain. Regarding osseous tumors of the spine, characteristic morphology is encountered in osteoid osteoma and nonaggressive osteoblastomas (giant osteoid osteomas), and in these cases, radiological imaging can make a specific diagnosis, especially when the radiologist has chosen thin-sliced computed tomography (CT) as imaging modality of choice to establish the diagnosis in suspected osteoid osteoma. In osteoid osteoma, CT reveals the typical radiolucent nidus surrounded by a sclerotic reaction. Magnetic resonance imaging (MRI) typically demonstrates a nidal contrast enhancement and perifocal edema. Especially in spinal osteoid osteomas, the diagnosis is often delayed by more than 1 year. The radiologist plays a crucial role in the clinical pathway by "choosing wisely" the imaging approach, by narrowing the differential diagnosis list, and, when characteristic morphology is encountered, by establishing the diagnosis. Having shown excellent success rates, radiofrequency ablation has become the treatment of choice, which allows minimally invasive and precise destruction of nidal tumor tissue. By using thermal protection techniques and multiple ablation positions, successful therapy of perineural tumors and niduses with diameters of more than 2 cm (giant osteoid osteomas) are possible.

1 Introduction

Imaging has a pivotal role in the detection and characterization of the spine bone tumors, especially using magnetic resonance (MR) and computed tomography (CT). In conjunction with clinical history, imaging is generally used to differentiate benign from malignant lesions and narrow the list of differential diagnoses by searching usual signs of aggressiveness of the lesion itself, evaluating cortical destruction, neighboring bone and periosteal reaction (e.g., by CT), or bone marrow edema and soft tissue extension (e.g., by MRI) (Albano et al. 2019). Moreover, MRI is indispensable to determine the extension and relationship of the spinal bone tumor with the spinal canal and nerve roots, and thus determine the plan of management (Orguc and Arkun 2014). Furthermore, with the available more advanced imaging techniques such as hybrid imaging, dynamic contrast-enhanced MRI, chemical-shift and diffusion-weighted MRI, Dixon MR sequences, and dual-energy CT (Albano et al. 2019), the differential diagnosis list may be narrowed in an extent that no biopsy is needed, for instance in vertebral hemangiomas, bone islands, and osteoid osteomas. However, since imaging features of benign and malignant spinal bone tumors may overlap, even when a multimodality imaging approach has been sought and the diagnosis may remain uncertain, a bone biopsy should be performed to reach the final diagnosis (Albano et al. 2019; Thawait et al. 2012; Weber et al. 2022). The radiologist can really influence patient's management by ascertaining that a lesion is benign and thus prevent a possibly non-diagnostic biopsy (Weber et al. 2022). Thus, the aim and learning objectives of this book chapter are first to describe the characteristic morphology of osteoid osteomas and giant osteoid osteomas as examples of osseous tumors of the spine with characteristic morphology; in these entities, radiological imaging can make a specific diagnosis and thereby avoid biopsy; hence, the radiologist has to "choose wisely" the specific imaging modality to make the diagnosis, for instance thin-sliced CT in suspected osteoid osteoma (Weber et al. 2022). Therefore, so-called safety features of osteoid osteoma (OO) are summarized as well.

2 Pathologic Features

OO is a benign bone-forming tumor characterized by a nidus of vascularized osteoid tissue surrounded by a variable amount of reactive sclerotic bone. The nidus mean size is less than 1.5 cm and is always located on the concave side of the apex (Tepelenis et al. 2021).

3 Epidemiology

OO accounts for 10–14% of all benign bone tumors and 2–3% of all primary bone tumors (Tepelenis et al. 2021). It commonly occurs in the second decade of life with a male predominance (male-to-female ratio 2–3:1) (Riahi et al. 2018; Tepelenis et al. 2021). Spinal OO accounts for 1% of all spinal tumors.

4 Localization

About 10% (6–20%) of all OO are located in the spine, mainly in the posterior elements. The lumbar spine is most commonly affected (59%), followed by the cervical, thoracic, and sacral spine (Riahi et al. 2018; Tepelenis et al. 2021).

5 Clinical Presentation

Eighty to hundred percent of patients present with neck or back pain, usually localized but occasionally radicular or nocturnal (Riahi et al. 2018). Stiff and/or painful scoliosis is observed in up to 70% of cases and constitutes the most suggestive clinical presentation. OO should be mainly suspected in atypical scoliosis (male patient, left convex thoracic scoliosis, or right convex lumbar scoliosis) although hyperlordosis, kyphoscoliosis, and torticollis may also occur. From a clinical perspective, persisting back pain in children, adolescents, and young adults should always lead to an extended diagnostic workup until the final diagnosis of OO is made. The chronic perinidal inflammation due to prostaglandins (cyclooxygenase-2) is thought to explain either spinal pain (by nerve irritation, close to the nidus) or scoliosis (subsequent muscle spasms, which are initially reducible and non-rotational and progressively lead to a structured scoliosis) (Zairi and Nessib 2023). Additional clinical features may include nerve root irritation, night pain, and dramatic pain relief with aspirin or nonsteroidal anti-inflammatory drugs (14–90% of cases). Neurologic deficits are uncommon (less than 30% of cases) compared with patients who have osteoblastomas (25–70%) (Riahi et al. 2018; Kan and Schmidt 2008).

6 Imaging

Since 10% of all osteoid osteomas (OOs) are located in the spine, the key message here is to think of an OO, when encountering a lytic lesion, surrounded by a sclerotic osseous reaction, located in the posterior elements of the thoracic and lumbar spine in a child, adolescent, or young adult (Weber et al. 2015; Beyer et al. 2019). In our experience, the diagnosis is often delayed (delayed correct diagnosis by 2 years has been reported (Goldstein et al. 1977)), since the nidus, i.e., the tumor itself, may be hardly discernible, either on radiographs or when solely using MRI. The reactive edema surrounding the nidus may obscure visualization of the nidus, which has a low to intermediate signal on T1- and an intermediate to high signal on T2-weighted images (Orguc and Arkun 2014). Thus, in case of suspicion, a thin-sliced CT will definitely help in identifying the radiolucent, vascular nidus with or without intranidal calcification that is often associated with cortical thickening and bony sclerosis to establish the diagnosis (Fig. 1) (Orguc and Arkun 2014).

6.1 Radiographs

Superposition of reactive bone sclerosis makes the nidus difficult to detect on radiographs. However, in our experience, subtle radiographic signs are present in up to 60% of cases (Fig. 1), including localized posterior arch bone sclerosis, regional osteoporosis, and solid or laminated periosteal reaction. Even if radiographs are inferior to CT to demonstrate the nidus within the spine due to superimposing structures, these aforementioned radiographic signs should be looked for at the scoliosis apex and should indicate further assessment by MRI, thin-sliced CT, or scintigraphy.

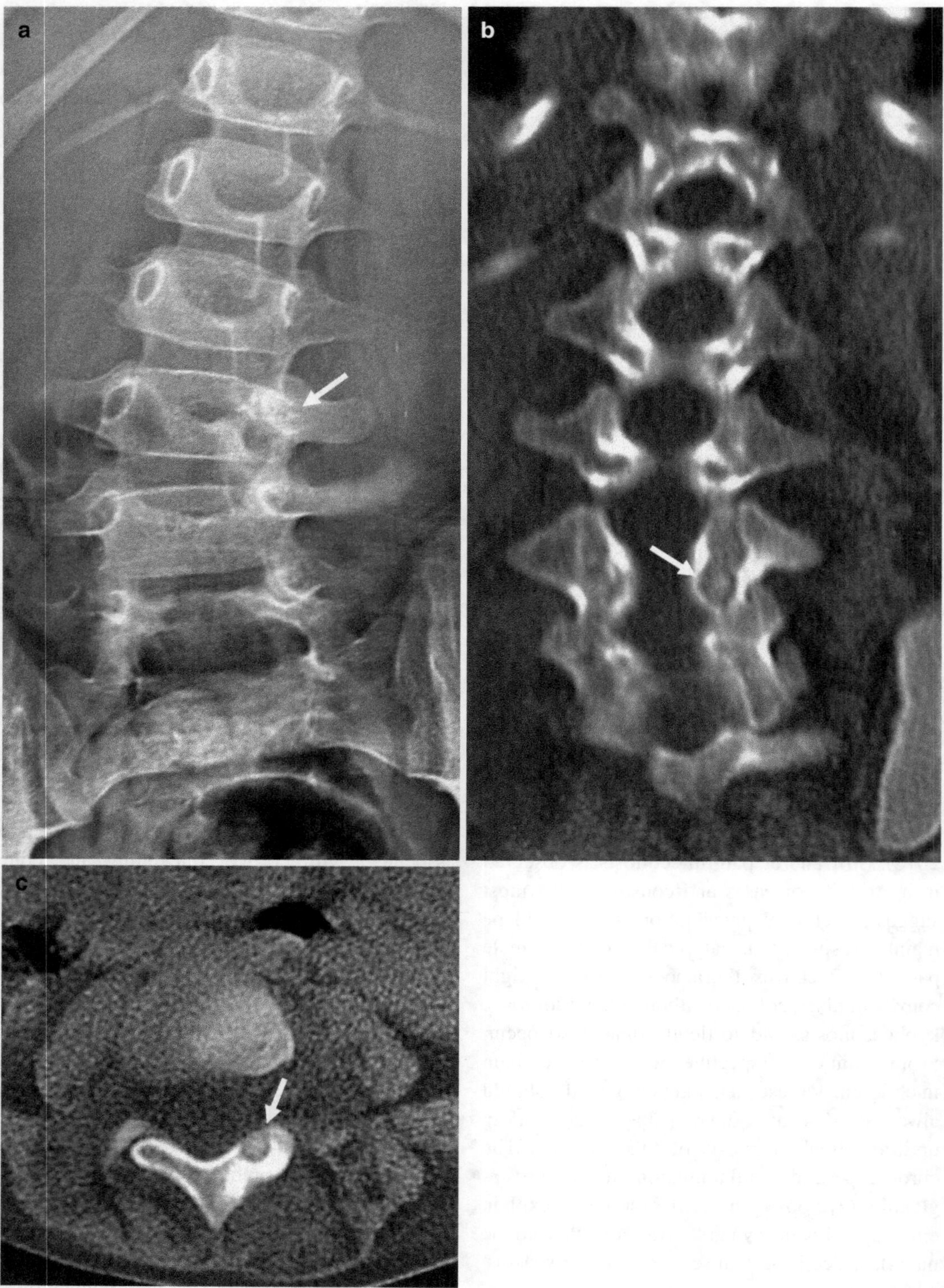

Fig. 1 L3 neural arch osteoid osteoma in a 4-year-old boy presenting with painful scoliosis. (**a**) AP radiograph of the lumbar spine shows a sclerosis and lamination of the left pedicle (at the concave side of scoliosis apex, arrow). (**b**) Thin-sliced coronal and (**c**) axial CT images demonstrate the nidus and the surrounding bone sclerosis (arrows)

6.2 Computed Tomography

CT is the modality of choice to detect a spinal OO. It is more sensitive than radiographs and MRI. The CT detection rate of spinal osteoid osteomas is almost 100% (Tepelenis et al. 2021). Typically, OO appears on CT as a well-defined round or oval area of soft tissue attenuation surrounded by a variable amount of bone sclerosis (Fig. 2). Calcifications of the nidus center (also known as "bull's-eye" appearance) are visible on CT in about 50% of cases and are typically punctate, amorphous, or ringlike (Tepelenis et al. 2021).

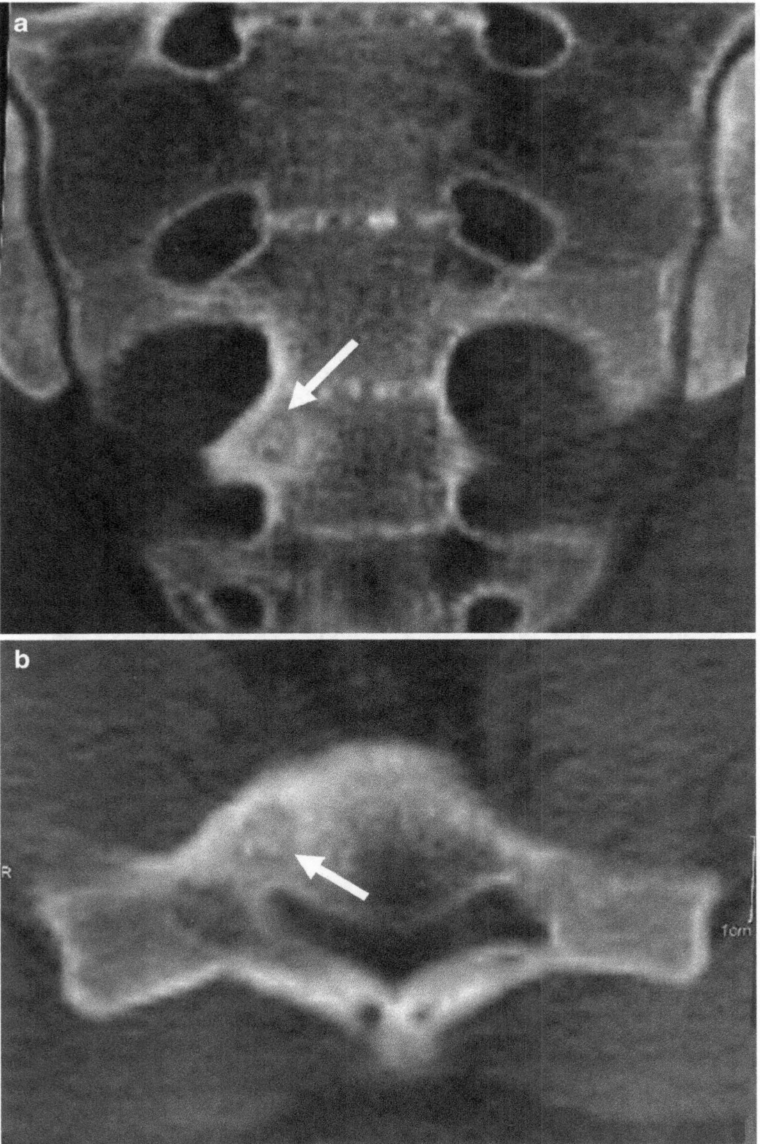

Fig. 2 Vertebral body osteoid osteoma of the sacrum (S3) in a 19-year-old man, treated by percutaneous excision. Coronal (**a**) and axial (**b**) CT reformations show the calcified nidus of the vertebral body (arrows) surrounded by sclerotic bone. Needle introduction under CT guidance (**c**), and subsequent percutaneous excision of the nidus (**d**)

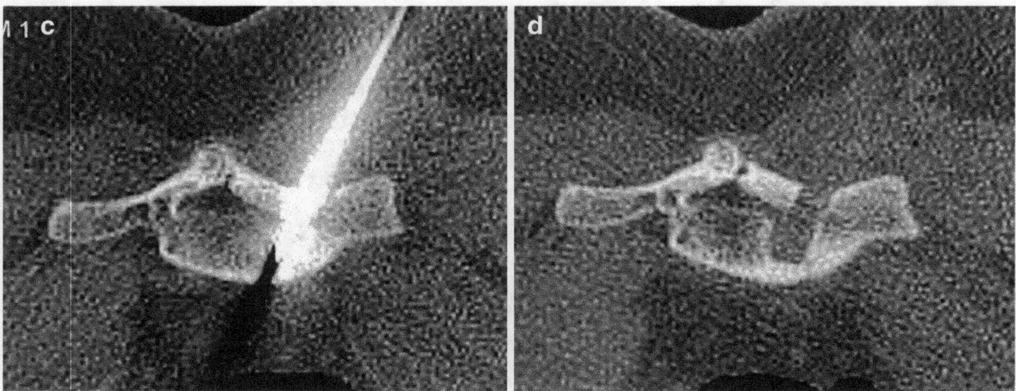

Fig. 2 (continued)

6.3 Magnetic Resonance Imaging

MRI appearance varies along with the amount of calcification within the nidus, size of the fibrovascular zone, amount of reactive sclerosis, and bone marrow edema (Fig. 3). Besides standard MRI and focused thin-sliced CT, advanced MRI techniques may be very helpful. For detecting the nidus itself and also to judge the nidus vitality posttreatment, the dynamic contrast-enhanced (DCE) MRI is very useful. As the nidus is highly vascularized, it appears hyperintense on early arterial perfusion images and thus greatly enhances nidus visibility (Fig. 4). On the other hand, on regular (late) postcontrast images, the nidus is often less visible due to lower contrast affinity and lower contrast to surrounding structures (Fig. 5). A vascular groove sign is a highly specific sign for distinguishing OO from other radiolucent bone lesions on CT (Liu et al. 2011), while DCE MRI has been shown to depict the nidus more clearly than unenhanced MRI or static postcontrast MR sequences. Most OOs show arterial phase enhancement and rapid partial washout because of hypervascularity of the nidus (Davies et al. 2002).

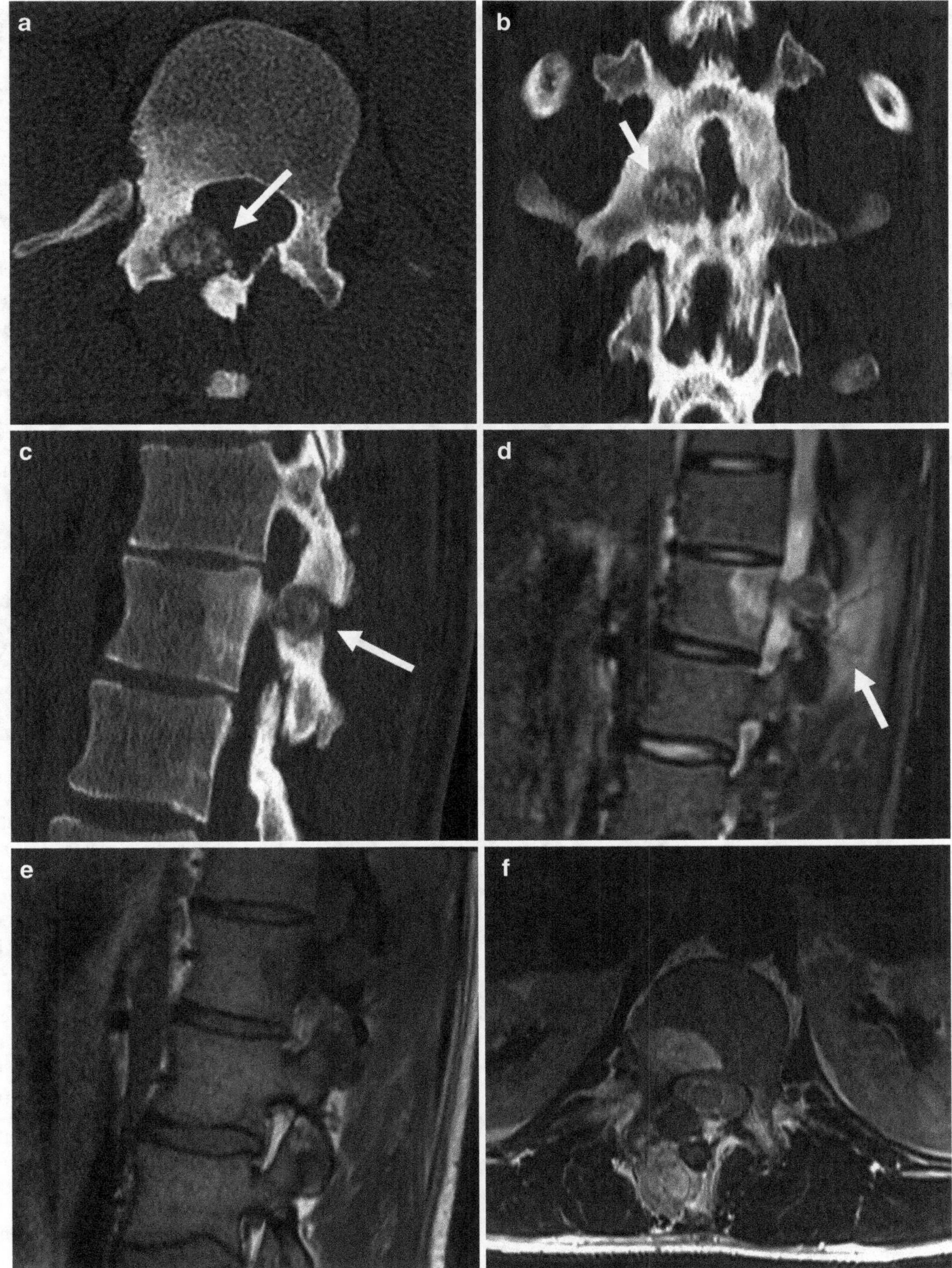

Fig. 3 Osteoid osteoma (OO) of the spine in a 22-year-old man with daily pain (8 of 10 by using a visual analogue scale). (**a–c**) CT in axial, sagittal, and coronal reformation. The OO (arrows) within the lamina of the first lumbar vertebra presents as centrally calcified osteolytic nidus and is surrounded by a zone of bony sclerosis. (**d–f**) 1.5 T MRI of the lumbar spine demonstrates the perifocal edema (arrow) on the short-tau inversion recovery sequence (**d**). The nidus is barely visible on unenhanced sagittal T1-weighted images (WI) (**e**) and appears isointense to the paravertebral muscles on axial T2-WI (**f**)

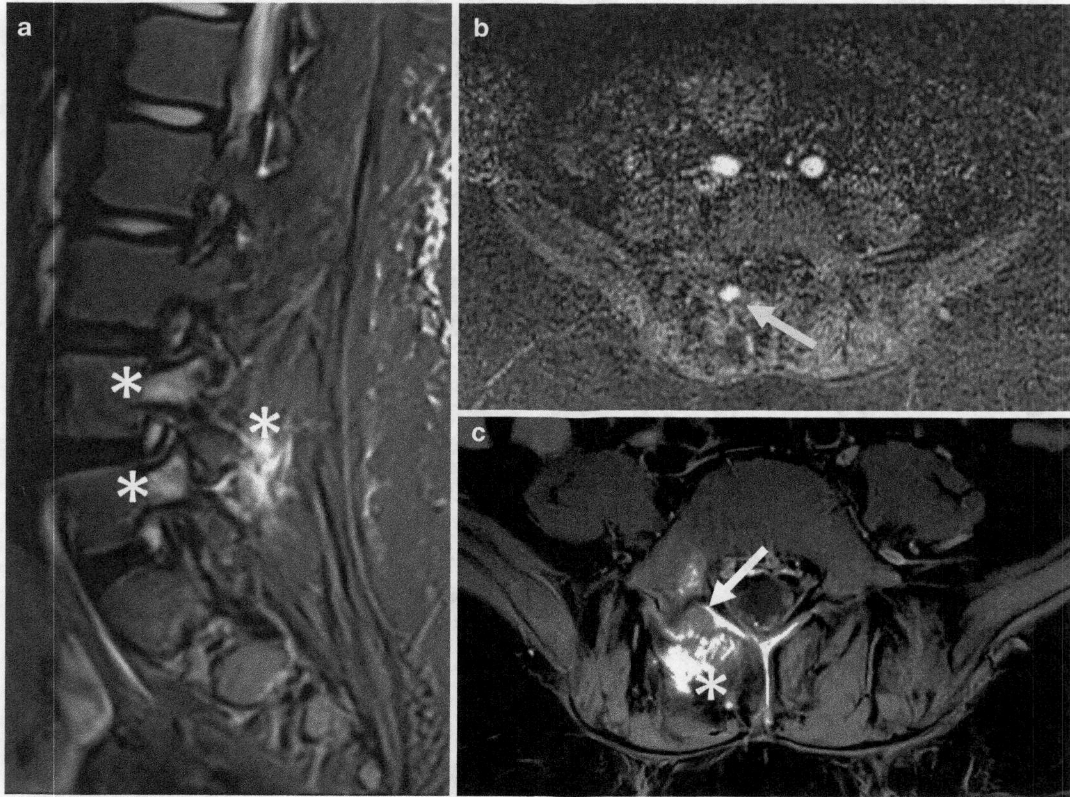

Fig. 4 Lumbar spinal osteoid osteoma (OO) evidenced by multimodal imaging and treated by RF ablation. Twelve-year-old boy with severe lower back pain. Several previous MR examinations at external institutions were either "unremarkable" or reported as "unclear edema." 3 T MRI at our institution: (**a**) STIR sagittal; (**b**) dynamic contrast-enhanced (DCE) axial in arterial phase; (**c**) static contrast-enhanced, T1-weighted fat-saturated axial sequence; and (**d**) static contrast-enhanced, T1-weighted fat-saturated sagittal sequence show bone marrow edema (asterisks) and contrast enhancement (asterisks) of the right pedicles L4 and L5 with posterior adjacent soft tissue edema. DCE MRI at the arterial phase reveals a focal highly contrast-enhancing spot at the right facet joint L4/L5, highly suspicious of the nidus of an OO (yellow arrow). Note that this nidus appears not avidly contrast-enhancing on regular (late) postcontrast T1-weighted fat-saturated MR imaging (white arrows), highlighting the value of DCE for nidus detection on MRI and vice versa the difficulties in nidus detection on regular static post-contrast MR images. The zoomed CT images of the lumbar spine (**e**) axial view and (**f**) sagittal view confirm a tiny partially sclerotic nidus of an (articular) osteoid osteoma at the inferior part of the right facet joint L4/L5 (arrows). Low-dose CT during radiofrequency ablation to localize the nidus (arrow) followed by needle placement (7 mm active tip) in the nidus (**g**) axial view and (**h**) sagittal view. Ablation was carried out for 6 min at 90 °C. Three months after the intervention, 3 T MRI shows markedly reduced bone and soft tissue edema (asterisks) on the sagittal STIR image (**i**). DCE in axial plane (**j**) reveals no contrast agent enhancement of the nidus itself during arterial phase (yellow arrow) but only an expected peripheral rim enhancement surrounding the ablation zone while there is no contrast enhancement of the nidus (white arrows) in the static contrast-enhanced fat-saturated T1-weighted sagittal (**k**) and axial (**l**) sequence, compatible with complete nidus devitalization. This rim-like enhancement in the absence of nidus enhancement should not be mistaken for nidus vitality or OO recurrence as it is an expected reactive finding post-ablation. The DCE is a helpful tool to detect arterial nidus enhancement and to judge possible nidus vitality, especially in patients with (partially) persisting or recurring pain after radiofrequency ablation

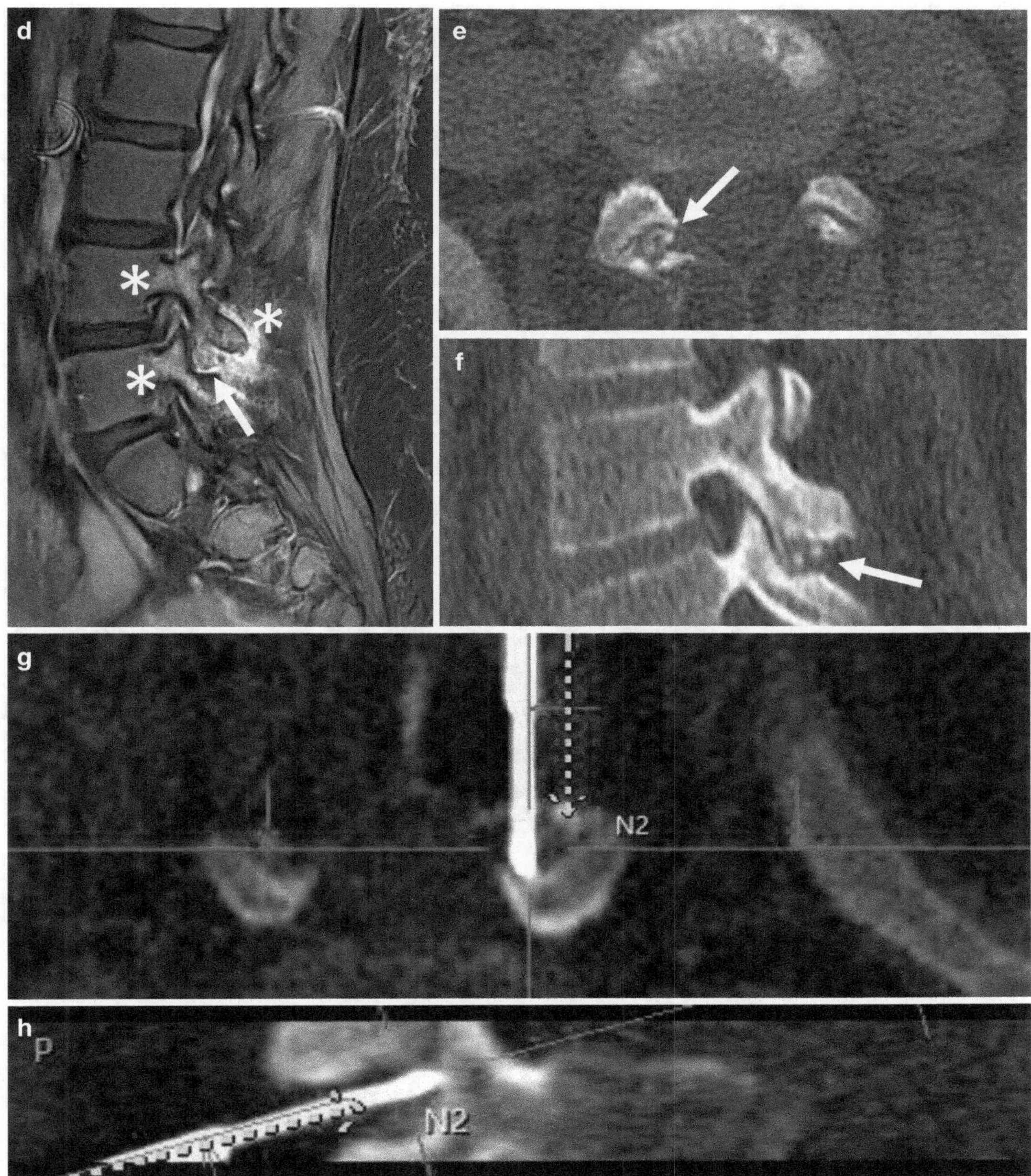

Fig. 4 (continued)

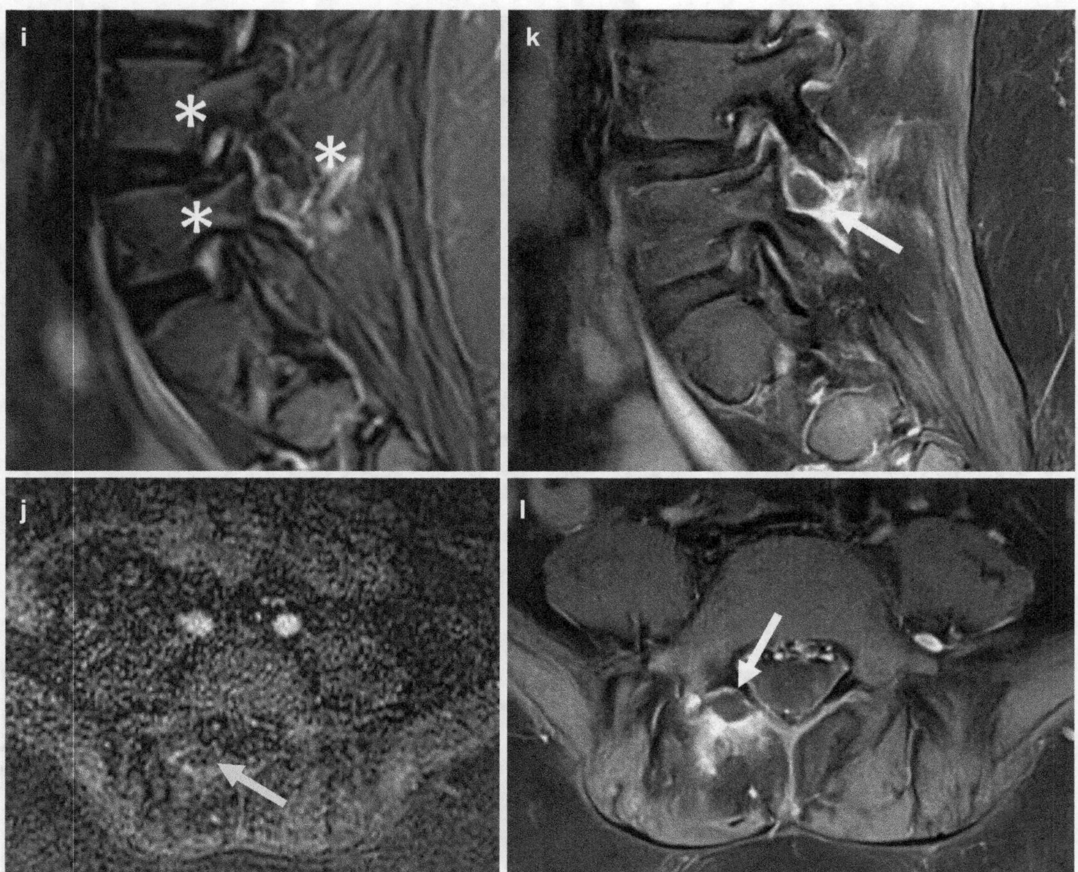

Fig. 4 (continued)

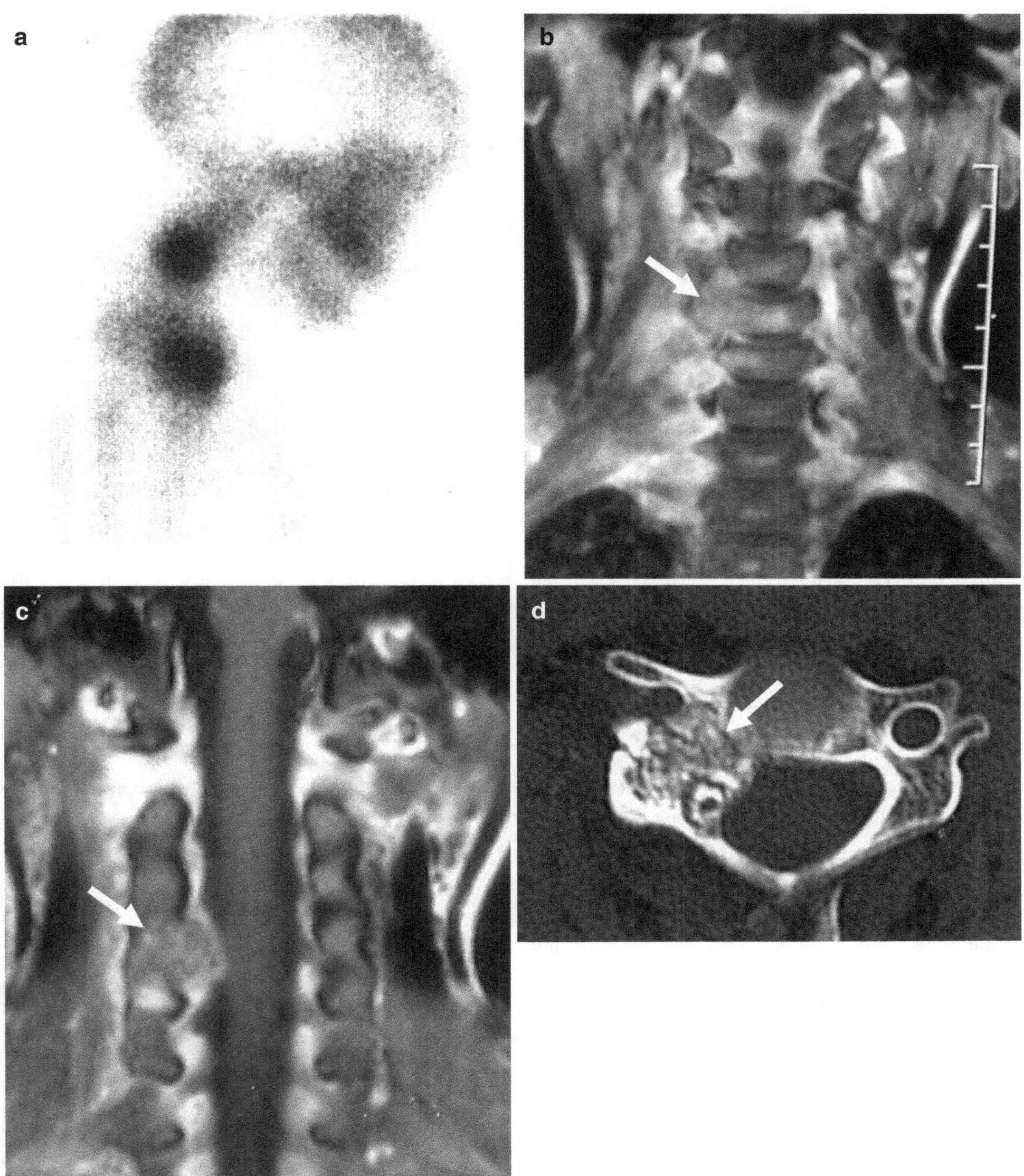

Fig. 5 Cervical spine osteoid osteoma in an 8-year-old girl presenting with torticollis. Bone scintigraphy (**a**) shows avid uptake of the cervical spine. Coronal contrast-enhanced T1-weighted MR images in different planes show bone marrow edema of C4 vertebral body and adjacent soft tissues (**b**) (arrow) and a well-vascularized lesion of the right neural arch (**c**) (arrow). Axial CT image shows the calcified nidus (arrow in **d**) and confirms the diagnosis

6.4 Nuclear Bone Scan, PET, and PET/CT

Triple scintigraphy is useful to detect and localize a radiographically occult nidus, as OO typically has early avid uptake (Fig. 5) (Riahi et al. 2018; Zairi and Nessib 2023). Hybrid imaging (SPECT/CT with 99mTc-labeled bisphosphonates or PET/CT with 18F-NaF) is also highly accurate and provides either morphological or functional information for diagnosis and treatment. Currently, the hybrid imaging technique PET/CT has no routine use in OO of the spine.

7 Histopathology

Macroscopically, OO is a well-circumscribed tumor. OO typically is red in color with soft and friable composition and a diameter of 1.5–2 cm. Its consistency rises, and its reddish color lessens due to the central part of the nidus' osseous maturation, either spontaneously or after treatment. These changes are in proportion to the degree of bone tissue maturation (Ghanem 2006; Tepelenis et al. 2021). Histologically, it is composed of a central nidus, which contains sheets of immature woven bone, occasionally with osteoblastic rimming, scattered osteoclasts in the fibrous connecting tissue that separates the osteoid trabeculae, and vascular spaces of small and intermediate size. There is a zone of solid, mature bone in the periphery of the lesion that surrounds the nidus (Ghanem 2006; Tepelenis et al. 2021).

8 Differential Diagnosis

Regarding solitary "true" bone tumors of the vertebral column (i.e., no mimickers and secondary bone tumors), OO is the only entity that enables the skip of biopsy. All other primary bone tumors of the spine must be finally diagnosed by an intraprocedural biopsy, and any specimens obtained during the procedure would be sent off for histological evaluation to obtain a definitive diagnosis. This is necessary to achieve best practices and optimize patient care. Biopsies are performed prior to planning therapeutic procedures in all "indeterminate," "suspicious," "probably malignant," and/or "definitely malignant" tumors for histological diagnosis and grading (Dalili et al. 2020). The results should be discussed in multidisciplinary tumor board meetings consisting of at least a tumor or spine surgeon, a pathologist, and an experienced MSK radiologist prior to any subsequent intervention (Lalam et al. 2017; Cazzato et al. 2020). Of note, the diagnosis is also often delayed in intra-articular OO. For these, MRI is excellently suited for establishing the diagnosis and for distinguishing intra- from extra-articular OOs (Germann et al. 2020). Joint effusion and synovitis are the most helpful imaging findings to distinguish both forms (Germann et al. 2020). Also, from a clinical perspective, persisting back pain in children, adolescents, and young adults should always lead to an extended diagnostic workup until the final diagnosis is made. Besides standard MRI and focused thin-sliced CT, advanced MRI techniques may be very helpful. Some skeletal lesions may mimic radiological and clinical appearance of spinal OO. The main differential diagnoses are osteoblastoma (OB), osteoblastic metastasis, enostosis, infection, and reactive sclerosis caused by facet degeneration or malformation (Fig. 6), as well as stress fracture (Riahi

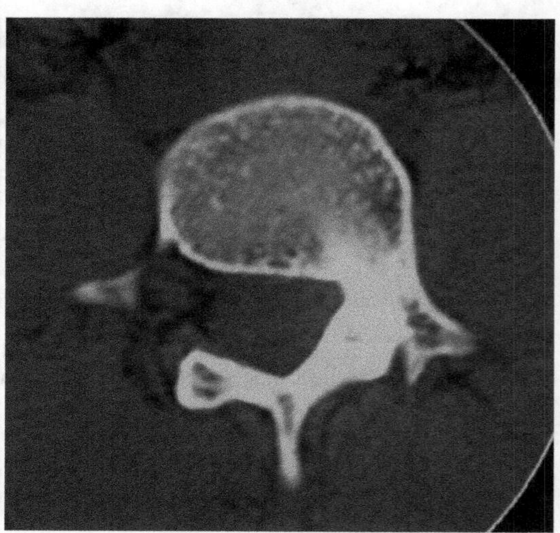

Fig. 6 Reactive bone sclerosis mimicking osteoid osteoma. Axial CT image of a lumbar vertebra showing aplasia of the right pedicle and reactive bone condensation of the left neural arch

et al. 2018; Bhure et al. 2019) or the rare unilateral arch hypertrophy associated with contralateral deficiency (Maldague and Malghem 1976).

8.1 Osteoblastoma of the Spine

OB is a good example of indeterminate lesions. In general, OO larger than 15 mm is denominated giant OO or OB (Lucas 2010). This entity is four times less frequent than OO, appears more expansive, and has less sclerotic borders. OB in 30–40% of all cases affects the vertebral column and in 85% originates from the posterior elements with 42% extending into the vertebral body (Orguc and Arkun 2014). In addition, OB may have more aggressive imaging (and histologic) features than OO. In these cases, the denomination as giant OO is misleading and thus OB should be rather used than giant OO. Malignant transformation into osteosarcoma of OB is rare but possible. Consequently, histologic sampling is mandatory in all cases of presumed OB (Orguc and Arkun 2014; Papaioannou et al. 2009). Radiographic presentation of OB may vary. The most common appearance of spinal OB is an expansile lesion with a prominent sclerotic rim and multiple small calcifications (Figs. 7 and 8), while the more aggressive type demonstrates in addition bone destruction and paravertebral extension (Orguc and Arkun 2014). As with OO, the radiological examination of choice is CT showing the multifocal matrix calcifications (as opposed to central in OO), sclerotic margin, expansile bone remodeling, or thin osseous shell around its margins (Fig. 7), while MRI better depicts the surrounding soft tissue involvement (Orguc and Arkun 2014) (Fig. 8). The radiologist can only avoid unnecessary biopsy by exactly measuring the nidus size on thin-sliced CT datasets with multiplanar reconstructions, because a nidus size less than 1.5 cm in maximum diameter turns per definition an OB into an OO that needs no biopsy before the intervention. Of note, likewise to OO, osteoblastoma is an infrequent but important cause of pain in the back and neurological findings in children and young adults and its diagnosis may be difficult and often delayed (Elder et al. 2016; Wu et al. 2019) (in one series, 23% of patients had not been diagnosed after 2 years of symptoms (Paige et al. 1991)). In addition to CT, MRI may be useful to noninvasively demonstrate both the lesion and its soft tissue and bony extent and its relationship, if any, to the spinal cord. The MRI features of spinal OB are generally nonspecific and depend on the degree of tumor mineralization. The tumor exhibits a low T1 and mixed T2 signal intensity with surrounding bone and soft tissue edema. After contrast administration, the lesions enhance intensely as well as surrounding edema, often resulting in overestimation of size of lesion (Fig. 8) (Riahi et al. 2018). The radiologist plays a crucial role in the clinical pathway because his role is to "choose wisely" the imaging approach, to narrow the differential diagnosis list, and to perform the image-guided biopsy after interdisciplinary case discussion. As a rule of thumb, histological verification or confirmation of suspected diagnosis by short-term follow-up should be sought in any case of doubt regarding the benignity of the lesion or when metastases or myeloma lesions are of utmost probability and no histologic verification is necessary to optimize therapy (Weber et al. 2022). Biopsy can be avoided, and a follow-up examination within 6 weeks or 3 months may be reasonable (in an "image wisely" setting), when the lesion is small, for instance smaller than 5 mm. Because then, both all available imaging biomarkers and biopsy may not be diagnostic (Weber et al. 2022). For instance, the diagnostic yield of CT-guided biopsy of bone tumors is significantly lower for lesions with size smaller than 20 mm, compared to bigger lesions. Several reports showed that the size of the lesion is important for the success of the imaging-guided biopsy of skeletal tumors, because of the amount of the obtained material and the possibility of sampling error. The optimal size of the lesion for successful imaging-guided biopsy should be 20 mm or more, according to the authors (Rimondi et al. 2011; Wu et al. 2008; Virayavanich et al. 2011; Li et al. 2014; Yang et al. 2018).

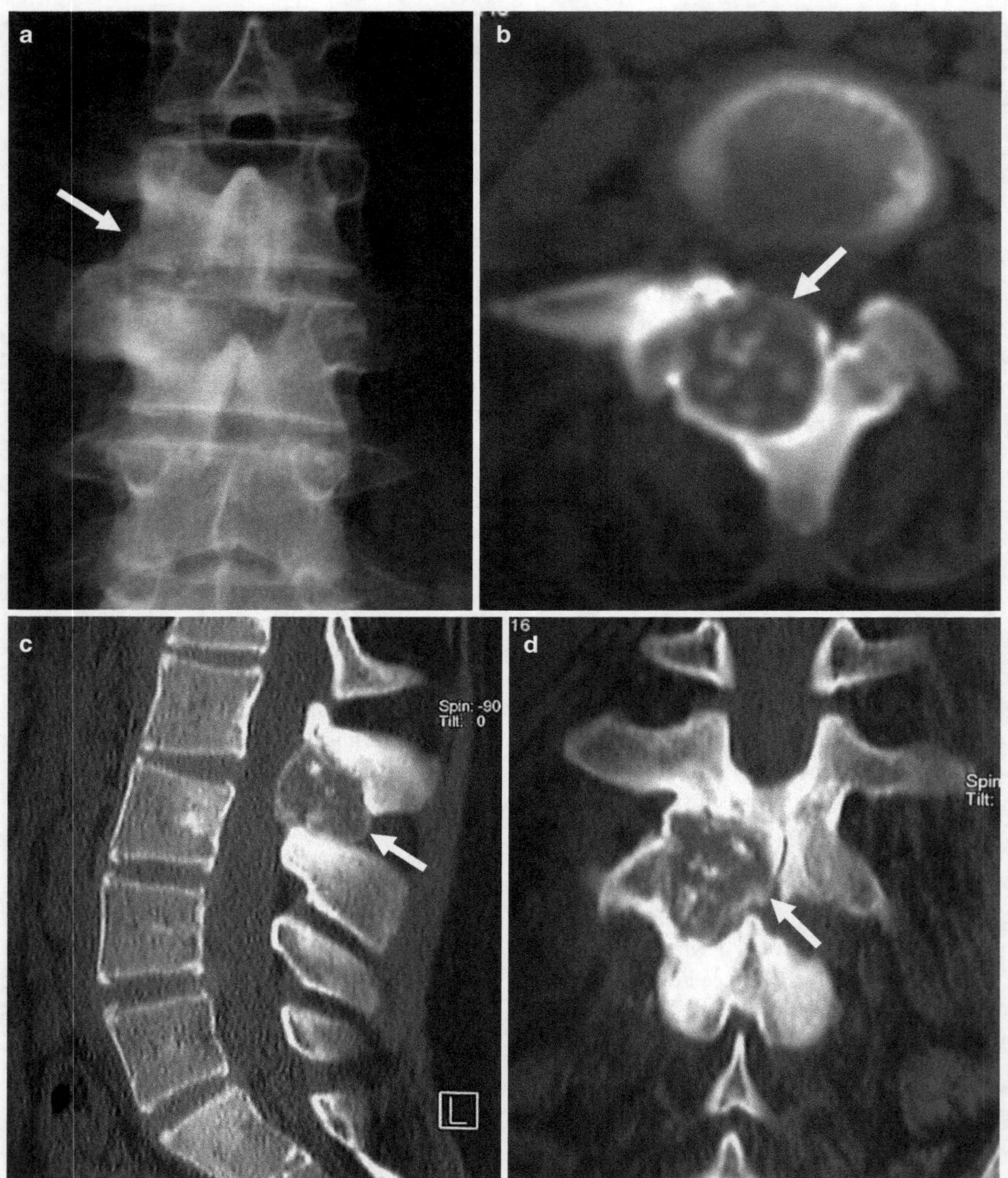

Fig. 7 Osteoblastoma of the lumbar spine (L3) in a 14-year-old girl. AP radiograph (**a**) shows an osteolysis of the right neural arch (arrow), with peripheral sclerosis and inner calcifications. Axial (**b**), sagittal (**c**), and coronal (**d**) CT images better depict the expansile osteolytic lesion (arrows) of the neural arch with bone remodeling, sclerotic margins, and multifocal matrix calcifications. (*With courtesy of Prof. M.-S. Daghfous*)

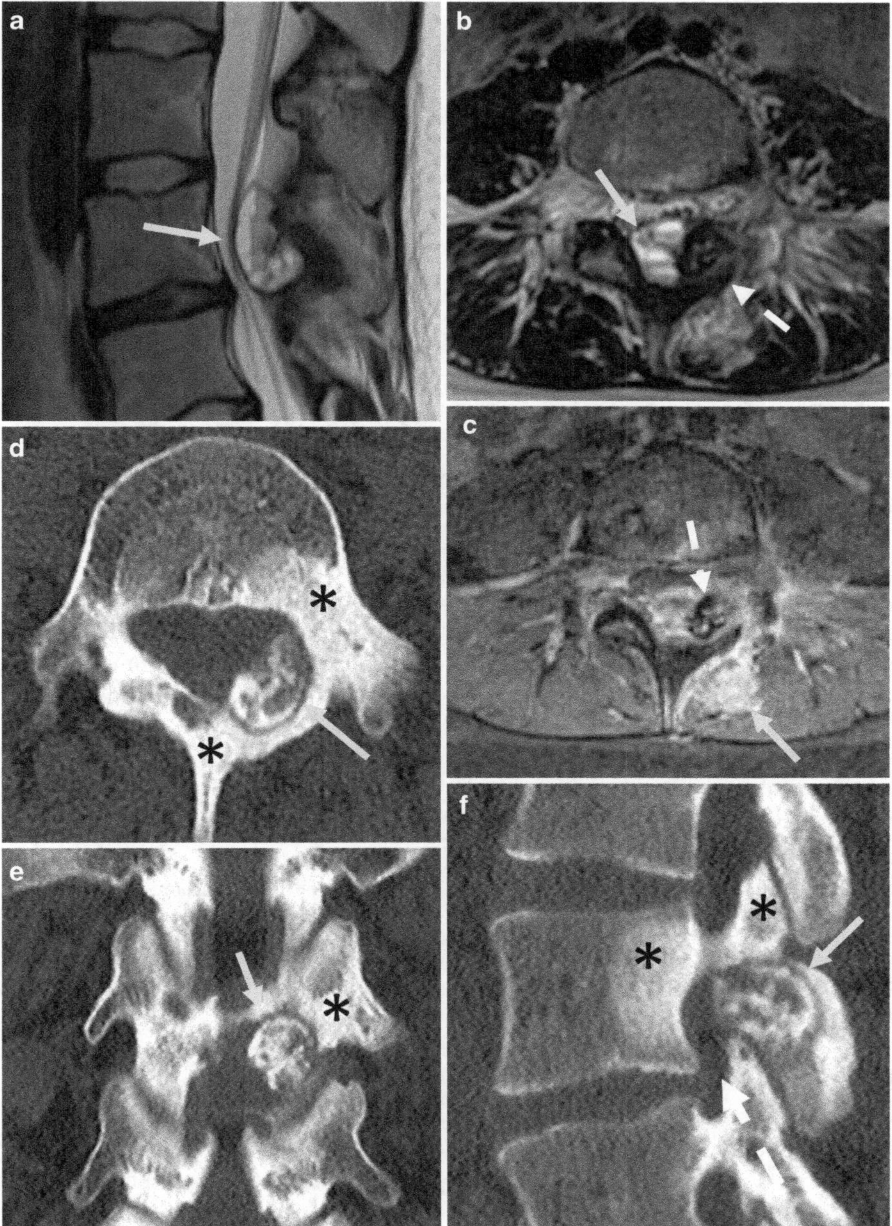

Fig. 8 Osteoblastoma of the spine with adjacent aneurysmal bone cyst (ABC). Seventeen-year-old female with lower back pain. Sagittal T2-WI (**a**) of the lumbar spine reveals a multicystic lesion with blood-fluid levels (yellow arrow) adjacent to the posterior structures at the level L4. Axial T2-WI (**b**) additionally shows a hypointense lesion (dashed white arrow) of the posterior arc near the facet joint and directly adjacent to the cystic lesion (yellow arrow). The dorsal adjacent arc is hypointense, compatible with sclerosis. After intravenous gadolinium administration, this lesion is mainly hypointense (dashed white arrow) with avid surrounding contrast enhancement (yellow arrow) in the axial contrast-enhanced fat-saturated sequence (**c**). This pattern is highly suggestive of an osteoblastoma with an associated ABC. The focused lumbar CT (**d–f**) at the L4 level shows a centrally ossified oval-shaped lesion adjacent to the dorsolateral spinal canal and the posterior arc with involvement of the inferior articular process and the facet joint L4/L5 (yellow arrows). There is also a stenosis of the left neuroforamen (dashed white arrow) as well as surrounding reactive sclerosis of the surrounding bone (asterisks). This patient subsequently underwent CT-guided biopsy followed by surgical resection combined with decompression and hemilaminectomy, and the diagnosis of an osteoblastoma with secondary aneurysmal bone cyst was confirmed by histopathology

8.2 Other Differential Diagnoses

Enostosis and pseudotumoral lesions will be discussed in other chapters of this book.

9 Local and Distant Staging

CT is the best modality to detect as well as to assess the extent of the nidus. We have not encountered patients with more than one OO nidus, and thus distant staging is not necessary in typical OO cases.

10 Treatment

The establishment of an early diagnosis of spinal OO is important because it has been demonstrated that late-diagnosed vertebral OO can be the cause of structural scoliosis (Zhang et al. 2016; Zairi and Nessib 2023). Spontaneous resolution of OO has been rarely reported. However, prompt treatment is preferred to avoid treatment delay and permanent structural scoliosis. Alternative treatment options to surgical excision include CT-guided percutaneous resection of the nidus, percutaneous CT-guided thermocoagulation, cryoablation, microwave ablation, and percutaneous CT-guided interstitial laser thermotherapy (Lidar et al. 2021; Riahi et al. 2018; Tepelenis et al. 2021). Regrowth of OO is generally due to incomplete removal rather than multiple nidus. In our centers, we use local ablative treatment options such as radiofrequency ablation of the nidus without biopsy (Weber et al. 2015; Beyer et al. 2019), when there is a typical OO morphology in imaging together with a typical clinical presentation. We share the prevailing opinion that a histological confirmation is not necessary in the typical constellation of OO (Weber et al. 2015; Rehnitz et al. 2012). In a recent trans-European multicenter study with a large cohort of 77 patients with spinal OO and 10 patients with spinal osteoblastoma (OB), radiofrequency ablation was proven to be a safe and efficient method to treat spinal OO and OB with technical and clinical success rates of 94.8%/89.6% for spinal OO and 90.0%/90.0% for spinal OB (Beyer et al. 2019). Other local ablative techniques have also been described to be efficient in OO, such as radiofrequency ablation, or other techniques like interstitial laser ablation (Gangi et al. 2007), microwave ablation (Kostrzewa et al. 2019), cryoablation (Cazzato et al. 2019), or high-intensity focused ultrasound ablation (Napoli et al. 2017; Tepelenis et al. 2021); for an overview of available thermal ablation procedures, see Dalili et al. (2020). Thus, in our opinion (Weber et al. 2022), a typical OO in the spine can be treated without prior biopsy with local ablative techniques.

11 Prognosis

Regrowth of OO is rare, usually due to incomplete removal rather than multiple nidus. CT is the preferred follow-up technique after treatment (Riahi et al. 2018).

12 Summary

In conclusion, characteristic morphology is encountered in osteoid osteoma of the spine and nonaggressive osteoblastomas (giant osteoid osteomas), and in these cases, radiological imaging can make a specific diagnosis, especially when the radiologist has chosen thin-sliced CT in suspected OO as imaging modality of choice to establish the diagnosis (Fig. 9). Although spine OO is clinically rare, it shall not be overlooked when young patients present with scoliosis first. Radiological results including CT and MRI shall be taken carefully as reference when making diagnosis. Minimal invasive treatment options are available, and successful ablation of the nidus could well improve scoliosis and relieve back pain. Suspicion of an aggressive OB or even a malignancy should be raised in spinal lesions with heterogeneous, disordered matrix, distinct signal decrease in T1-weighted MRI (many cells), blurred border, perilesional edema, cortex erosion, and large soft tissue component (fast

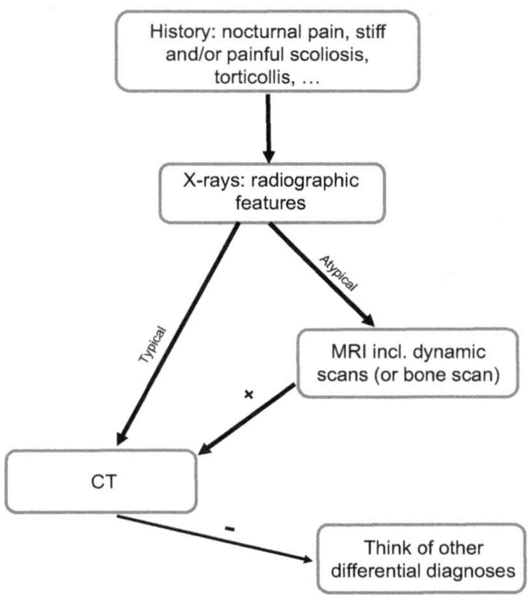

Fig. 9 Osteoid osteoma of the spine: Proposal of a diagnostic algorithm that helps to "choose imaging wisely"

growth). Biopsy is mandatory in presumed malignancy, such as any Lodwick grade II or III osteolytic lesion in the vertebral column. Especially in osteoid osteomas, the diagnosis is often delayed by more than 1 year. The radiologist plays a crucial role in the clinical pathway by "choosing wisely" the imaging approach, by narrowing the differential diagnosis list, and, when characteristic morphology is encountered, by establishing the diagnosis. Since especially at the vertebral column, due to projection effects, bone neoplasms with remarkably normal-appearing radiographs may show distinct abnormalities on CT, MRI, or bone scintigraphy, further assessment with a more sensitive modality is essential in patients with persisting symptoms but negative radiographs ("image wisely"), and in suspected OO and OB, thin-sliced CT is the modality of choice (Fig. 9).

13 Key Points

1. Ten percent of all osteoid osteomas are located in the spine.
2. Osteoblastomas affect the vertebral column in 30–40% of all cases and mainly originate from the posterior elements.
3. Especially in spinal osteoid osteomas, the establishment of the final diagnosis is often delayed.
4. In suspected osteoid osteoma and osteoblastoma, thin-sliced CT is the diagnostic modality of choice.
5. Radiofrequency ablation is a safe and efficient method to treat spinal osteoid osteomas and osteoblastomas with high technical and clinical success rates.

Conflicts of Interest The authors declare no conflicts of interest. All images appear in original publication.

References

Albano D, Messina C, Gitto S et al (2019) Differential diagnosis of spine tumors: my favorite mistake. Semin Musculoskelet Radiol 23:26–35

Beyer T, van Rijswijk CSP, Villagrán JM et al (2019) European multicentre study on technical success and long-term clinical outcome of radiofrequency ablation for the treatment of spinal osteoid osteomas and osteoblastomas. Neuroradiology 61:935–942

Bhure U, Roos JE, Strobel K (2019) Osteoid osteoma: multimodality imaging with focus on hybrid imaging. Eur J Nucl Med Mol Imaging 46:1019–1036

Cazzato RL, Auloge P, Dalili D et al (2019) Percutaneous image-guided cryoablation of osteoblastoma. Am J Roentgenol 213:1157–1162

Cazzato RL, Garnon J, De Marini P et al (2020) French multidisciplinary approach for the treatment of MSK tumors. Semin Musculoskelet Radiol 24:310–322

Dalili D, Isaac A, Bazzocchi A et al (2020) Interventional techniques for bone and musculoskeletal soft tissue tumors: current practices and future directions - Part I. Ablation. Semin Musculoskelet Radiol 24:692–709

Davies M, Cassar-Pullicino VN, Davies AM et al (2002) The diagnostic accuracy of MR imaging in osteoid osteoma. Skeletal Radiol 31:559–569

Elder BD, Goodwin CR, Kosztowski TA et al (2016) Surgical management of osteoblastoma of the spine: case series and review of the literature. Turk Neurosurg 26:601–617

Gangi A, Alizadeh H, Wong L et al (2007) Osteoid osteoma: percutaneous laser ablation and follow-up in 114 patients. Radiology 242:293–301

Germann T, Weber MA, Lehner B et al (2020) Intraarticular osteoid osteoma: MRI characteristics and clinical presentation before and after radiofrequency ablation compared to extraarticular osteoid osteoma. Fortschr Röntgenstr 192:1190–1199

Ghanem I (2006) The management of osteoid osteoma: updates and controversies. Curr Opin Pediatr 18:36–41

Goldstein GS, Dawson EG, Batzdorf U (1977) Cervical osteoid osteoma: a cause of chronic upper back pain. Clin Orthop Relat Res 129:177–180

Kan P, Schmidt MH (2008) Osteoid osteoma and osteoblastoma of the spine. Neurosurg Clin N Am 19:65–70

Kostrzewa M, Henzler T, Schoenberg SO et al (2019) Clinical and quantitative MRI perfusion analysis of osteoid osteomas before and after microwave ablation. Anticancer Res 39:3053–3057

Lalam R, Bloem JL, Noebauer-Huhmann IM et al (2017) ESSR consensus document for detection, characterisation, and referral pathway for tumors and tumorlike lesions of bone. Semin Musculoskelet Radiol 21:630–647

Li Y, Du Y, Luo TY et al (2014) Factors influencing diagnostic yield of CT-guided percutaneous core needle biopsy for bone lesions. Clin Radiol 69:e43–e47

Lidar Z, Khashan M, Ofir D et al (2021) Resection of benign osseous spine tumors in pediatric patients by minimally invasive techniques. World Neurosurg 152:758–764

Liu PT, Kujak JL, Roberts CC et al (2011) The vascular groove sign: a new CT finding associated with osteoid osteomas. AJR Am J Roentgenol 196:168–173

Lucas DR (2010) Osteoblastoma. Arch Pathol Lab Med 134:1460–1466

Maldague BE, Malghem JJ (1976) Unilateral arch hypertrophy with spinous process tilt: a sign of arch deficiency. Radiology 121:567–574

Napoli A, Bazzocchi A, Scipione R et al (2017) Noninvasive therapy for osteoid osteoma: a prospective developmental study with MR imaging-guided high-intensity focused ultrasound. Radiology 285:186–196

Orguc S, Arkun R (2014) Primary tumors of the spine. Semin Musculoskelet Radiol 18:280–299

Paige ML, Michael AS, Brodin A (1991) Case report 647: Benign osteoblastoma causing spinal cord compression and spastic paresis. Skeletal Radiol 20:54–57

Papaioannou G, Sebire NJ, McHugh K (2009) Imaging of the unusual pediatric 'blastomas'. Cancer Imaging 9:1–11

Rehnitz C, Sprengel SD, Lehner B et al (2012) CT-guided radiofrequency ablation of osteoid osteoma and osteoblastoma: clinical success and long-term follow up in 77 patients. Eur J Radiol 81:3426–3434

Riahi H, Mechri M, Barsaoui M et al (2018) Imaging of benign tumors of the osseous spine. J Belg Soc Radiol 102:13

Rimondi E, Rossi G, Bartalena T et al (2011) Percutaneous CT-guided biopsy of the musculoskeletal system: results of 2027 cases. Eur J Radiol 77:34–42

Tepelenis K, Skandalakis GP, Papathanakos G et al (2021) Osteoid osteoma: an updated review of epidemiology, pathogenesis, clinical presentation, radiological features, and treatment option. In Vivo 35:1929–1938

Thawait SK, Marcus MA, Morrison WB et al (2012) Research synthesis: what is the diagnostic performance of magnetic resonance imaging to discriminate benign from malignant vertebral compression fractures? Systematic review and meta-analysis. Spine (Phila Pa 1976) 37:E736–E744

Virayavanich W, Ringler MD, Chin CT et al (2011) CT-guided biopsy of bone and soft-tissue lesions: role of on-site immediate cytologic evaluation. J Vasc Interv Radiol 22:1024–1030

Weber MA, Sprengel SD, Omlor GW et al (2015) Clinical long-term outcome, technical success, and cost analysis of radiofrequency ablation for the treatment of osteoblastomas and spinal osteoid osteomas in comparison to open surgical resection. Skeletal Radiol 44:981–993

Weber MA, Bazzocchi A, Nöbauer-Huhmann IM (2022) Tumors of the spine: when can biopsy be avoided? Semin Musculoskelet Radiol 26:453–468

Wu JS, Goldsmith JD, Horwich PJ et al (2008) Bone and soft-tissue lesions: what factors affect diagnostic yield in image guided core needle biopsy? Radiology 248:962–970

Wu M, Xu K, Xie Y et al (2019) Diagnostic and management options of osteoblastoma in the spine. Med Sci Monit 25:1362–1372

Yang SY, Oh E, Kwon JW et al (2018) Percutaneous image-guided spinal lesion biopsies: factors affecting higher diagnostic yield. AJR Am J Roentgenol 211:1068–1074

Zairi M, Nessib MN (2023) Structural scoliosis secondary to thoracic osteoid osteoma: a case report of delayed diagnosis. Spine Deform 11:247–251

Zhang H, Niu X, Wang B et al (2016) Scoliosis secondary to lumbar osteoid osteoma: a case report of delayed diagnosis and literature review. Medicine (Baltimore) 95:e5362

Giant Cell Tumor of the Spine

Sebnem Orguc, Çağdaş Rıza Açar, and Remide Arkun

Contents

S. Orguc (✉) · Ç. R. Açar
Department of Radiology, Manisa Celal Bayar University Medical School, Manisa, Türkiye
e-mail: sebnem.orguc@cbu.edu.tr

R. Arkun
Star Imaging Center, Izmir, Türkiye

Abstract

Giant cell tumor (GCT) of the spine is a rare condition characterized by locally aggressive osteolytic tumors. While GCTs commonly occur in the epiphysiometaphysis of long bones, spinal lesions are relatively uncommon. The pathologic features of GCTs involve a vascularized stroma composed of spindle-shaped mononuclear cells and multinucleated giant cells. Although GCTs are typically considered benign, approximately 10% may exhibit malignant behavior. Spinal GCTs can present with pain, weakness, and neurological deficits due to compression of neural elements. Imaging techniques such as conventional radiography, computed tomography (CT), magnetic resonance imaging (MRI), and PET/CT can help in diagnosis and staging. The solid portions of GCTs typically demonstrate low signal intensity on T2-weighted images (WI) and intermediate signal intensity on T1-WI, due to the presence of collagen within the fibrous components and hemosiderin deposition. Treatment typically involves complete resection of the tumor, preferably with en bloc resection for better prognosis. However, surgery may be challenging due to the soft and easily ruptured nature of GCTs. In cases where complete surgical resection is not feasible or the tumor exhibits aggressive behavior, adjuvant treatments such as radiotherapy may be considered to control

Med Radiol Diagn Imaging (2023)
https://doi.org/10.1007/174_2023_445,
Published Online: 26 September 2023

local disease progression, while the use of denosumab has shown promise in reducing tumor size and inhibiting osteolysis in unresectable or recurrent giant cell tumors of the spine. Histopathological verification is essential for a definitive diagnosis, and differential diagnoses include other bone tumors and cystic lesions. Various classification systems exist to assess the aggressiveness and guide treatment decisions, although their correlation with local recurrence and metastases is uncertain.

1 Introduction

Giant cell tumors (GCTs) of the bone are locally aggressive osteolytic primary tumors. Cooper and Travers originally described GCT of the bone in 1818, while Jaffe et al. later provided a formal definition in 1940 (Cooper and Travers 1818; Jaffe et al. 1940).

They usually arise in the epiphysiometaphysis of the long bones and are eccentric in location. While the radiological features of GCTs in the extremities are well documented, there are relatively few reports on spinal lesions due to their rarity.

2 Pathologic Features

Although GCTs are typically considered benign tumors, they can exhibit locally aggressive behavior. The estimated frequency of malignant giant cell tumors or malignant transformation of benign giant cell tumors, which is often associated with radiotherapy, is approximately 10% (Seider et al. 1986).

Macroscopically, GCTs appear as soft, friable, fleshy, red-brown masses with yellowish areas. Hemorrhage, hemosiderin, cyst formation, and necrosis may also be present in GCTs. Secondary aneurysmal bone cysts may be present. The bony cortex may be expanded or destroyed.

Microscopically, GCTs are characterized by a vascularized stroma composed of oval or plump, spindle-shaped mononuclear cells uniformly interspersed with multinucleated giant cells (Dorfman and Czerniak 1995). The spindle-shaped mononuclear cells in GCTs have poorly defined cytoplasm, spindle-shaped nuclei, and variable degrees of mitotic activity and are considered the neoplastic cell population. On the other hand, the multinucleated giant cells, resembling osteoclasts, have eosinophilic cytoplasm and vesicular nuclei and are believed to be a reactive cell population within the tumor (Mavrogenis et al. 2017).

3 Epidemiology

GCTs of the bone typically affect individuals between the ages of 20 and 40 years, with a slightly higher incidence in females. Spinal GCTs have been reported to affect younger patients compared to extremity GCTs (Dahlin 1977). An increase in the lesion size can be seen with pregnancy (Murphey et al. 1996).

4 Localization

Spinal location of GCT is rare with only 2.7% of cases in a review of 1277 cases (Shankman et al. 1988). GCT of the sacrum is the most common location with thoracic, cervical, and lumbar levels in decreasing frequency (Bidwell et al. 1987).

The tumor usually develops in the vertebral body, and the posterior elements are frequently involved in patients with advanced lesions.

Generally, GCT of the vertebrae is limited to a single segment. Various structures in the spine, including the intervertebral disk, periosteum, anterior and posterior longitudinal ligaments, hyaline cartilage of the facet joint, and dura mater, have been suggested to act as barriers to preventing tumor spread (Tomita et al. 1997). Lesions originating from the vertebral body can be either centrally or eccentrically located. Typically, larger lesions tend to be centrally located (Shi et al. 2015). Spinal GCTs usually present as a solitary lesion, although multicentric lesions have been documented before (Kos et al.

1997). Due to their locally aggressive nature, GCT of the bone can extend into the paravertebral soft tissues and compress the spinal cord or nerve roots.

5 Clinical Presentation

Cortical destruction and expansion into the spinal canal and neural foramina may cause compression of the neural elements. Pain often with radicular distribution is the most common clinical symptom. Patients may present with weakness and neurological deficits.

6 Imaging

6.1 Conventional Radiography (CR)

Starting with CR is recommended as the initial step in imaging for evaluation. Unlike GCTs in long bones, the absence of epiphyseal-metaphyseal landmarks in the spine and sacrum makes radiographic diagnosis of GCTs in these areas less clear. GCT typically appears as a radiolucent-osteolytic lesion, exhibiting geographic bone lysis, a narrow zone of transition, abutment of the articular margin, and a lack of surrounding sclerotic rim (Fig. 1a). The cortex in the lytic areas appears indistinct with an associated soft tissue component. Any soft tissue shadow in the psoas muscle should be noted. The oval-shaped pedicle of the vertebra may be deformed or not visible due to destruction. Spine GCTs can cause collapse of the vertebral body, ranging from mild collapse to complete vertebra plana. Unless there is a fracture, GCT does not cause a periosteal reaction. GCTs typically demonstrate a characteristic pattern of prominent trabeculation and a loculated appearance.

GCTs in the sacrum typically exhibit characteristics such as larger size, central location, and a destructive nature. Invasion of sacroiliac joint can be seen (Batnitzky et al. 1982; Jong et al. 2007).

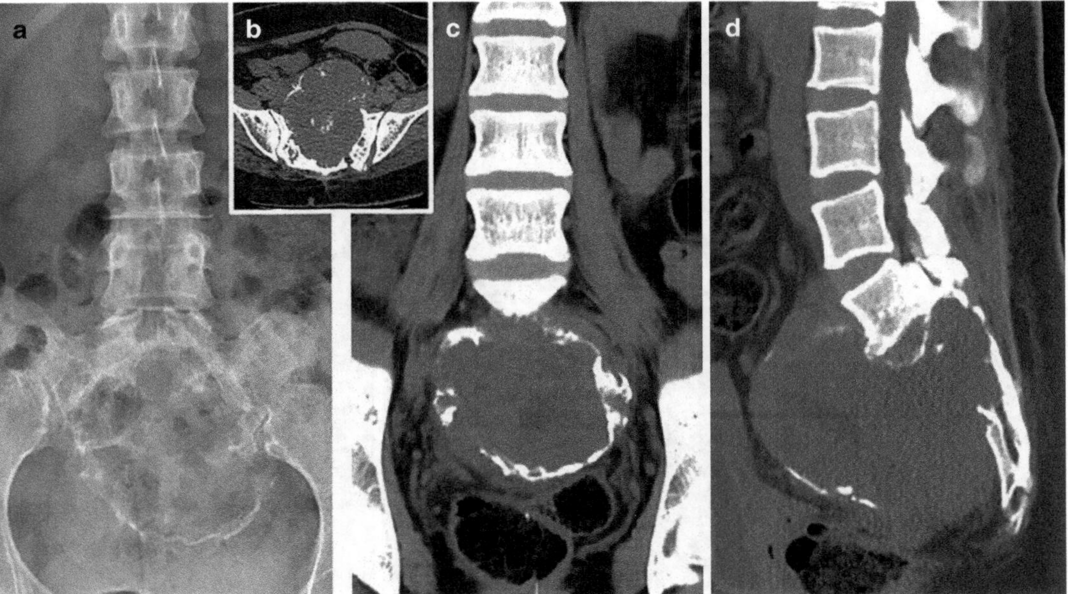

Fig. 1 (**a**–**d**) Giant cell tumor of sacrum in an 18-year-old female patient. (**a**) AP radiograph, (**b**) axial CT scan, and (**c**) coronal and (**d**) sagittal MIP reconstruction CT images demonstrate a lytic expansile mass lesion with prominent trabeculation originating from the midsacral segment. The bony cortex of the corpus vertebra is destructed with extension of the lesion to the posterior elements. No matrix calcification is detected

During the evaluation of follow-up radiographs after resection, any new developing lucency should be noted as a possible sign of recurrence.

6.2 Computed Tomography (CT)

Computed tomography is superior to CR for detecting cortical thinning, pathological fractures, periosteal reaction, and degree of osseous expansile remodeling and confirming the absence of mineralization (Fig. 1). Low attenuation areas, which may represent hemorrhage and necrosis, can be seen (Murphey et al. 1996). Additionally, bony septations arising from the border of the lesion and extending into the lesion may produce a characteristic "soap bubble" (Si et al. 2014). The remaining bony trabecula may be thickened secondary to a compensatory response to weakened bone. This appearance can also be seen in other bone lesions such as plasmacytomas and hemangiomas (see chapters "Plasmacytoma" and "Vertebral Hemangioma and Angiomatous Neoplasms") (Shi et al. 2015). Nonaggressive GCTs typically exhibit prominent trabeculation, while aggressive tumors often lack this feature.

6.3 Magnetic Resonance Imaging (MRI)

CT and especially MRI can provide information on the extent of bony and soft tissue involvement in GCT (Fig. 2). The solid portions of GCTs typically demonstrate low signal intensity on T2-weighted images (WI) and intermediate signal intensity on T1-WI, due to the presence of collagen within the fibrous components and hemosiderin deposition. Hemosiderin deposition may show nodular, zonal, whorled, or diffuse low signal intensity. The low signal on T2-WI in GCTs is very helpful in differentiating these lesions from most other spinal lesions, which may have high T2-weighted signal intensity, such as metastases, lymphoma, and chordoma.

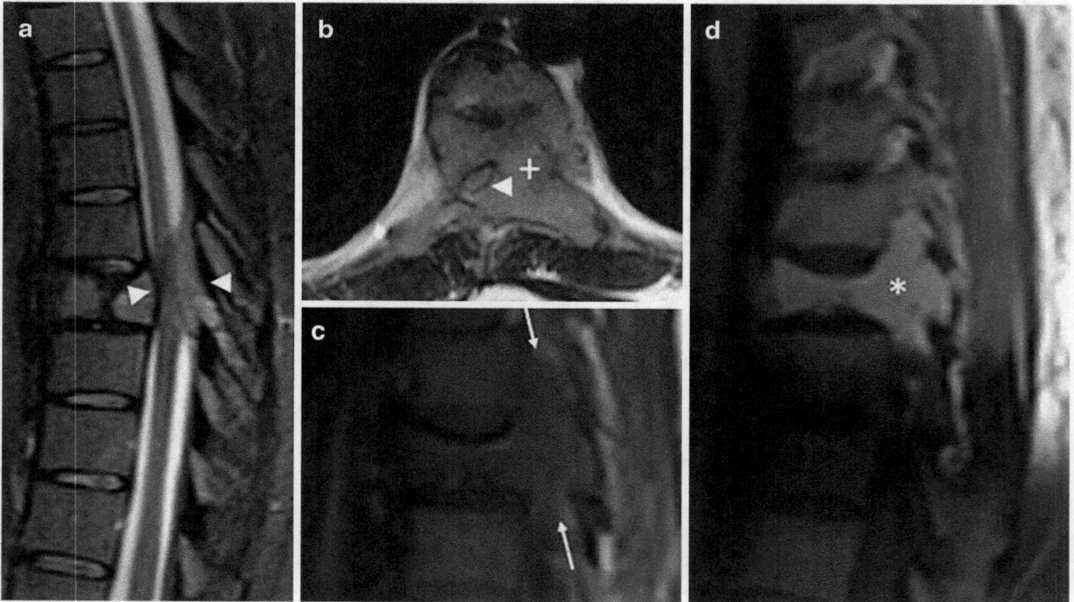

Fig. 2 (**a–d**) Thoracal giant cell tumor in a 26-year-old female patient. (**a**) Sagittal STIR, (**b**) axial T2-WI, (**c**) sagittal T1-WI, and (**d**) postcontrast sagittal T1-WI. Expansile, destructive mass lesion of eighth dorsal vertebra with low T2 signal (+) compresses the spinal cord (arrowheads), infiltrates the left pedicle (arrow), and enhances after contrast administration (asterisk)

Enhancement after IV gadolinium-based contrast agents may be helpful to differentiate between solid and cystic components in the tumor. On dynamic contrast-enhanced MRI, the solid portions of GCTs typically exhibit early and rapid progressive enhancement, followed by a contrast washout. Another feature to consider is the presence of a fluid-fluid level, which can indicate intralesional hemorrhage or development of a secondary aneurysmal bone cyst. With an incidence of 19–39%, GCTs are the most common lesions associated with secondary aneurysmal bone cysts (Chakarun et al. 2013; Kransdorf and Sweet 1995; Murphey et al. 2001; Turcotte 2006). The presence of a secondary aneurysmal bone cyst is associated with an increased risk of recurrence (Kransdorf and Sweet 1995; Wang et al. 2013). Curvilinear low-signal areas on both T1- and T2-WI can be observed within the lesion, which may represent thickened trabeculae, fibrous septa, or hemosiderin deposits (Jong et al. 2007). A sclerotic border or fibrous capsule may accompany the tumor, causing low signal on MR images (Si et al. 2014).

6.4 PET and PET/CT

Contrary to most benign tumors, the majority of GCTs show intense uptake of F18-FDG, which can be explained by their high cellularity (Muheremu et al. 2017).

7 Histopathology

Although clinical and imaging findings can limit the number of possible diagnoses, histopathological verification remains essential for a definitive diagnosis of spinal GCTs. Tissue samples can be obtained with either open or imaging-guided biopsy. Image-guided biopsy used with CT or US is a minimally invasive technique with low cost and a low risk of tumor spread and contamination.

GCTs consist of three distinct cell types: round mononuclear stromal cells, spindle-shaped mononuclear stromal cells, and multinucleated giant cells (Wülling et al. 2001). Destructive osteolysis caused by osteoclasts is responsible for the morbidity associated with GCTs (Morgan et al. 2005). Since other lesions such as brown tumors, aneurysmal bone cysts, and giant cell reparative granulomas also contain giant cells, a detailed histopathological examination and correlation with clinical and imaging findings are crucial in distinguishing GCTs from these other conditions (Greenspan and Remagen 1998). While the distribution of giant cells is even in GCTS, they are not evenly distributed in brown tumors.

Primary malignant GCT of the bone may demonstrate malignant pleomorphic spindle cells along with the normal GCT areas (Yin et al. 2015).

8 Differential Diagnosis

The differential diagnosis for GCT includes brown tumor of hyperparathyroidism, metastatic disease, hematologic malignancies, aneurysmal bone cyst, giant cell reparative granuloma, chordoma, chondroblastoma, sarcoma, and fibrous histiocytoma (Greenspan and Remagen 1998; Chakarun et al. 2013).

Plasmacytoma is usually associated with older age (over 40 years of age) and lack of cystic changes (see chapter "Plasmacytoma").

Pathological compression of vertebral bodies and destruction of cortex are not common findings in hemangiomas. Other imaging features of hemangiomas such as prominent hyperintensity on T2-weighted images can aid in the diagnosis (see chapter "Vertebral Hemangioma and Angiomatous Neoplasms").

If there is a sacral lesion suspected to be a GCT, chordomas should also be considered in the differential diagnosis. Sacral chordomas typically present as midline lesions that may contain calcifications or sequestered bony fragments and have a very high T2 signal (see chapter "Notochordal Tumors").

When associated with secondary aneurysmal bone cysts, differential diagnosis with primary aneurysmal bone cysts should be considered. In primary aneurysmal bone cysts, the tumor is mostly located at the posterior elements and lacks a soft tissue component, and the patients are typically below the age of 20 years (see chapter "Aneurysmal Bone Cyst and Other Cystic Lesions") (Sanjay et al. 1993).

9 Local and Distant Staging

The incidence of metastasis in GCTs is reported to be 1% of cases (Abernethy et al. 2015; Thomas et al. 2010). Similar to GCTs in long bones, spinal GCTs can also lead to the development of "benign lung metastasis," with an incidence rate of 13.7% reported (Sanjay et al. 1993). The occurrence of histologically identical benign lesions at sites distant from the primary location can provide an explanation for benign metastases. Usually, pulmonary metastases remain stable or show regression after the treatment.

Histological, radiographic, and clinico-radiological staging systems have been suggested for GCTs. Jaffe et al. proposed a histological classification system composed of three stages: benign, aggressive, and malignant (Mavrogenis et al. 2017). This classification system is based on histological appearance of the stromal cells, as well as the number of giant cells and mitotic activity.

Enneking et al. proposed a clinico-radiological classification system for all benign bone tumors, which can also be used for GCTs (Enneking et al. 1980). This system consists of three stages. Stage 1 describes a lesion that is completely confined within the bone, being asymptomatic, histologically benign, and inactive on bone scan. Stage 2 refers to a lesion with an expanded cortex and no breakthrough, being symptomatic, histologically benign, and active on bone scan. Stage 3 refers to a rapidly growing symptomatic mass with cortical perforation and a soft tissue mass, which may metastasize, become histologically benign, and show extensive activity on bone scan.

Campannacci et al. proposed a radiographic classification system for GCTs, which consists of three grades (Campanacci et al. 1987). Grade 1 refers to a lesion with a well-defined margin and an intact cortex. Grade 2 refers to a lesion with a relatively well-defined margin but no radiopaque rim, and the cortex is thinned and moderately expanded. Grade 3 refers to a lesion with indistinct borders and cortical destruction.

The Weinstein-Boriani-Biagini surgical staging system was developed to create a comprehensive method for managing spinal tumors, utilizing 12 radiating zones and 5 concentric layers to classify tumors based on their location. The classification of tumor involvement in this classification system enables surgeons to distinguish between three treatment options: vertebrectomy, sagittal resection, and resection of the posterior arch (Boriani et al. 1997).

The accuracy and reliability of GCT classifications in assessing aggressiveness, providing prognostic significance, and guiding surgical decision-making are uncertain. Furthermore, there is no clear correlation between these classifications and the incidence of local recurrence or metastases (Mavrogenis et al. 2017).

10 Treatment

The primary management strategy for GCTs is complete resection of the tumor. For spinal GCTs, removal of the vertebral body is recommended (Ozaki et al. 2002; Sanjay et al. 1993). Spinal GCTs are often asymptomatic and typically remain undiagnosed until the later stages of the disease, by which time the tumor has grown considerably, and surgery could lead to severe neurological deficits (Martin and McCarthy 2010). En bloc resection with wide margins is suggested to be associated with a lower recurrence rate and better prognosis (Luksanapruksa et al. 2016). En bloc resection could not be applied in all spinal GCT patients because of inherent risk of operation. The soft and easily ruptured nature of GCTs can make en bloc resection more challenging. Intralesional resection is associated with lower functional morbidity and fewer complications but high recurrence rate (Lin et al. 2018) (Fig. 3).

To eliminate the tumor and decrease the recurrence rate, high-speed burring, phenol, cement-

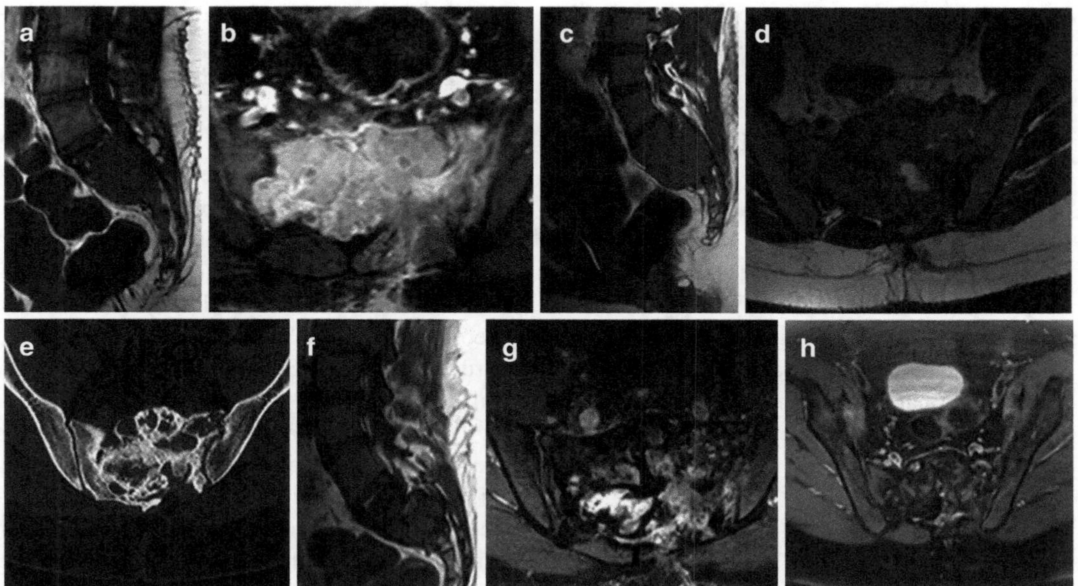

Fig. 3 (**a**–**h**) Sacral giant cell tumor in a 26-year-old male patient. (**a**) Sagittal T1-WI and (**b**) postcontrast axial fat-suppressed (FS) T1-WI demonstrating expansile, destructive, and enhancing solid mass. (**c**) Sagittal T1w and (**d**) axial T2-WI taken 1 year after intralesional resection, depicting tumor recurrence. (**e**) Axial CT scan, (**f**) sagittal T1-WI, and (**g**) postcontrast axial FS T1-WI taken 3 years later, showing regression of the lesion after initiating denosumab treatment. (**h**) Postcontrast axial FS T1-WI taken after 5 years, indicating further regression of the lesion. (Courtesy of Dr. Ipek Tamsel and Ege University Musculoskeletal Tumor Board)

ing, electrocoagulation, and cryotherapy were suggested (Lin et al. 2018).

Radiotherapy after resection is suggested to reduce the recurrence rate and can also be used for spinal GCT patients who are not suitable for resection (Khan et al. 1999; Ma et al. 2015; Sharma et al. 2002). Some authors suggested that there is no benefit of adjuvant radiotherapy after conservative management of sacral GCTs, while others still recommend it (Donthineni et al. 2009; Hart et al. 1997; Shi et al. 2013; Thangaraj et al. 2010). It is important to note the potential side effects of radiation therapy, such as radiation-induced spinal cord myelitis and malignant transformation (Luksanapruksa et al. 2016).

Selective angiography and embolization can be performed as the main treatment in inoperable cases and before surgery to reduce intraoperative bleeding since GCTs are vascular lesions (Refai et al. 2009).

Since the recruitment of osteoclasts depends on several factors, including the receptor activator of nuclear factor kappa B ligand (RANKL), denosumab, a human monoclonal antibody that inhibits RANKL, can be used as a treatment (Fig. 3). By inhibiting RANKL, denosumab prevents osteoclast-driven bone destruction (Thomas et al. 2010). Denosumab can be used as a standalone or adjuvant treatment. Preoperative use of denosumab for 6 months has been shown to reduce tumor burden and develop clear cortical margins (Palmerini et al. 2020). However, there is no consensus on the optimal duration for standalone treatment. Although lifelong treatment is an option, it carries the risk of adverse events such as mandible osteonecrosis (Aghaloo et al. 2010).

While there is no strong evidence supporting bisphosphonate treatment for GCTs, Maurice et al. reported that bisphosphonates may be useful in controlling disease progression due to their inhibition of osteoclast resorption (Balke et al. 2010). Additionally, Tse et al. reported that bisphosphonates can reduce tumor recurrence when used as adjuvant therapy to intralesional curettage or excision (Tse et al. 2008).

GCTs have been found to overexpress angiogenic growth factors. In cases of metastatic or unresectable disease, interferon (IFN), which targets angiogenic growth factors, has been suggested as a treatment option (López-Pousa et al. 2015).

For pulmonary metastases, surgical resection is usually recommended especially if the patient is symptomatic or has tumor-related pulmonary morbidity (Balke et al. 2008). For unresectable or recurrent metastasis, nonsurgical options such as radiotherapy and denosumab can be considered. Also, pulmonary metastases may be managed with regular surveillance (Tsukamoto et al. 2020).

11 Prognosis

Treatment for tubular bone lesions typically results in complete cure in 85–90% of cases. However, when it comes to axial skeleton lesions, particularly those in the sacrum, the prognosis is often poorer due to their larger size and the difficulty in achieving complete excision (Randall 2003). The recurrence rate reported is between 22% and 44% for spinal GCTs (Figs. 4 and 5) (Xu et al. 2013). The higher recurrence rate of spinal GCTs in younger patients has been reported in previous studies (Sanjay et al. 1993; Boriani et al. 2012). Postirradiation sarcoma is another concern for patients with GCTs. According to the literature, there is a reported rate of 17% for secondary sarcoma in patients with GCTs of the spine, sacrum, and pelvis (Sanjay et al. 1993; Turcotte et al. 1990).

After treatment, patients need to follow up for at least 10 years. During the first 2 years, clinical and radiographic surveillance should be conducted every 3 months, followed by a 3-year period during which follow-up visits can be spaced out to every 6 months. After that, yearly follow-up visits are recommended for the next 5 years. CT or MRI can be used to assess local recurrence, and chest CT scans can be used to assess possible pulmonary metastases (Boriani et al. 2012).

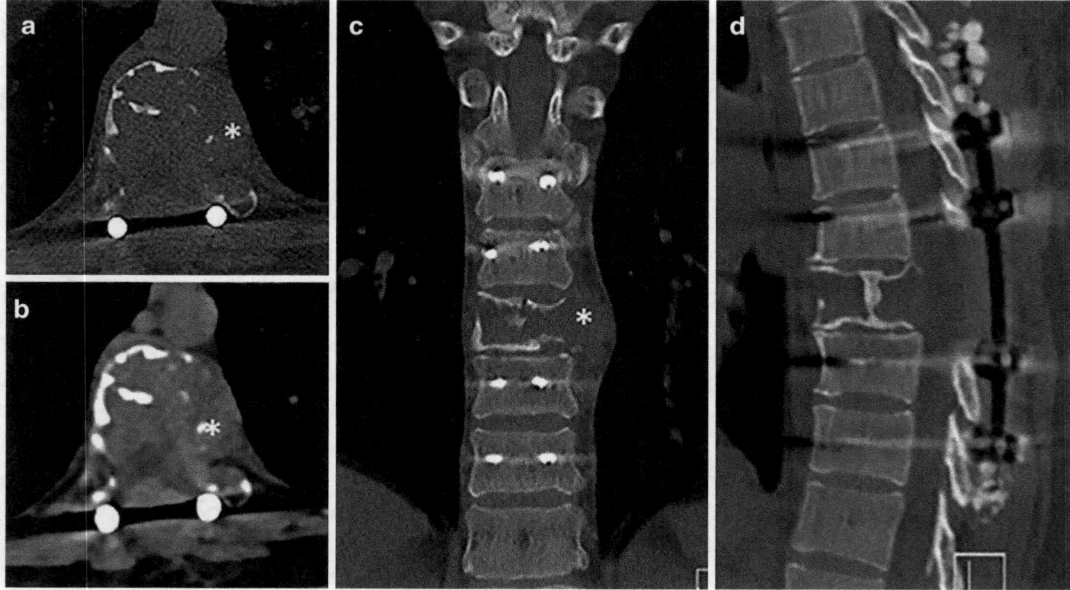

Fig. 4 (**a**–**d**) CT of the case in Fig. 2. Residual-recurrent dorsal giant cell tumor in a 26-year-old female patient. (**a**, **b**) Axial CT scan, (**c**) coronal and (**d**) sagittal reformatted images. Expansile, destructive mass lesion of eighth dorsal vertebra showing coarse trabecular pattern with paravertebral soft tissue (asterisk) 3 months post-surgery. The patient was treated with radiation therapy and a second operation subsequently

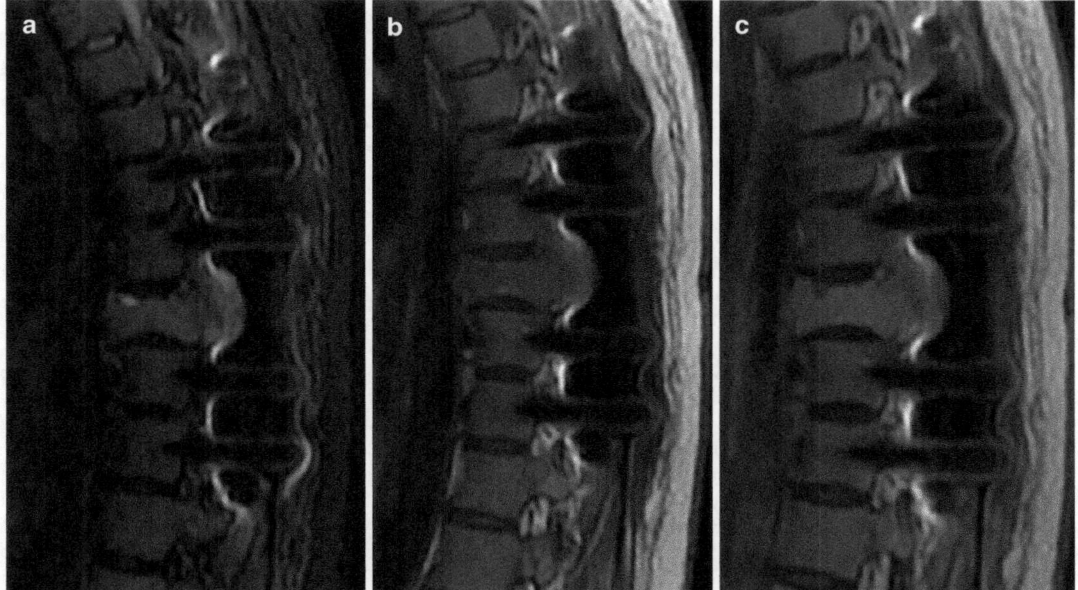

Fig. 5 (**a–c**) Postoperative MRI of the same case. Residual-recurrent thoracal giant cell tumor in a 26-year-old female patient. (**a**) Sagittal FSE T2-WI, (**b**) sagittal T1-WI, and (**c**) sagittal postcontrast T1-WI. Expansile, destructive mass lesion of eighth dorsal vertebra with mild enhancement 3 months after intralesional resection

12 Key Points

- Giant cell tumors (GCTs) of the bone typically originate in the epiphysiometaphysis of long bones and exhibit an eccentric location. Although the radiological characteristics of GCTs in the extremities have been extensively documented, there is a scarcity of reports on spinal lesions due to their rare occurrence.
- GCTs of the bone typically affect individuals in the age range of 20–40 years, with a slightly higher incidence observed in females. It has been noted that spinal GCTs tend to affect younger patients when compared to GCTs in the extremities.
- GCT of the bone often develops in the vertebral body and can involve the posterior elements. It may extend into the paravertebral soft tissues, compressing the spinal cord or nerve roots. Common symptoms include pain with radicular distribution, weakness, and neurological deficits.
- GCTs often exhibit low signal intensity on T2-WI and intermediate signal intensity on T1-WI due to collagen and hemosiderin deposition. A fluid-fluid level may also be observed, suggesting intralesional hemorrhage or formation of an aneurysmal bone cyst. Surgical resection is the primary treatment option for GCTs; however, in cases where complete resection is not possible or the tumor is unresectable or recurrent, adjuvant therapies like radiotherapy and denosumab may be considered.

References

Abernethy A, Appelbaum F, Buckner J, Clurman B, Cohen H, Gandara D et al (2015) ASCO-SEP, 4th edn. American Society of Clinical Oncology, Alexandria, VA, p 369

Aghaloo TL, Felsenfeld AL, Tetradis S (2010) Osteonecrosis of the jaw in a patient on denosumab. J Oral Maxillofac Surg 68(5):959–963. https://doi.org/10.1016/j.joms.2009.10.010

Balke M, Schremper L, Gebert C, Ahrens H, Streitbuerger A, Koehler G, Hardes J, Gosheger G (2008) Giant cell tumor of bone: treatment and outcome of 214 cases. J Cancer Res Clin Oncol 134(9):969–978. https://doi.org/10.1007/s00432-008-0370-x

Balke M, Campanacci L, Gebert C, Picci P, Gibbons M, Taylor R, Hogendoorn P, Kroep J, Wass J, Athanasou N (2010) Bisphosphonate treatment of aggressive primary, recurrent and metastatic giant cell tumour of bone. BMC Cancer 10:462. https://doi.org/10.1186/1471-2407-10-462

Batnitzky S, Soye I, Levine E, Price HI, Hart KZ (1982) Computed tomography in the evaluation of lesions arising in and around the sacrum. Radiographics 2(4):500–528. https://doi.org/10.1148/radiographics.2.4.500

Bidwell JK, Young JW, Khalluff E (1987) Giant cell tumor of the spine: computed tomography appearance and review of the literature. J Comput Tomogr 11(3):307–311. https://doi.org/10.1016/0149-936x(87)90104-4

Boriani S, Weinstein JN, Biagini R (1997) Primary bone tumors of the spine: terminology and surgical staging. Spine 22(9):1036–1044

Boriani S, Bandiera S, Casadei R, Boriani L, Donthineni R, Gasbarrini A, Pignotti E, Biagini R, Schwab JH (2012) Giant cell tumor of the mobile spine: a review of 49 cases. Spine 37(1):37–45. https://doi.org/10.1097/BRS.0b013e3182233ccd

Campanacci M, Baldini N, Boriani S, Sudanese A (1987) Giant-cell tumor of bone. J Bone Joint Surg Am 69(1):106–114

Chakarun CJ, Forrester DM, Gottsegen CJ, Patel DB, White EA, Matcuk GR (2013) Giant cell tumor of bone: review, mimics, and new developments in treatment. Radiographics 33(1):197–211. https://doi.org/10.1148/rg.331125089

Cooper A, Travers B (1818) Surgical essays, 3rd edn. Cox & Son, London, England

Dahlin DC (1977) Giant-cell tumor of vertebrae above the sacrum: a review of 31 cases. Cancer 39(3):1350–1356. https://doi.org/10.1002/1097-0142(197703)39:3<1350::aid-cncr2820390351>3.0.co;2-1

Donthineni R, Boriani L, Ofluoglu O, Bandiera S (2009) Metastatic behaviour of giant cell tumour of the spine. Int Orthop 33(2):497–501. https://doi.org/10.1007/s00264-008-0560-9

Dorfman HD, Czerniak B (1995) Bone cancers. Cancer 75(1 Suppl):203–210. https://doi.org/10.1002/1097-0142(19950101)75:1+<203::aid-cncr2820751308>3.0.co;2-v

Enneking WF, Spanier SS, Goodman MA (1980) A system for the surgical staging of musculoskeletal sarcoma. Clin Orthop Relat Res 153:106–120

Greenspan A, Remagen R (1998) Differential diagnosis of tumors and tumorlike lesions of bones and joints. Lippincott-Raven, Philadelphia

Hart RA, Boriani S, Biagini R, Currier B, Weinstein JN (1997) A system for surgical staging and management of spine tumors. A clinical outcome study of giant cell tumors of the spine. Spine 22(15):1773–82; discussion 1783. https://doi.org/10.1097/00007632-199708010-00018

Jaffe HL, Lichtenstein L, Portis RB (1940) Giant cell tumor of bone: its pathologic appearance, grading, supposed variants and treatment. Arch Pathol 30:993–1031

Jong WK, Chung HW, Eun YC, Sung HH, Choi SH, Young CY, Sang KY (2007) MRI findings of giant cell tumors of the spine. AJR Am J Roentgenol 189(1):246–250. https://doi.org/10.2214/AJR.06.1472

Khan DC, Malhotra S, Stevens RE, Steinfeld AD (1999) Radiotherapy for the treatment of giant cell tumor of the spine: a report of six cases and review of the literature. Cancer Invest 17(2):110–113

Kos CB, Taconis WK, Fidler MW, ten Velden JJ (1997) Multifocal giant cell tumors in the spine. A case report. Spine 22(7):821–822. https://doi.org/10.1097/00007632-199704010-00022

Kransdorf MJ, Sweet DE (1995) Aneurysmal bone cyst: concept, controversy, clinical presentation, and imaging. AJR Am J Roentgenol 164(3):573–580. https://doi.org/10.2214/ajr.164.3.7863874

Lin P, Lin N, Teng W, Wang SD, Pan WB, Huang X, Yan XB, Liu M, Li HY, Li BH, Sun LL, Wang Z, Zhou XZ, Ye ZM (2018) Recurrence of giant cell tumor of the spine after resection: a report of 10 cases. Orthop Surg 10(2):107–114. https://doi.org/10.1111/os.12375

López-Pousa A, Martín Broto J, Garrido T, Vázquez J (2015) Giant cell tumour of bone: new treatments in development. Clin Transl Oncol 17(6):419–430. https://doi.org/10.1007/s12094-014-1268-5

Luksanapruksa P, Buchowski JM, Singhatanadgige W, Bumpass DB (2016) Systematic review and meta-analysis of en bloc vertebrectomy compared with intralesional resection for giant cell tumors of the mobile spine. Global Spine J 6(8):798–803. https://doi.org/10.1055/s-0036-1579746

Ma Y, Wei X, Yin H, Huang Q, Liu T, Yang X, Wei H, Xiao J (2015) Therapeutic radiotherapy for giant cell tumor of the spine: a systemic review. Eur Spine J 24(8):1754–1760. https://doi.org/10.1007/s00586-015-3834-0

Martin C, McCarthy EF (2010) Giant cell tumor of the sacrum and spine: series of 23 cases and a review of the literature. Iowa Orthop J 30:69–75

Mavrogenis AF, Igoumenou VG, Megaloikonomos PD, Panagopoulos GN, Papagelopoulos PJ, Soucacos PN (2017) Giant cell tumor of bone revisited. SICOT-J 3:54. https://doi.org/10.1051/sicotj/2017041

Morgan T, Atkins GJ, Trivett MK, Johnson SA, Kansara M, Schlicht SL, Slavin JL, Simmons P, Dickinson I, Powell G, Choong PFM, Holloway AJ, Thomas DM (2005) Molecular profiling of giant cell tumor of bone and the osteoclastic localization of ligand for receptor activator of nuclear factor KB. Am J Pathol 167(1):117–128. https://doi.org/10.1016/S0002-9440(10)62959-8

Muheremu A, Ma Y, Huang Z, Shan H, Li Y, Niu X (2017) Diagnosing giant cell tumor of the bone using positron emission tomography/computed tomography: a retrospective study of 20 patients from a single center. Oncol Lett 14(2):1985–1988. https://doi.org/10.3892/ol.2017.6379

Murphey MD, Andrews CL, Flemming DJ, Temple HT, Smith WS, Smirniotopoulos JG (1996) From the archives of the AFIP. Primary tumors of the spine: radiologic pathologic correlation. Radiographics 16(5):1131–1158. https://doi.org/10.1148/radiographics.16.5.8888395

Murphey MD, Nomikos GC, Flemming DJ, Gannon FH, Thomas Temple H, Kransdorf MJ (2001) Imaging of giant cell tumor and giant cell reparative granuloma of bone: radiologic-pathologic correlation. Radiographics 21(5):1283–1309. https://doi.org/10.1148/radiographics.21.5.g01se251283

Ozaki T, Liljenqvist U, Halm H, Hillmann A, Gosheger G, Winkelmann W (2002) Giant cell tumor of the spine. Clin Orthop Relat Res 401:194–201. https://doi.org/10.1097/00003086-200208000-00022

Palmerini E, Staals EL, Jones LB, Donati DM, Longhi A, Lor Randall R (2020) Role of (neo)adjuvant denosumab for giant cell tumor of bone. Curr Treat Options Oncol 21(8):68. https://doi.org/10.1007/s11864-020-00766-4

Randall RL (2003) Giant cell tumor of the sacrum. Neurosurg Focus 15(2):E13. https://doi.org/10.3171/foc.2003.15.2.13

Refai D, Dunn GP, Santiago P (2009) Giant cell tumor of the thoracic spine: case report and review of the literature. Surg Neurol 71(2):228–233. https://doi.org/10.1016/j.surneu.2007.07.056

Sanjay BK, Sim FH, Unni KK, McLeod RA, Klassen RA (1993) Giant-cell tumours of the spine. J Bone Joint Surg Br 75:148–154. https://doi.org/10.1302/0301-620X.75B1.8421014

Seider MJ, Rich TA, Ayala AG, Murray JA (1986) Giant cell tumors of bone: treatment with radiation therapy. Radiology 161(2):537–540. https://doi.org/10.1148/radiology.161.2.3763928

Shankman S, Greenspan A, Klein MJ, Lewis MM (1988) Giant cell tumor of the ischium. A report of two cases and review of the literature. Skeletal Radiol 17(1):46–51. https://doi.org/10.1007/BF00361455

Sharma RR, Mahapatra AK, Pawar SJ, Sousa J, Dev EJ (2002) Craniospinal giant cell tumors: clinicoradiological analysis in a series of 11 cases. J Clin Neurosci 9(1):41–50. https://doi.org/10.1054/jocn.2001.0963

Shi W, Indelicato DJ, Reith J, Smith KB, Morris CG, Scarborough MT, Gibbs CP, Mendenhall WM, Zlotecki RA (2013) Radiotherapy in the management of giant cell tumor of bone. Am J Clin Oncol 36(5):505–508. https://doi.org/10.1097/coc.0b013e3182568fb6

Shi LS, Li YQ, Wu WJ, Zhang ZK, Gao F, Latif M (2015) Imaging appearance of giant cell tumour of the spine above the sacrum. Br J Radiol 88(1051):2–5. https://doi.org/10.1259/bjr.20140566

Si MJ, Wang CG, Wang CS, Du LJ, Ding XY, Zhang WB, Lu Y, Zu JY (2014) Giant cell tumours of the mobile spine: characteristic imaging features and differential diagnosis. Radiol Med 119(9):681–693. https://doi.org/10.1007/s11547-013-0352-1

Thangaraj R, Grimer RJ, Carter SR, Stirling AJ, Spilsbury J, Spooner D (2010) Giant cell tumour of the sacrum: a suggested algorithm for treatment. Eur Spine J 19(7):1189–1194. https://doi.org/10.1007/s00586-009-1270-8

Thomas D, Henshaw R, Skubitz K, Chawla S, Staddon A, Blay J-Y, Roudier M, Smith J, Ye Z, Sohn W, Dansey R, Jun S (2010) Denosumab in patients with giant-cell tumour of bone: an open-label, phase 2 study. Lancet Oncol 11(3):275–280. https://doi.org/10.1016/S1470-2045(10)70010-3

Tomita K, Kawahara N, Baba H, Tsuchiya H, Fujita T, Toribatake Y (1997) Total en bloc spondylectomy. A new surgical technique for primary malignant vertebral tumors. Spine 22(3):324–333. https://doi.org/10.1097/00007632-199702010-00018

Tse LF, Wong KC, Kumta SM, Huang L, Chow TC, Griffith JF (2008) Bisphosphonates reduce local recurrence in extremity giant cell tumor of bone: a case–control study. Bone 42(1):68–73. https://doi.org/10.1016/j.bone.2007.08.038

Tsukamoto S, Ciani G, Mavrogenis AF, Ferrari C, Akahane M, Tanaka Y, Rocca M, Longhi A, Errani C (2020) Outcome of lung metastases due to bone giant cell tumor initially managed with observation. J Orthop Surg Res 15(1):510. https://doi.org/10.1186/s13018-020-02038-1

Turcotte RE (2006) Giant cell tumor of bone. Orthop Clin North Am 37(1):35–51. https://doi.org/10.1016/j.ocl.2005.08.005

Turcotte RE, Biagini R, Sim FH, Unni KK (1990) Giant cell tumor of the spine and sacrum. Chir Organi Mov 75(1 Suppl):104–107

Wang CS, Lou JH, Liao JS, Ding XY, Du LJ, Lu Y, Yan L, Chen KM (2013) Tumore Osseo a Cellule Giganti Recidivante: Caratteristiche Radiologiche e Fattori Di Rischio. Radiol Med 118(3):456–464. https://doi.org/10.1007/s11547-012-0860-4

Wülling M, Engels C, Jesse N, Werner M, Delling G, Kaiser E (2001) The nature of giant cell tumor of bone. J Cancer Res Clin Oncol 127(8):467–474. https://doi.org/10.1007/s004320100234

Xu W, Li X, Wending Huang Y, Wang SH, Chen S, Xu L, Yang X, Liu T, Xiao J (2013) Factors affecting prognosis of patients with giant cell tumors of the mobile spine: retrospective analysis of 102 patients in a single center. Ann Surg Oncol 20(3):804–810. https://doi.org/10.1245/s10434-012-2707-6

Yin H, Cheng M, Li B, Li B, Wang P, Meng T, Wang J, Zhou W, Yan W, Xiao J (2015) Treatment and outcome of malignant giant cell tumor in the spine. J Neurooncol 124(2):275–281. https://doi.org/10.1007/s11060-015-1835-9

Spinal Osteosarcoma

Mohamed Chaabouni, Hend Riahi, Mouna Chelli Bouaziz, and Mohamed Fethi Ladeb

Contents

M. Chaabouni (✉) · H. Riahi · M. Chelli Bouaziz
M. F. Ladeb
Department of Radiology, MT Kassab Institute of Orthopaedics, Ksar Said, Tunisia

Faculty of Medicine of Tunis, Tunis-El Manar University, Tunis, Tunisia
e-mail: dr.chaabounimed@gmail.com; hendriahi@gmail.com; bouaziz_mouna@yahoo.fr; fethiladeb@hotmail.fr

Abstract

Spinal involvement of osteosarcoma is rare, accounting for 3–5% of all osteosarcomas. The most frequent symptom of spinal osteosarcoma is pain, whereas neurologic deficit is frequent, indicating a locally advanced disease at presentation. The diagnosis is made by histology. MRI is the imaging modality of choice for local staging. Chest CT and bone scintigraphy is the classic combination for distant staging. Whole-body MRI, 18-FDG-PET/CT, and 18-FDG-PET/MRI are interesting alternatives. Treatment is based on en bloc tumor removal, chemotherapy, and radiotherapy, although curative surgery is technically difficult due to anatomical particularities of the spine. Overall prognosis remains poor.

1 Introduction

Osteosarcoma is a rare malignancy characterized by the direct formation of immature bone or osteoid tissue by the tumor cells (Picci 2007).

Spinal osteosarcoma (SO) represents only 3–5% of all osteosarcomas, and the sacrum is the most common location (Kelley et al. 2007).

Age of onset follows a bimodal distribution, being more common in young adults (mean age of 38 years) with a second peak in the elderly population (seventh decade of life) (Katonis et al. 2013).

Med Radiol Diagn Imaging (2023)

https://doi.org/10.1007/174_2023_435,
Published Online: 23 May 2023

SO presents almost always with pain, and neurologic impairment is frequent, due to spinal canal invasion.

According to the World Health Organization (WHO) classification, conventional osteoblastic osteosarcoma is the most common histological subtype and is always high grade (Baumhoer et al. 2020).

Radical surgery without major patient morbidity is usually challenging.

We herein review the epidemiology, imaging features, up-to-date staging means, treatment, and prognosis of SO.

2 Pathologic Features

The pathogenesis and cell of origin of osteosarcoma are unclear. Many potential driver genes have been identified (Behjati et al. 2017). Unknown triggers initiate massive chromosomal rearrangements grouped under the name of "chromoanagenesis" resulting in chromosomal instability and subsequent tumor development.

Pleomorphic spindle cells that produce disorganized osteoid are the defining and unifying characteristic of osteosarcoma.

The WHO histological classification recognizes central and surface osteosarcoma types with different subtypes depending on the dominant component (Baumhoer et al. 2020).

Subtypes of central or medullary osteosarcoma include:

- Conventional central osteosarcoma (COS), such as osteoblastic, chondroblastic, fibroblastic, and mixed subtypes
- Telangiectatic osteosarcoma (TAEOS)
- Small cell osteosarcoma (SCOS)
- Low-grade central osteosarcoma

Subtypes of surface or peripheral osteosarcoma include:

- Parosteal osteosarcoma that is well differentiated or low grade
- Periosteal osteosarcoma that is low grade to intermediate grade
- High-grade surface osteosarcoma

Secondary osteosarcomas include:

- Osteosarcoma in Paget's disease of bone
- Radiation-associated sarcoma
- Infarct-related osteosarcoma
- Osteosarcoma due to chronic osteomyelitis
- Implant-related osteosarcoma
- Osteosarcoma secondary to early postzygotic disorders such as fibrous dysplasia

Studies on the histology and molecular biology of SO are limited due to the rarity of the disease: The most common histologic type is osteoblastic COS; others include chondroblastic COS, fibroblastic COS, TAEOS, and SCOS types.

Only one case of low-grade SO was reported in the literature (Kim et al. 2007).

There are no reports of surface SO (Colman and Schwab 2017).

3 Epidemiology

SO accounts for 4–15% of primary spinal tumors and 3–5% of all osteosarcomas (Katonis et al. 2013).

Although predilection for males is admitted in appendicular osteosarcoma, reviews show no significant sex difference in spinal osteosarcoma (Ozaki et al. 2002; Dekutoski et al. 2016).

There are two frequency peaks of age of onset of SO: It is most common in adolescents and young adults with tendency to occur in older age groups (mean of 38 years) (Green et al. 1996) compared to appendicular osteosarcoma (Ottaviani and Jaffe 2009).

The late peak is seen in the seventh decade of life (Katonis et al. 2013) with osteosarcoma more likely resulting from malignant degeneration of predisposing bone conditions.

In the majority of cases, no risk factor is identified. Furthermore, the number of proven risk factors associated with osteosarcoma is limited, including Paget's disease of bone and previous radiotherapy for a different cancer (Savage and Mirabello 2011).

Germline genetic abnormalities associated with Li-Fraumeni syndrome, Werner syndrome,

Rothmund-Thomson syndrome, Bloom syndrome, and hereditary retinoblastoma are considered risk factors for the occurrence of osteosarcoma (Hameed and Mandelker 2018).

Histologically proven malignant transformation of osteoblastoma into SO was rarely reported (Mesfin et al. 2020).

4 Localization

SO is most commonly located in the sacrum followed by the lumbar and thoracic spine segments (Katonis et al. 2013).

There is no consensus on the location within the vertebra in the literature.

However, according to a large-scale study (Ilaslan et al. 2004), the tumor arises from the posterior elements, with partial involvement of the vertebral body in 79% of cases.

The involvement of two vertebral levels (17%) appears to be higher than in other malignant and benign spinal tumors.

Sacral tumors most commonly involve the body and sacral ala (Ilaslan et al. 2004). Tumor spread across the sacroiliac joint is possible, most commonly through the interosseous ligamentous portion (Chhaya et al. 2005).

5 Clinical Presentation

The most common symptom at presentation is persistent nonmechanical bone pain, predominantly at night, with insidious onset and becoming gradually intolerable, reported in 81–95% of cases (Green et al. 1996; Ozaki et al. 2002; Feng et al. 2013; Dekutoski et al. 2016).

Neurologic deficit is also common, accounting for 55–77% of cases (Green et al. 1996; Ozaki et al. 2002; Feng et al. 2013).

A palpable mass is rare at presentation (Green et al. 1996).

The disease is rarely revealed by a vertebral collapse.

New pain and an enlarging mass in a patient with a history of predisposing bone condition suggest the diagnosis of secondary osteosarcoma. Occasionally, the underlying condition is unknown.

6 Imaging

6.1 Radiographs

Radiography is the first-line radiological investigation for any spinal symptoms (Strauss et al. 2021). The examination includes two orthogonal views of the symptomatic spinal segment supplemented by images centered on the suspect vertebra(e).

Abnormalities may be subtle or obscured by overlying visceral anatomy and intestinal gas.

Radiographs usually show osteosclerotic or mixed osteosclerotic-osteolytic lesion (Ilaslan et al. 2004).

A purely lytic pattern is less common, seen in subtypes such as TAEOS (Mechri et al. 2018).

A tumor that develops in a posterior vertebral segment may manifest on an anteroposterior view as a “winking owl” sign because of an obliterated pedicle (Colman and Schwab 2017).

A tumor with marked mineralization arising in the vertebral body may rarely manifest as an “ivory vertebra.”

A vertebral collapse may be associated (Lefebvre et al. 2013).

A heterogeneous soft tissue opacity with ossified and nonossified components is commonly associated (Mechri et al. 2018).

6.2 CT

Computed tomography (CT) is more sensitive than radiography for detecting spinal bone lesions and identifying the vertebral segment(s) involved. It is also superior in analyzing tumor matrix and bone changes: presence of calcification, cortical destruction, and periosteal bone formation.

Soft tissue paravertebral and extradural extension is assessed as well.

The most common pattern is a solitary aggressive mixed tumor, both osteolytic and sclerotic, affecting the posterior arch and extending into the vertebral body (Fig. 1a). The extra-osseous extension is frequent, both epidural and paravertebral, with mineralized matrix (Fig. 2).

In Paget’s disease of bone, findings suggestive of malignant transformation comprise osteolysis,

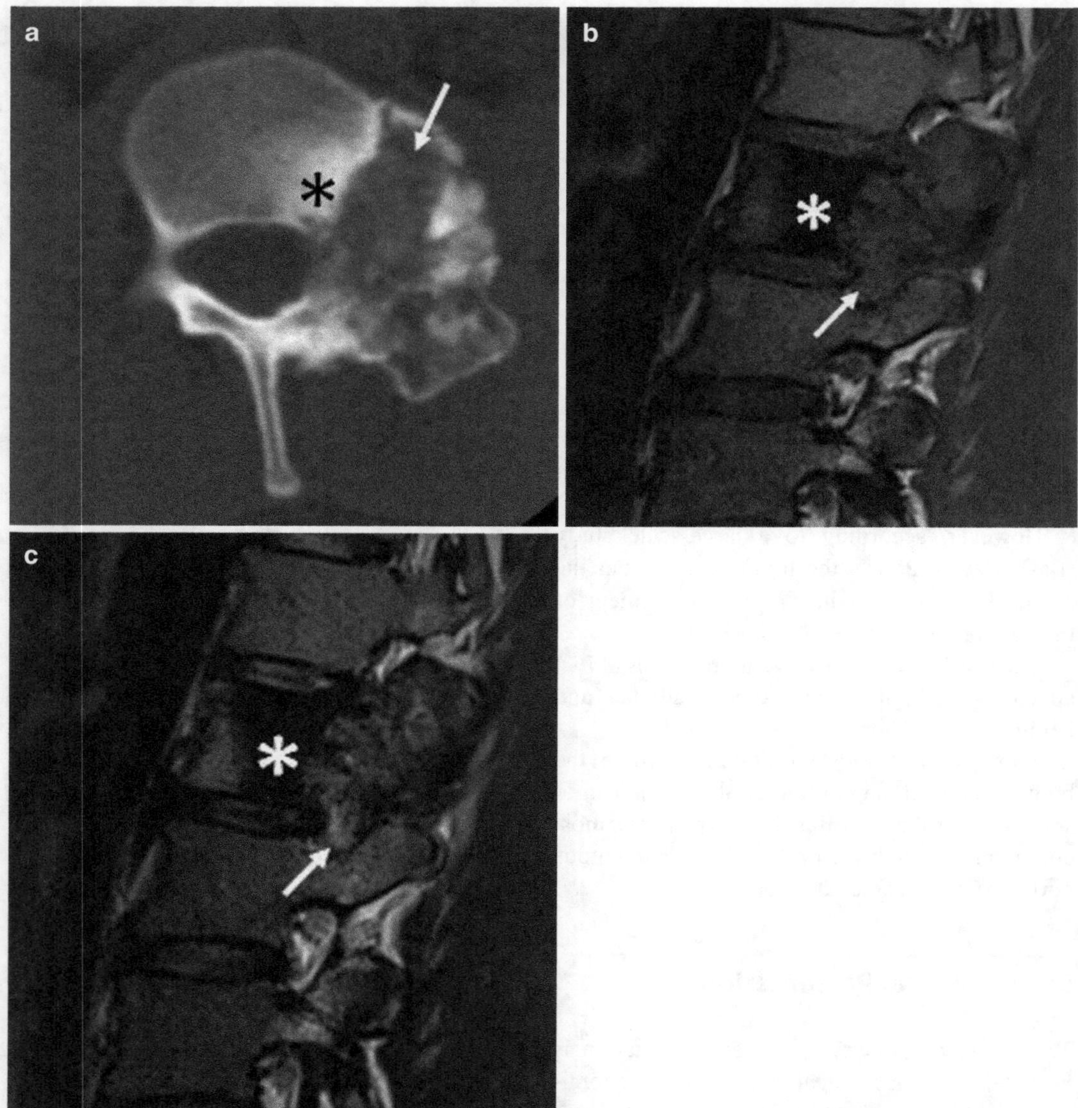

Fig. 1 Spinal osteosarcoma in a 25-year-old male patient: (**a**) CT scan axial image with bone window: A mixed osteolytic (arrow) and sclerotic (asterisk) mass affecting the left posterior arch of L1 and extending into the vertebral body. (**b**, **c**) MRI sagittal T1-WI (**b**) and T2-WI (**c**): The mineralized component has a low signal on T1-WI and T2-WI (asterisks), whereas the less mineralized areas show an intermediate signal on T1-WI and a high signal on T2-WI (arrows). (Images courtesy of Pr. Filip Vanhoenacker, Belgium)

cortical destruction, and a soft tissue mass. The presence of fatty foci within the bone marrow and the soft tissue mass (on CT or MRI) is very useful to rule out malignancy (Davies et al. 2009).

Chest CT is the most sensitive imaging modality for identifying pulmonary nodules.

Intravenous (IV) contrast is not recommended (Strauss et al. 2021) since it does not improve the detection of pulmonary nodules and may lead to equivocal assessment of mineralization, which can be a useful morphologic feature to distinguish benign from malignant pulmonary nodules.

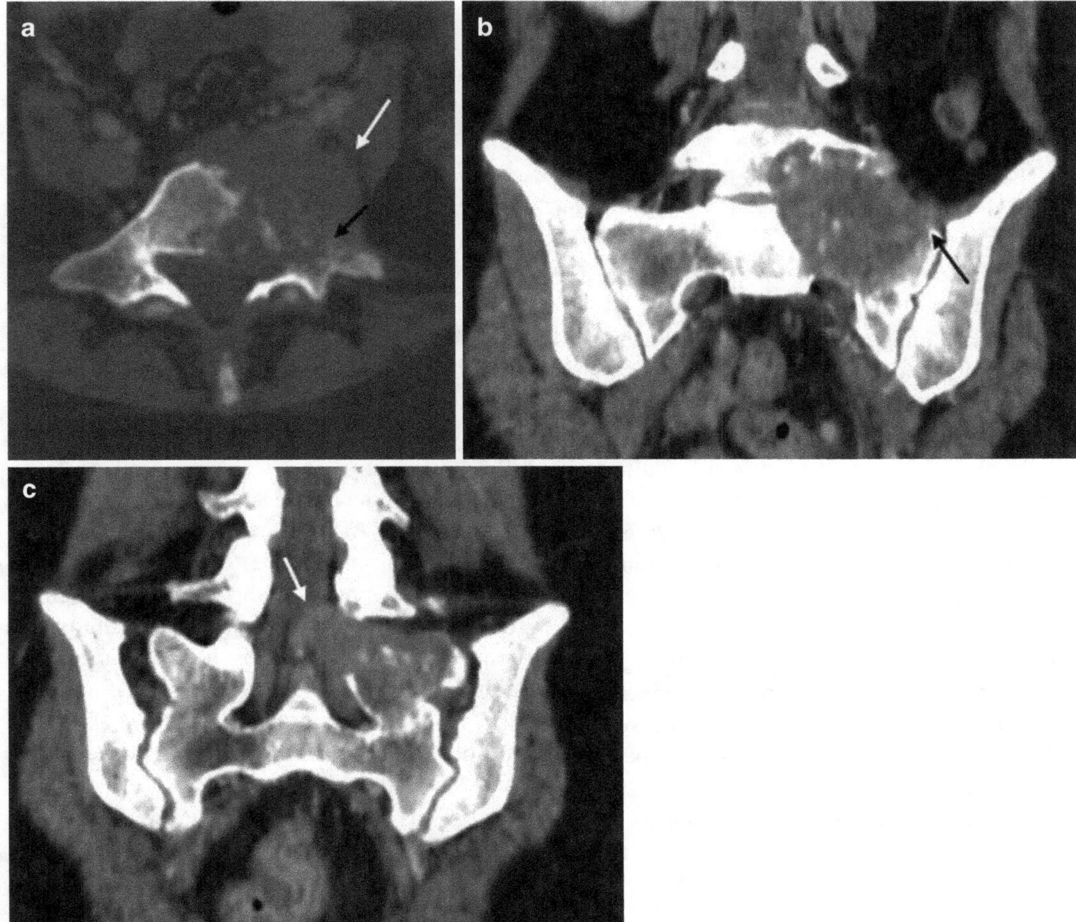

Fig. 2 Spinal osteoblastic osteosarcoma in a 36-year-old female patient: CT scan axial image with bone window (**a**) and coronal images with soft tissue window (**b**, **c**): Eccentric osteolytic mass involving the anterior and posterior elements of two vertebrae (L5 and S1). The mass is aggressive with bone destruction, cortical breakthrough (black arrows), and soft tissue paravertebral and epidural extension (white arrows). Calcifications are seen within the mass

Chest CT scan without IV is recommended in the initial assessment in search of pulmonary metastases and in subsequent monitoring (Strauss et al. 2021).

CT-guided core needle biopsy is an appropriate alternative to open biopsy.

The biopsy should be carried out by a dedicated interventional radiologist after discussing with the biopsy trajectory with surgeon (Blay et al. 2017), as the biopsy trajectory must be considered potentially contaminated and must be removed later, with the resection specimen, to minimize the risk of a local recurrence (Strauss et al. 2021).

Contamination of surrounding tissue should be minimized, using a coaxial system, and multiple sampling of representative tumoral areas should be performed.

6.3 MRI

MRI, with its unparalleled soft tissue resolution and contrast, is the imaging modality of choice for accurate local staging of SO.

The examination should include the primary tumor site and the entire spine to identify distant lesions.

The imaging protocol combines anatomic and functional or multiparametric sequences.

Anatomic images are obtained by T1-weighted images (WI) and T2-WI sequences. For fat suppression, Dixon provides more homogeneous signal intensity than STIR or fat-suppressed T1-WI and T2-WI, with additional quantification of fat content (Guerini et al. 2015).

SO features on anatomic MRI images are nonspecific compared to appendicular osteosarcoma. The unmineralized component displays a low to intermediate signal on T1-WI with variable enhancement following IV gadolinium and a high signal on T2-WI, whereas the mineralized component shows low signal on T1-WI and T2-WI (Fig. 1b, c). Fluid-fluid level appearance is associated with TAEOS (Mechri et al. 2018).

Anatomic MRI images accurately assess the lesion extent within the bone and to the surrounding soft tissue, especially epidural, nerve, and spinal cord involvement (Fig. 3) (Patnaik et al. 2016).

Axial T2-WI predicts invasion of arteries, veins, and nerves if the contact between tumor and vascular or neural circumference exceeds 180°. MR angiography is useful for the mapping of major arteries and helps to evaluate vascular invasion.

Diffusion-WI (DWI) with different *b* values (0, 500, 800, or 1000 s/mm^2) and apparent diffusion coefficient (ADC) mapping is a functional MRI technique that provides quantitative evaluation of tumor cellularity (Inarejos Clemente et al. 2022).

High cellular tumors show high signal on DWI and low ADC values and are likely malignant (Guirguis et al. 2022).

DWI also improves the MRI assessment of treatment response by monitoring the signal intensity and ADC values before, during, and after chemotherapy (Saleh et al. 2020).

Dynamic contrast-enhanced (DCE) 3D T1-WI is another functional MRI technique that assesses tumor vascularization.

Analysis of DCE-MRI sequence can be done in a quantitative or qualitative manner.

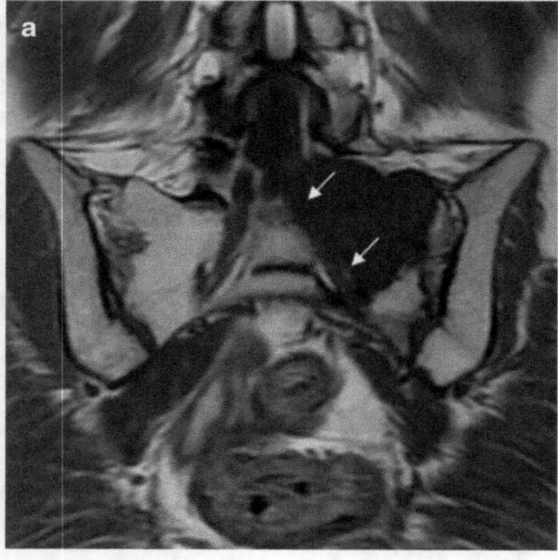

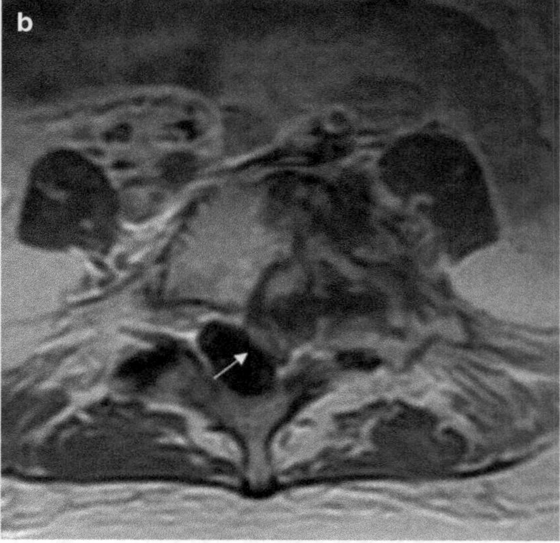

Fig. 3 Spinal osteoblastic osteosarcoma (same patient as in Fig. 2): MRI coronal T1-WI (**a**) and axial T1 post-gadolinium contrast image (**b**): The mass of L5 and S1 vertebrae has a low signal on T1-WI (**a**) with a heterogeneous enhancement pattern after gadolinium contrast administration (**b**). Local extension, especially central and nerve involvement, is better assessed by MRI (arrows)

Quantitative assessment allows the measurement of tissue microvasculature parameters such as contrast agent transfer rate between blood and tissue (K^{trans}), contrast agent back-flux rate constant (K_{ep}), and extracellular fractional volume (V_e). These parameters values are significantly higher not only in malignancies, but also in progressive disease patients on posttreatment assessment (Xia et al. 2022).

A qualitative analysis approach relies on signal intensity-time curve (ITC) profile. Curves that show delayed plateau (type 3) or a delayed washout (type 4) correlate with malignancy (Lavini et al. 2007).

The slope of the ITC shows speed of enhancement and is useful for the assessment of treatment response after chemotherapy in osteosarcoma (Kubo et al. 2016).

Other semiquantitative values measure the relative signal intensity (higher postcontrast signal intensity/precontrast signal ratio) or the area under the intensity-time curve (AUC) (Vilanova et al. 2016).

MRI helps to select target viable tumor areas for biopsy. These areas are iso/hyperintense on T2-WI, enhance following IV gadolinium contrast, and show high signal on high *b* DWI and low ADC values and avid arterial contrast enhancement with type 3 and 4 ITC.

Whole-body MRI is regarded as a new alternative to the combination of chest CT and bone scintigraphy for the evaluation of pulmonary and bone metastases, respectively (Strauss et al. 2021). Protocol consists of acquisition from head to toes of T1-WI, STIR, and DWI in the coronal or axial planes. Additional sagittal T1-WI and T2-WI or STIR-WI are recommended for the spine (Lecouvet 2016).

6.4 PET and PET/CT

Positron emission tomography (PET) is an emerging modality in musculoskeletal tumor imaging (Blodgett et al. 2008).

Fusion of PET-acquired images with CT scans and more recently with MRI has significantly improved the overall diagnostic accuracy (Choi et al. 2014).

Viable malignant primary bone tumors are usually avid for 18F-fluorodeoxyglucose (FDG).

PET using FDG as a radiotracer produces images that allow diagnosis of these neoplasms, initial staging, selection of biopsy sites, evaluation of treatment response, and assessment for tumor recurrence.

Metabolic activity, based on the maximum standardized uptake value (SUV_{max}), is a useful marker for differentiating between benign and malignant lesions.

Uptake time (duration between radiopharmaceutical administration and imaging) is an important factor, and the acquisition should be performed using a 60-min uptake period, with less than 10-min variation between studies (Boellaard et al. 2008).

Dual-time-point imaging is a technique that adds a second delayed acquisition (2-h uptake period) to help further distinguish malignant from benign bone lesions: The FDG uptake in malignancies tends to increase for several hours, whereas it typically undergoes an early plateau or clearance in benign lesions (Parghane and Basu 2017).

PET assesses nodal staging well, whereas PET and MRI are highly accurate for the detection of metastases. The CT/MRI component of this hybrid imaging modality significantly improves localization of the metabolic abnormalities (Behzadi et al. 2018).

Hence, whole-body PET/MRI with concurrent MRI local assessment of the primary spinal osteosarcoma allows complete TNM staging in a single session.

FDG-PET scanning in osteosarcoma also defines the metabolic response to treatment: A reduction of SUV_{max} after chemotherapy correlates well with the degree of tumor necrosis and subsequent patient outcome (Davis et al. 2018).

On PET/MR imaging, changes in SUV_{max} and ADC significantly correlate with the histologic response. The combination of the two variables increases the sensitivity, specificity, and accuracy of either value alone (Batouli et al. 2019).

7 Histopathology

Biopsy samples should be quickly submitted for histopathological assessment to an experienced bone tumor pathologist and discussed in a multidisciplinary team.

It is necessary to decalcify the bone tumor biopsy. Ethylenediaminetetraacetic acid (EDTA) is preferred over acid-based methods. In the latter case, sampling frozen tissue is essential to allow molecular diagnostics (Strauss et al. 2021).

Tumor type must be diagnosed according to the most recent version of the WHO classification of bone tumors (Baumhoer et al. 2020).

For surgical specimens, tumor size, site, local extent of spread, status of surgical margins, and percentage of pathological response to preoperative chemotherapy should be described (Strauss et al. 2021).

Histologic assessment is the most accurate method to determine the response to preoperative chemotherapy. Tumor mapping assesses percentage area occupied by necrosis and viable malignant cells. Huvos criteria (>90% necrosis—good response) are most commonly used (Wadhwa 2014).

7.1 Macroscopic Appearance

COS usually presents as a large mass arising in the cancellous bone. The cut surface is heterogeneous, depending on the type and degree of mineralization of the predominant matrix. Heavily mineralized tumors are tan white/yellow and densely solid, whereas non-mineralized components are either gray and rubbery (hyaline) or mucoid (myxoid degeneration). Areas of hemorrhage, necrosis, and cystic change are common. Extra-osseous infiltration is frequent, with an eccentric soft tissue mass that displaces the periosteum peripherally.

TAEOS shows a hemorrhagic multicystic lesion filled with blood clots.

The gross features of SCOS are indistinguishable from those of COS (Baumhoer et al. 2020).

7.2 Microscopic Appearance

Identification of neoplastic bone formation is essential to the diagnosis. The tumor grows with a permeative pattern, replacing the marrow space, eroding preexisting trabeculae, and filling and expanding haversian systems within cortical bone (Baumhoer et al. 2020).

The neoplastic cells typically demonstrate severe anaplasia and pleomorphism, usually spindle shaped (fusiform), plasmacytoid, or epithelioid. They often become small and normalized in appearance when surrounded by bone matrix mimicking benign osteocytes.

Mitotic activity is usually brisk, and abundant atypical mitotic figures are often present.

Bone formation varies in quantity.

On hematoxylin-eosin staining, bone matrix is eosinophilic if unmineralized and basophilic/purple if mineralized. Distinguishing unmineralized matrix (osteoid) from other eosinophilic extracellular materials such as collagen or compacted fibrin matrices may be difficult.

On the basis of the predominant matrix, COSs are divided into osteoblastic (76–80%), chondroblastic (10–13%), and fibroblastic (10%) subtypes. There is no relationship between these histological patterns, treatment, and prognosis (Hauben et al. 2002).

Ultrastructurally, osteosarcoma cells have the features of mesenchymal cells with abundant dilated rough endoplasmic reticulum. The nuclei may be eccentric and the Golgi apparatus prominent. The matrix contains collagen fibers, which may show calcium hydroxyapatite crystal deposition. These findings can be helpful in excluding Ewing's sarcoma, metastatic carcinoma, melanoma, and lymphoma (Baumhoer et al. 2020).

TAEOS is composed of blood-filled or empty cystic spaces. Unlike aneurysmal bone cyst, the septa are populated by pleomorphic cells showing nuclear hyperchromasia and atypical mitoses. Some malignant cells can be seen floating in the hemorrhagic areas. Osteoid formation is usually focal. Permeation into normal bone trabeculae is often observed at the edges of the lesion.

SCOS is composed of small cells with scant cytoplasm, associated with osteoid production. Nuclei are most frequently round to oval, and the chromatin may be fine to coarse with atypical mitoses.

The histological features of secondary osteosarcoma are not distinguishable from those of primary osteosarcoma (Baumhoer et al. 2020).

Immunohistochemistry lacks diagnostic specificity, and no specific diagnostic molecular pathology tests are available (Baumhoer et al. 2020).

8 Differential Diagnosis

The differential diagnosis of SO includes osteomyelitis, benign tumors, other bone sarcomas, lymphoma, myeloma, and metastases. The diagnosis suspicion should be strongly oriented by patients' age. For patients less than 5 years old, a destructive bone lesion could be interpreted predominantly as either metastatic neuroblastoma or Langerhans cell histiocytosis. For young patients aged more than 5 years, the likelihood of a primary bone sarcoma is higher. After 40 years of age, bone metastases and myeloma are the most common diagnoses (Strauss et al. 2021).

An expansile multiloculated lytic lesion with a thin peripheral bony rim and fluid-fluid levels on MRI may suggest the diagnoses of aneurysmal bone cyst (ABC), giant cell tumor (GCT), and chondroblastoma. ABCs occur in the first two decades of life, with slight female predominance, and present with pain, rarely with neurologic deficit. They typically involve the posterior elements and rarely the vertebral body (Zileli et al. 2013).

Spinal GCTs affect patients in their second to fourth decades of life and are more frequently found in women. Only the vertebral body is usually involved, and the most common location is the sacrum (Kwon et al. 2007).

Osteoblastomas, unlike most other primary osseous tumors, typically arise in the spine, with cervical and lumbar segments being most commonly involved. Almost all patients present by 30 years of age, predominantly males. Osteoblastoma usually results in a lytic, expansile lesion of the posterior elements, commonly extending to the vertebral body, with a well-defined, sclerotic margin. The matrix may be partially or completely mineralized (Galgano et al. 2016).

More aggressive lesions may break through the cortex with adjacent soft tissue mass, making differentiation from SO particularly difficult.

Malignant lesions that must be considered in the differential diagnosis of SO include metastases, lymphoma, myeloma, chordoma, and Ewing's sarcoma.

Metastases usually occur in patients older than 40 years of age. Lymphoma occurs in an age group similar to SO, and bone involvement is almost always secondary to lymph node disease. Myeloma occurs in patients older than 50 years of age and mainly produces lytic lesions within the vertebral body.

Myeloma, lymphoma, and metastases usually present as multiple lesions, while SO is often solitary.

Chordoma may occur at any age, typically 40–60-year-old age group. Chordoma produces a large lytic area of bone destruction with a well-defined margin and a large soft tissue mass. It typically occurs centrally within the sacrum (Tenny and Varacallo 2022).

Spinal Ewing's sarcoma occurs in a much younger age group, and it has no mineralization.

The involvement of several contiguous vertebrae is more frequent in SO than in other benign or malignant spinal tumors (Ilaslan et al. 2004).

9 Local and Distant Staging

The European Society for Medical Oncology-European Reference Network for Rare Adult Solid Cancers-European Reference Network for Genetic Tumour Risk Syndromes (ESMO-EURACAN-GENTURIS) guidelines for bone sarcomas recommend MRI for local staging.

Chest CT and bone scintigraphy and/or whole-body MRI and/or FDG-PET/CT/MRI are recommended for distant staging (Strauss et al. 2021).

Baseline serum analysis should include Alcaline Phosphatase (AP) and Lactate Dehydrogenase (LDH) serum levels given their proven prognostic value and their use as response monitoring during treatment (Kamal et al. 2021).

SO staging has been assessed according to the Enneking (Enneking et al. 1980) and the Weinstein-Boriani-Biagini (WBB) (Boriani et al. 1997) staging systems.

However, the Enneking system was designed for appendicular tumors rather than spine tumors.

The WBB system is a surgical local staging system for primary spine tumors that does not specify tumor grade or presence or absence of distant spread. Experts of the Spine Oncology Study Group found that it has only modest interobserver agreement (Chan et al. 2009).

The cancer staging system developed by the Union for International Cancer Control and the American Joint Committee on Cancer (AJCC) in the 1950s and which is regularly updated is used at nearly all American and many international cancer centers. The eighth edition staging manual (Kniesl et al. 2018) is the current standard oncologic staging system for primary malignant bone tumors (except lymphoma and myeloma).

It separates, for the first time, axial from peripheral skeletal tumors and provides a new distinct classification for spine tumors integrating tumor location and traditional anatomic criteria (tumor size (T), presence of lymph node (N), or distant metastases (M)).

The vertebra is divided into five segments (right and left hemibodies, right and left pedicles, and posterior element); tumors in two segments are generally resectable with proper margins by experienced surgeons; tumors in three segments are likely resectable with a negative margin in many cases. More advanced tumors or those with significant epidural or retroperitoneal extension are challenging to resect with a true oncologic margin (Rose et al. 2019).

The new TNM categories for spine tumors are based on expert experience and opinion and imply resectability and margin status (Rose et al. 2019).

It is of note that the eighth edition of the AJCC lacks prognostic stage groupings for spine tumors. Further data collection and analysis will indicate if the new TNM classification improves discrimination of patient outcome, with possible subsequent prognostic stage group release in the upcoming staging manual updates.

10 Treatment

Curative treatment of SO consists of chemotherapy and surgery (Strauss et al. 2021).

Chemotherapy generally relies on combinations of four active drugs (doxorubicin, cisplatin, high-dose methotrexate, and ifosfamide) and is administered before and after surgery (Wagner et al. 2016).

Preoperative chemotherapy allows the assessment of histological response, which predicts survival (Smeland et al. 2019).

Curative en bloc resection with clear margins (R0) may be challenging due to either anatomical/functional particularities of the occipitocervical, cervicothoracic, thoracolumbar, and lumbosacral junctional zones or a locally advanced disease with soft tissue extension and neurologic and/or vascular involvement (Colman and Schwab 2017).

Clear margins (R0) are the first goal of surgery because microscopic (R1) and macroscopic (R2) positive margins both increase the local recurrence rate, with reduced overall survival.

Surgery will also strive to remove all metastases if they are resectable (Strauss et al. 2021).

In case of unresectable primary or metastatic disease, chemotherapy with or without radiotherapy is recommended (Strauss et al. 2021).

Radiotherapy may also be used in case of positive resection margins or recurrent unresectable disease.

11 Prognosis

The axial skeleton tumor site is a well-known adverse prognostic factor for osteosarcoma (Smeland et al. 2019).

Although surgery improves the outcome of SO (Tang et al. 2022), the prognosis remains poor with median overall survival of 15 months and 5-year overall survival of 17% (Wang et al. 2023).

Poor prognosis risk factors for SO include age ≥60 years, high grade, regional advanced stage, metastasis stage, and no-surgery treatment (Wang et al. 2023).

12 Conclusion

Spinal osteosarcoma is a rare disease. Its management from diagnosis to follow-up under treatment can only be conceived in a specialized center comprising a team of experienced radiologists, pathologists, oncologists, and surgeons.

The prognosis remains poor despite progress in diagnostic and therapeutic methods.

13 Key Points

- The initial workup of a suspected spinal osteosarcoma should be carried out at a reference center and should include medical history, physical examination, radiological assessment, and biopsy.
- Pathological diagnosis should be made by a bone tumor pathologist according to the 2020 WHO classification. The diagnosis is based on morphological findings, and no specific diagnostic molecular tests are available.
- MRI is the imaging modality of choice for local staging. Anatomic sequences localize the tumor and describe anatomical boundaries. Functional MR imaging adds value in the detection, characterization, staging, and post-therapy assessment.
- Whole-body MRI and PET/CT/MRI are an alternative to the combination of chest CT and bone scintigraphy for metastasis screening.
- Radical surgery of the tumor and possible metastases with neoadjuvant or adjuvant chemotherapy and radiotherapy are the base of treatment.

References

Batouli A, Gholamrezanezhad A, Petrov D et al (2019) Management of primary osseous spinal tumors with PET. PET Clin 14(1):91–101

Baumhoer D, Böhling TO, Cates JMM et al (2020) Osteosarcoma. In: WHO Classification of tumours Editorial Board (ed) WHO classification of soft tissue and bone tumours, 5th edn. IARC Press, Lyon, pp 403–409

Behjati S, Tarpey PS, Haase K et al (2017) Recurrent mutation of IGF signalling genes and distinct patterns of genomic rearrangement in osteosarcoma. Nat Commun 8:15936

Behzadi AH, Raza SI, Carrino JA et al (2018) Applications of PET/CT and PET/MR imaging in primary bone malignancies. PET Clin 13(4):623–634

Blay JY, Soibinet P, Penel N et al (2017) Improved survival using specialized multidisciplinary board in sarcoma patients. Ann Oncol 28(11):2852–2859

Blodgett TM, Meltzer CC, Townsend DW (2008) PET/CT: form and function. Radiology 242:360–385

Boellaard R, Oyen WJ, Hoekstra CJ et al (2008) The Netherlands protocol for standardisation and quantification of FDG whole body PET studies in multi-centre trials. Eur J Nucl Med Mol Imaging 35:2320–2333

Boriani S, Weistein JN, Biagini R (1997) Primary bone tumors of the spine. Terminology and surgical staging. Spine 22:1036–1044

Chan P, Boriani S, Fourney DR et al (2009) An assessment of the reliability of the Enneking and Weinstein-Boriani-Biagini classifications for staging of primary spine tumors by the Spine Oncology Study Group. Spine 34:384–391

Chhaya S, White LM, Kandel R et al (2005) Transarticular invasion of bone tumours across the sacroiliac joint. Skeletal Radiol 34(12):771–777

Choi YY, Kim JY, Yang SO (2014) PET/CT in benign and malignant musculoskeletal tumors and tumor-like conditions [review]. Semin Musculoskelet Radiol 18(2):133–148

Colman MW, Schwab JH (2017) Current concepts in primary benign, primary malignant, and metastatic tumors of the spine. In: Grauer JN (ed) Orthopaedic knowledge update, 12th edn. American Academy of Orthopaedic Surgeons, USA, pp 655–672

Davies A, Pluot E, James S (2009) Tumour and tumour-like conditions associated with Paget's disease of bone. In: Davies A, Sundaram M, James S (eds) Imaging of bone tumors and tumor-like lesions, Medical radiology. Springer, Berlin

Davis JC, Daw NC, Navid F et al (2018) ^{18}F-FDG uptake during early adjuvant chemotherapy predicts histologic response in pediatric and young adult patients with osteosarcoma. J Nucl Med 59(1):25–30

Dekutoski MB, Clarke MJ, Rose P et al (2016) Osteosarcoma of the spine: prognostic variables for local recurrence and overall survival, a multicenter ambispective study. J Neurosurg Spine 25(1):59–68

Enneking WF, Spanier SS, Goodman MA (1980) A system for the surgical staging of musculoskeletal sarcoma. Clin Orthop Relat Res 153:106–120

Feng D, Yang X, Liu T et al (2013) Osteosarcoma of the spine: surgical treatment and outcomes. World J Surg Oncol 11(1):89

Galgano MA, Goulart CR, Iwenofu H et al (2016) Osteoblastomas of the spine: a comprehensive review. Neurosurg Focus 41(2):E4

Green R, Saifuddin A, Cannon S (1996) Pictorial review: Imaging of primary osteosarcoma of the spine. Clin Radiol 51:325–329

Guerini H, Omoumi P, Guichoux F et al (2015) Fat suppression with Dixon techniques in musculoskeletal magnetic resonance imaging: a pictorial review. Semin Musculoskelet Radiol 19(4):335–347

Guirguis M, Sharan G, Wang J et al (2022) Diffusion-weighted MR imaging of musculoskeletal tissues: incremental role over conventional MR imaging in bone, soft tissue, and nerve lesions. BJR Open 4(1):20210077

Hameed M, Mandelker D (2018) Tumor syndromes predisposing to osteosarcoma. Adv Anat Pathol 25(4):217–222

Hauben EI, Weeden S, Pringle J et al (2002) Does the histological subtype of high-grade central osteosarcoma influence the response to treatment with chemotherapy and does it affect overall survival? A study on 570 patients of two consecutive trials of the European Osteosarcoma Intergroup. Eur J Cancer 38(9):1218–1225

Ilaslan H, Sundaram M, Unni KK et al (2004) Primary vertebral osteosarcoma: imaging findings. Radiology 230(3):697–702

Inarejos Clemente EJ, Navarro OM, Navallas M et al (2022) Multiparametric MRI evaluation of bone sarcomas in children. Insights Imaging 13(1):33

Kamal AF, Abubakar I, Salamah T (2021) Alkaline phosphatase, lactic dehydrogenase, inflammatory variables and apparent diffusion coefficients from MRI for prediction of chemotherapy response in osteosarcoma. A cross sectional study. Ann Med Surg (Lond) 64:102228

Katonis P, Datsis G, Karantanas A et al (2013) Spinal osteosarcoma. Clin Med Insights Oncol 18(7):199–208

Kelley SP, Ashford RU, Rao AS et al (2007) Primary bone tumours of the spine: a 42-year survey from the Leeds Regional Bone Tumour Registry. Eur Spine J 16(3):405–409

Kim YC, Suh JS, Kim MI et al (2007) Low-grade osteosarcoma of the spine: a case report. J Korean Radiol Soc 56:575–578

Kniesl JS, Rosenberg AE, Anderson PM et al (2018) Bone. In: Amin MB, Edge S, Greene D et al (eds) AJCC Cancer Staging Manual, 8th edn. Springer, Chicago

Kubo T, Furuta T, Johan MP et al (2016) Percent slope analysis of dynamic magnetic resonance imaging for assessment of chemotherapy response of osteosarcoma or Ewing sarcoma: systematic review and meta-analysis. Skeletal Radiol 45(9):1235–1242

Kwon JW, Chung HW, Cho EY et al (2007) MRI findings of giant cell tumors of the spine. AJR Am J Roentgenol 189(1):246–250

Lavini C, de Jonge MC, van de Sande MGH et al (2007) Pixel-by-pixel analysis of DCE MRI curve patterns and an illustration of its application to the imaging of the musculoskeletal system. Magn Reson Imaging 25(5):604–612

Lecouvet FE (2016) Whole-body MR imaging: musculoskeletal applications. Radiology 279(2):345–365

Lefebvre G, Renaud A, Rocourt N et al (2013) Primary vertebral osteosarcoma: five cases. Joint Bone Spine 80(5):534–537

Mechri M, Riahi H, Sboui I et al (2018) Imaging of malignant primitive tumors of the spine. J Belg Soc Radiol 102(1):56

Mesfin A, Boriani S, Gambarotti M et al (2020) Can osteoblastoma evolve to malignancy? A challenge in the decision-making process of a benign spine tumor. World Neurosurg 136:150–156

Ottaviani G, Jaffe N (2009) The epidemiology of osteosarcoma. Cancer Treat Res 152:3–13

Ozaki T, Flege S, Liljenqvist U et al (2002) Osteosarcoma of the spine: experience of the Cooperative Osteosarcoma Study Group. Cancer 94(4):1069–1077

Parghane RV, Basu S (2017) Dual-time point ^{18}F-FDG-PET and PET/CT for differentiating benign from malignant musculoskeletal lesions: opportunities and limitations. Semin Nucl Med 47(4):373–391

Patnaik S, Jyotsnarani Y, Uppin SG et al (2016) Imaging features of primary tumors of the spine: a pictorial essay. Indian J Radiol Imaging 26(2):279–289

Picci P (2007) Osteosarcoma (osteogenic sarcoma). Orphanet J Rare Dis 2:6

Rose PS, Holt GE, Kneisl JS (2019) Changes to the American Joint Committee on Cancer staging system for spine tumors-practice update. Ann Transl Med 7(10):215

Saleh MM, Abdelrahman TM, Madney Y et al (2020) Multiparametric MRI with diffusion-weighted imaging in predicting response to chemotherapy in cases of osteosarcoma and Ewing's sarcoma. Br J Radiol 93(1115):20200257

Savage SA, Mirabello L (2011) Using epidemiology and genomics to understand osteosarcoma etiology. Sarcoma 2011:548151

Smeland S, Bielack SS, Whelan J et al (2019) Survival and prognosis with osteosarcoma: outcomes in more than 2000 patients in the EURAMOS-1 (European and American Osteosarcoma Study) cohort. Eur J Cancer 109:36–50

Strauss SJ, Frezza AM, Abecassis N et al (2021) Bone sarcomas: ESMO-EURACAN-GENTURIS-ERN PaedCan Clinical Practice Guideline for diagnosis, treatment and follow-up. Ann Oncol 32(12):1520–1536

Tang C, Wang D, Wu Y et al (2022) Surgery has positive effects on spinal osteosarcoma prognosis: a population-based database study. World Neurosurg 164:e367–e386

Tenny S, Varacallo M (2022) Chordoma. In: StatPearls [Internet]. StatPearls Publishing, Treasure Island, FL

Vilanova JC, Baleato-Gonzalez S, Romero MJ et al (2016) Assessment of musculoskeletal malignancies with functional MR imaging. Magn Reson Imaging Clin N Am 24(1):239–259

Wadhwa N (2014) Osteosarcoma: diagnostic dilemmas in histopathology and prognostic factors. Indian J Orthop 48(3):247–254

Wagner MJ, Livingston JA, Patel SR et al (2016) Chemotherapy for bone sarcoma in adults. J Oncol Pract 12(3):208–216

Wang J, Ni XZ, Yang ML et al (2023) Prognostic factors and treatment outcomes of spinal osteosarcoma: surveillance, epidemiology, and end results database analysis. Front Oncol 13:1083776

Xia X, Wen L, Zhou F et al (2022) Predictive value of DCE-MRI and IVIM-DWI in osteosarcoma patients with neoadjuvant chemotherapy. Front Oncol 12:967450

Zileli M, Isik HS, Ogut FE et al (2013) Aneurysmal bone cysts of the spine. Eur Spine J 22(3):593–601

Fibrous Dysplasia of the Spine

Miriana Rosaria Petrera,
Maria Pilar Aparisi Gómez,
Adriano Novais de Carvalho,
and Alberto Bazzocchi

Contents

M. R. Petrera · A. Bazzocchi (✉)
Diagnostic and Interventional Radiology, IRCCS Istituto Ortopedico Rizzoli, Bologna, Italy
e-mail: abazzo@inwind.it

M. P. Aparisi Gómez
Department of Radiology, Te Toka Tumai Auckland (Auckland City Hospital - Greenlane Clinical Centre), Auckland, New Zealand

Department of Radiology, IMSKE, Valencia, Spain

A. Novais de Carvalho
Diagnostic and Interventional Radiology, IRCCS Istituto Ortopedico Rizzoli, Bologna, Italy

IPO-Porto, Porto, Portugal

Abstract

Fibrous dysplasia is a benign, nonhereditary bone tumor-like disease that can involve one (monostotic) or multiple (polyostotic) bones, affecting the entire skeleton.

It is caused by a mutation of the gene GNAS1 resulting in a maturation defect of bone-forming mesenchymal tissue, leading to poorly mineralized woven bone trabeculae surrounded by fibrous tissue.

Involvement of the spine is uncommon and may involve any vertebral element at every vertebral level, more frequently at the lumbar spine.

Most monostotic lesions are asymptomatic and incidentally found. Expansile lesions tend to clinically manifest with pain, fractures, and deformities. Scoliosis is an important manifestation in polyostotic FD with multilevel involvement.

Imaging plays a pivotal role in the diagnosis, identifying typical features, in the surveillance and follow-up, and therapeutic management. Additionally, it helps to guide the biopsy procedures required in case of atypical non-diagnostic radiologic findings.

The radiographic presentation varies based on the histopathologic features.

Med Radiol Diagn Imaging (2023)
https://doi.org/10.1007/174_2023_443,
Published Online: 02 August 2023

On plain radiograph and CT, FD may appear as pure osteolytic, or ground glass lesions surrounded by a sclerotic rim. CT allows a better assessment of lesion extension, cortical boundaries, and endosteal scalloping.

On MRI, signal intensity is heterogeneous, mostly hypo/isointense on T1-weighted images (WI) and hyperintense on T2-WI.

Contrast enhancement is usually present in variable intensity and distribution.

PET-CT and SPECT are used in the evaluation of FD lesion burden, especially in the polyostotic form, and may be helpful in monitoring bisphosphonate therapy.

Treatment options range from conservative approach and observation in asymptomatic monostotic lesions, bisphosphonate administration in painful polyostotic form, to surgical augmentation procedures in the case of vertebral fractures and surgical fixation for severe scoliosis deformities.

1 Introduction

Fibrous dysplasia (FD) is a genetic, benign tumor-like disease which was first reported by Von Recklinghausen (1891) and later described by Lichtenstein (1938).

It is a developmental defect of bone tissue characterized by the inability of mesenchymal tissue to form mature lamellar bone, which is replaced by fibrous tissue and poorly mineralized woven bone.

It can be subclassified into monostotic or polyostotic according to the number of bones involved and may be associated with metabolic and endocrine dysfunction in McCune-Albright syndrome (Adetayo et al. 2015).

The spine is an uncommon localization for FD lesions.

Imaging plays a pivotal role in the detection and identification of typical findings, helping with the differential diagnosis from other malignant and benign lesions, avoiding unnecessary invasive biopsy, and guiding the clinical and therapeutic management.

2 Pathologic Features

Fibrous dysplasia is a congenital and nonhereditary disease caused by a postzygotic mutation of the GNAS1 gene, located on chromosome 20q.13.2–13.3 and encoding the alpha subunit of the stimulatory G protein, which induces the adenylyl cyclase activation responsible for the exchange of guanosine triphosphate to guanosine diphosphate. A gain of function mutation of this subunit results in a constitutive activation of adenylyl cyclase leading to an excess of cyclic adenosine monophosphate (Weinstein et al. 1991).

These mutations of genetic and enzymatic activity translate at bony level in the inhibition of maturation of osteoprogenitor cells into osteoblasts resulting in undifferentiated and immature mesenchymal cells.

Failure in the maturation process results in the replacement of bone marrow with fibro-osseous tissue, consisting of immature isolated trabeculae entangled in dysplastic fibrous tissue, which does not mineralize normally (Bianco et al. 2003).

The structural changes may result in loss of mechanical strength, inducing pain, deformity, and pathologic fractures.

The clinical presentation, severity, and subtype of FD are variable according to the expression of the mosaic genetic mutation.

Severe disease may be caused by early mutation events that result in a large number of mutant cells (Dicaprio and Enneking 2005).

3 Epidemiology

Fibrous dysplasia accounts for 7% of all benign tumor-like bone lesions and 2.5% of all bone lesions, without a specific gender prevalence (Gogia et al. 2007).

It can affect any bone, but the most frequently involved sites are the proximal femur, tibia, ribs, and skull.

FD may be subdivided into monostotic and polyostotic form.

The monostotic form accounts for 70–80% of cases, affecting one bone, more frequently the long tubular ones, most commonly the femur and ribs, and presents between the second and the third decade (Favus and Vokes 2018).

The polyostotic form, occurring in 20–30% of cases, affects two or multiple bones, frequently craniofacial bones, the femur, tibia, and ribs, and presents earlier than the monostotic one, usually in the first decade, with a more severe prognosis.

Spine involvement ranges from 1.4% to 5.5% and has been reported in both monostotic and polyostotic form, more frequently in the latter (Rahim et al. 2021).

Polyostotic FD is seen in 3% of cases in association with McCune-Albright syndrome, which is prevalent in females (10:1), particularly young females, and characterized by the classic triad of fibrous dysplasia, cafè-au-lait skin pigmentation, and endocrine dysfunction, consisting of phosphate depletion with or without hypophosphatemia, vitamin D deficiency, hyperthyroidism, growth hormone excess, and precocious puberty (Favus and Vokes 2018).

Mazabraud syndrome is another rare disease in which fibrous dysplasia, more frequently the polyostotic form, is associated with intramuscular myxomas (Dicaprio and Enneking 2005).

4 Localization

The axial bones can be affected by the monostotic and polyostotic forms, but the latter is more frequent.

Spinal localization of FD is more common in patients with lesions in the skull and pelvis, suggesting an axial pattern of distribution throughout the skeleton (Mancini et al. 2009).

FD has been described in each segment of the spine, but the lumbar spine is most frequently affected followed by the thoracic, cervical, and less frequently the sacrum, with only few cases reported in literature (Leet et al. 2004; Liu et al. 2021).

FD lesions can be localized in a single vertebra, or spread along multiple levels, and any component of the vertebra may be involved (Wu et al. 2013).

There is no predilection for any particular element of the vertebral metamer. Lesions may be confined to the vertebral body, extend to the pedicles and posterior arch, or involve the elements of the posterior arch solely (Wright and Stoker 1988).

Contiguous invasion of the posterior arc of the ribs is possible in case of thoracic vertebral localization (Nabarro and Giblin 1994).

5 Clinical Presentation

The majority of monostotic lesions are asymptomatic and represent an incidental finding in radiographs performed for other clinical purposes.

If large, lesions can result in vertebral deformities and enlargement of the affected bone, manifesting with neck or back pain.

Monostotic lesions tend to increase in size in proportion to skeletal growth, stabilizing when bone maturity is reached.

Polyostotic FD lesions, instead, appear in the early adolescence and often continue to grow after skeletal maturity (Dicaprio and Enneking 2005).

FD of the spine may present with pain localized in the involved metamers, inducing progressive deformities due to its expansile nature. This may manifest as atlantoaxial dislocation and torticollis when the cervical spine is involved, kyphosis if the thoracic spine and deviation of physiological curves (Wu et al. 2013).

Pathologic fractures may occur when lesions become voluminous, with subsequent myelopathy and neurological manifestations caused by spinal cord and nerve root compression with clinical deficits that vary according to the implicated level.

Scoliosis is an important clinical aspect in the range of polyostotic FD with multilevel vertebral involvement.

There is a high prevalence (40–52%) of scoliosis and pelvic asymmetry in the polyostotic forms associated with McCune-Albright syndrome.

Since most lesions are localized in the lumbar and thoracic segments, patients may have a combination of thoracolumbar curves, or lumbar or thoracic curves only (Leet et al. 2004).

Given the strong association, patients with FD in the spine should be monitored for the occurrence of scoliosis.

Moreover, progression of the curves may continue after the end of skeletal growth, since lesions in polyostotic FD can progress for years even in adulthood (Mancini et al. 2009).

6 Imaging

Imaging plays a key role in the diagnosis, allowing the identification of the typical radiological features, narrowing the differential from other benign or malignant conditions, and avoiding unnecessary biopsy procedures.

Furthermore, it is a fundamental tool in the surveillance and follow-up of the lesions, guiding the therapeutic management.

Imaging findings of spine FD in both monostotic and polyostotic forms are consistent with the typical findings of extraspinal FD.

6.1 Radiographs

Radiographic features may vary. Indeed, plain radiographs may show no abnormal findings, but typically FD lesions appear as oval or round areas of geographic osteolysis surrounded by a sclerotic rim (Figs. 1 and 2).

The normal bone is replaced by more radiolucent tissue consisting of a solid fibro-osseous component that shows a grayish "ground glass" pattern without visible trabeculae. Cystic components may be present in more radiolucent areas.

A shell of reactive bone surrounds the lesions, and variation of the cortical thickness may be due to endosteal scalloping following the expansile behavior, but without periosteal reaction.

Decrease of vertebral body height is a common finding when extensive intravertebral lesion causes vertebral collapse.

Intervertebral spaces are always normal.

Monostotic lesions mature with the end of skeletal growth, showing a thicker sclerotic rim and increased density of the lesion, as features of stability (Dicaprio and Enneking 2005).

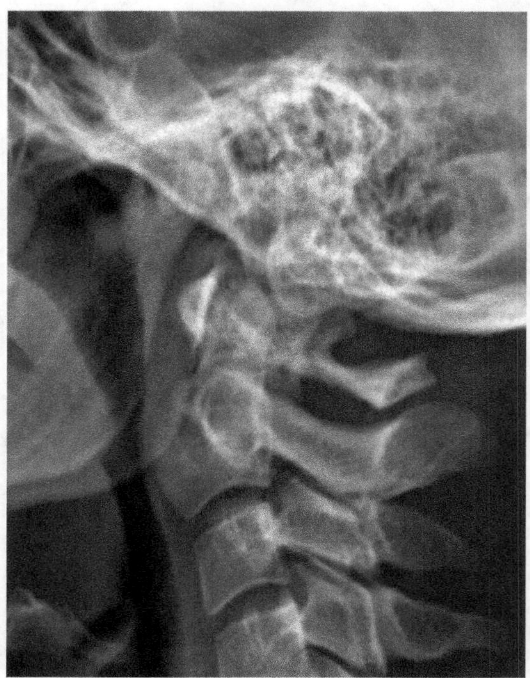

Fig. 1 Lateral radiograph in a 33-year-old woman, complaining about cervicalgia. Note a lucent, lytic lesion in the base of the dens, with bulging of the anterior cortex, consistent with expansile behavior, typical of slow growth

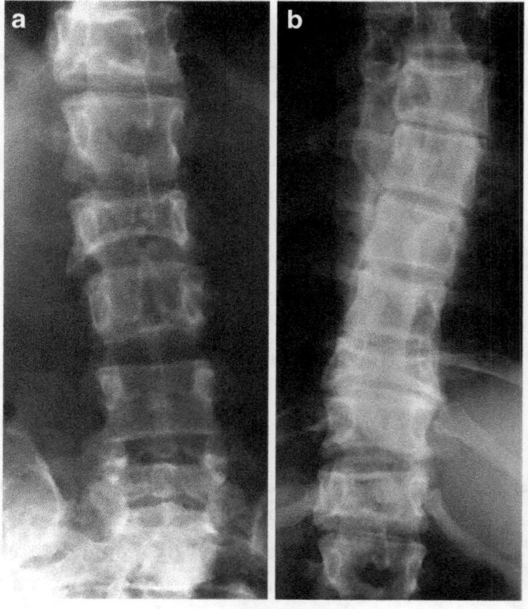

Fig. 2 Lumbar spine AP radiograph (**a**) demonstrates a lytic lesion in the body of L1. Note the compression fracture of L2. AP radiograph in the same patient including the lower thoracic segment (**b**) shows thoracolumbar scoliosis and a T10 vertebral fracture. (Courtesy of Prof. Mohamed Fethi Ladeb)

6.2 CT

Computed tomography is the best technique to assess the radiographic features of FD, with more detailed definition than the plain radiographs of lesion extension, cortical boundaries, in particular reactive bone rim and endosteal scalloping (Fig. 3).

CT imaging features depend on the underlying histopathologic changes, resulting in a spectrum of radiographic densities depending on the amount of fibrous tissue with interposed trabeculae of woven bone.

Purely fibrous structures appear as osteolytic lesions, acquiring the typical "ground glass" appearance with the deposition of irregular bone spicules (Wright and Stoker 1988).

The remodeling of the affected bone with consequent endosteal scalloping and thinning of the adjacent cortex is evident because of the expanding fibro-osseous mass. Markedly expansile lesions may also induce deformities in the contour of the vertebrae (Park et al. 2012) (Fig. 4).

Lesions are typically surrounded by a rim of reactive sclerotic bone, more sharply defined in

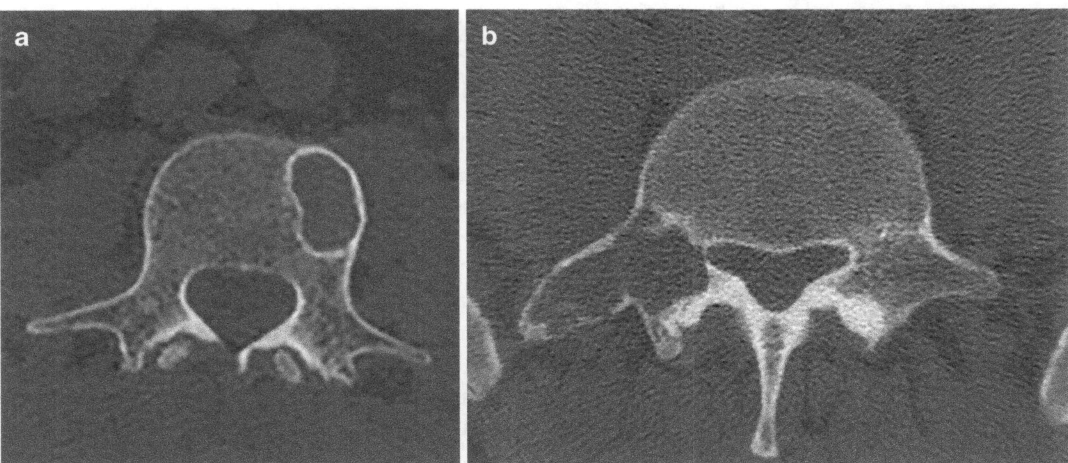

Fig. 3 FD lesions involving different vertebral components. (**a**) Axial acquisition CT image through the L4 vertebral body of 46-year-old woman with polyostotic form. Note the sclerotic rim and subtle bulging of the left anterolateral cortex. (**b**) Axial acquisition CT image through the L5 vertebral body of 30-year-old man with monostotic FD. Note involvement of the right pedicle and transverse process, with expansile characteristics. There are foci of cortical thinning, mineralization within the lesion and a subtle sclerotic rim

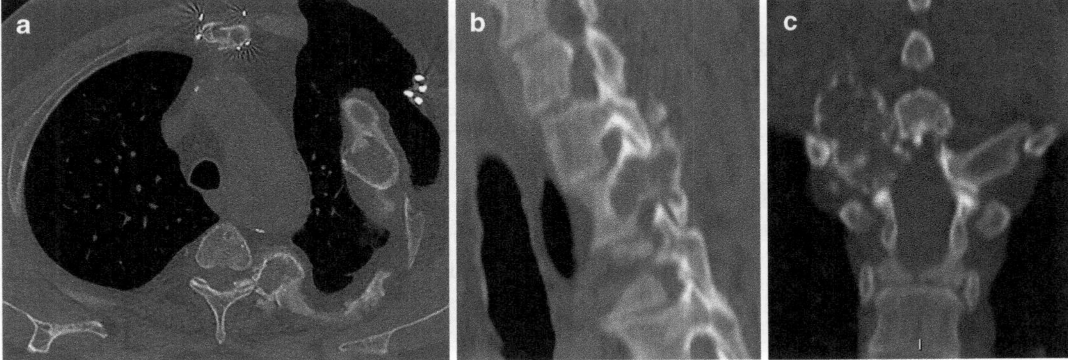

Fig. 4 Two different examples of thoracic FD involvement on CT. Axial acquisition (**a**) in 66-year-old male, with polyostotic FD demonstrates expansile lesions, with deforming characteristics on the left ribs, note also right scapular and minimal vertebral body involvement. Sagittal (**b**) and coronal (**c**) CT reconstructions in 55-year-old with monostotic FD demonstrate involvement of the posterior elements at the T3 level

its inner than its outer border, which may also be incomplete or interrupted (Zhang et al. 2018).

In addition, CT allows the assessment of the degree of mineralization of the lesion, and the possible encroachment of the spinal canal (Fig. 5).

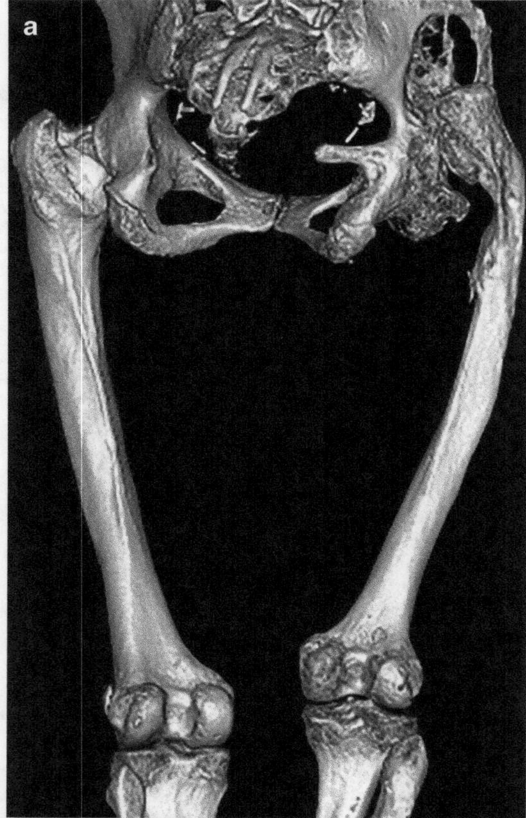

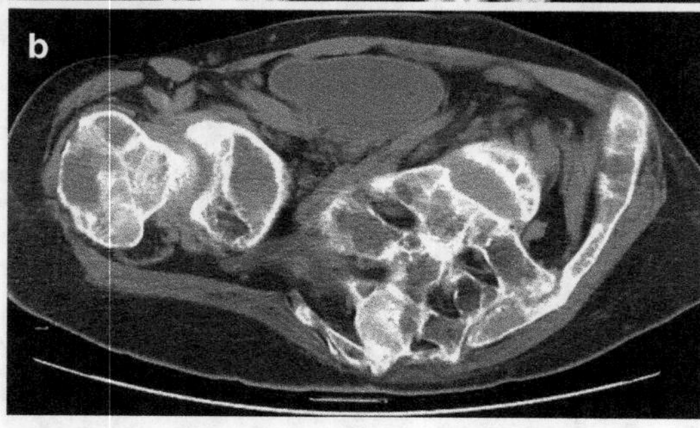

Fig. 5 Polyostotic FD with sacral involvement in a 68-year-old patient. (**a**) 3D CT reformat, showing different regions of lytic and deforming FD lesions, including sacrum, iliac bones, and femora. (**b**) Axial CT acquisition in the same patient demonstrates the typical ground glass appearances in the multiples sites of involvement and severe scoliosis

As these are vascularized lesions, contrast enhancement is present after contrast medium administration (Dicaprio and Enneking 2005).

6.3 MRI

MRI is a sensitive technique to define lesion size and content, as well as the extension in the involved bone, providing complementary information to CT examination. MRI is particularly useful in the evaluation of spinal cord and nerve root compression (Dicaprio and Enneking 2005).

Signal intensity and contrast enhancement are highly variable in FD.

On T1-weighted imaging (WI), signal has been reported to be mostly iso- or hypointense or a combination of these two; increased signal intensity or partially increased signal intensity has been reported in a lower percentage of cases, often related to the presence of hemorrhagic foci and methemoglobin content.

On T2-WI, signal is highly variable, frequently resulting in heterogeneous appearances.

FD lesions are not only composed by pure fibrous tissue, which would result in hypointense signal, but also contain spindle cells, trabeculae of immature woven bone and scattered osteoblasts, resulting in a metabolic active tissue, which manifests a prolonged T2 relaxation time, which in addition to the water content result in globally increased signal intensity on T2w imaging (Figs. 6 and 7).

The heterogeneous hyperintense signal on T2-WI can be attributed to the presence of bony trabeculae, cellularity, collagen fibers, cystic changes, and hemorrhage within the lesion.

The rim of sclerotic bone is hypointense in both T1 and T2-WI (Jee et al. 1996).

Various patterns of gadolinium enhancement have been reported in literature (Utz et al. 1989), from none to central or peripheral enhancement according to the distribution and number of small vessels and peripheral sinusoids, in addition to homogeneous or heterogeneous distribution and variable enhancement degree (mild, moderate, or marked).

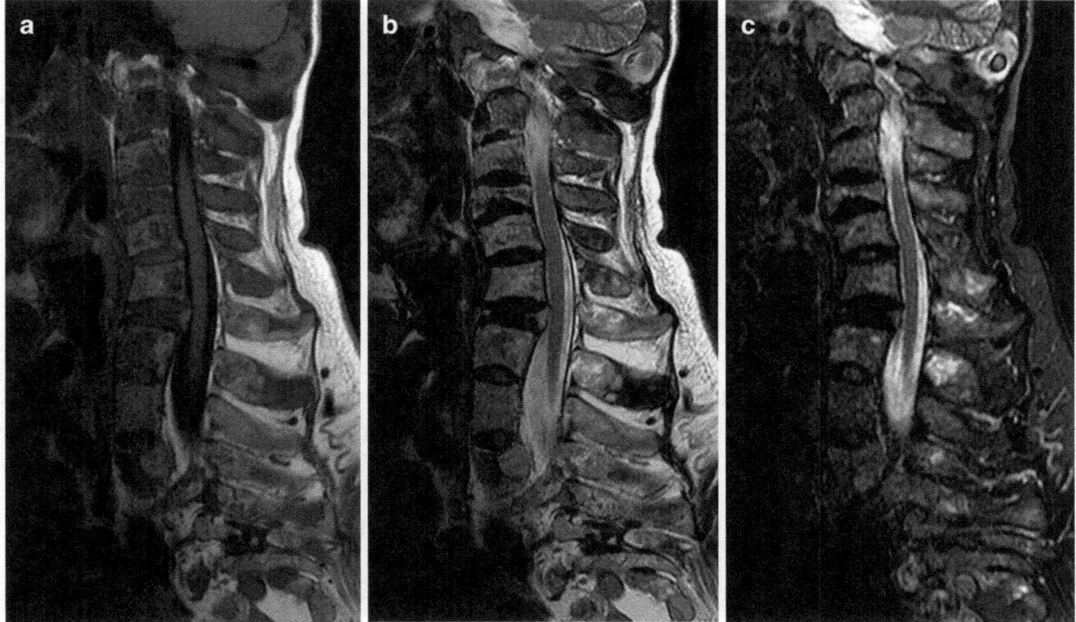

Fig. 6 Polyostotic FD in a 40-year-old man. Different sequences in the sagittal plane (**a**) T1-weighted, (**b**) T2-weighted, (**c**) STIR demonstrate multiple lesions in different vertebral locations in the cervical spine segment. Note the concomitant straightening of the cervical lordosis and scoliosis involving the thoracic segment, as well as compression fractures of the C4 and C7 vertebral bodies

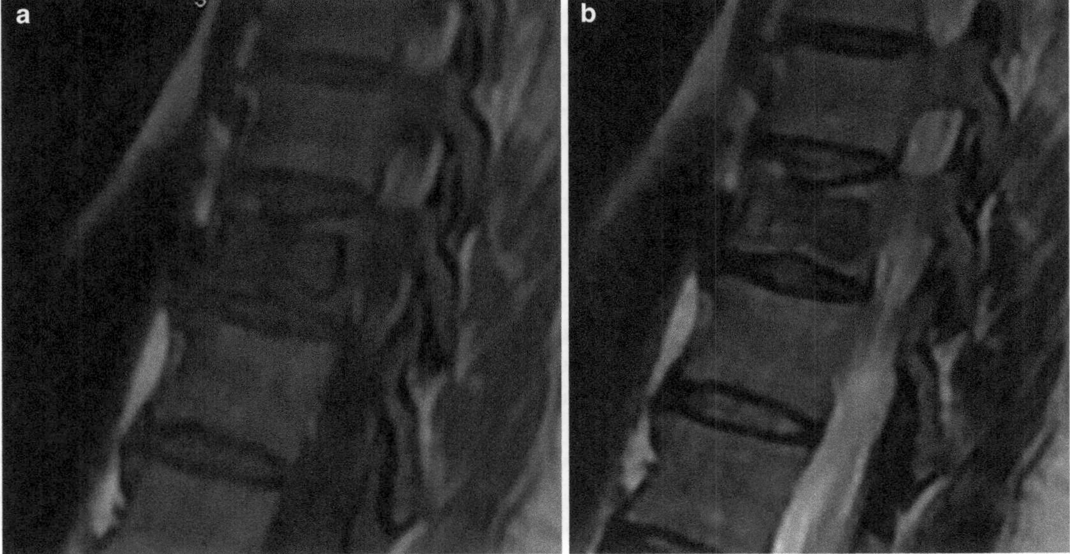

Fig. 7 MRI images of a thoracic FD vertebral lesion, revealing hypointense signal on T1-WI (**a**) with heterogeneously hyperintense signal on T2-WI (**b**). Note the compression fracture of the vertebral body. (Courtesy of Prof. Mohamed Fethi Ladeb)

Malignant degeneration in the form of sarcomatous transformation is rare in extraspinal FD, and even more in spine lesions.

Prevalence of malignant transformation has been reported to range from 0.4% to 6.7%, but only few cases of spine FD degeneration have been described.

This should be suspected if rapid radiological changes occur, in particular, if there is development of osteolytic lesions within or near the area of ground glass.

These osteolytic lesions are typically poorly marginated, with cortical destruction and periosteal reaction, and may present an associated soft tissue mass, better depicted on CT or MRI. The development of bone marrow edema is well identified with MRI (Kinnunen et al. 2020).

There is also usually an increase in contrast enhancement. All these signs are suggestive of sarcomatous transformation (Qu et al. 2015).

6.4 PET, PET-CT, and Scintigraphy

Bone scintigraphy with radionuclide agents displays the biological activity of the lesion, with strong isotope uptake in actively forming lesions, usually in young patients at the initial FD presentation, and less intense uptake in mature lesions.

The size of the uptake area on scintigraphy typically corresponds to the size of the lesions on radiographs (Zhibin et al. 2004).

Bone scintigraphy with ^{99}Tc-methylene-diphosphonate is recommended by the present guidelines as an imaging technique able to define the extent of FD and should be performed in patients starting from age of 5 (Javaid et al. 2019).

The skeletal burden score (SBS) is a useful tool for the assessment of skeletal FD burden in clinical practice (Collins et al. 2004). It is a semi-quantitative parameter, obtained by a weighted sum of percentage of segments involved in selected anatomical regions, that highly correlates with metabolic markers of bone formation, in particular ALP, P1NP, and bone reabsorption, like pyridinoline.

However, it has several limitations. First of all, it is based on planar imaging, which is particularly limited in the assessment of spine, pelvis, and thorax (van der Bruggen et al. 2020). It is unable to quantify bone turnover activity of one specific lesion and doesn't change during bisphosphonate treatment, thus not allowing therapeutic monitoring.

A combination of ^{99}Tc-DPD uptake in single photon emission computed tomography (SPECT) with whole-body CT is emerging as a valid technique for clinical assessment of skeletal FD burden since the SBS multiplied for SUV_{max} and SUV_{mean} allows a better correlation between imaging and disease activity, with higher spatial resolution (Jreige et al. 2022).

On the other hand, PET-CT using sodium fluoride provides whole body, 3D quantitative data on osteoblastic activity (van der Bruggen et al. 2020).

PET has higher resolution than planar scintigraphy and whole-body SPECT, and shorter incubation time of the radiopharmaceutical.

Na ^{18}F-PET-CT can discriminate healthy bone metabolism from FD lesions using standardized uptake values (SUV) cutoffs (SUV max and SUV peak). The parameter total bone fluorination (TLF) has been proven to show high correlation with bone formation markers, especially ALP and P1NP, providing important clinical information on FD burden (Fig. 8).

Furthermore, unlike SBS which stays stable, TLF in Na ^{18}F-PET-CT has a higher level in baseline evaluation before bisphosphonate therapy administration, being able to serve as a tool in the quantitative evaluation of treatment efficacy.

PET-CT and SPECT are used in the evaluation of FD lesion burden and could represent a useful tool in monitoring the efficacy of bisphosphonate treatment. Additionally, in patients affected by spine FD and scoliosis, it is well correlated with the severity of scoliosis, serving as a marker of spine deformity progression and potentially predictive of the development of complications (Berglund et al. 2018).

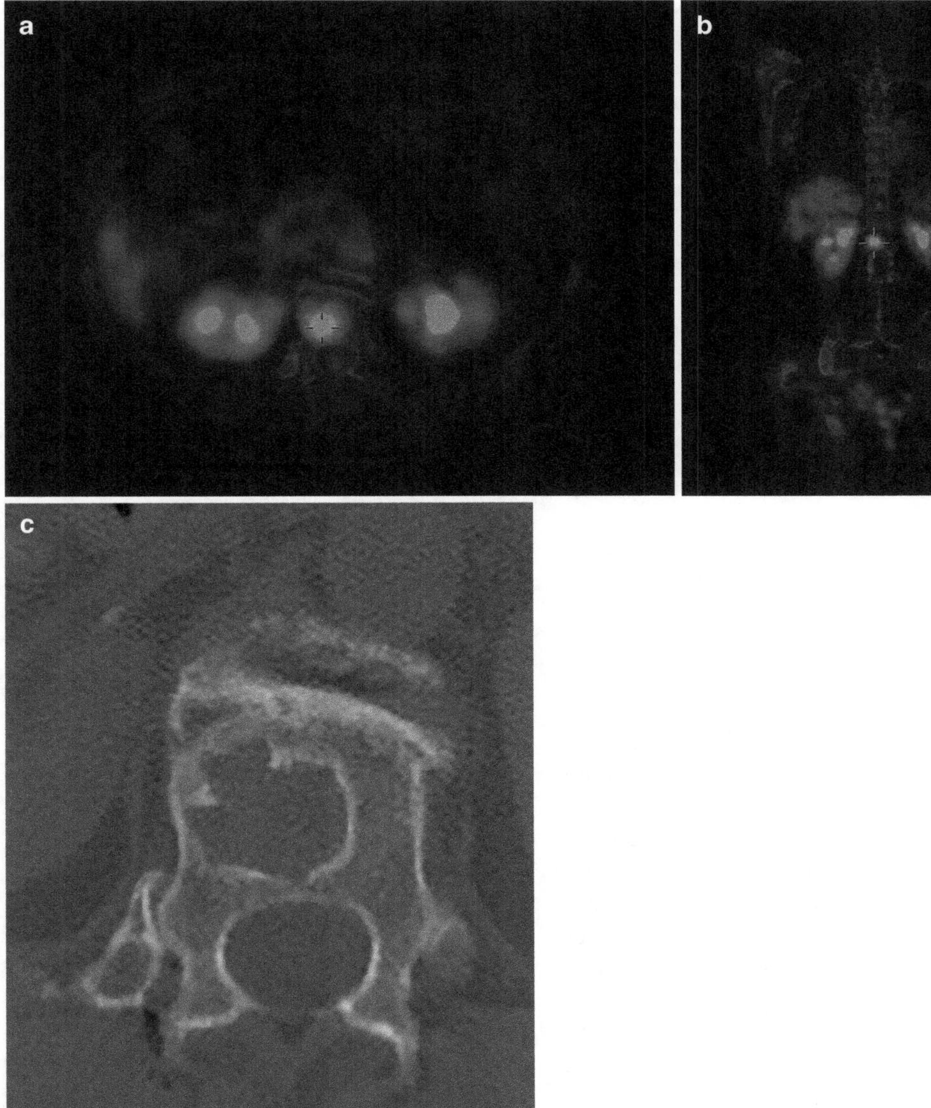

Fig. 8 Na ^{18}F-PET-CT imaging in a 68-year-old woman with polyostotic FD. (**a**) Axial acquisition and (**b**) coronal reconstruction demonstrating avid uptake of the T12 vertebral body. The lesion has lytic characteristics and presents a thin sclerotic rim on the corresponding axial CT image (**c**)

7 Histopathology

The pathogenetic mechanism behind the development of fibrodysplasia is the focal or multifocal inability of bone—forming mesenchymal tissue to form mature lamellar bone resulting in slender irregular trabeculae of woven bone surrounded by bland spindle cells in the medullary canal.

Different histological patterns of fibrodysplasia in atypical sites have been identified:

1. Conventional bone deposition pattern composed of discrete, irregular spicules of woven bone.
2. Complex/anastomosing pattern composed of long interconnecting trabeculae of woven bone with less interposed stroma.

3. Psammomatoid/cementum-like pattern composed of small round spicules or nodules of calcified bone.
4. Matrix-poor consisting of fibroblastic spindle to stellate shaped cells in a fibrous background without bone interposed in a 10x field region.

The conventional pattern is the most common, followed by the complex/anastomosing and psammomatoid/cementum-like ones in a quarter of cases.

In 21% of cases in the main background pattern, there may be interposed matrix-poor areas. In a smaller subset, there may be stromal hypercellularity, osteoclast-type giant cells, and myxoid changes may be present (Olson et al. 2021).

8 Differential Diagnosis

The diagnosis of spinal FD based solely on imaging findings may be challenging (Table 1). A spectrum of both benign and malignant entities is included in the differential diagnosis. The most frequent entities are metastasis, multiple myeloma, and osteoblastoma.

Metastases are the most frequently occurring bone tumors, and the spine represents the main skeletal localization. They may present as osteoblastic or osteolytic lesions, usually multiple, but eventually solitary, involving mostly the posterior vertebral aspect and the posterior arch.

On plain radiographs and CT (with higher sensitivity), metastases appear as osteolytic lesions with geographical or moth-eaten appearance, ill-defined margins, and wide transition zone due to the rapid growth, resulting in cortical destruction, posterior wall convexity, vertebral collapse, and soft-tissue invasion, in contrast to to the expansile nature of FD.

Osteolytic bone metastases are usually low on T1-WI, high signal in T2-WI and fat suppressed images and enhance after gadolinium administration (Guillevin et al. 2007).

Multiple myeloma usually involves the vertebral body more extensively, with consequent vertebral collapse rather than being expansile (Kumar et al. 1988).

Table 1 Summary of typical features of Fibrous Dysplasia

	Fibrous dysplasia
Behavior	Benign
Associated syndrome	McCune-Albright Mazabraud
Form	Monostotic Polyostotic
Locations	Extra-vertebral: Femur, ribs, lower extremities, craniofacial bones Spinal: Lumbar, thoracic, cervical, sacral No preference: Vertebral body/posterior elements
Histological findings	Irregular trabeculae of woven bone surrounded by immature mesenchymal cells
X-ray/CT findings	Intramedullary lytic lesion Lytic Ground glass appearance Well-defined margin and sclerotic rim Thinning of cortical bone Endosteal scalloping in expansive lesion
MRI	T1w: Hypo- to isointensity signal T2w: Heterogeneous hyperintense signal Variable contrast enhancement
Nuclear medicine	Tracer uptake in metabolic active lesions
Treatment options	Conservative/observation Vertebral augmentation procedure (curettage, vertebroplasty) Vertebral resection Surgical fixation

In the cases in which FD presents as lytic lesions, the differential diagnosis could also be made with hemangioma, aneurysmal bone cyst (ABC), and giant cell tumor (GCT).

ABC is a benign tumor-like lesion which appears as an expansile lytic lesion surrounded by a thin bone rim, that can grow quickly and extend over the cortical as a soft-tissue mass.

Features suggestive of ABC are multiloculated cystic appearance, with internal septations and involvement of posterior arch; enhancing solid components may be present (Rodallec et al. 2008).

ABCs are blood-filled lesions, and therefore MRI signal intensity is variable, and fluid-fluid levels common, representing different stages of hemoglobin degradation products (Sebaaly et al. 2015). ABC is further discussed in the chapter "Aneurysmal Bone Cyst and Other Cystic Lesions."

On radiographs and CT, GCT of the spine appears as expansile, osteolytic, "soap bubble-like" lesions; the presence of a sclerotic rim is infrequent, unlike cortical destruction, which is commonly seen.

On MRI, GCT is iso- or hypointense on T1-WI, heterogeneous (hypo- to hyperintense) on T2-WI, and variable enhancement is present after gadolinium administration. GCT of the spine presents as a benign tumor but are frequently locally aggressive, invading the epidural space (Si et al. 2014). Giant cell tumor is further discussed in the chapter "Giant Cell Tumor."

Hemangioma, in its typical form, is characterized by the polka-dot sign appearance on CT scan, which represents the thickened vertical trabecular on the axial plane, and demonstrated high signal intensity on MRI on T1-WI and T2-WI, due to the high fat content.

Atypical forms, with less fat and more vascular content, may enter in the differential diagnosis with FD. These appear iso- or hypointense on T1-WI and hyperintense on T2-WI and fat suppressed images and show different degrees of enhancement after gadolinium administration.

Moreover, aggressive hemangiomas may show rapid growth, and expansile appearance with soft tissue protruding in the epidural space mimicking bony malignancies.

The identification of vertebral trabeculae as the classic "polka dot sign" on CT, more difficult to see in the atypical form, helps guide the differential diagnosis (Gaudino et al. 2015) (see chapter "Vertebral Haemangioma and Angiomatous Neoplasms").

Paget disease and osteoblastoma should be considered in cases of mainly osteoblastic FD.

Paget disease is characterized by focal bone resorption and new formation of woven bone, with the succession of three phases: an osteolytic one, with wedge-shaped osteolytic areas, followed by osteoblastic response in which the radiographic lucent areas become more radiopaque, and the osteosclerotic phase with bone formation and enlargement of the involved bone (see chapter "Paget of the Spine") (Weber et al. 2022).

Osteoblastoma usually originates in the vertebral arch and extends into the vertebral body. Histologically composed of osteoid and woven bone, osteoblastoma appears as expansive lesion, usually greater than 2 cm, with sclerotic shell and multifocal matrix mineralization (Rodallec et al. 2008). Osteoblastoma is further discussed in the chapter "Osteoid Osteoma and Osteoblastoma."

Spine tuberculosis, as an infectious disease, could enter into differential diagnosis with FD since it involves mostly the thoracic and upper lumbar tract of the spine.

The posterior vertebral elements are rarely involved, instead the anterior aspect of the vertebral body, adjacent to endplates are frequently sites of demineralization, focal areas of erosions and bony destruction in the early stage of the disease allowing intervertebral disc spread. This results into the pathogen dissemination through the anterior and posterior longitudinal ligaments to multiple contiguous vertebral levels followed by intervertebral disc destruction, vertebral collapse, and the typical gibbous deformity of the spine (Shanley 1995).

A single vertebral body involvement is rare, but may lead to collapse and vertebra plana deformation.

Sclerotic reaction is infrequent, but paravertebral abscess often calcified is a typical feature (Burrill et al. 2007).

The thoracic and upper lumbar tract of the spine is typically site of sarcoidosis vertebral localization, which although rare may be considered as a differential diagnosis of FD.

Lesions can be either osteolytic or osteosclerotic, and the MRI appearance is heterogeneous showing low signals in T1-W1, and mainly high signal in T2-W1 due to granulomatous infiltration. However osseous involvement in sarcoidosis usually manifest in association with pulmonary symptoms, facilitating the differential diagnosis (Saad et al. 2022).

9 Local and Distant Staging

Imaging plays a key role in the local and distant assessment of extent of FD.

Spine CT and MRI, with high spatial and tissue contrast resolution, are useful in local staging, providing information about the number and size of the lesions, vertebra/vertebrae affected, vertebral elements involved (body, posterior arch), cortical involvement, extent into the spinal canal or into vertebral foramina, intervertebral discs, and paravertebral soft tissues.

Total body CT is the method of choice for the identification of extraspinal FD lesions. Furthermore PET-CT and SPECT provide information on the total skeletal burden that correlates well with the activity status of the lesions.

In case of malignant degeneration, further information regarding the nodal and metastatic involvement should be provided, in accordance with the 2020 WHO update of staging and classification of primary musculoskeletal bone and soft-tissue tumors (Murphey and Kransdorf 2021).

10 Treatment

Treatment options may vary based on the clinical presentation and symptoms, including conservative approach/observation, biopsy, surgical resection, and vertebral augmentation procedures, such as vertebroplasty and kyphoplasty.

In patients with asymptomatic, incidentally found monostotic lesions that remain stable over years, no treatment is required.

In polyostotic and symptomatic disease, oral or intravenous bisphosphonate administration, especially pamidronate, has been proven to be effective in decreasing pain and preventing pathologic fracture development. Since pamidronate and other second- and third-generation biphosphonates affect bone turnover by inhibiting resorption, they induce progressive ossification, with cortical thickening and lesion diameter reduction, resulting in radiological improvement (Dicaprio and Enneking 2005).

CT-guided percutaneous biopsy is a safe and effective interventional procedure, with about 90% of accuracy (Lis et al. 2004). Biopsy is needed when radiological findings are atypical or confounding.

Surgery is indicated in case of persistent pain, neurological deficits due to spinal cord compression/injury, pathologic fractures, and instability (Stanton et al. 2012).

For lesions involving the posterior arch, laminectomy and fusion with or without internal fixation may be performed (Xin et al. 2019; Wu et al. 2013; Arantes et al. 2008).

For vertebral body invasion, three types of treatments are available:

(a) Curettage of the lesion followed by bone grafting to increase mechanical bone resistance.

    The use of autogenous cancellous bone grafts has been shown to be limited by its high rate of resorption. This is replaced by dysplastic tissue when the remodeling process occurs, leading to lesion recurrence (Leet et al. 2016).

    Cortical autogenous grafts tend to persist longer with lower rates of replacement, hence biological allografts are preferred in FD (Dicaprio and Enneking 2005).

(b) Vertebroplasty is a valid therapeutic option for FD with pathologic fractures and in patients without neurological deficits since it has shorter hospitalization and faster recovery times compared to other techniques (Xin et al. 2019).

    The use of cement has several advantages. Firstly, cement provides vertebral mechanical stability relieving pain, which is further eased by the heat released in the solidification process that destroys nerve endings, providing an analgesic effect (Evans et al. 2003).

    Furthermore, the cemental agent, with its cytotoxic effect reduces the cellular metabolic activity of the lesion cemented (San Millán Ruíz et al. 1999).

    In addition, vertebroplasty does not present the problem of adsorption, and the typical sclerotic rim of FD lesion prevents cement leaking (Wu et al. 2013).

(c) Complete surgical resection with corpectomy and instrumented fusion should be avoided as long as there are no signs of cord compression and aggressive progression, and chosen in case of malignant transformation (Meredith and Healey 2011).

    In the management of scoliosis, bisphosphonate administration shows no efficacy in reducing the progression of curves, and a surgical fixation should be considered for Cobb angles greater than 30° (Javaid et al. 2019; Berglund et al. 2018).

11 Prognosis and Follow-Up

The prognosis depends on the type of FD, ranging from very good in incidental asymptomatic isolated monostotic lesions to variable or poor in cases of diffuse polyostotic spinal and skeletal involvement resulting in scoliosis and bone deformity, inducing limitation of movements and progressively debilitating neurological deficits (Boyce et al. 1993).

FD and in particular polyostotic DF may be seen in association with McCune-Albright syndrome, which is characterized by endocrine dysfunction.

In case of newly diagnosed FD lesions, a CT scan is suggested to exclude polyostotic involvement (Fig. 6). If a single lesion is confirmed, follow-up radiographs should be periodically made to verify the stability or eventual progression (Boyce et al. 1993).

Lesions in monostotic FD tend to enlarge until the end of skeletal growth, but in case of stability and no correlated symptoms, only clinical monitoring is required.

Since most cases of monostotic FD do not progress and are not associated with increased risk of deformity and pathologic fracture, long-term outcome is satisfactory regardless of treatment (Dicaprio and Enneking 2005).

When multiple FD lesions are detected and McCune-Albright syndrome is suspected, it is important to determine the extent of bone involvement and associated metabolic and endocrinological conditions, in particular the serum phosphate levels, which tend to be depleted during the skeletal growth (coinciding with major lesion activity), the presence of hyperthyroidism, growth hormone excess, and gonadic functional and morphological abnormalities.

Clinically, significative FD is frequently associated with high lesion burden, including spine, craniofacial, and femoral involvement (Collins et al. 2004).

As surveillance, radiographs should be periodically carried out to evaluate the evolution of pre-existing lesions, occurrence of new ones, and the quality of the bone structure (Javaid et al. 2019).

In particular, strict monitoring of scoliosis is mandatory, because untreated and progressive scoliosis results in increased morbidity, and severe cases may be potentially lethal due to complications of restrictive lung disease (Berglund et al. 2018). From the moment of diagnosis, an early multidisciplinary approach is recommended.

In case of craniofacial involvement, periodic CT examination along with annual hearing and visual testing should be performed, to assess the neurological involvement, as this is an important cause of morbidity (Javaid et al. 2019).

Malignant transformation of FD is rare, with prevalence reported ranging from 0.4% to 6.7% (Qu et al. 2015), but only few cases of spine FD degeneration have been described (Yalniz et al. 1995).

In general, malignancy can occur in both monostotic and polyostotic FD, but mainly occurs in the latter, when associated with McCune-Albright syndrome. The most frequent forms of malignant degeneration are osteosarcoma (53.4%), followed by fibrosarcoma (17.8%) and chondrosarcoma (8.9%).

Irradiation of FD seems to induce sarcomatous transformation, thus radiotherapy should never be used as treatment option for FD lesions (Ruggieri et al. 1994).

Malignant transformation usually occurs over longstanding lesions (over a decade) and should be suspected with the onset of rapidly increasing pain and swelling without trauma and radiological progression. Poor prognosis is always associated (Qu et al. 2015).

12 Key Points

1. Fibrous dysplasia is a benign tumor-like disease that affects either a single bone (monostotic form) or multiple bones (polyostotic form) and may be associated with syndromic endocrine dysfunction.
2. Every tract of the spine could be involved, presenting as incidental finding, totally asymptomatic, to pain, vertebral deformity, and collapse. Scoliosis is an important clinical feature in case of multilevel polyostotic form.

3. Imaging plays a pivotal role in diagnosis and follow-up, allowing the radiological features identification, the lesion burden definition and monitoring the evolution and extension of the disease.
4. Biopsy should be performed in case of undefined or suspected findings, and every biopsy tract should be reviewed with the oncologic spine surgeon involved in the definitive surgical management.
5. Treatment ranges from conservative approach in asymptomatic patients to surgical management in case of pain, instability, fracture, and neurological symptoms.

References

Adetayo OA, Salcedo SE, Borad V, Richards SS, Workman AD, Ray AO (2015) Fibrous dysplasia: an overview of disease process, indications for surgical management, and a case report fibrous dysplasia: an overview of disease process, indications for surgical management, and a case report. Eplasty 15:e6

Arantes M, Vaz AR, Honavar M et al (2008) Fibrous dysplasia of the first cervical vertebra. Spine 33:E933–E935. https://doi.org/10.1097/BRS.0b013e318186b31a

Berglund JA, Tella SH, Tuthill KF et al (2018) Scoliosis in fibrous dysplasia/McCune-Albright syndrome: factors associated with curve progression and effects of bisphosphonates: scoliosis in FD/MAS. J Bone Miner Res 33:1641–1648. https://doi.org/10.1002/jbmr.3446

Bianco P, Robey PG, Wientroub S (2003) Fibrous dysplasia. In: Glorieux FH, Pettifor J, Juppner H (eds) Pediatric bone—biology and disease. Academic Press, New York, pp 509–539

Boyce AM, Florenzano P, de Castro LF, Collins MT (1993) Fibrous dysplasia/McCune-Albright syndrome. In: Adam MP, Mirzaa GM, Pagon RA et al (eds) GeneReviews®. University of Washington, Seattle, WA

Burrill J, Williams CJ, Bain G et al (2007) Tuberculosis: a radiologic review. Radiographics 27:1255–1273. https://doi.org/10.1148/rg.275065176

Collins MT, Kushner H, Reynolds JC et al (2004) An instrument to measure skeletal burden and predict functional outcome in fibrous dysplasia of bone. J Bone Miner Res 20:219–226. https://doi.org/10.1359/JBMR.041111

Dicaprio MR, Enneking WF (2005) Fibrous dysplasia. Pathophysiology, evaluation, and treatment. J Bone Joint Surg Am 87:1848

Evans AJ, Jensen ME, Kip KE et al (2003) Vertebral compression fractures: pain reduction and improvement in functional mobility after percutaneous polymethylmethacrylate vertebroplasty—retrospective report of 245 cases. Radiology 226:366–372. https://doi.org/10.1148/radiol.2262010906

Favus MJ, Vokes TJ (2018) Paget's disease and other dysplasias of bone. In Jameson J, Fauci AS, Kasper DL, Hauser SL, Longo DL, Loscalzo J (eds) Harrison's Principles of Internal Medicine, 20e. McGraw Hill. https://accessmedicine.mhmedical.com/content.aspx?bookid=2129§ionid=192530772

Gaudino S, Martucci M, Colantonio R et al (2015) A systematic approach to vertebral hemangioma. Skelet Radiol 44:25–36. https://doi.org/10.1007/s00256-014-2035-y

Gogia N, Marwaha V, Atri S et al (2007) Fibrous dysplasia localized to spine: a diagnostic dilemma. Skelet Radiol 36:19–23. https://doi.org/10.1007/s00256-006-0102-8

Guillevin R, Vallee J-N, Lafitte F et al (2007) Spine metastasis imaging: review of the literature. J Neuroradiol 34:311–321. https://doi.org/10.1016/j.neurad.2007.05.003

Javaid MK, Boyce A, Appelman-Dijkstra N et al (2019) Best practice management guidelines for fibrous dysplasia/McCune-Albright syndrome: a consensus statement from the FD/MAS international consortium. Orphanet J Rare Dis 14:139. https://doi.org/10.1186/s13023-019-1102-9

Jee WH, Choi KH, Choe BY et al (1996) Fibrous dysplasia: MR imaging characteristics with radiopathologic correlation. Am J Roentgenol 167:1523–1527. https://doi.org/10.2214/ajr.167.6.8956590

Jreige M, Hall N, Becce F et al (2022) A novel approach for fibrous dysplasia assessment using combined planar and quantitative SPECT/CT analysis of Tc-99m-diphosphonate bone scan in correlation with biological bone turnover markers of disease activity. Front Med 9:1050854. https://doi.org/10.3389/fmed.2022.1050854

Kinnunen A-R, Sironen R, Sipola P (2020) Magnetic resonance imaging characteristics in patients with histopathologically proven fibrous dysplasia—a systematic review. Skelet Radiol 49:837–845. https://doi.org/10.1007/s00256-020-03388-x

Kumar R, Guinto FC, Madewell JE et al (1988) Expansile bone lesions of the vertebra. Radiographics 8:749–769. https://doi.org/10.1148/radiographics.8.4.3175086

Leet AI, Magur E, Lee JS et al (2004) Fibrous dysplasia in the spine: prevalence of lesions and association with scoliosis. J Bone Joint Surg 86:531–537. https://doi.org/10.2106/00004623-200403000-00011

Leet AI, Boyce AM, Ibrahim KA et al (2016) Bone-grafting in polyostotic fibrous dysplasia. J Bone Joint Surg 98:211–219. https://doi.org/10.2106/JBJS.O.00547

Lichtenstein L (1938) Polyostotic fibrous dysplasia. Arch Surg 36:874

Lis E, Bilsky MH, Pisinski L et al (2004) Percutaneous CT-guided biopsy of osseous lesion of the spine in patients with known or suspected malignancy. AJNR Am J Neuroradiol 25:1583–1588

Liu X-X, Xin X, Yan Y-H, Ma X-W (2021) Imaging characteristics of a rare case of monostotic fibrous dysplasia of the sacrum: a case report. WJCC 9:1111–1118. https://doi.org/10.12998/wjcc.v9.i5.1111

Mancini F, Corsi A, De Maio F et al (2009) Scoliosis and spine involvement in fibrous dysplasia of bone. Eur Spine J 18:196–202. https://doi.org/10.1007/s00586-008-0860-1

Meredith DS, Healey JH (2011) Twenty-year follow-up of monostotic fibrous dysplasia of the second cervical vertebra: a case report and review of the literature. J Bone Joint Surg 93:e74. https://doi.org/10.2106/JBJS.J.01881

Murphey MD, Kransdorf MJ (2021) Staging and classification of primary musculoskeletal bone and soft-tissue tumors according to the 2020 WHO update, from the AJR special series on cancer staging. Am J Roentgenol 217:1038–1052. https://doi.org/10.2214/AJR.21.25658

Nabarro MN, Giblin PE (1994) Monostotic fibrous dysplasia of the thoracic spine. Spine (Phila Pa 1976) 19(4):463–5. https://doi.org/10.1097/00007632-199402001-00016. PMID: 8178238.

Olson NJ, Inwards CY, Wenger DE, Fritchie KJ (2021) Fibrous dysplasia at unusual anatomic sites: a series of 86 cases with emphasis on histologic patterns. Int J Surg Pathol 29:704–709. https://doi.org/10.1177/1066896921997141

Park SK, Lee IS, Choi J-Y et al (2012) CT and MRI of fibrous dysplasia of the spine. BJR 85:996–1001. https://doi.org/10.1259/bjr/81329736

Qu N, Yao W, Cui X, Zhang H (2015) Malignant transformation in monostotic fibrous dysplasia: clinical features, imaging features, outcomes in 10 patients, and review. Medicine 94:e369. https://doi.org/10.1097/MD.0000000000000369

Rahim AH, Hidajat NN, Ramdan A, Magetsari RMSN (2021) Fibrous dysplasia of the spine—a case involving the polyostotic form isolated to the thoracolumbar spine. Int J Spine Surg 14:S46–S51. https://doi.org/10.14444/7164

Rodallec MH, Feydy A, Larousserie F et al (2008) Diagnostic imaging of solitary tumors of the spine: what to do and say. Radiographics 28:1019–1041. https://doi.org/10.1148/rg.284075156

Ruggieri P, Sim FH, Bond JR, Krishnan Unni K (1994) Malignancies in fibrous dysplasia. Cancer 73:1411–1424. https://doi.org/10.1002/1097-0142(19940301)73:5<1411::AID-CNCR2820730516>3.0.CO;2-T

Saad E, Agab M, Zhang Q et al (2022) Multisystemic sarcoidosis presenting with widespread vertebral osseous and visceral lesions masquerading as metastatic disease: a case report and literature review. Am J Case Rep 23:10.12659/AJCR.935158

San Millán Ruíz D, Burkhardt K, Jean B et al (1999) Pathology findings with acrylic implants. Bone 25:85S–90S. https://doi.org/10.1016/S8756-3282(99)00140-4

Sebaaly A, Ghostine B, Kreichati G et al (2015) Aneurysmal bone cyst of the cervical spine in children: a review and a focus on available treatment options. J Pediatr Orthop 35:693–702. https://doi.org/10.1097/BPO.0000000000000365

Shanley DJ (1995) Tuberculosis of the spine: imaging features. Am J Roentgenol 164:659–664. https://doi.org/10.2214/ajr.164.3.7863889

Si M-J, Wang C-G, Wang C-S et al (2014) Giant cell tumours of the mobile spine: characteristic imaging features and differential diagnosis. Radiol Med 119:681–693. https://doi.org/10.1007/s11547-013-0352-1

Stanton RP, Ippolito E, Springfield D et al (2012) The surgical management of fibrous dysplasia of bone. Orphanet J Rare Dis 7:S1. https://doi.org/10.1186/1750-1172-7-S1-S1

Utz JA, Kransdorf MJ, Jelinek JS et al (1989) MR appearance of fibrous dysplasia. J Comput Assist Tomogr 13:845–851. https://doi.org/10.1097/00004728-198909000-00018

van der Bruggen W, Hagelstein-Rotman M, de Geus-Oei L-F et al (2020) Quantifying skeletal burden in fibrous dysplasia using sodium fluoride PET/CT. Eur J Nucl Med Mol Imaging 47:1527–1537. https://doi.org/10.1007/s00259-019-04657-1

Von Recklinghausen. Festschrift Rudolf Virchow on the 13th Berlin, Germany: Georg Reimer Verlag; 1891. Fibrous or deforming osteitis, osteomalacia, and osteoplastic carcinosis in their mutual relations.

Weber M-A, Bazzocchi A, Nöbauer-Huhmann I-M (2022) Tumors of the spine: when can biopsy be avoided? Semin Musculoskelet Radiol 26:453–468. https://doi.org/10.1055/s-0042-1753506

Weinstein LS, Shenker A, Gejman PV et al (1991) Activating mutations of the stimulatory G protein in the McCune–Albright syndrome. N Engl J Med 325:1688–1695. https://doi.org/10.1056/NEJM199112123252403

Wright JFC, Stoker DJ (1988) Fibrous dysplasia of the spine. Clin Radiol 39(5):523–527. https://doi.org/10.1016/s0009-9260(88)80222-8

Wu FL, Jiang L, Liu C et al (2013) Fibrous dysplasia of the mobile spine: report of 8 cases and review of the literature. Spine 38:2016–2022. https://doi.org/10.1097/BRS.0b013e3182a8cc05

Xin X, Feng J, Yue C et al (2019) Monostotic fibrous dysplasia at C7 treated with vertebroplasty: a case report and review of the literature. World J Surg Oncol 17:186. https://doi.org/10.1186/s12957-019-1717-2

Yalniz E, Er T, Ozyilmaz F (1995) Fibrous dysplasia of the spine with sarcomatous transformation: a case report and review of the literature. Eur Spine J 4:372–374. https://doi.org/10.1007/BF00300303

Zhang Y, Zhang C, Wang S et al (2018) Computed tomography and magnetic resonance imaging manifestations of spinal monostotic fibrous dysplasia. J Clin Imaging Sci 8:23. https://doi.org/10.4103/jcis.JCIS_20_18

Zhibin Y, Quanyong L, Libo C et al (2004) The role of radionuclide bone scintigraphy in fibrous dysplasia of bone. Clin Nucl Med 29:177–180. https://doi.org/10.1097/01.rlu.0000113856.77103.7e

Aneurysmal Bone Cyst and Other Cystic Lesions

Emna Labbène and Mohamed Fethi Ladeb

Contents

E. Labbène (✉) · M. F. Ladeb
Department of Radiology, M T Kassab Institute of Orthopedics, Tunis, Tunisia

Faculty of Medicine of Tunis, Tunis-El Manar University, Tunis, Tunisia
e-mail: emnasensei@gmail.com; fethiladeb@hotmail.fr

Abstract

Aneurysmal bone cyst (ABC) is a benign tumor that can be locally aggressive with a risk of recurrence after treatment. It mainly affects children and young adults and generally occurs in long bones. The spine is involved in 8.7–19% of cases with a predilection for the posterior arch. ABC presents typically as a lytic and expansile lesion with internal bony septa. MRI is the modality of choice to show the blood-filled cavities with fluid-fluid levels and to evaluate paravertebral and spinal canal extension. Some tumors can present with similar imaging features (ABC-area changes), and histologic study is mandatory to confirm the diagnosis. Many treatment modalities are available but there is a lack of consensus regarding the management of spinal ABC.

1 Introduction

The name of aneurysmal bone cyst (ABC) was first suggested by Jaffe and Lichtenstein in 1942 to describe two cases of "peculiar blood-containing cysts of large size," and the lesion was definitely identified as a distinctive entity by the same authors in 1950 (Jaffe and Lichtenstein 1942; Jaffe 1950). Its nature was uncertain for a long time but now it is recognized as a true neoplasm. Although it is a benign tumor, ABC can be

Med Radiol Diagn Imaging (2023)
https://doi.org/10.1007/174_2023_432,
Published Online: 23 May 2023

locally aggressive with a risk of recurrence after treatment. It mainly occurs in children and young adults and involves most frequently long bones. The spine is involved in 8.7–19% of cases with a predilection for the posterior arch (Vergel De Dios et al. 1992; Papagelopoulos et al. 1998; de Kleuver et al. 1998; Cottalorda et al. 2004). The typical aspect of ABC consists of a lytic and expansile lesion composed of blood-filled cavities with fluid-fluid levels (Restrepo et al. 2022). The presence of fluid-fluid levels is characteristic but not pathognomonic. It can be found in other lesions among which the telangiectatic osteosarcoma. Histological confirmation of ABC is thus recommended (WHO Classification of Tumours Editorial Board 2020). Many treatment modalities are available but there is a lack of consensus regarding the management of spinal ABC.

2 Pathologic Features

ABC can develop de novo (70% of cases) or occur in association with other tumors (30% of cases). The first condition was called "primary ABC" while the second one was referred to as "secondary ABC." Nowadays, it is recommended to replace these terms, respectively, by "ABC" and "ABC-like changes." The main tumors that can be associated with ABC-like changes are giant cell tumor, osteoblastoma, chondroblastoma, fibrous dysplasia, and telangiectatic osteosarcoma (Restrepo et al. 2022).

ABC was previously considered as a tumor-like lesion and not a true neoplasm. However, since the discovery of recurrent chromosomal abnormalities involving the USP6 gene, ABC is considered a true bone tumor (Oliveira and Chou 2014). The USP6 gene rearrangement is found in 70% of ABC while it is absent in lesions with ABC-like changes (WHO Classification of Tumours Editorial Board 2020).

3 Epidemiology

ABC is rare and represents about 1.4% of all bone tumors (Hay et al. 1978; Boriani et al. 2001).

It can occur in any bone of the body but it is most frequently seen in long bones of lower limb. The spine is involved in 8.7–19% of cases (Vergel De Dios et al. 1992; Papagelopoulos et al. 1998; de Kleuver et al. 1998; Cottalorda et al. 2004).

ABC represents 15% of primary bone tumors of the spine (Unni and Inwards 2010).

A slight female predominance is generally reported in the literature (Vergel De Dios et al. 1992; Leithner et al. 1999). However, in spinal location, some authors reported female predominance with a male to female ratio between 0.75 and 0.95 (Hay et al. 1978; De Kleuver et al. 1998; Boriani et al. 2001) while others reported male predominance with a male to female ratio between 1.47 and 2 (Papagelopoulos et al. 1998; Ozaki et al. 1999; Zileli et al. 2013; Boriani et al. 2014; Sayago et al. 2020).

Similarly to the appendicular location, spinal ABC occurs mainly in children and young adults with about 80% of cases discovered during the first two decades of life and with a mean age between 13 and 16.6 years (Hay et al. 1978; Papagelopoulos et al. 1998; De Kleuver et al. 1998; Boriani et al. 2001).

4 Localization

ABC distribution among spine segments differs in literature. In some studies, the lumbar spine is the most frequent location, involved in 40–45%, followed by the cervical (10–30%) and the thoracic segments (25–35.5%) (De Kleuver et al. 1998; Boriani et al. 2001; Cottalorda et al. 2004).

In a study including 92 spinal ABC, the thoracic spine was the most frequent location (34%) followed by the lumbar spine (31%) and the cervical spine (22%) (Hay et al. 1978).

In some studies, cervical and thoracic segments were involved with the same frequency (Papagelopoulos et al. 1998; Cottalorda et al. 2004).

The sacrum is involved in 13–21% of cases (Hay et al. 1978; Papagelopoulos et al. 1998; De Kleuver et al. 1998; Ozaki et al. 1999).

ABC presents generally as a solitary bone lesion, and multiple or metachronous lesions are extremely rare (Donigan et al. 2003; AlYami et al. 2022).

However, involvement of two or more contiguous vertebrae is not rare and found in 7–44% of cases. In these cases, intervertebral disc is generally preserved (Papagelopoulos et al. 1998; De Kleuver et al. 1998; Boriani et al. 2001).

Within vertebra, involvement of the posterior arch is almost constant and reported in 100% of cases in different studies. Vertebral body is involved in 63–83% of cases in association with posterior arch (Papagelopoulos et al. 1998; De Kleuver et al. 1998; Boriani et al. 2001; Zileli et al. 2013). The distribution among posterior elements differs between studies with pedicles, lamina and spinous process being the most involved elements (Hay et al. 1978; Papagelopoulos et al. 1998).

ABC has generally an eccentric position developing mainly on one side of the vertebra (Zileli et al. 2013).

5 Clinical Presentation

The two main clinical symptoms are pain and neurologic symptoms (Hay et al. 1978; Papagelopoulos et al. 1998; Boriani et al. 2001, 2014; Chan et al. 2002).

Pain is the most frequent complaint, consisting of either local axial pain or radicular pain.

Neurological symptoms are the result of spinal cord or nerve root compression and include paresthesia, motor weakness, paraplegia, and bowel and bladder dysfunction.

Acute neurological symptoms result from vertebral body collapse with neurologic structures compression.

Vertebral body collapse, muscle spasm, and back pain can cause spinal deformities such as scoliosis, kyphosis, and torticollis (Papagelopoulos et al. 1998; Boriani et al. 2001).

Reduced spine motion, stiffness, swelling, and palpable mass were also reported (Hay et al. 1978).

The mean duration of symptoms varies between 4 and 9.4 months (Hay et al. 1978; Ameli et al. 1985; Papagelopoulos et al. 1998; Zileli et al. 2013).

6 Imaging

6.1 Radiographs

Conventional Radiography (CR) is generally the first imaging modality used to explore patients but in some cases, it can have a limited contribution in characterizing spinal tumors due to the complex anatomy of the vertebral column.

The typical aspect of ABC on radiographs consists of a geographic lytic and expansile lesion either limited to the posterior elements or extending to the vertebral body (Fig. 1a) (Papagelopoulos et al. 1998; Boriani et al. 2001; Sans and Perroncel 2014; Restrepo et al. 2022). Nevertheless, the appearance depends on the growth rate and the phase at which is discovered the tumor. At an early phase and during active growing phase, ABC appears as a purely lytic lesion with possible ill-defined margins, no internal septation nor surrounding periosteal rim and can be associated with a cortical destruction mimicking a malignant tumor. During intermediate phase (phase of stabilization), a process of ossification begins. A surrounding reactive rim is seen at the periphery of the tumor and internal bony septation can appear giving a "soap bubble" appearance. At a late reparative phase (healing phase), the process of ossification extends progressively with possible decrease in tumor size (Dabska and Buraczewski 1969; Malghem et al. 1989) (Fig. 1b).

6.2 CT

CR and CT share the same radiological semiology but the latter allows a more detailed analysis of different imaging features in this location. The different aspects described on plain radiographs can be seen: the typical aspect of a lytic and expansile lesion with a surrounding shell egg periosteal reaction (Figs. 2 and 3); the aspect of an aggressive lytic lesion with ill-defined borders and cortical destruction; the internal bony septation with a "soap bubble" appearance; a healing lesion with peripheral and internal ossification (Figs. 3 and 4). The tumor is generally eccentric and involves one side of the vertebra (Zileli et al. 2013; Sans and Perroncel 2014) (Fig. 2).

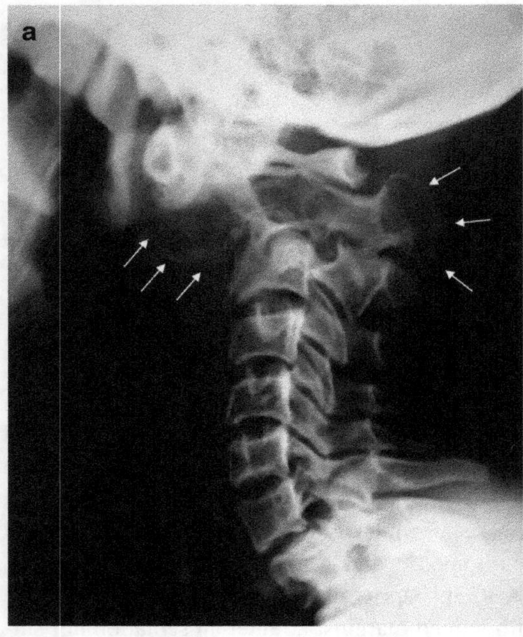

Fig. 1 Aneurysmal bone cyst of C2 (lateral view radiographs of the cervical spine). (**a**) Expansile and lytic lesion of C2 involving the posterior arch and extending to the body and dens (white arrows). (**b**) One year later: extensive ossification of the tumor consisting with a process of healing (open arrows)

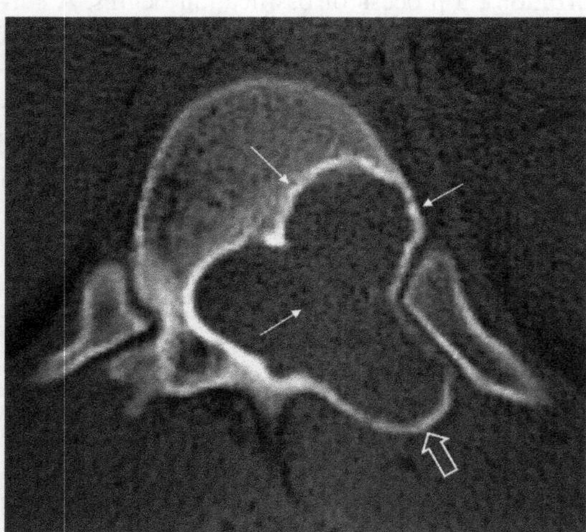

Fig. 2 Aneurysmal bone cyst of T12 vertebra on an axial CT image appearing as an expansile and lytic lesion (arrows) with an eggshell periosteal reaction (open arrow). The tumor involves the posterior arch and the vertebral body and has a characteristic eccentric location, limited to the left side of the vertebra

CT can also show additional radiological findings not seen on radiographs such as the presence of fluid-fluid levels composed of a lower layer of high-density hemorrhagic fluid relative to an upper layer of lower-density liquid (Sans and Perroncel 2014) (Fig. 3d) and limited by enhancing septa (Fig. 5). This finding is characteristic but not specific and can be seen in other lesions. Areas of fat density can also be found and orient to the benign nature of the tumor (Fig. 4).

Although less performant than MRI, CT can assess the extension of the tumor in paravertebral soft tissues and into the spinal canal (Fig. 3).

Involvement of the vertebral body can result in fracture and vertebral collapse (Fig. 6).

6.3 MRI

Similar to CT, MRI shows a tumor with fluid-fluid levels and internal septa limiting the blood-filled cavities (Mahnken et al. 2003; Zileli et al. 2013). The signal inside the cavities is variable both on T1- and on T2-weighted images (WI) depending on the age of blood. It can appear as low, intermediate, or high signal (Figs. 7 and 8). Following intravenous gadolinium contrast administration, ABC shows peripheral and septal enhancement (Fig. 7) and in some cases enhancing of a solid

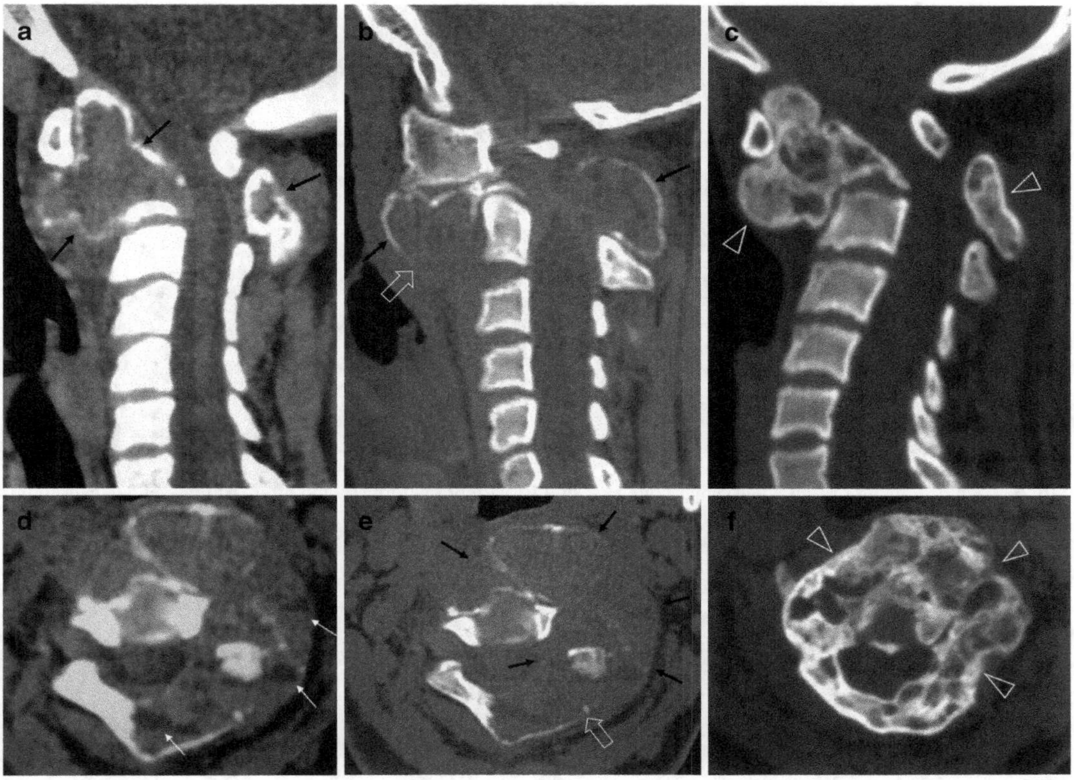

Fig. 3 Aneurysmal bone cyst of C2 (same patient in Fig. 1). Sagittal (**a, b**) and axial (**d, e**) CT images show an expansile and lytic lesion of C2 (black arrows) with cortical destruction, interrupted eggshell periosteal reaction (open arrows) and fluid-fluid levels (white arrows in image **d**). Extensive ossification of the tumor on follow-up (**c, f**) with well-defined margins (arrowheads) consisting with a process of healing

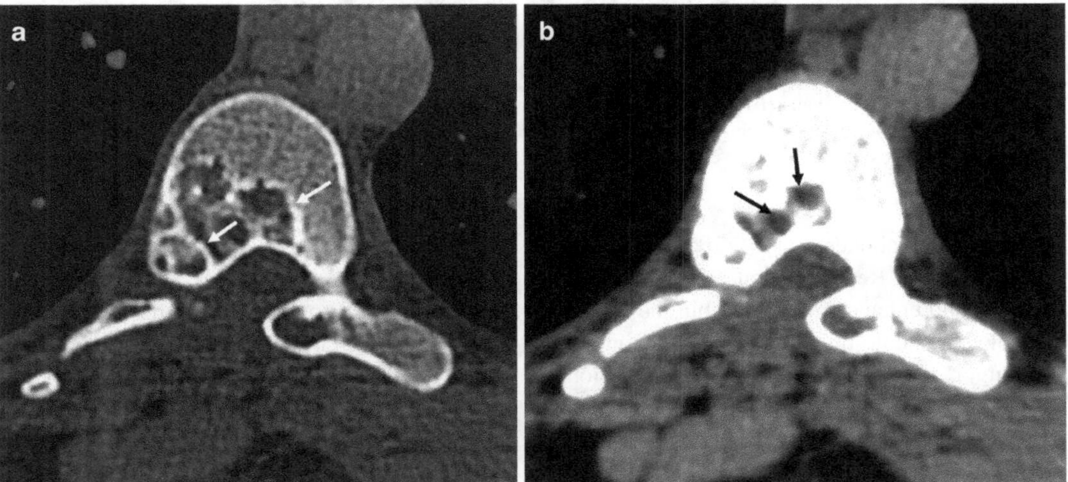

Fig. 4 Axial CT images of a vertebral aneurysmal bone cyst showing (**a**) peripheral and internal ossification (white arrows) and (**b**) fatty areas within the tumor (black arrows)

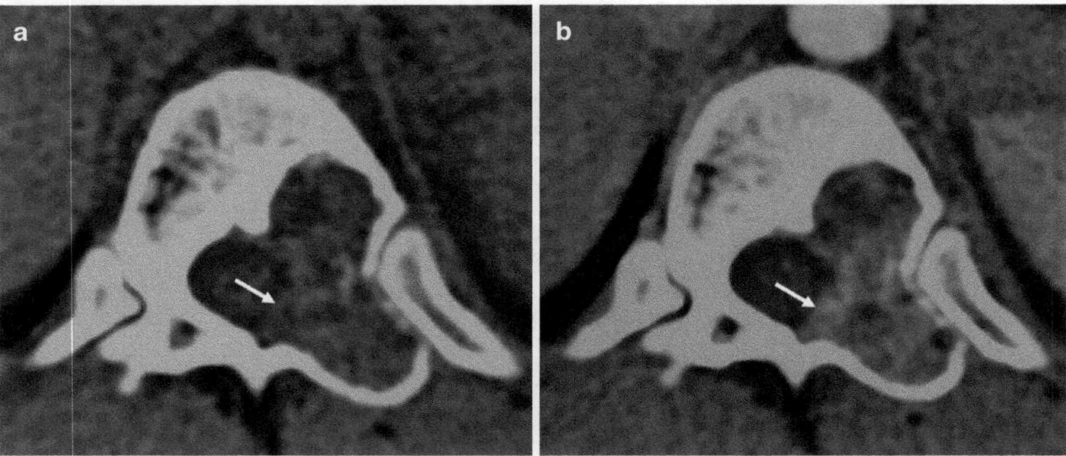

Fig. 5 Axial CT images of an aneurysmal bone cyst of T12 vertebra before (**a**) and after (**b**) intravenous gadolinium administration show septal enhancement within the tumor (white arrow)

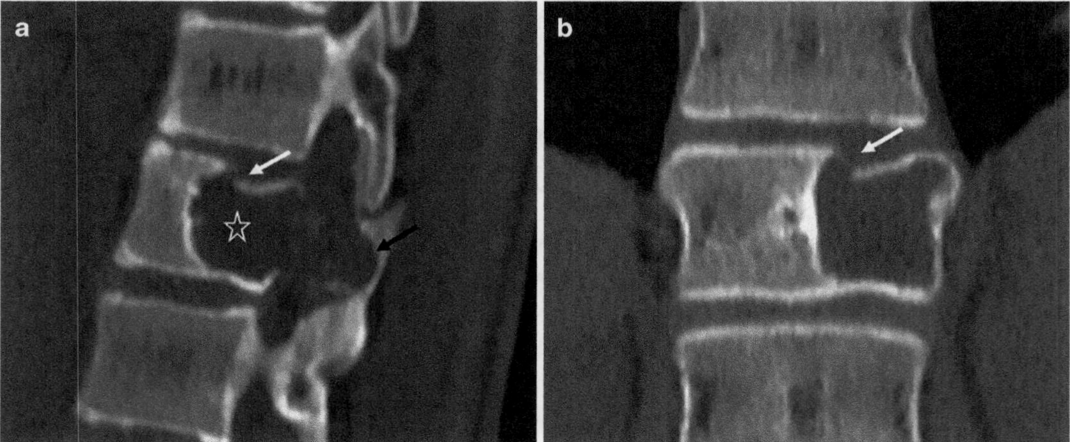

Fig. 6 Sagittal (**a**) and coronal (**b**) CT images of a vertebral aneurysmal bone cyst involving the posterior arch (black arrow) and extending to the vertebral body (star) resulting in a fracture of the superior endplate (white arrow) with a mild vertebral body collapse

component (Mahnken et al. 2003; Sans and Perroncel 2014; Restrepo et al. 2022). The presence of solid enhancing areas within the tumor is possible but should raise suspicion of an underlying tumor with ABC-like changes and biopsy should target these areas to confirm the diagnosis. The solid variant of ABC is a rare subtype in which the solid enhancing component is predominant over the cystic component (Suzuki et al. 2004).

The presence of perilesional edema in surrounding soft tissues and bone marrow has been reported (Zileli et al. 2013; Restrepo et al. 2022).

Involvement of adjacent vertebrae (two or more consecutive vertebrae) is possible with preservation of intervertebral disc height (De Kleuver et al. 1998; Boriani et al. 2001). Extension to adjacent ribs has also been reported (Al-Shamy et al. 2011).

MRI is the modality of choice to assess tumor extension into paravertebral soft tissues, spinal canal, and neural foramen and to evaluate its impact on neurological structures (Fig. 7).

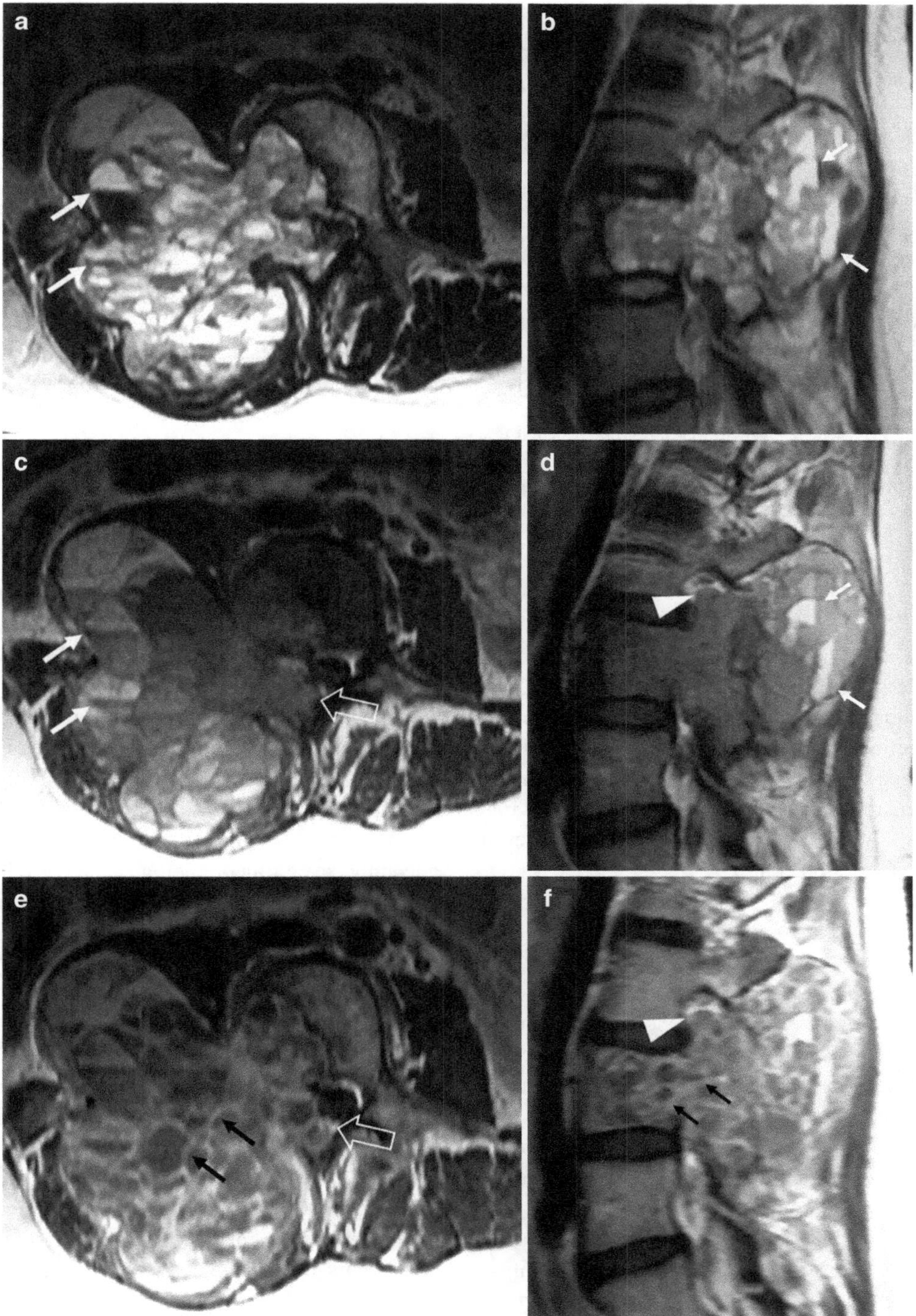

Fig. 7 MRI of a vertebral aneurysmal bone cyst. Axial (left images) and sagittal (right images) T2-weighted images (WI) (**a**, **b**), T1 (**c**, **d**) and enhanced T1-WI (**e**, **f**) images: the tumor is composed of blood-filled cavities with fluid-fluid levels (white arrows) surrounded by enhancing septa (black arrows). The tumor extends into the spinal canal (open arrow) and the right foramen (arrowhead)

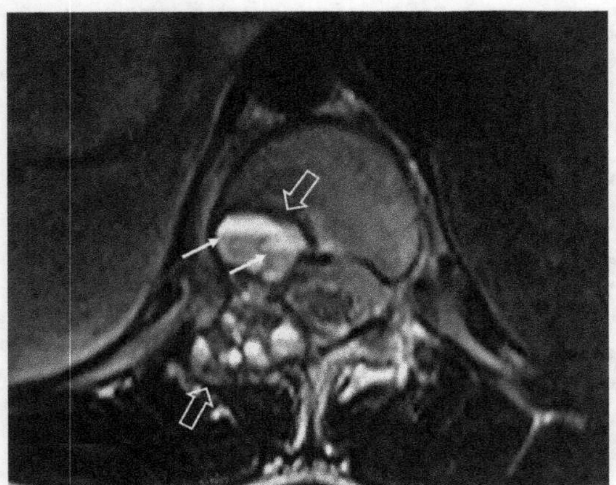

Fig. 8 Axial MR T2-WI of a vertebral aneurysmal bone cyst. The tumor involves the right side of the posterior arch with extension to the vertebral body (open arrows). It is composed of blood-filled cavities with fluid-fluid levels (arrows)

6.4 PET and PET CT

There is lacking data in literature concerning the characteristic features of ABC in PET and PET CT.

Studies including ABC are mainly focused on evaluating the value of PET in distinguishing between benign and malignant bone tumors and staging them. ABC can exhibit an increased FDG uptake without being specific (Schulte et al. 2000; Costelloe et al. 2014).

7 Histopathology

ABC is a true neoplasm and not a pseudo-tumor. It is a benign tumor belonging to the osteoclastic giant cell-rich tumors (WHO Classification of Tumours Editorial Board 2020).

It is composed of blood-filled cavities of different size, separated by connective-tissue septa. The septa are composed of osteoclast-like giant cells, fibroblasts, and reactive woven bone rimmed by osteoblasts. The presence of mitoses is common but there are no atypical forms. A solid component can be present and is composed of the same elements as the septa. Necrosis is rarely found unless there is a fracture (Papagelopoulos et al. 1998; De Kleuver et al. 1998; WHO Classification of Tumours Editorial Board 2020). In rare cases, solid areas are the predominant component of the tumor consisting with a solid variant of ABC.

Although imaging features can be characteristic of ABC, histologic confirmation is necessary. The search for USP6 gene rearrangement is desirable but not necessary for the diagnosis (WHO Classification of Tumours Editorial Board 2020).

8 Differential Diagnosis

Table 1 summarizes the main characteristic imaging features common to ABC and other bone lesions.

8.1 Benign Tumors

Blood-filled cavities with fluid-fluid levels are characteristic but not pathognomonic of ABC. Indeed, similar areas can be found within tumors that have undergone hemorrhagic cystic changes and are termed ABC-like changes. The main benign tumors that can be associated with similar changes are **giant cell tumor, osteoblastoma, chondroblastoma, and fibrous dysplasia** (Riahi et al. 2018; Gutierrez et al. 2020; WHO Classification of Tumours Editorial Board 2020). These lesions can mimic ABC (Fig. 9) but they generally have further radiological and histological findings characteristic of the underlying primary tumor. They also lack the USP6 gene alterations.

8.2 Malignant Tumors

ABC can mimic malignant bone tumors such as Ewing's sarcoma and osteosarcoma when it has the appearance of an aggressive lesion. The presence of cysts with fluid-fluid levels points rather to ABC. Nevertheless, the **telangiectatic osteosarcoma**, a rare subtype of osteosarcoma that occurs in the same age group as ABC, can also have fluid-fluid levels and mimic ABC on imaging. It represents the most important differential diagnosis. Histologic examination confirms the diagnosis by showing blood-filled cavities limited by septa containing atypical malignant cells. This tumor also lacks the USP6 gene rearrangement and exhibits other cytoge-

Table 1 Differential diagnosis of aneurysmal bone cyst of spine based on some characteristic imaging features

Imaging feature	Diagnosis
Expansile lytic bone lesion (eggshell periosteal reaction)	Giant cell tumor
	Osteoblastoma
	Chondroblastoma
	Aggressive hemangioma
	Plasmacytoma
	Telangiectatic osteosarcoma
	Metastases (kidney, thyroid, breast)
	Hydatidosis
	Fibrous dysplasia
	Brown tumor
Involvement of adjacent vertebrae with preservation of intervertebral disc	Osteosarcoma
	Chondrosarcoma
	Ewing's sarcoma
	Plasmacytoma
Involvement of the adjacent rib	Fibrous dysplasia
	Hydatidosis
Fluid–fluid levels	Giant cell tumor
	Osteoblastoma
	Chondroblastoma
	Fibrous dysplasia
	Unicameral cyst (associated with fracture)
	Telangiectatic osteosarcoma
	Hemorrhagic metastases
	Brown tumor
Internal bony septa	Giant cell tumor
	Hemangioma (thickened vertical trabeculae)
	Plasmacytoma
	Fibrous dysplasia
	Chordoma
	Telangiectatic osteosarcoma
Lesions arising frequently in the posterior arch	Osteosarcoma
	Chondrosarcoma
	Ewing's sarcoma
	Osteoblastoma

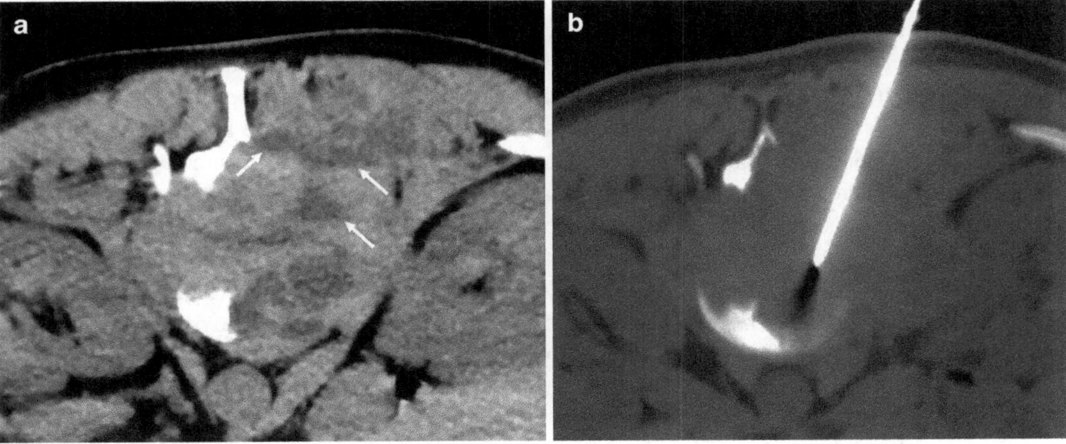

Fig. 9 Giant cell tumor with ABC-like changes. (**a**) Axial CT image shows a vertebral lytic lesion with cortical destruction, including an area with fluid-fluid levels (arrows). (**b**) Percutaneous biopsy concludes to the diagnosis of giant cell tumor

netic abnormalities associated with osteosarcoma (WHO Classification of Tumours Editorial Board 2020; Restrepo et al. 2022).

Based on imaging appearance, ABC can mimic other malignant tumors such as plasmacytoma, chordoma, and metastasis but these tumors generally occur in older people.

8.3 Other Cystic Lesions of Spine

Solitary bone cyst (unicameral or simple bone cyst) is a benign tumor consisting of a cystic bone lesion filled with serous or serosanguinous liquid and lined by a fibrous membrane (WHO Classification of Tumours Editorial Board 2020). It mainly occurs in the metaphysis of long bones with proximal humerus and proximal femur being the most frequent sites (Safaei et al. 2021). Spinal location is rare, with limited data provided in case reports (Funayama et al. 2017; Safaei et al. 2021). Back pain is the main clinical presentation reported in spinal solitary bone cysts. Fracture and mild vertebral body collapse may occur but no neurological symptoms nor acute spinal cord compression were reported. Lumbar and cervical segments are more frequently involved than thoracic spine. Vertebral body and spinous process are the most involved parts of the vertebra (Funayama et al. 2017; Safaei et al. 2021). Radiographs and CT show a geographic lytic lesion with well-defined margins and surrounding sclerosis. The lesion can be expansile with thinning of the cortical bone especially when it develops in posterior elements. MRI confirms the cystic nature of the tumor by showing a low signal intensity on T1-weighted images and a high signal intensity on T2-weighted images with no or only peripheral enhancement following intravenous gadolinium injection (Ha and Kim 2003). There is no uptake on bone scan outside the cases associated with fracture. There are no reported cases of recurrence after treatment (Funayama et al. 2017; Safaei et al. 2021). Solitary bone cyst can undergo hemorrhagic cystic changes when associated with fracture and appears with fluid-fluid levels, mimicking an ABC (Burr et al. 1993; Maas et al. 1998).

Giant cystic Schmorl's node: Schmorl's node is frequent and consists of disk material herniation in the vertebral body. In rare cases, it may present as a giant and cystic-like lesion (Hauger et al. 2001). On radiographs and CT, it appears as an inactive benign lytic lesion with well-defined margins and surrounded by a sclerotic rim. Communication with intervertebral disc through a focal interruption of the vertebral endplate is seen. On MRI, it has a fluid signal with peripheral enhancement (Hauger et al. 2001).

Intraosseous epidermoid cyst is extremely rare and occurs mainly in the skull and in phalanges of fingers and toes. The distal phalanx is the most frequent location (Gibson and Prayson 2007; Simon et al. 2011; Sasaki et al. 2017). Vertebral location is exceedingly rare, related in case reports (Doğanavşargil et al. 2015). This non-neoplastic lesion consists of a unilocular cyst containing keratin and limited by a squamous epithelium. It presents as a geographic lytic lesion with well-defined margins, inconstantly surrounded by a sclerotic rim. It can also appear as an expansile lytic lesion with cortical thinning or destruction, mimicking an aggressive lesion. There is no enhancement after intravenous contrast media administration (Simon et al. 2011; Sasaki et al. 2017).

Cystic angiomatosis of bone is a rare disease characterized by the presence of multifocal and disseminated hemangiomatous and/or lymphangiomatous lesions involving the skeletal and possibly soft tissues and viscera (most commonly the spleen). It mainly occurs during the first three decades of life with men being more frequently affected than women. Patients are often asymptomatic, and the lesions are incidentally discovered. The spine is frequently involved along with the ribs, the pelvis, and proximal appendicular skeleton. The lesions are lytic and sharply marginated with possible surrounding sclerotic rim. A honeycomb or latticework appearance is also possible. On MRI, the lesions have a low or intermediate signal intensity on T1-weighted images and a markedly hyperintense signal on T2-weighted images with no or variable enhancement following intravenous gadolinium administration. Fatty areas can be found within the lesions (Murphey et al. 1995; Lateur et al. 1996; Soler et al. 1996; Boyse and Jacobson 2002) (Fig. 10).

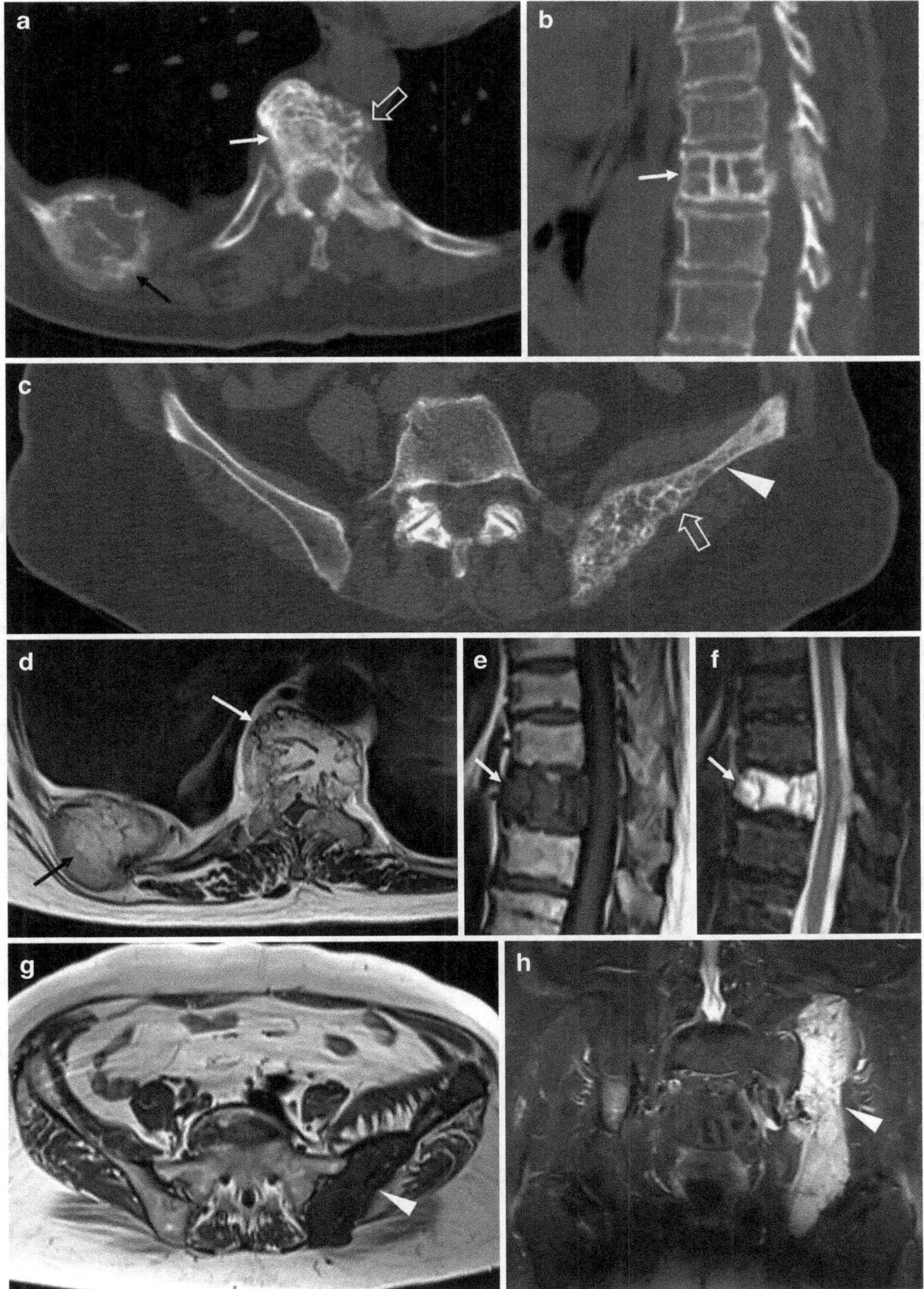

Fig. 10 Cystic angiomatosis of bone with spine, pelvis, and rib involvement. (**a**–**c**) CT images show lytic lesions of T10 vertebra (white arrows), the right ninth rib (black arrow) and the left coxal bone (arrowhead) with a honeycomb pattern (open arrows). On axial T2-WI (**d**), sagittal T1 (**e**), sagittal STIR (**f**), axial T1-WI (**g**), and coronal STIR (**h**) MR images, the lesions of T10 vertebra (white arrows), the right ninth rib (black arrow) and the left iliac bone (arrowhead) have a low T1 signal intensity (**e**, **g**) and a markedly high T2 signal intensity (**d**, **f**, **h**)

8.4 Other Pseudo-Tumors

Brown tumor is a non-neoplastic lesion that can occur in patients with primary or secondary hyperparathyroidism. Spinal location is rare. It can present as a lytic and expansile lesion. Intralesional hemorrhage can cause fluid-fluid levels mimicking an ABC. This lesion has also histological similarities with giant cell tumor and ABC, namely the presence of osteoclast-like giant cells and hemosiderin. Other skeletal manifestations of hyperparathyroidism such as subperiosteal bone resorption, the multiplicity of brown tumors and laboratory tests (elevated parathyroid hormone levels) lead to the diagnosis (Tayfun et al. 2014; Sonmez et al. 2015) (see also chapter on other pseudotumoral lesions of the spine).

Hydatidosis is a parasitic infection caused by *Echinococcus granulosus*. The spine is involved in more than half of the cases of bone hydatidosis. On radiographs and CT, the infection can have a similar appearance to ABC (Fig. 11). On MRI, the multivesicular lesion can mimic the blood-filled cavities of ABC but there are no fluid-fluid levels nor enhancement of the cystic masses. Serological tests can help make the diagnosis (Ladeb et al. 2021) (see also chapter on other pseudotumoral lesions of the spine).

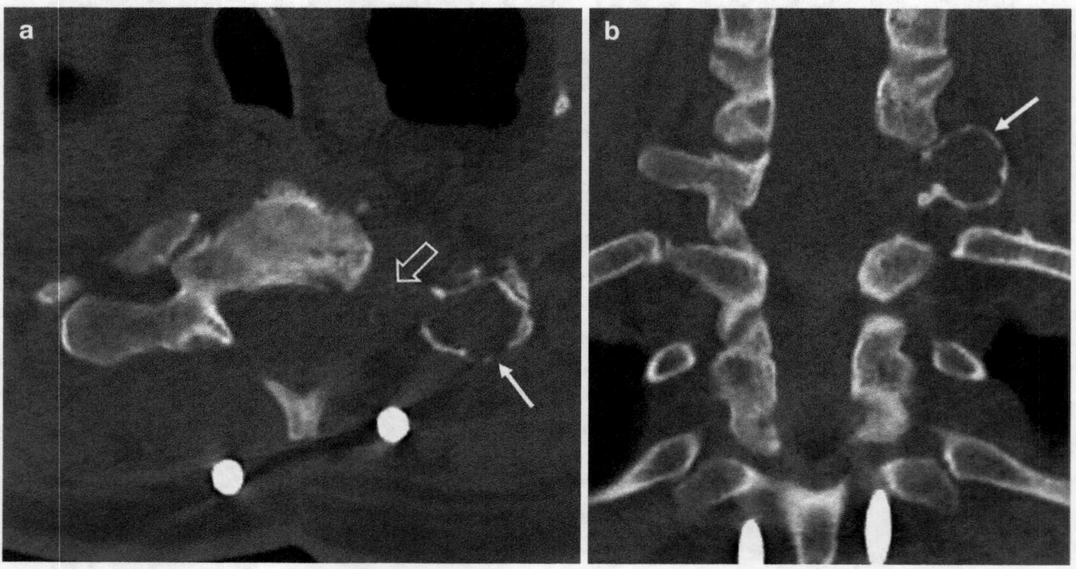

Fig. 11 Postoperative bone hydatidosis recurrence. Axial (**a**) and coronal (**b**) CT images show a lytic and expansile lesion of the posterior arch of T1 vertebra (arrows) with cortical breach and left pedicle destruction (open arrow)

9 Local and Distant Staging

According to the Enneking/MSTS staging system (refer to the chapter "Local and Distant Staging" in this book), benign musculoskeletal tumors can be classified as stage 1 (inactive), stage 2 (active), or stage 3 (aggressive) depending on their biological activity and aggressiveness (Musculoskeletal tumor society and Enneking 1985).

ABC can have different growth rates and thus can appear as a stage 1, 2, or 3 lesion.

For spinal location, it is mainly a stage 2 or 3 lesion, the aggressive form being more frequent. ABC presents rarely as a stage 1 tumor (Boriani et al. 2001, 2014; Sayago et al. 2020).

CT can be useful, in addition to MRI, to delineate the tumor margins and define the Enneking staging.

ABC is a benign tumor that does not metastasize although one case with pulmonary and extrapulmonary metastases has been reported in the literature (Van de Luijtgaarden et al. 2009).

10 Treatment

Compared to ABC of extremities, special considerations need to be taken into account in the treatment of ABC of spine, namely the proximity to the spinal cord and nerve roots and the risk of spinal instability.

Many treatment modalities have been reported in literature, used separately or in association (surgery, radiation therapy, selective arterial embolization, sclerotherapy) but there is a lack of consensus regarding the management of spinal ABC (Papagelopoulos et al. 1998; Boriani et al. 2001).

Surgical resection options include "en bloc" resection and intralesional resection (curettage with or without bone grafting). Surgical fixation may be needed if there is a risk of spinal instability.

Selective arterial embolization can be used alone, or as a neoadjuvant treatment before surgery. When used alone, it has been shown to be successful and to be as effective as surgical treatment. Nevertheless, it may require many treatment sessions with some patients needing more than ten embolization procedures, 88% of patients requiring at least two embolization procedures (Boriani et al. 2014). This is due to persistence of feeding arteries or development of a collateral circulation and exposes the patient to repeated anesthesia, repeated arterial catheterization, and radiation exposure (Patsalides et al. 2016).

Another non-surgical procedure is percutaneous sclerotherapy but similar to embolization, it generally requires many treatment sessions and takes time to show bone healing (Doyle et al. 2015; Desai et al. 2019).

Radiation therapy should no longer be used. Its side effects, including the rare but serious risk of sarcoma induced tumor, do not justify its use for a benign tumor in pediatric population (Papagelopoulos et al. 1998; Boriani et al. 2001).

11 Prognosis

ABC is a benign tumor that has generally an excellent prognosis.

However, because it can be locally aggressive and because clinical course in unpredictable, recurrence after treatment is possible and reported in 6–20% of cases (Capanna et al. 1985; Papagelopoulos et al. 1998; Boriani et al. 2001). Recurrence occurs early, within the first and less frequently the second year following treatment (Papagelopoulos et al. 1998; Gibbs et al. 1999; Boriani et al. 2001, 2014).

Nevertheless, healing of the lesion is nearly constant and 96–100% of patients end up being free of disease, even those that are treated again for recurrence (Papagelopoulos et al. 1998; De Kleuver et al. 1998; Boriani et al. 2001).

Some cases of spontaneous healing of spinal ABC have been reported (Malghem et al. 1989) while in some series, healing was reported in patients treated with incomplete surgical removal (De Kleuver et al. 1998).

Malignant transformation is extremely rare and consists mainly of radiation-induced sarcoma (Papagelopoulos et al. 1998; Boriani et al. 2001).

Death was reported in few cases and was related to malignant transformation, surgical complications (intraoperative hemorrhage), and cervical vertebral collapse with spinal cord compression (Papagelopoulos et al. 1998; Desai et al. 2019).

12 Key Points

- Aneurysmal bone cyst is a benign tumor that can be locally aggressive with a risk of recurrence after treatment.
- The typical radiological aspect is a lytic and expansile lesion composed of blood-filled cavities with fluid-fluid levels involving the posterior elements of vertebra with possible extension to vertebral body, paravertebral soft tissues, and spinal canal.
- The presence of fluid-fluid levels is characteristic but not pathognomonic and can be seen in other tumors with ABC-like changes such as telangiectatic osteosarcoma and giant cell tumor.
- The diagnosis of aneurysmal bone cyst should always include a histological proof.

References

Al-Shamy G, Relyea K, Adesina A et al (2011) Solid variant of aneurysmal bone cyst of the thoracic spine: a case report. J Med Case Rep 5:261

AlYami AH, AlMaeen BN, AlMuraee M et al (2022) Multiple primary aneurysmal bone cysts: a case report and literature review. Cureus 14:e26509

Ameli NO, Abbassioun K, Saleh H, Eslamdoost A (1985) Aneurysmal bone cysts of the spine. Report of 17 cases. J Neurosurg 63:685–690

Boriani S, De Iure F, Campanacci L et al (2001) Aneurysmal bone cyst of the mobile spine: report on 41 cases. Spine (Phila Pa 1976) 26:27–35

Boriani S, Lo SL, Puvanesarajah V et al (2014) Aneurysmal bone cysts of the spine: treatment options and considerations. J Neurooncol 120:171–178

Boyse TD, Jacobson JA (2002) Case 45: cystic angiomatosis. Radiology 223:164–167

Burr BA, Resnick D, Syklawer R, Haghighi P (1993) Fluid-fluid levels in a unicameral bone cyst: CT and MR findings. J Comput Assist Tomogr 17:134–136

Capanna R, Albisinni U, Picci P et al (1985) Aneurysmal bone cyst of the spine. J Bone Joint Surg Am 67:527–531

Chan MSM, Wong Y-C, Yuen M-K, Lam D (2002) Spinal aneurysmal bone cyst causing acute cord compression without vertebral collapse: CT and MRI findings. Pediatr Radiol 32:601–604

Costelloe CM, Chuang HH, Madewell JE (2014) FDG PET/CT of primary bone tumors. AJR Am J Roentgenol 202:521–531

Cottalorda J, Kohler R, Sales de Gauzy J et al (2004) Epidemiology of aneurysmal bone cyst in children: a multicenter study and literature review. J Pediatr Orthop B 13:389–394

Dabska M, Buraczewski J (1969) Aneurysmal bone cyst. Pathology, clinical course and radiologic appearances. Cancer 23:371–389

De Kleuver M, van der Heul RO, Veraart BE (1998) Aneurysmal bone cyst of the spine: 31 cases and the importance of the surgical approach. J Pediatr Orthop B 7:286–292

Desai SB, O'Brien C, Shaikh R et al (2019) Multidisciplinary management of spinal aneurysmal bone cysts: a single-center experience. Interv Neuroradiol 25:564–569

Doğanavşargil B, Ayhan E, Argin M et al (2015) Cystic bone lesions: histopathological spectrum and diagnostic challenges. Turk Patoloji Derg 31:95–103

Donigan JA, Kebaish KM, McCarthy EF (2003) Metachronous aneurysmal bone cysts with involvement of the humerus and the thoracic vertebrae. Skeletal Radiol 32:468–471

Doyle A, Field A, Graydon A (2015) Recurrent aneurysmal bone cyst of the cervical spine in childhood treated with doxycycline injection. Skeletal Radiol 44:609–612

Funayama T, Gasbarrini A, Ghermandi R et al (2017) Solitary bone cyst of a lumbar vertebra treated with percutaneous steroid injection: a case report and review of literature. Eur Spine J 26:58–62

Gibbs CPJ, Hefele MC, Peabody TD et al (1999) Aneurysmal bone cyst of the extremities. Factors related to local recurrence after curettage with a high-speed burr. J Bone Joint Surg Am 81:1671–1678

Gibson SE, Prayson RA (2007) Primary skull lesions in the pediatric population: a 25-year experience. Arch Pathol Lab Med 131:761–766

Gutierrez LB, Link TM, Horvai AE et al (2020) Secondary aneurysmal bone cysts and associated primary lesions: imaging features of 49 cases. Clin Imaging 62:23–32

Ha K-Y, Kim Y-H (2003) Simple bone cyst with pathologic lumbar pedicle fracture: a case report. Spine (Phila Pa 1976) 28:129–131

Hauger O, Cotten A, Chateil J et al (2001) Giant cystic Schmorl's nodes: imaging findings in six patients. AJR Am J Roentgenol 176:969–972

Hay MC, Paterson D, Taylor TKF (1978) Aneurysmal bone cysts of the spine. J Bone Joint Surg 6:406–411

Jaffe HL (1950) Aneurysmal bone cyst. Bull Hosp Joint Dis 11:3–13

Jaffe HL, Lichtenstein L (1942) Solitary unicameral bone cyst: with emphasis on the roentgen picture, the pathologic appearance and the pathogenesis. Arch Surg 44:1004–1025

Ladeb MF, Riahi H, Mechri M et al (2021) Imaging of spinal hydatidosis. In: Ladeb MF, Peh WCG (eds) Imaging of spinal infection. Springer Nature, Switzerland, pp 237–250

Lateur L, Simoens CJ, Gryspeerdt S et al (1996) Skeletal cystic angiomatosis. Skeletal Radiol 25:92–95

Leithner A, Windhager R, Lang S et al (1999) Aneurysmal bone cyst. A population based epidemiologic study and literature review. Clin Orthop Relat Res 363:176–179

Maas EJ, Craig JG, Swisher PK et al (1998) Fluid-fluid levels in a simple bone cyst on magnetic resonance imaging. Australas Radiol 42:267–270

Mahnken A, Nolte-Ernsting C, Wildberger J et al (2003) Aneurysmal bone cyst: value of MR imaging and conventional radiography. Eur Radiol 13:1118–1124

Malghem J, Maldague B, Esselinckx W et al (1989) Spontaneous healing of aneurysmal bone cysts. A report of three cases. J Bone Joint Surg Br 71:645–650

Murphey MD, Fairbairn KJ, Parman LM et al (1995) From the archives of the AFIP. Musculoskeletal angiomatous lesions: radiologic-pathologic correlation. Radiographics 15:893–917

Musculoskeletal Tumor Society, Enneking WF (1985) Staging of musculoskeletal neoplasms. Skeletal Radiol 13:183–194

Oliveira AM, Chou MM (2014) USP6-induced neoplasms: the biologic spectrum of aneurysmal bone cyst and nodular fasciitis. Hum Pathol 45:1–11

Ozaki T, Halm H, Hillmann A et al (1999) Aneurysmal bone cysts of the spine. Arch Orthop Trauma Surg 119:159–162

Papagelopoulos PJ, Currier BL, Shaughnessy WJ et al (1998) Aneurysmal bone cyst of the spine. Management and outcome. Spine (Phila Pa 1976) 23:621–628

Patsalides A, Leng LZ, Kimball D et al (2016) Preoperative catheter spinal angiography and embolization of cervical spinal tumors: outcomes from a single center. Interv Neuroradiol J 22:457–465

Restrepo R, Zahrah D, Pelaez L et al (2022) Update on aneurysmal bone cyst: pathophysiology, histology, imaging and treatment. Pediatr Radiol 52:1601–1614

Riahi H, Mechri M, Barsaoui M et al (2018) Imaging of benign tumors of the osseous spine. J Belg Soc Radiol 102:1–11

Safaei S, Athari M, Azimi P et al (2021) Simple bone cyst of spinal vertebrae: two case reports and literature review. J Surg Case Rep 11:1–5

Sans N, Perroncel G (2014) Kyste anévrysmal. In: Sans N, Perroncel G (eds) Imagerie des tumeurs osseuses. Sauramps Médical, Montpellier, pp 425–438

Sasaki H, Nagano S, Shimada H et al (2017) Intraosseous epidermoid cyst of the distal phalanx reconstructed with synthetic bone graft. J Orthop Surg 25:1–4

Sayago LR, Remondino RG, Tello CA et al (2020) Aneurysmal bone cysts of the spine in children: a review of 18 cases. Global Spine J 10:875–880

Schulte M, Brecht-Krauss D, Heymer B et al (2000) Grading of tumors and tumorlike lesions of bone: evaluation by FDG PET. J Nucl Med 41:1695–1701

Simon K, Leithner A, Bodo K, Windhager R (2011) Intraosseous epidermoid cysts of the hand skeleton: a series of eight patients. J Hand Surg Eur 36:376–378

Soler R, Pombo F, Bargiela A et al (1996) Diffuse skeletal cystic angiomatosis: MR and CT findings. Eur J Radiol 22:149–151

Sonmez E, Tezcaner T, Coven I, Terzi A (2015) Brown tumor of the thoracic spine: first manifestation of primary hyperparathyroidism. J Korean Neurosurg Soc 58:389–392

Suzuki M, Satoh T, Nishida J et al (2004) Solid variant of aneurysmal bone cyst of the cervical spine. Spine (Phila Pa 1976) 29:376–381

Tayfun H, Metin O, Hakan S et al (2014) Brown tumor as an unusual but preventable cause of spinal cord compression: case report and review of the literature. Asian J Neurosurg 9:40–44

Unni KK, Inwards CY (2010) Cystic lesions of bone. In: Unni KK, Inwards CY (eds) Dahlin's bone tumors: general aspects and data on 10,165 cases, 6th edn. Lippincott Williams & Wilkins, Philadelphia, pp 333–340

Van de Luijtgaarden ACM, Veth RPH, Slootweg PJ et al (2009) Metastatic potential of an aneurysmal bone cyst. Virchows Arch 455:455–459

Vergel De Dios AM, Bond JR, Shives TC et al (1992) Aneurysmal bone cyst. A clinicopathologic study of 238 cases. Cancer 69:2921–2931

WHO Classification of Tumours Editorial Board (2020) Soft tissue and bone tumours, 5th edn. International Agency for Research on Cancer, Lyon, pp 437–439

Zileli M, Isik HS, Ogut FE et al (2013) Aneurysmal bone cysts of the spine. Eur Spine J 22:593–601

Spinal Cartilaginous Tumors

Mohamed Chaabouni, Emna Labbène, Mouna Chelli Bouaziz, and Mohamed Fethi Ladeb

Contents

M. Chaabouni (✉) · E. Labbène · M. Chelli Bouaziz
M. F. Ladeb
Department of Radiology, MT Kassab Institute of Orthopaedics, Ksar Said, Tunisia

Faculty of Medicine of Tunis, Tunis-El Manar University, Tunis, Tunisia

Abstract

Osteochondroma is the most common benign bone tumor, and its spinal location is well documented, although uncommon. Spinal osteochondroma most commonly arises in the cervical segment and is usually asymptomatic.

Spinal location of other types of cartilaginous tumors including chondroma and chondroblastoma is extremely rare, and the available literature is restricted to case reports.

Spinal involvement of chondrosarcoma is rare, accounting for less than 15% of all chondrosarcomas. It affects adults in the fifth decade of life or older, predominantly males. The most frequent symptom of spinal chondrosarcoma is pain, whereas neurologic deficit is frequent, indicating a locally advanced disease at presentation. Differentiating spinal chondrosarcoma from benign cartilaginous tumors can be challenging on both imaging and histology. MRI is the imaging modality of choice for local staging. Treatment is based on en bloc tumor removal. Overall prognosis is poor compared to appendicular skeleton chondrosarcoma and varies with tumor subtype, grade, and stage.

Med Radiol Diagn Imaging (2023)
https://doi.org/10.1007/174_2023_447,
Published Online: 27 October 2023

1 Introduction

Benign cartilaginous tumors are classified into four histological types: osteochondroma (OC), chondroma, chondroblastoma, and chondromyxoid fibroma.

OC is a surface bone lesion composed of both cortex and medulla in continuity with those of the underlying bone, capped by hyaline cartilage (Bovée et al. 2020c). It accounts for 20–50% of benign bone tumors, and the spine is involved in only 1–4% of cases (García-Ramos et al. 2015).

Spinal OC (SOC) most commonly arises in the cervical segment and is usually asymptomatic. CT and MRI are usually required for SOC detection, complication screening, and surgical planning.

Spinal location of other benign cartilaginous tumors is extremely rare, and the available literature is restricted to case reports.

Chondrosarcoma (CS) is a malignant cartilaginous neoplasm accounting for about 20% of all primary malignant tumors of the bone and usually arises in the pelvis or long bones. Primary CS arises in preexisting normal bone and is distinguished from the rarer secondary CS, which occurs within a preexisting enchondroma or OC (Thorkildsen et al. 2019). The spine is involved in 6.5–15% of cases (Arshi et al. 2017), and the thoracic segment is the site of predilection. It is typically a tumor of adulthood and older age with male predominance.

Spinal CS usually presents with pain, and neurologic impairment is frequent.

The imaging features of the most common conventional CS are well described, but discrimination between benign and low-grade malignant cartilaginous tumors remains both an imaging and a histological challenge. High-grade chondrosarcoma (HGCS) exhibits distinct malignant imaging features that allow the discrimination from enchondroma.

The current standard of care is en bloc resection of the tumor with negative margins.

Prognosis of spinal CS is worse compared with appendicular skeleton CS.

We herein review the epidemiology, imaging features, up-to-date staging means, treatment, and prognosis of benign and malignant spinal cartilaginous tumors.

2 Pathologic Features

The diagnosis of cartilaginous lesions of the skeleton is one of the most challenging dilemmas in bone pathology. Although histological patterns for enchondroma and CS have been well described, they are not easy to recognize in small samples, and the diagnosis is usually made with the support of clinical and radiological findings. Not only the distinction between benign and malignant cartilaginous tumors can be misleading, but also the grading of malignant lesions may differ significantly, even among experts (Roitman et al. 2017).

2.1 Osteochondroma

OC is caused by biallelic inactivation of the *EXT1, EXT2,* or *EXT3* gene, found within the cartilage cap, supporting the tumoral nature of this lesion. The cell of origin is either a chondrocyte within the growth plate or a mesenchymal progenitor cell from the perichondrium (Bovée et al. 2020c).

OC is the result of progressive enchondral ossification of aberrant cartilage that migrates from the growth plate. The exact cause of this aberrant growth is not known, but congenital defects and traumatic injuries are likely implicated in the pathogenesis (Srikantha et al. 2008). No OC develops or enlarges after skeletal maturity.

OC has three layers. The outer layer is a fibrous perichondrium in continuity with the periosteum of the underlying bone. The second layer is a cartilage cap that mimics a disorganized growth plate cartilage with enchondral ossification. Cellularity gradually decreases with age, and nuclear atypia and mitoses are absent. Extensive coarse calcification may be seen. Binucleated cells, focal necrosis, and cystic or mucoid changes are possible findings. The deepest layer is represented by a bone stalk with cortex and medullary cavity continuous with those of the underlying bone (Bovée et al. 2020c).

2.2 Chondroblastoma

Chondroblastoma is a well-defined tumor composed of sheets of chondroblastic cells that are ovoid to polygonal with small singular grooved nuclei and eosinophilic cytoplasm. Epithelioid cells may be present. There are interspersed osteoclast-like giant cells and islands of eosinophilic chondroid matrix. Pericellular lacelike or chickenwire calcification is characteristic. Nuclear atypia and/or mitoses may be found. Aneurysmal bone cyst-like change is common (Armany et al. 2020).

2.3 Chondroma/Chondrosarcoma

Chondroma is labeled as enchondroma when it arises from the medullary cavity of bone, and as periosteal chondroma when the cortical surface is the site of origin. It may be caused by heterozygous somatic mutations in the isocitrate dehydrogenase genes *IDH1* and *IDH2*, leading to promoted chondrogenic differentiation of mesenchymal stem cells, presumed precursor cells of chondroma (Bovée et al. 2020b).

CS consists of a heterogeneous group of malignant bone tumors that produce cartilaginous matrix without tumor osteoid (Sundaresan et al. 2009).

It is debated whether CS originates from a cartilage remnant of preexistent growth plate or from a mesenchymal stem cell (Cleton-Jansen 2015).

CS most commonly arises de novo in normal bone, rarely in a predisposing bone condition such as enchondroma or OC.

The World Health Organization (WHO) histological classification categorizes CS into histologic subtypes (Baumhoer et al. 2020; Bovée et al. 2020a; Fanburg-Smith et al. 2020; Inwards et al. 2020) including:

- Conventional central chondrosarcoma (primary or secondary to enchondroma)
- Peripheral chondrosarcoma (secondary to osteochondroma)
- Dedifferentiated chondrosarcoma (DCS)
- Mesenchymal chondrosarcoma (MCS)
- Clear cell chondrosarcoma (CCC)
- Extraskeletal myxoid chondrosarcoma

CS is further classified by a grading system that ranges from low grade (grade I, corresponding to the "atypical cartilaginous tumor" in the appendicular skeleton) to high grade (grade III). The grade is based on histologic features such as tumor cellularity, nuclear atypia, number of mitoses, and stromal content.

Conventional subtype is the most common (80–90%). It is usually low grade with low cellularity, little nuclear atypia, absent mitoses, and a large amount of hyaline cartilage matrix. A lobular pattern is common, and areas of calcifications are often seen. It may be difficult to differentiate from benign enchondroma. Distinguishing features of low-grade chondrosarcoma (LGCS) include replacing the marrow space, eroding preexisting trabeculae, penetration of the bony cortex, and invasion of surrounding tissues. Less than 10% are high-grade lesions with increased cellularity, multinucleated cells with prominent nucleoli, and frequent mitoses within a scarce, mostly myxoid matrix (Bovée et al. 2020a).

DCS (3.5%) is a high-grade subtype that occurs when a conventional LGCS undergoes a malignant degeneration. It has a bimorphic histological appearance of a conventional CS component with abrupt transition to a high-grade, non-cartilaginous sarcoma (Inwards et al. 2020).

MCS represents less than 10% of all CS (Elmajee et al. 2022). It is a high-grade subtype and, similarly to DCS, has two cellular components of low-grade chondrocytes and undifferentiated mesenchymal cells, which are interspersed without clear margins (Fanburg-Smith et al. 2020).

CCC is a rare form (1.6–5.4%) of spinal CS (Elmajee et al. 2022). It is a low-grade subtype characterized by lobules of cells with abundant clear vacuolated cytoplasm containing large amounts of glycogen (Baumhoer et al. 2020).

Accurate pathologic diagnosis is mandatory for prognostic assessment and management decisions. Interpretation of a CT-guided biopsy must be cautious because pockets of high-grade tumor may reside within a LGCS, and a nonrepresentative sampling may mistake a MCS or a DCS for a conventional LGCS.

3 Epidemiology

3.1 Osteochondroma

OC is the most common benign bone tumor accounting for 20–50% of benign bone tumors and 9% of all bone tumors. 85% of OCs occur sporadically as solitary exostoses (SEs), while 15% occur in the context of hereditary multiple exostoses (HMEs), an autosomal dominant inherited genetic disorder (Tepelenis et al. 2021).

OC is most commonly found in the appendicular skeleton. The spine is involved in only 1–4% of cases (García-Ramos et al. 2015). SOC is most commonly SE. However, 68% of patients with HME have SOC (Roach et al. 2009). SOC generally presents within the first four decades of life with male preponderance. The average age of presentation is younger in patients with HME (21 years) compared with SE (36 years) (Fowler et al. 2021; Tepelenis et al. 2021). Radiation-induced OC is a well-documented phenomenon, accounting for 12–15% of all OCs. It occurs in children who had received radiation doses of 15–55 Gy for neuroblastoma or Wilms' tumor between the ages of 8 months and 11 years. Prevalence is higher after total-body irradiation as opposed to localized irradiation. The lesions can occur anywhere in the radiation field, and the latency period is 3–17 years (Murphey et al. 2000; Srikantha et al. 2008).

3.2 Chondroma

Chondroma represents approximately 5% of all primary bone tumors. It mainly occurs in the small bones of the hands and feet, and fewer than 4% originate within the spine. Men are twice more likely to have a chondroma than women, and lesions typically present between the third and fifth decades of life (McLoughlin et al. 2008).

3.3 Chondroblastoma

Chondroblastoma accounts for less than 1% of all bone tumors. This tumor most commonly arises in the epiphysis of the growing long bones. Spinal chondroblastoma has been the subject of case reports in the literature, occurring predominantly in males, with mean age of 29 years, a decade later than in its appendicular counterpart (Ilaslan et al. 2003).

3.4 Chondrosarcoma

CS occurs in 5 per million patients/year (Giuffrida et al. 2009), of which 6.5–10% arise from the mobile spine and 5% arise from the sacrum (Arshi et al. 2017).

It is the second most common non-lymphomyeloproliferative primary malignant tumor of the spine in adults after chordoma.

Spinal CS represents 7–12% of all primary spine tumors and accounts for up to 25% of malignant spine tumors (van den Hauwe et al. 2021).

Men are affected two to four times more frequently than women.

The mean age of patients is 45–51 years (Arshi et al. 2017; van den Hauwe et al. 2021).

Most spinal CSs are primary (85%); however, secondary spinal CS (15%) may arise from a pre-existing benign cartilaginous tumor such as enchondroma and OC.

Secondary central CS occurs in up to 4% of sporadic enchondroma, 10–30% of Ollier disease, and 57% of Maffucci syndrome cases (Herget et al. 2014). Secondary peripheral CS occurs in OC, and underlying HME syndrome is found in up to 41% of cases (Thorkildsen et al. 2019).

Malignant degeneration of Paget's disease of bone into CS is rarely reported (Ferreira et al. 2019).

4 Localization

4.1 Osteochondroma

SOC involves the cervical spine in 50% of cases, most frequently C2 vertebra followed by C3 and C6. The second most frequent location is the thoracic spine, particularly T8 vertebra followed by T4 (Tepelenis et al. 2021).

Sacrum is involved less commonly than mobile spine, with an occurrence of about 0.5% of all SOC.

The predominance of the cervical spine location is explained by the fact that this segment is prone to microtrauma due to its increased mobility and flexibility, thus leading to displacement of cartilage and formation of abnormal growth (Albrecht et al. 1992).

Another theory suggests that secondary ossification centers in the cervical spine ossify during adolescence, faster than in thoracic or lumbar spine, with greater probability of aberrant cartilage formation (Fiumara et al. 1999).

Although any part of the vertebral column can be affected, the posterior elements where most of the ossification centers are located are often involved (Tepelenis et al. 2021).

Tumors that cause cord compression are found in adolescents and young adults with HME and often arise from the posterior vertebral elements, especially the neural arch (Thiart and Herbst 2010).

4.2 Chondrosarcoma

Spinal CS has a predilection for the thoracic segment (60%) but can arise anywhere in the spine (Arshi et al. 2017; Zhou et al. 2017).

The sacrum may be affected in 16–20% of cases, and the tumor is usually eccentric and involves the proximal part of the sacrum, destroying the sacroiliac joint (Angelini et al. 2017).

Spinal CS typically arises in the posterior elements with extension to the vertebral body (45% of cases) and may be confined to the posterior elements (40%) or to the vertebral body (15%) (van den Hauwe et al. 2021).

About 35% of spinal CSs extend across the intervertebral disk into adjacent vertebral levels, and adjacent ribs may be affected in thoracic locations (Mechri et al. 2018).

Sacral CSs are often eccentric in the upper to mid-sacrum and may extend to the sacroiliac joint (Stuckey and Marco 2011).

5 Clinical Presentation

5.1 Osteochondroma

OC arising from the vertebral posterior elements tends to grow outside the spinal canal and is therefore often asymptomatic, presenting as an incidental finding (Sciubba et al. 2015). It may manifest at an early age as a cosmetic deformity or a palpable mass (Fiechtl et al. 2003).

The main symptom is pain by pressure on adjacent soft tissue structures or rarely secondary to fracture (García-Ramos et al. 2015).

OC encroaching into intervertebral foramina or the spinal canal and compressing neural elements may present with radiculopathy (29.5%) or myelopathy (27%) (Yakkanti et al. 2018).

When located anteriorly, cervical OC may cause dysphagia, Horner syndrome, sleep apnea, and hoarseness (Fowler et al. 2021).

Lesions that grow or cause pain after skeletal maturity should be suspected of malignant transformation. Bursitis is another complication that may present with an enlarging painful mass, mimicking malignant transformation.

5.2 Chondrosarcoma

The most common symptom at presentation is insidious focal paravertebral pain (Pennington et al. 2021).

Neurologic deficit is more frequent in sacral location (36%) than in the mobile spine (8%) (Bergh et al. 2001).

A palpable mass is identified in 34–40% of patients (Stuckey and Marco 2011).

The disease may be asymptomatic at the diagnosis in 8% of cases (Zhou et al. 2017).

6 Imaging

6.1 Osteochondroma

Pathognomonic findings of OC on imaging are the corticomedullary continuity with the underlying bone and the cartilaginous cap.

6.1.1 Radiographs

Diagnosis of SOC is difficult on radiographs, with inconclusive interpretation in up to 79% of cases (Rajakulasingam et al. 2020) due to the superimposition of the various spinal elements on the lesion area.

When the tumor is large and outside the projection superimpositions, the pathognomonic continuity between its cortical and medullary bone and those of the bearing vertebra may not be apparent on radiographs (Fig. 1a).

The chondroid nature of the hyaline cartilage cap is suggested when arcs and rings calcifications are identified. Its thickness is not well evaluated with radiography unless there is extensive mineralization (Murphey et al. 2000).

Radiographic features that suggest malignancy include growth of a previously unchanged OC in a skeletally mature patient, irregular or indistinct lesion surface, focal regions of radiolucency in the interior of the bone stalk, erosion or destruction of the underlying bone, and a large soft tissue opacity containing irregular calcifications scattered away from the bone stalk suggesting a thick cartilage cap (Murphey et al. 2000).

6.1.2 CT

CT scan is the imaging modality that offers the best spatial resolution to detect OC in the anatomically complex spine and to depict the pathognomonic cortical and marrow continuity with the underlying vertebra (Figs. 1b and 2a), thus ruling out the differential diagnoses of other juxta-osseous lesions.

CT scan is necessary to clarify the zone of attachment of the tumor to the spine, contributing to preoperative planning (Gille et al. 2005).

Differentiating a non-mineralized cartilage cap from the surrounding muscle or bursa is difficult, making its thickness measurement often inaccurate (Fig. 2a) (Murphey et al. 2000).

6.1.3 Ultrasound

Ultrasound enables accurate measurement of the hyaline cartilage cap thickness when it has a superficial posterior development, with a mean measurement error of less than 2 mm in cartilage caps less than 2 cm thick (Fig. 1c) (Murphey et al. 2000). The non-mineralized cartilage cap appears as a hypoechoic layer and is easily distinguished from the echoic surrounding fat and muscle. Areas of mineralization in the cartilage cap and the underlying osseous component show posterior acoustic shadowing (Murphey et al. 2000).

An adjacent bursa appears as an anechoic area, compressible under the probe and limited by a wall that can be thickened or vascularized on color Doppler in the event of a complication.

Limitations of this technique in SOC include operator dependence and inability to evaluate deep cartilage cap as well as the osseous component of the lesion (Murphey et al. 2000).

6.1.4 MRI

With its unmatched tissue contrast, MRI is the imaging modality of choice for the evaluation of the cartilaginous cap, and for the assessment of the tumor effect on surrounding structures, especially intraspinal extension, spinal cord compression, and myelomalacia.

MRI also demonstrates cortical and medullary continuity between the OC and the parent vertebra.

The signal of OC depends on the size of the lesion, amount of bone marrow, and degree of cartilage calcification.

The fatty marrow of the medulla has a high signal intensity on T1-weighted images (WI) and T2-WI with a peripheral low signal intensity rim representing the cortex (Riahi et al. 2018).

The covering cap is identified by typical signal of hyaline cartilage: low to intermediate signal intensity on T1-WI and high signal intensity on T2-WI, related to the high water content. It is often outlined by a superficial zone of low signal intensity, representing the perichondrium.

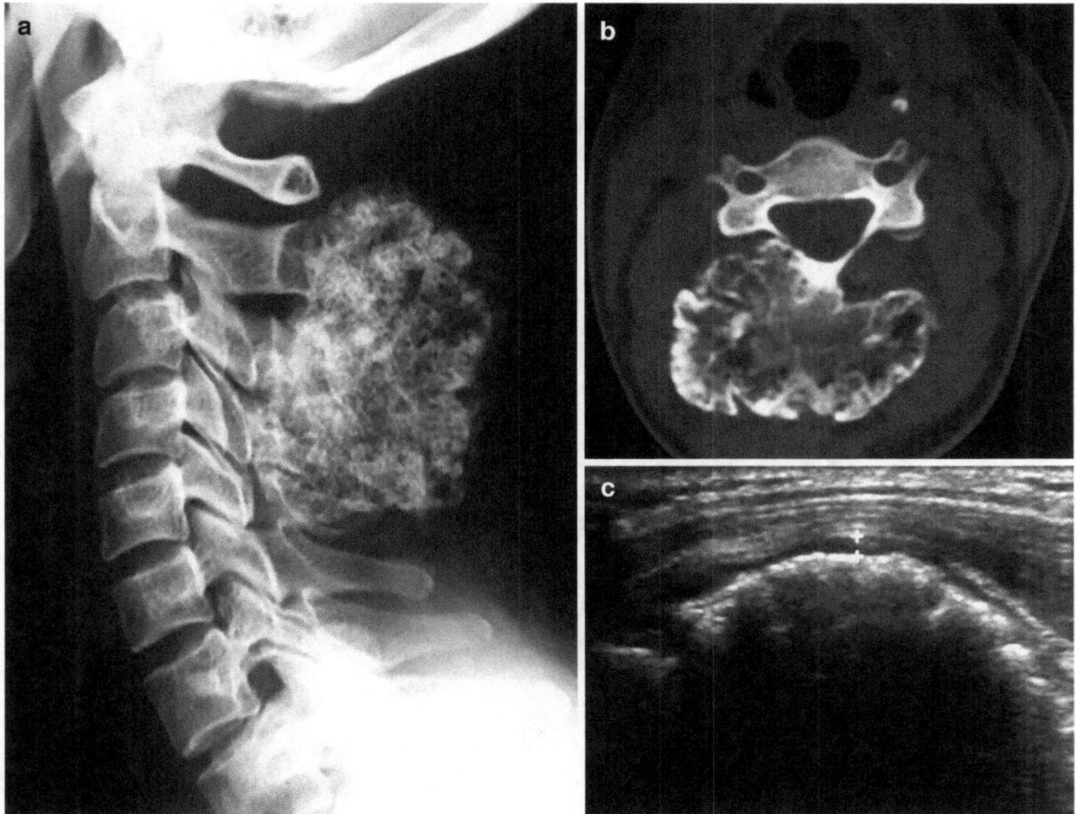

Fig. 1 Osteochondroma of the cervical spine. (**a**) Radiograph shows an osseous mass projecting on the spinous processes of C2–C5 vertebrae. (**b**) CT better depicts the cortical and medullary continuity with the spinous process. (**c**) The superficial mass is accessible to ultrasound, which finds a thin hypoechoic cartilaginous cap (+)

Calcifications of the cartilaginous matrix present as regions of signal void on all sequences (Fig. 2b, c). Gadolinium-enhanced T1-WI may show a thin peripheral enhancement, corresponding to fibrovascular tissue covering the nonenhancing hyaline cartilage (Murphey et al. 2000; Riahi et al. 2018).

MRI is the most accurate imaging modality for measurement of cartilage cap thickness, and malignancy should be suspected, if it exceeds 2 cm in adults and 3 cm in children (Fig. 2c) (Murphey et al. 2000).

A reactive bursa presents as a localized fluid collection adjacent to the OC, with similar signal features to those of the cartilaginous cap on T1-WI and T2-WI, hence the difficulty in distinguishing their respective limits. Due to the presence of fibrin or methemoglobin deposits, the bursa fluid may have a high signal intensity on T1-WI. Bursal wall thickening with marked synovial enhancement and edema of surrounding soft tissues is observed in cases of inflammation, infection, and hemorrhage. Loose bodies within the bursa may be observed in case of synovial chondromatosis (Woertler et al. 2000).

6.1.5 PET and PET/CT

OC generally shows no or faint fluorodeoxyglucose uptake. During childhood and adolescence, an uptake higher than that of the background could be found due to the growth of OC, making

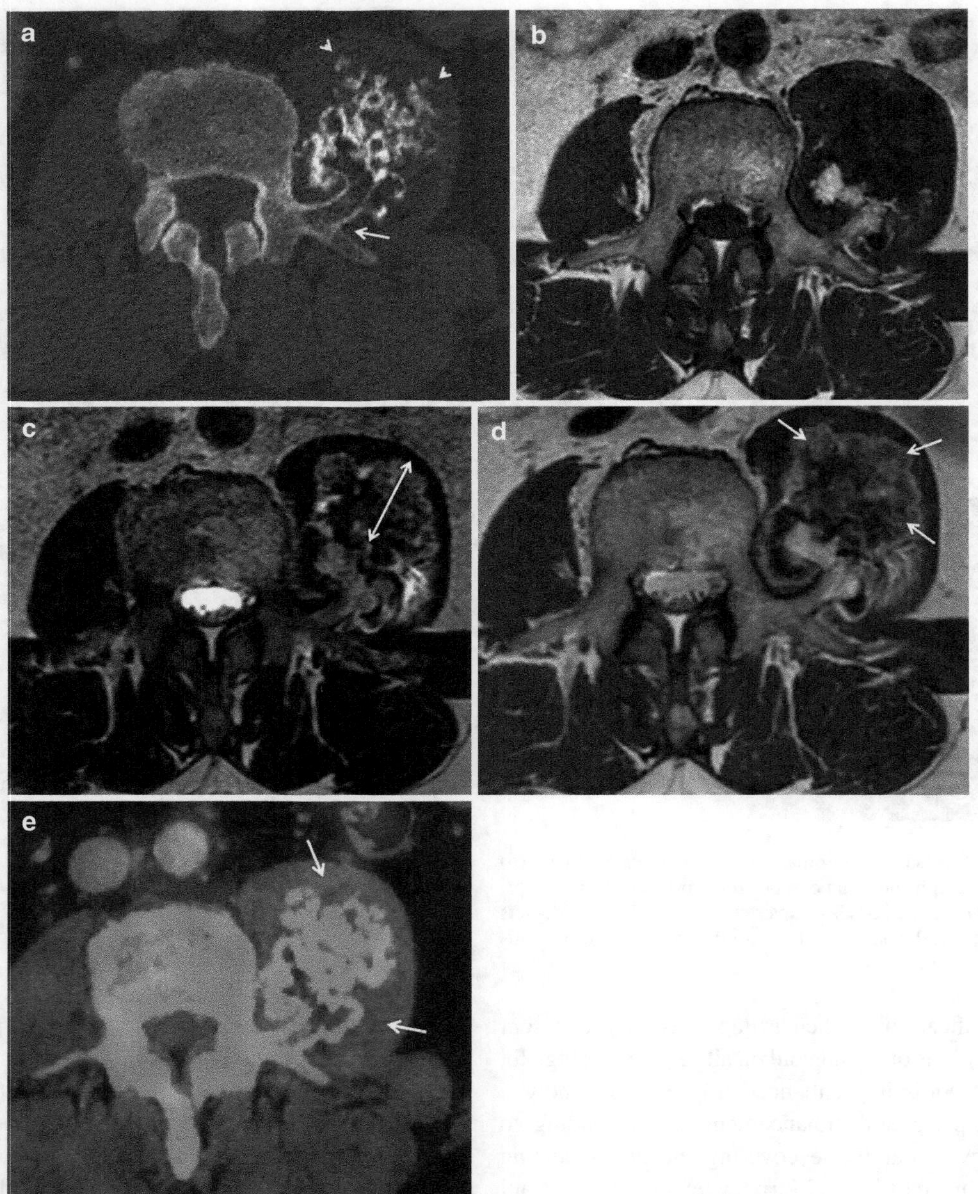

Fig. 2 Osteochondroma of L3 vertebra with malignant degeneration (secondary chondrosarcoma grade I). (**a**) CT shows a bone stalk with cortex and medullary cavity continuous with those of the underlying left transverse process (arrow). The outer limits of the cartilaginous cap are indistinguishable from the surrounding psoas muscle. This cap is the seat of cartilaginous rings and arcs calcifications that are extensive (arrowheads), suggesting its thickening. (**b–d**) MRI with axial T1-WI (**b**), axial T2-WI (**c**), and axial post-gadolinium T1-WI (**d**): MRI shows the continuity of the fatty signal medullary bone and the hypointense linear cortex between the osteochondroma and the bearing bone. The cartilaginous cap has a low signal on T1-WI and intermediate signal intensity on T2-WI due to heavy mineralization. On T2-WI (**c**), the tissue contrast between the bone stalk, the cartilaginous cap, and the surrounding muscle allows a precise measurement of the cartilaginous cap's thickness (double arrow). The thickening of the cartilaginous cap (**c**) and the diffuse and nodular enhancement pattern (**d**) suggest malignancy. (**e**) PET scan shows areas of hypermetabolic activity within the cartilaginous cap. (Images courtesy of Dr Hannes Devos, Belgium)

the distinction from low-grade peripheral chondrosarcoma difficult (Cheung et al. 2022).

Shortcomings of FDG-PET are limited availability and high cost.

6.2 Chondroblastoma

Unlike the appendicular counterpart, spinal chondroblastoma appears aggressive on imaging, with a destructive bony lesion, a large soft tissue mass, and significant spinal cord compression. The characteristic surrounding bone edema is usually not found in the spinal location (Ilaslan et al. 2003).

6.3 Enchondroma/ Chondrosarcoma

Although the large number of pathologic subtypes may lead to some variability in the appearance of spinal CS, the imaging features of the most common conventional CS are well described.

6.3.1 Radiographs

Radiography is the first-line radiological investigation for any spinal symptoms (Strauss et al. 2021).

The examination includes two orthogonal views on the symptomatic spinal segment with or without additional views centered on the suspected level.

Radiography may identify bone destruction and chondroid mineralization in up to 70% of cases (Golden et al. 2018).

It usually shows a well-defined osteolytic mass. The chondroid matrix mineralization appears as characteristic "ring and arc" calcifications (Fig. 3a) (Mechri et al. 2018).

When the posterior vertebral segment is involved, the tumor may manifest as a "winking owl" sign on an anteroposterior view (Colman and Schwab 2017).

A tumor with marked mineralization arising in the vertebral body may manifest as an "ivory vertebra" (Fig. 4a, b).

Occasionally, the lytic lesion involves the vertebral body and may be complicated by a compression fracture of the superior or inferior end plate (Mechri et al. 2018).

6.3.2 CT

Computed tomography (CT) is more sensitive than radiography for detecting spinal bone lesions and identifying the vertebral segment(s) involved (Fig. 4b, c). It allows more optimal detection and characterization of chondroid matrix mineralization.

The characteristic "ring and arc" appearance usually allows confident radiologic diagnosis of a cartilaginous lesion (Figs. 2a and 5a) (Murphey et al. 2003).

Spinal CS usually manifests as a large (>5 cm) lobulated, calcified mass with bone destruction. Cortical scalloping without breakthrough is often present.

The non-mineralized portion of the tumor has low attenuation on CT images (Fig. 2a).

True ossification may be seen, corresponding to residual OC in cases of secondary CS (Fig. 2a) (van den Hauwe et al. 2021).

Soft tissue paravertebral and extradural extension is also well assessed.

Chest CT is the most sensitive imaging modality for identifying pulmonary nodules and is recommended without intravenous contrast in the initial screening for pulmonary metastases and in subsequent monitoring (Strauss et al. 2021).

CT guides core needle biopsy. This percutaneous approach is strongly recommended instead of surgical open biopsy, which increases local recurrence and mortality (Yamazaki et al. 2009).

The biopsy should be carried out by a dedicated interventional radiologist after discussing with the surgeon (Blay et al. 2017).

Contamination of surrounding tissue should be minimized, using a coaxial system, and multiple sampling of representative tumoral areas should be performed.

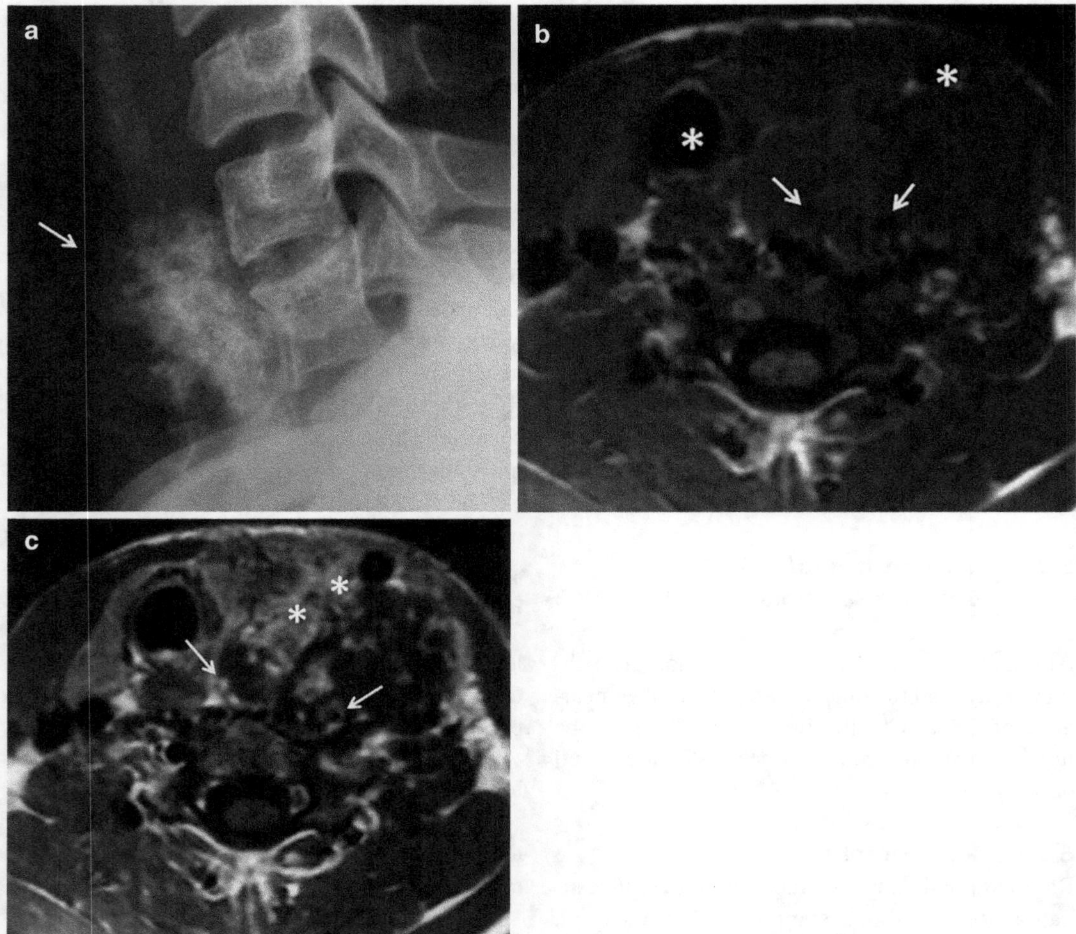

Fig. 3 Chondrosarcoma of C7 in a 23-year-old male patient. (**a**) Radiograph lateral view: a large prevertebral mass with matrix calcifications with "rings and arcs" morphology. (**b**) MRI axial T1-WI: the mass has low signal intensity with dark spots corresponding to calcifications (arrows). Note the displaced trachea and left carotid artery (asterisks). (**c**) MRI post-gadolinium T1-WI: enhancement is heterogeneous: the characteristic septa-like and rings and arcs enhancement pattern is seen in some areas (arrows). Other areas show diffuse heterogeneous enhancement (asterisks)

The biopsy tract has to be considered potentially contaminated and must be removed later, with the resection specimen, to minimize the risk of a local recurrence (Strauss et al. 2021).

Concordance between the preoperative needle biopsy and the final histologic diagnosis on resection specimen is much higher in long-bone CS (90% accuracy rate) than in axial pelvic CS (67%) when categorizing the lesions as low grade or high grade (Roitman et al. 2017).

6.3.3 MRI

MRI is the imaging modality of choice for accurate local staging of spinal CS. It completely evaluates the internal tumor architecture and its relationship to critical structures such as spinal cord, nerve roots, and adjacent soft tissues and organs.

The examination includes the primary tumor site and the entire spine to identify distant lesions.

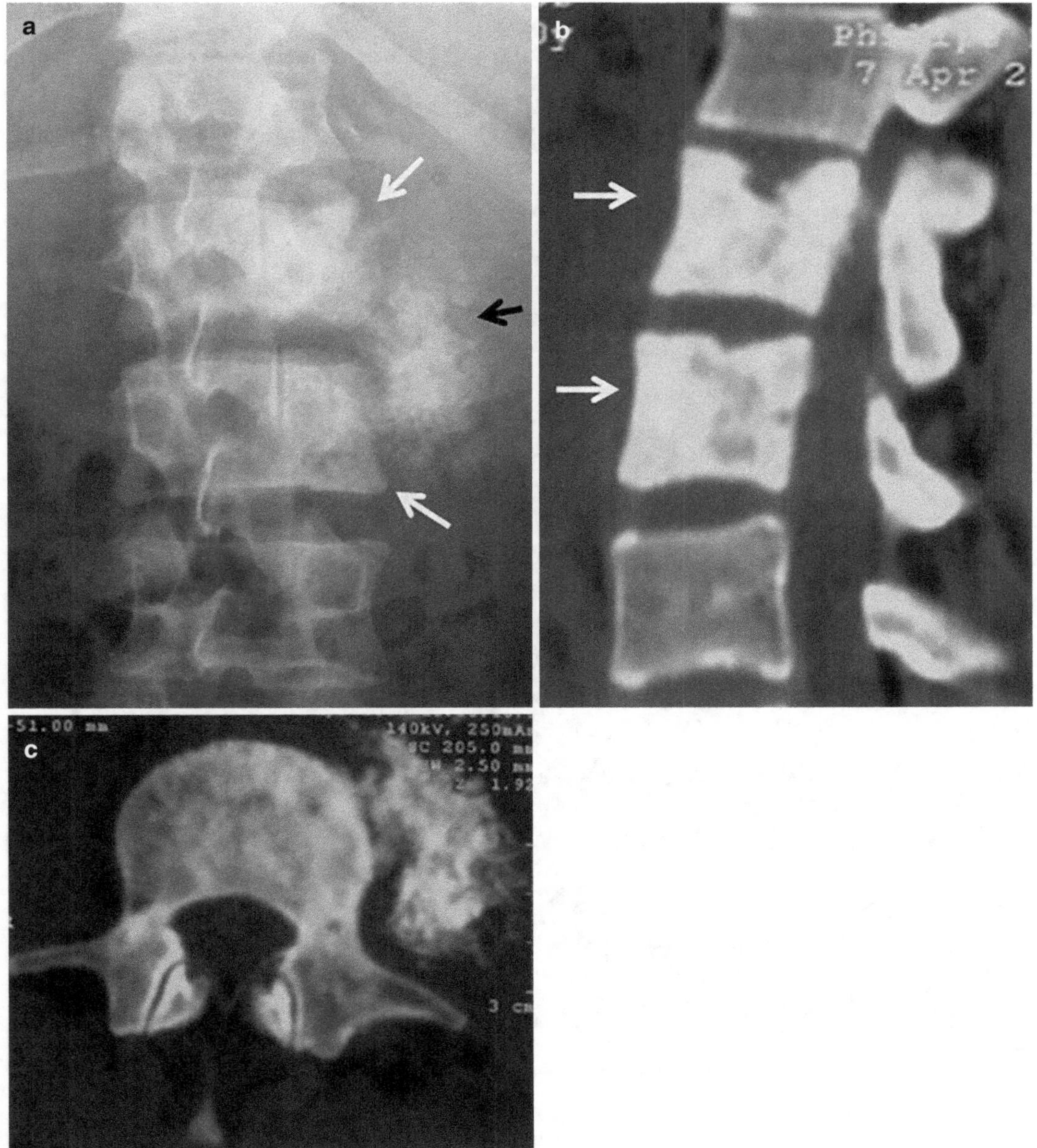

Fig. 4 Chondrosarcoma in a 20-year-old male patient. (**a**) Frontal view radiograph: marked osteocondensation of the vertebral body of L1 and L2 (white arrows) with a paravertebral calcified mass (black arrow). (**b**) CT scan sagittal reformatted image: The ivory vertebrae appearance is well depicted by CT (arrows). (**c**) CT scan axial image with bone window: bone changes and matrix mineralization of the mass are best assessed by CT. (Images courtesy of Dr. Hossam Salah, Egypt)

Anatomic images are obtained by T1- and T2-weighted images (WI). For fat suppression, DIXON provides more homogeneous signal intensity than STIR or fat-suppressed T1- and T2-WI, with additional information on fat content (Guerini et al. 2015).

The high water content of CS makes it appear hypointense on T1-WI and hyperintense on

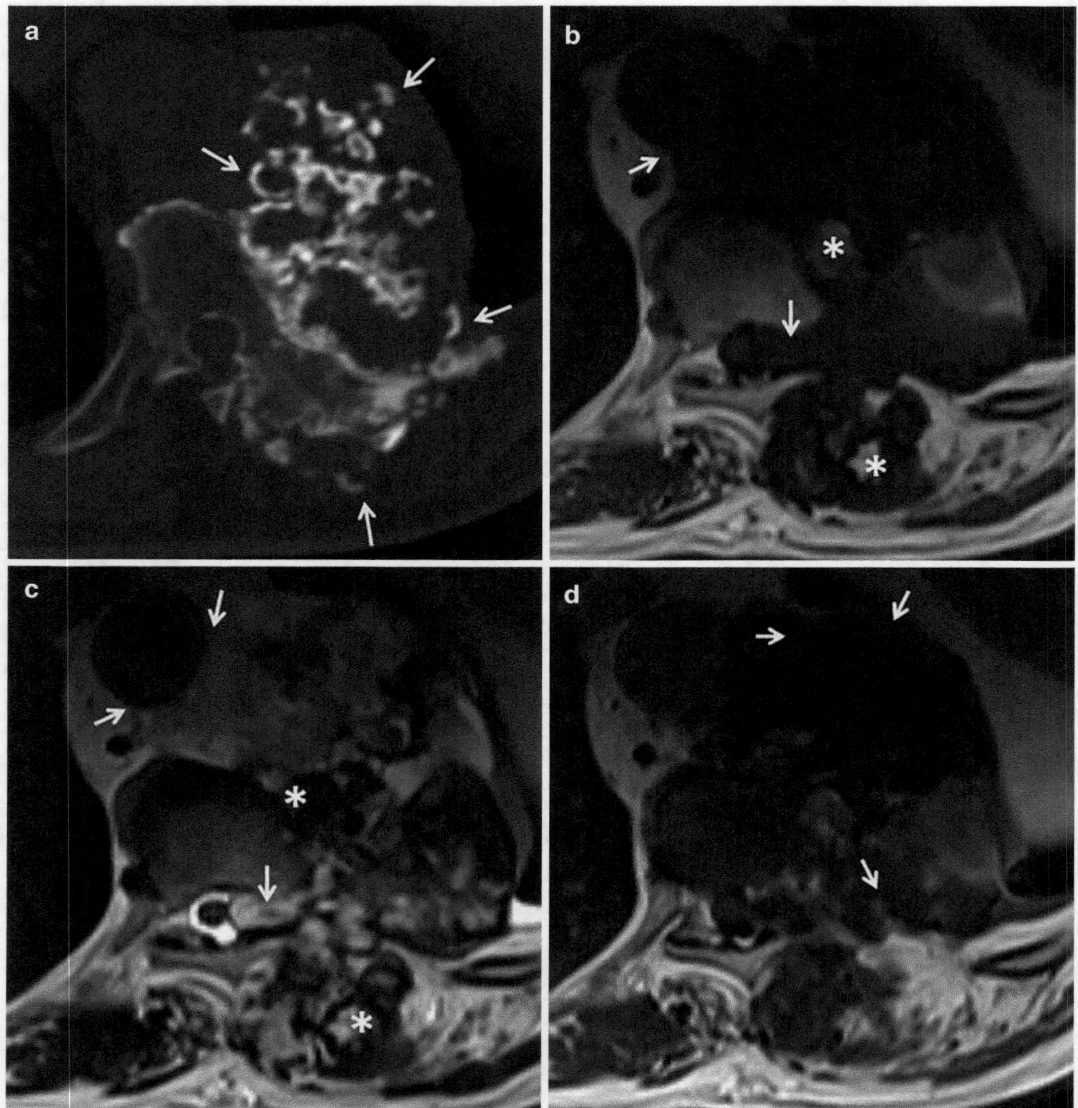

Fig. 5 Chondrosarcoma of the thoracic spine. (**a**) CT scan axial image with bone window: a large mass arising from the posterior and anterior vertebral elements with characteristic cartilaginous ring and arc calcifications (arrows). (**b**, **c**) MRI axial T1-WI (**b**) and T2-WI (**c**): the mass is lobulated and has a heterogeneous signal with unmineralized areas being hypointense on T1-WI and hyperintense on T2-WI. Calcifications have low signal intensity on all sequences. Some residual trabecular bone areas are recognizable by the high signal on T1-WI and T2-WI corresponding to fat signal (asterisks). Note the transforaminal epidural extension with spinal cord contact and the contact of the aorta of less than 180°, better depicted on the axial T2-WI (arrows). (**d**) On post-gadolinium contrast T1-WI, peripheral and lobulated septa-like enhancement pattern is seen

T2-WI (Figs. 3, 5, 6, and 7). Entrapped foci of fat are frequently observed in LGCS (Murphey et al. 2003).

Mineralized cartilage appears as dark signal voids on all sequences. Low-signal septa may be seen (Figs. 3, 5, 6, and 7).

Peripheral and lobulated rim (linear or septa-like) enhancement on contrast-enhanced T1-WI is characteristic (Figs. 3c and 5d). Other patterns such as diffuse and heterogeneous enhancement may be seen (Figs. 2d and 3c) (Murphey et al. 2003).

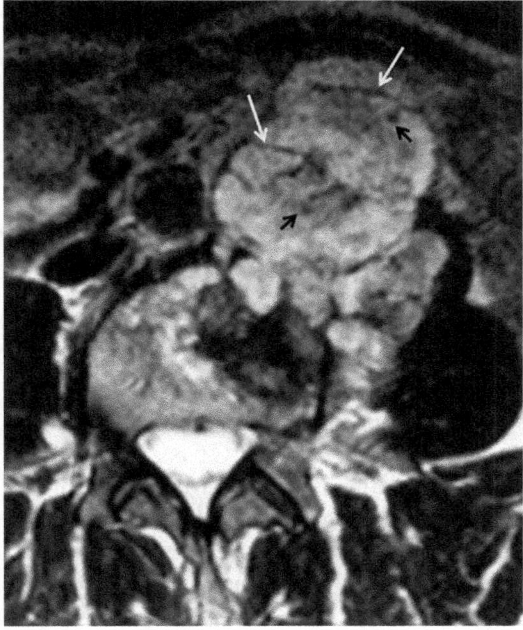

Fig. 6 Chondrosarcoma of the lumbar spine. MRI axial T2-WI: a lobulated mass arising in the vertebral body with anterior soft tissue extension. It has a high signal intensity. Mineralization appears as multiple dark signal voids (black arrows). Low-signal septa are seen (white arrows)

Conventional LGCS imaging features overlap with those of enchondroma (Crim et al. 2015) but are useful in the distinction from HGCS.

HGCS (conventional grade III, MCS, DCS) lacks the lobular growth pattern and shows aggressive features of bone destruction and large soft tissue masses. The signal intensity on T2-WI is intermediate, less than in LGCS, because the increased cellularity reduces water content. They often contain less extensive areas of matrix mineralization (better assessed by radiography or CT), and entrapped fat is a less common finding. Contrast enhancement is more prominent, diffuse, or nodular (Alhumaid et al. 2020).

Axial T2-WI predicts invasion of arteries, veins, and nerves if the contact between tumor and vascular or neural circumference exceeds 180° (Fig. 5c). MR angiography is useful for the mapping of major arteries and helps evaluate vascular invasion.

MRI is the best validated modality to detect peripheral CS arising from OC. A 2 cm cutoff point for cartilage cap thickness is used to indicate malignant degeneration in adults (Fig. 2c) (Bernard et al. 2010).

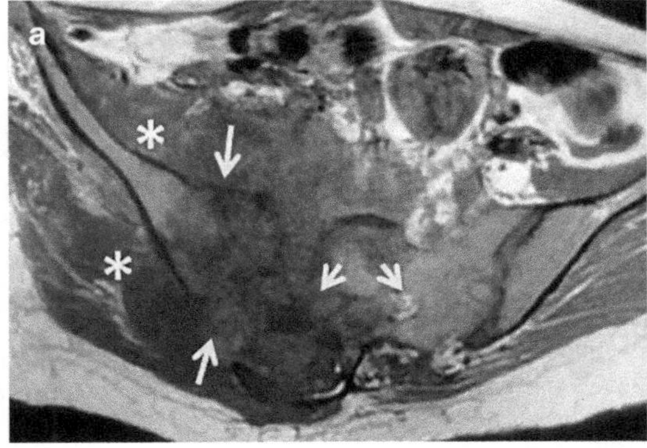

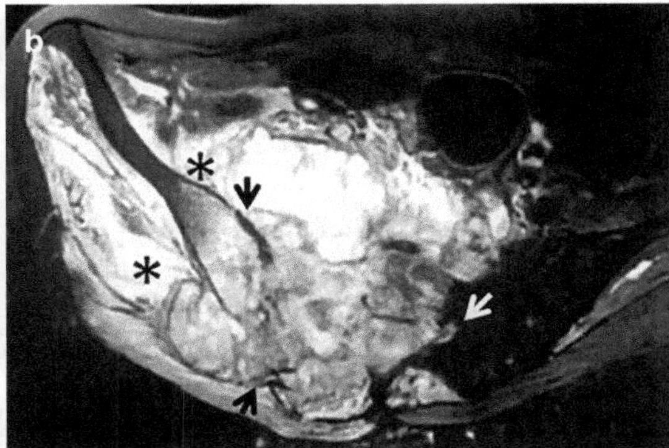

Fig. 7 Chondrosarcoma of the sacrum. MRI axial T1-WI (**a**) and STIR-WI (**b**): a right-sided lobulated eccentric sacral mass with extension to the sacral foramen and iliac bone through the synovial and ligamentous portions of the right sacroiliac joint, and to the exo- and endopelvic soft tissues (arrows). Characteristic features of chondrosarcoma are seen, namely the lobulated structure, the low to intermediate signal intensity on T1-WI, the high signal intensity on T2-WI, and the calcifications and hypointense septa on all sequences. Note the edema-like signal abnormalities in the adjacent exo- and endopelvic soft tissues (asterisks)

Anatomic MRI directs percutaneous biopsy toward the aggressive areas and helps minimize sampling errors within the usually heterogeneous CS.

Dynamic contrast-enhanced MRI may help distinguish CS (as a whole entity) from enchondroma: Early enhancement, within 10 s of arterial enhancement, with greater slope of the uptake curve would favor the diagnosis of CS (Geirnaerdt et al. 2000). But it is not reliable in the differentiation between enchondroma and LGCS (Douis et al. 2018).

Diffusion-WI (DWI) with different *b* values and apparent diffusion coefficient (ADC) mapping is a functional MRI technique that provides quantitative evaluation of tumor cellularity (Inarejos Clemente et al. 2022). DWI cannot differentiate between enchondroma and CS and does not aid in the distinction of LGCS from HGCS (Douis et al. 2015). Among the malignant primary bone tumors, CS has the highest ADC values (Rao et al. 2019).

New advanced tools including texture analysis and radiomics have shown promising diagnostic performances for CS grading (Li et al. 2023).

Whole-body MRI is regarded as a new alternative to the classic chest CT and bone scintigraphy combination for metastasis screening (Strauss et al. 2021). It is especially important for patients with known history of Maffucci syndrome, Ollier disease, or another enchondromatosis, as these patients may develop multiple secondary CS. Protocol consists of an acquisition from head to toes of T1-WI, STIR, and DWI in the coronal or axial planes.

6.3.4 PET and PET/CT

Positron emission tomography (PET) has emerged as a modality in musculoskeletal tumor imaging. Fusion of PET-acquired images with CT scans and more recently with MRI has significantly improved the overall diagnostic accuracy (Choi et al. 2014).

Viable malignant primary bone tumors are usually avid for 18F-fluorodeoxyglucose (FDG), which is used as a radiotracer.

Metabolic activity, based on the maximum standardized uptake value (SUV_{max}), may correlate with histologic grade in intra-osseous chondroid neoplasms. Very low SUV_{max} supports the diagnosis of benign tumor, while elevated SUV_{max} is suggestive of higher grade CS (Fig. 2e) (Subhawong et al. 2017; Zhang et al. 2020).

7 Differential Diagnosis

The differential diagnosis of CS includes both primary and metastatic neoplasms, as well as benign tumors of the spine.

The identification of chondroid matrix calcifications on radiography or CT enables the diagnostic orientation toward a cartilaginous tumor.

Unlike its appendicular counterpart, spinal chondroblastoma appears aggressive on imaging, making it virtually indistinguishable from spinal CS.

The distinction between enchondroma and LGCS is difficult histologically and radiologically. Clinical presentation and presence or absence of aggressive behavior on imaging and histology guide the diagnosis. As a rule of thumb, cartilaginous tumors in the axial skeleton should be considered as CS.

Chondroblastic osteosarcoma is a rare subtype of conventional osteosarcoma that occurs in younger patients and involves the sacrum rather than the thoracic spine (see chapter "Spinal Osteosarcoma"). Besides a cartilaginous component, it contains an osteoid more or less mineralized component, demonstrated as fluffy and cloudy opacities on radiography and CT, characteristic of bone production. The presence of the latter component on histology rules out CS.

Chordoma (see chapter "Notochordal Tumors") is the most common primary malignant spinal bone tumor, excluding hematologic malignancies, and mimics CS on imaging. It may occur at any age, typically 40–60-year-old age group, predominantly in males. Chordoma typically arises in the midline because it originates from remnants of the primitive notochord in the intervertebral regions and nucleus pulposus, with predilection for the lower sacrum and sacrococcygeal regions. Radiographs and CT usually show a lytic lesion of a vertebral body and a soft tissue mass with a "mushroom" appearance, spanning several segments and sparing the disks. Calcifications are frequently present and are distributed in an amorphous or punctuate pattern. Bone sequestra may also be seen. On MRI, chordoma characteristically has low to intermediate signal on T1-WI, high signal on T2-WI, reflecting of mucoid and high water content, and mild-to-moderate enhancement after gadolinium contrast. They may contain internal septations, with low-signal bands (Golden et al. 2018; Mechri et al. 2018).

Spinal giant cell tumor may appear similar to CS (see chapter "Giant Cell Tumor"). It affects patients in their second to fourth decades of life and is more frequently found in women. Only the vertebral body is usually involved, and the most common location is the upper sacrum. It is then more likely to extend laterally to involve the sacroiliac joint and more likely to have fluid levels than CS. Giant cell tumor typically lacks internal calcifications and is of low to intermediate signal intensity on T2-WI rather than the high T2 signal that is typical of chordoma or CS (Golden et al. 2018; Riahi et al. 2018).

Myeloma (see chapter "Plasmacytoma"), lymphoma (see chapter "Lymphoma"), and metastases usually occur in patients older than 40 years of age and present as multiple lytic lesions within vertebral bodies, while CS is often solitary.

Hydatidosis, a parasitic disease of tapeworms of the Echinococcus type, is another less known differential diagnosis of chondrosarcoma on imaging. Spinal hydatidosis occurs in more than 50% of the 0.5–4% of cases affecting bones and most commonly involves the thoracic spine (50%) followed by lumbar (20%), sacral (20%), and cervical spine (Ladeb 2019). Radiography shows nonspecific pure osteolysis of the vertebral body with possible extension to the posterior vertebral elements. Paravertebral soft tissue extension is frequent and presents as paraspinal opacities with well-defined rounded or polycyclical, sometimes calcified contours. CT assesses bone destruction. It shows vertebral hypodense multivesicular cystic masses with cortical scalloping and interruption (Fig. 8a). There is typically no modification of the surrounding normal bone. MRI is the best imaging modality for diagnosis confirmation: It best depicts the pathognomonic multivesicular appearance with low signal intensity on T1-WI and high signal intensity on T2-WI without enhancement after gadolinium administration (Fig. 8b, c). MRI is also the modality of choice for local extension assessment: it depicts the extension to the spinal canal and the relationship with spinal cord and nerve roots, as well as with paraspinal soft tissues (Ladeb 2019).

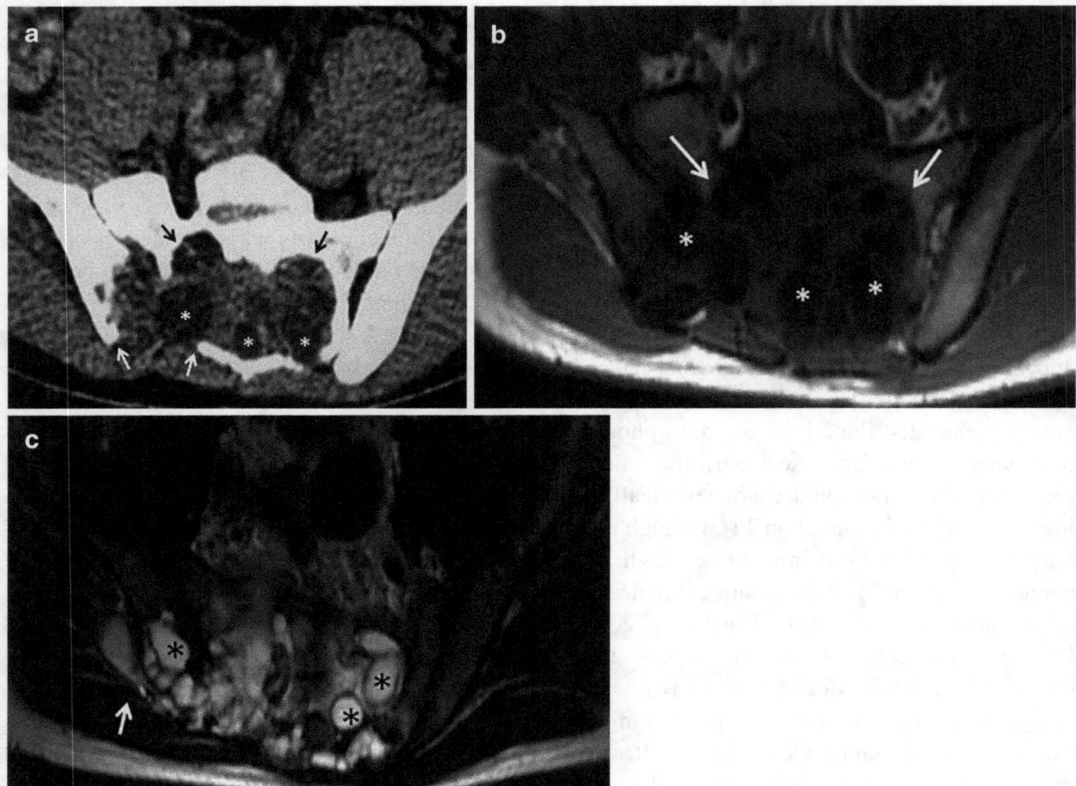

Fig. 8 Sacral hydatidosis in a 16-year-old male patient. (**a**) CT scan axial image: expansile osteolytic mass of the sacrum with multi-lobed contours. It enlarges the sacral foramina (black arrows) and interrupts the lateral cortex of the right sacral ala with extension through the posterior part of the right sacroiliac joint toward the right iliac bone (white arrows). Its density is heterogeneous with intralesional rounded hypodense areas (asterisks). (**b**, **c**) MRI axial T1-WI (**b**) and T2-WI (**c**): MRI confirms the diagnosis: endolesional vesicles are shown as well-delineated round-shaped lesions of hypointense signal on T1-WI and hyperintense signal on T2-WI (asterisks). MRI also better assesses the local extension to the sacral foramina, sacroiliac joint, iliac bone, and right gluteal muscles (arrows)

8 Local and Distant Staging

The European Society for Medical Oncology-European Reference Network on Rare Adult Solid Cancers-European Reference Network on Genetic Tumour Risk Syndromes (ESMO-EURACAN-GENTURIS) guidelines for bone sarcomas recommend MRI for local staging.

Chest CT and bone scintigraphy and/or whole-body MRI and and/or FDG-PET/CT/MRI are recommended for distant staging (Strauss et al. 2021).

Bone tumor staging has been assessed according to the Enneking (Enneking et al. 1980) and the Weinstein-Boriani-Biagini (WBB) (Boriani et al. 1997) staging systems.

However, the Enneking system was designed for appendicular tumors rather than spine tumors.

The WBB system is a surgical local staging system for primary spine tumors that does not specify tumor grade or presence or absence of distant spread. Experts of the Spine Oncology Study Group found that it has only modest interobserver agreement (Chan et al. 2009).

The eighth edition staging manual (Kniesl et al. 2018) is the current standard oncologic staging system for primary malignant bone tumors (except lymphoma and myeloma).

It separates, for the first time, axial from peripheral skeletal tumors and provides a new distinct classification for spine tumors integrating tumor location and traditional anatomic criteria (tumor size (T), presence of lymph node (N), or distant metastases (M)).

The new TNM categories for spine tumors are based on expert experience and opinion and imply resectability and margin status (Rose et al. 2019).

It is of note that the eighth edition of the AJCC lacks prognostic stage groupings for spine tumors. Further data collection and analysis will indicate if the new TNM classification improves discrimination of patient outcomes, with possible subsequent prognostic stage groups' release in the upcoming staging manual updates.

At diagnosis of spinal CS, the disease is usually locally invasive (71.6%) and may be confined (16.6%) or metastatic in 11.8% of cases (Arshi et al. 2017).

9 Treatment

Asymptomatic OC does not require treatment. However, if symptomatic, it is excised at its base. Surgical decompression via laminectomy and laminotomy is the most common treatment strategy.

The current standard of care of CS is curative en bloc resection. Clear margins (R0) are the first goal of surgery because microscopic (R1) and macroscopic (R2) positive margins both increase the local recurrence rate, with reduced overall survival. Local curettage almost always results in recurrence.

Metastatic disease is generally considered as a contraindication to surgery.

Adjuvant radiotherapy of at least 60 Gy equivalents is indicated when there has been incomplete resection or with intralesional margins. It improves local control and disease-free survival.

CS is generally resistant to chemotherapy, except for mesenchymal and dedifferentiated subtypes (Pennington et al. 2021).

10 Prognosis

OC is a benign tumor with excellent prognosis. The reported local recurrence is less than 2%.

Malignant transformation usually happens within the cartilage cap leading to secondary peripheral chondrosarcoma. It occurs in approximately 1% of SE and 10% of HME cases. Osteosarcoma arising in the bone stalk is rare. Malignancy commonly involves the axial skeleton (64%), mostly the pelvic girdle (Righi et al. 2022).

The prognosis of CS varies widely and is based on tumor subtype, grade, and stage.

Location in the axial skeleton has a worse outcome than location in the appendicular skeleton (van Praag Veroniek et al. 2018) probably due to the often late diagnosis with a locally advanced tumor and the anatomical complexity of the spine, which may hinder surgical oncology.

The histologic grade of spinal CS is an important prognostic factor. The 10-year survival rate for a grade I CS is 90%, which declines to 65–80% for grade II and to 30–40% for high grade III tumors (McLoughlin et al. 2008).

MCS has a poor prognosis with a 5-year survival rate of 50%. DDS is notoriously aggressive with frequent metastases at presentation and a 5-year survival rate of less than 10% (McLoughlin et al. 2008).

Other independent prognostic factors for tumor-related death include increasing age, tumor size >8 cm, metastatic disease, and intralesional or contaminated surgical margins (Arshi et al. 2017; van Praag Veroniek et al. 2018).

Regarding tumor recurrence, biopsy and treatment outside a reference tumor center and inadequate surgical margins are independent adverse prognostic factors (Katonis et al. 2011; Arshi et al. 2017).

A successful complete en bloc resection with clear oncologic margins is a major independent prognostic factor for a favorable course of the disease, affecting both local tumor control and patient survival (Katonis et al. 2011).

11 Key Points

- Osteochondroma is the most common benign bone tumor, and the spinal location is well documented although rare. Medullary and cortical continuity with the underlying vertebra is a pathognomonic imaging finding. MRI is the modality of choice for screening of complications.
- Unlike its appendicular counterpart, spinal chondroblastoma appears aggressive on imaging, and the characteristic surrounding bone edema is usually not found, making it virtually indistinguishable from spinal chondrosarcoma.
- Low-grade conventional chondrosarcoma accounts for 80–90% of the chondrosarcoma subtypes in the spine and may be difficult to distinguish from enchondroma. As a rule of thumb, cartilaginous tumors in the axial skeleton are probably chondrosarcomas.
- MRI is the imaging modality of choice for local staging and helps to differentiate enchondroma/low-grade from high-grade chondrosarcoma.
- Besides histological grade of the tumor, the prognosis depends on the possibility of performing en bloc resection with clear oncologic margins.

References

Albrecht S, Crutchfield JS, SeGall GK (1992) On spinal osteochondromas. J Neurosurg 77(2):247–252

Alhumaid SM, Alharbi A 4th, Aljubair H (2020) Magnetic resonance imaging role in the differentiation between atypical cartilaginous tumors and high-grade chondrosarcoma: an updated systematic review. Cureus 12(10):e11237

Angelini A, Mavrogenis AF, Ruggieri P (2017) Chondrosarcoma of the sacrum. In: Ruggieri P, Angelini A, Vanel D, Picci P (eds) Tumors of the sacrum. Springer, Cham, pp 237–244

Armany F, Bloem JL, Cleven AHG et al (2020) Chondroblastoma. In: WHO Classification of Tumours Editorial Board (ed) WHO classification of soft tissue and bone tumours, 5th edn. IARC Press, Lyon, pp 359–361

Arshi A, Sharim J, Park DY et al (2017) Chondrosarcoma of the osseous spine. An analysis of epidemiology, patient outcomes, and prognostic factors using the SEER Registry from 1973 to 2012. Spine (Phila Pa 1976) 42:644–652

Baumhoer D, Bloem JL, Oda Y (2020) Clear cell chondrosarcoma. In: WHO Classification of Tumours Editorial Board (ed) WHO classification of soft tissue and bone tumours, 5th edn. IARC Press, Lyon, pp 383–384

Bergh P, Gunterberg B, Meis-Kindblom JM et al (2001) Prognostic factors and outcome of pelvic, sacral, and spinal chondrosarcomas: a center-based study of 69 cases. Cancer 91(7):1201–1212

Bernard SA, Murphey MD, Flemming DJ et al (2010) Improved differentiation of benign osteochondromas from secondary chondrosarcomas with standardized measurement of cartilage cap at CT and MR imaging. Radiology 255(3):857–865

Blay JY, Soibinet P, Penel N et al (2017) Improved survival using specialized multidisciplinary board in sarcoma patients. Ann Oncol 28(11):2852–2859

Boriani S, Weistein JN, Biagini R (1997) Primary bone tumors of the spine. Terminology and surgical staging. Spine 22:1036–1044

Bovée JVMG, Bloem JL, Flanagan AM et al (2020a) Central and peripheral chondrosarcoma. In: WHO Classification of Tumours Editorial Board (ed) WHO classification of soft tissue and bone tumours, 5th edn. IARC Press, Lyon, pp 370–380

Bovée JVMG, Bloem JL, Flanagan AM et al (2020b) Enchondroma. In: WHO Classification of Tumours Editorial Board (ed) WHO classification of soft tissue and bone tumours, 5th edn. IARC Press, Lyon, pp 353–355

Bovée JVMG, Bloem JL, Heymann D et al (2020c) Osteochondroma. In: WHO Classification of Tumours Editorial Board (ed) WHO classification of soft tissue and bone tumours, 5th edn. IARC Press, Lyon, pp 356–358

Chan P, Boriani S, Fourney DR et al (2009) An assessment of the reliability of the Enneking and Weinstein-Boriani-Biagini classifications for staging of primary spine tumors by the Spine Oncology Study Group. Spine 34:384–391

Cheung H, Yechoor A, Behnia F et al (2022) Common skeletal neoplasms and nonneoplastic lesions at ^{18}F-FDG PET/CT. Radiographics 42(1):250–267

Choi YY, Kim JY, Yang SO (2014) PET/CT in benign and malignant musculoskeletal tumors and tumor-like conditions [review]. Semin Musculoskelet Radiol 18(2):133–148

Cleton-Jansen AM (2015) Role of mesenchymal stem cells in bone cancer: initiation, propagation and metastasis. In: Heymann D (ed) Bone cancer: primary bone cancers and bone metastases, 2nd edn. Academic Press, Amsterdam, pp 73–82

Colman MW, Schwab JH (2017) Current concepts in primary benign, primary malignant, and metastatic tumors of the spine. In: Grauer JN (ed) Orthopaedic Knowledge Update, 12th edn. American Academy of Orthopaedic Surgeons, USA, p 655–672

Crim J, Schmidt R, Layfield L et al (2015) Can imaging criteria distinguish enchondroma from grad 1 chondrosarcoma? Eur J Radiol 84(11):2222–2230

Douis H, Jeys L, Grimer R et al (2015) Is there a role for diffusion-weighted MRI (DWI) in the diagnosis of central cartilage tumors? Skelet Radiol 44(7):963–969

Douis H, Parry M, Vaiyapuri S et al (2018) What are the differentiating clinical and MRI-features of enchondromas from low-grade chondrosarcomas? Eur Radiol 28(1):398–409

Elmajee M, Osman K, Dermanis A et al (2022) A literature review: the genomic landscape of spinal chondrosarcoma and potential diagnostic, prognostic & therapeutic implications. Interdiscip Neurosurg Adv Techn Case Manag 30:101651

Enneking WF, Spanier SS, Goodman MA (1980) A system for the surgical staging of musculoskeletal sarcoma. Clin Orthop Relat Res 153:106–120

Fanburg-Smith JC, de Pinieux G, Ladanyi M (2020) Mesenchymal chondrosarcoma. In: WHO Classification of Tumours Editorial Board (ed) WHO classification of soft tissue and bone tumours, 5th edn. IARC Press, Lyon, pp p385–p387

Ferreira RM, Vieira L, Pimenta S et al (2019) Chondrosarcoma as inaugural manifestation of monostotic Paget's disease of bone. Acta Reumatol Port 44(2):163–164

Fiechtl JF, Masonis JL, Frick SL (2003) Spinal osteochondroma presenting as atypical spinal curvature: a case report. Spine (Phila Pa 1976) 28(13):E252–E255

Fiumara E, Scarabino T, Guglielmi G et al (1999) Osteochondroma of the L-5 vertebra: a rare cause of sciatic pain. Case report. J Neurosurg 91(2 Suppl):219–222

Fowler J, Takayanagi A, Fiani B et al (2021) Diagnosis, management, and treatment options: a cervical spine osteochondroma meta-analysis. World Neurosurg 149:215–225.e6

García-Ramos CL, Buganza-Tepole M, Obil-Chavarría CA et al (2015) Osteocondroma espinal: diagnóstico por imagen y tratamiento. Reporte de casos [Spinal osteochondroma: diagnostic imaging and treatment. Case reports]. Cir Cir 83(6):496–500

Geirnaerdt MJ, Hogendoorn PC, Bloem JL et al (2000) Cartilaginous tumors: fast contrast-enhanced MR imaging. Radiology 214(2):539–546

Gille O, Pointillart V, Vital JM (2005) Course of spinal solitary osteochondromas. Spine (Phila Pa 1976) 30(1):E13–E19

Giuffrida AY, Burgueno JE, Koniaris LG et al (2009) Chondrosarcoma in the United States (1973 to 2003): an analysis of 2890 cases from the SEER database. J Bone Joint Surg Am 91(5):1063–1072

Golden L, Pendharkar A, Fischbein N (2018) Chapter 8: Imaging chordoma and chondrosarcoma of the vertebrae and sacrum. In: Harsh GR, Vaz-Guimaraes F (eds) Chordomas and chondrosarcomas of the skull base and spine, 2nd edn. Academic Press, pp 79–86

Guerini H, Omoumi P, Guichoux F et al (2015) Fat suppression with Dixon techniques in musculoskeletal magnetic resonance imaging: a pictorial review. Semin Musculoskelet Radiol 19(4):335–347

Herget GW, Strohm P, Rottenburger C et al (2014) Insights into enchondroma, enchondromatosis and the risk of secondary chondrosarcoma. Review of the literature with an emphasis on the clinical behaviour, radiology, malignant transformation and the follow up. Neoplasma 61(4):365–378

Ilaslan H, Sundaram M, Unni KK (2003) Vertebral chondroblastoma. Skelet Radiol 32(2):66–71

Inarejos Clemente EJ, Navarro OM, Navallas M et al (2022) Multiparametric MRI evaluation of bone sarcomas in children. Insights Imaging 13(1):33

Inwards CY, Bloem JL, Hogendoorn PCW (2020) Dedifferentiated chondrosarcoma. In: WHO Classification of Tumours Editorial Board (ed) WHO classification of soft tissue and bone tumours, 5th edn. IARC Press, Lyon, pp 388–390

Katonis P, Alpantaki K, Michail K et al (2011) Spinal chondrosarcoma: a review. Sarcoma 2011:378957

Kniesl JS, Rosenberg AE, Anderson PM et al (2018) Bone. In: Amin MB, Edge S, Greene D et al (eds) AJCC cancer staging manual, 8th edn. Springer, Chicago

Ladeb MF (2019) Musculoskeletal hydatidosis. Centre de Publication Universitaire, Tunis. ISBN: 978-9973-37-998-6.

Li X, Lan M, Wang X et al (2023) Development and validation of a MRI-based combined radiomics nomogram for differentiation in chondrosarcoma. Front Oncol 13:1090229

McLoughlin GS, Sciubba DM, Wolinsky JP (2008) Chondroma/chondrosarcoma of the spine. Neurosurg Clin N Am 19(1):57–63

Mechri M, Riahi H, Sboui I et al (2018) Imaging of malignant primitive tumors of the spine. J Belg Soc Radiol 102(1):56

Murphey MD, Choi JJ, Kransdorf MJ et al (2000) Imaging of osteochondroma: variants and complications with radiologic-pathologic correlation. Radiographics 20(5):1407–1434

Murphey MD, Walker EA, Wilson AJ et al (2003) From the archives of the AFIP: imaging of primary chondrosarcoma: radiologic-pathologic correlation. Radiographics 23(5):1245–1278

Pennington Z, Ehresman J, Pittman PD et al (2021) Chondrosarcoma of the spine: a narrative review. Spine J 21(12):2078–2096

Rajakulasingam R, Murphy J, Botchu R et al (2020) Osteochondromas of the cervical spine-case series and review. J Clin Orthop Trauma 11(5):905–909

Rao A, Sharma C, Parampalli R (2019) Role of diffusion-weighted MRI in differentiating benign from malignant bone tumors. BJR Open 1(1):20180048

Riahi H, Mechri M, Barsaoui M et al (2018) Imaging of benign tumors of the osseous spine. J Belg Soc Radiol 102(1):13

Righi A, Pacheco M, Cocchi S et al (2022) Secondary peripheral chondrosarcoma arising in solitary osteochondroma: variables influencing prognosis and survival. Orphanet J Rare Dis 17(1):74

Roach JW, Klatt JW, Faulkner ND (2009) Involvement of the spine in patients with multiple hereditary exostoses. J Bone Joint Surg Am 91(8):1942–1948

Roitman PD, Farfalli GL, Ayerza MA et al (2017) Is needle biopsy clinically useful in preoperative grading of central chondrosarcoma of the pelvis and long bones? Clin Orthop Relat Res 475(3):808–814

Rose PS, Holt GE, Kneisl JS (2019) Changes to the American Joint Committee on Cancer staging system for spine tumors-practice update. Ann Transl Med 7(10):215

Sciubba DM, Macki M, Bydon M et al (2015) Long-term outcomes in primary spinal osteochondroma: a multicenter study of 27 patients. J Neurosurg Spine 22(6):582–588

Srikantha U, Bhagavatula ID, Satyanarayana S et al (2008) Spinal osteochondroma: spectrum of a rare disease. J Neurosurg Spine 8(6):561–566

Strauss SJ, Frezza AM, Abecassis N et al (2021) Bone sarcomas: ESMO-EURACAN-GENTURIS-ERN PaedCan Clinical Practice Guideline for diagnosis, treatment and follow-up. Ann Oncol 32(12):1520–1536

Stuckey RM, Marco RA (2011) Chondrosarcoma of the mobile spine and sacrum. Sarcoma 2011:274281

Subhawong TK, Winn A, Shemesh SS et al (2017) F-18 FDG PET differentiation of benign from malignant chondroid neoplasms: a systematic review of the literature. Skelet Radiol 46(9):1233–1239

Sundaresan N, Rosen G, Boriani S (2009) Primary malignant tumors of the spine. Orthop Clin North Am 40(1):21–36, v

Tepelenis K, Papathanakos G, Kitsouli A et al (2021) Osteochondromas: an updated review of epidemiology, pathogenesis, clinical presentation, radiological features and treatment options. In Vivo 35(2):681–691

Thiart M, Herbst H (2010) Lumbar osteochondroma causing spinal compression. SA Orthop J 9(2):44–47

Thorkildsen J, Taksdal I, Bjerkehagen B et al (2019) Chondrosarcoma in Norway 1990-2013; an epidemiological and prognostic observational study of a complete national cohort. Acta Oncol 58(3):273–282

van den Hauwe L, van Goethem JW, Balériaux D (2021) Spinal tumours. In: Adam A et al (eds) Grainger & Allison's diagnostic radiology, vol 49, 7th edn. Elsevier Ltd., pp 1267–1294

van Praag Veroniek VM, Rueten-Budde AJ, Ho V et al (2018) Incidence, outcomes and prognostic factors during 25 years of treatment of chondrosarcomas. Surg Oncol 27(3):402–408

Woertler K, Lindner N, Gosheger G, Brinkschmidt C, Heindel W (2000) Osteochondroma: MR imaging of tumor-related complications. Eur Radiol 10(5):832–840

Yakkanti R, Onyekwelu I, Carreon LY et al (2018) Solitary osteochondroma of the spine - a case series: review of solitary osteochondroma with myelopathic symptoms. Global Spine J 8(4):323–339

Yamazaki T, McLoughlin GS, Patel S et al (2009) Feasibility and safety of en bloc resection for primary spine tumors: a systematic review by the Spine Oncology Study Group. Spine (Phila Pa 1976) 34(22 Suppl):S31–S38

Zhang Q, Xi Y, Li D et al (2020) The utility of ^{18}F-FDG PET and PET/CT in the diagnosis and staging of chondrosarcoma: a meta-analysis. J Orthop Surg Res 15(1):229

Zhou Z, Wang X, Wu Z et al (2017) Epidemiological characteristics of primary spinal osseous tumors in eastern China. World J Surg Oncol 15(1):73

Notochordal Tumors

Simranjeet Kaur, Victor-Cassar Pullicino,
and Radhesh Lalam

Contents

S. Kaur (✉) · V.-C. Pullicino · R. Lalam
Department of Radiology, Robert Jones and Agnes Hunt Orthopaedic Hospital, Oswestry, UK
e-mail: Simranjeet.kaur5@nhs.net; victor.pullicino@nhs.net; Radhesh.lalam@nhs.net

Abstract

Notochordal tumors comprise a spectrum of tumors arising in the axial skeleton having notochordal differentiation characterized by the co-expression of cytokeratin and brachyury. Brachyury is the diagnostic hallmark and is the single most important immunohistochemical marker to differentiate notochordal tumors from chondrosarcoma, myoepithelial tumors, metastasis, and meningioma. The recent WHO classification divides notochordal tumors into benign notochordal cell tumors (BNCTs) and chordomas, which are further divided into three subtypes: (1) conventional chordoma, (2) poorly differentiated chordoma, and (3) dedifferentiated chordoma. BNCT and chordomas have defined histological and radiological criteria and differ significantly in terms of course of disease and management. BNCTs are benign tumors with limited intra-osseous growth, whereas chordomas are slow-growing malignant lesion with progressive destructive growth and capacity for metastasis. Patients with BNCT are generally followed up with serial imaging surveillance. On the other hand, chordomas are treated with surgical excision with negative surgical margin being the most important predictor for survival and recurrence. A distinction between BNCT and chordoma is very important, and it is imperative to detect any early transition of BNCT to chordoma. There

Med Radiol Diagn Imaging (2023)
https://doi.org/10.1007/174_2023_456,
Published Online: 21 October 2023

is growing evidence that BNCT has a potential for malignant transformation into chordoma, and therefore there is consensus that once identified, these lesions should be carefully followed up over a long period of time to detect any early transformation into chordomas.

1 Introduction

The notochord plays an important, although transient role in human embryology, by acting as the main structural organizer for the development of the spine by providing both signaling (Corallo et al. 2015) and mechanical cues to the developing embryo. It is located in the developing midline and defines the primitive longitudinal axis of the embryo. It also plays a pertinent role in the formation of the axial musculoskeletal system as it is surrounded by sclerotomes, which form the ossification centers of the vertebral column. The developing notochord secretes signaling proteins, which play an important role in the development of surrounding structures. As development progresses, the notochordal tissue fragments and involutes and persists in the intervertebral disks of fetus and infants as the nucleus pulposus till the age of 3 (Pazzaglia et al. 1989; Salisbury 1993). The notochordal tissue is characterized histologically by physaliferous or physaliphorous cells. The word physaliphorous comes from the combination of the word physalis which means "bubble" and phoros which means "bearing." Literally speaking, physaliphorous cells means cells having a bubbly appearance. These are large polygonal cells with vacuolated cytoplasm having a central or eccentric small round nucleus (Pandiar and Thammaiah 2018). Immunohistochemically, these cells show expression of pan-cytokeratin, S100, epithelial membrane antigen, and brachyury.

Notochordal tumors are very rare as the notochordal tissue has a purely embryonic role and disappears by 8 weeks of life. However, in a small percentage of individuals, notochordal cells persist embedded within the bones of the spine and base of skull and are the precursors of the notochordal tumors. Before 1996, until the first case presented from our institution at the International Skeletal Society (ISS) annual meeting, only malignant tumors of notochordal origin were recognized, known as chordomas. Autopsy studies by Yamaguchi et al. have shown a surprisingly high incidence of benign notochordal cell tumors with the same anatomical distribution as chordomas (Yamaguchi et al. 2004b). Tumors arising from the notochordal remnants arise exclusively in the axial skeleton in the midline.

2 Notochordal Remnants

There are some helpful important anatomical points to understand these notochordal tumors. Salisbury et al. demonstrated complex forking at the rostral and caudal ends of the notochord with fragments of chordal tissue (Salisbury et al. 1993). This would explain why notochordal cells persist at the basicranial and sacral region when the rest of the notochordal tissue undergoes involution. Secondly, the notochord is very small reaching complete maturation in an embryo measuring 11 mm before it starts to involute. Thus, the size of the notochordal remnants is bound correspondingly to be very small. Thirdly, Pazzaglia et al. found that the notochordal remnants did not contribute to the intervertebral disks in adults (Pazzaglia et al. 1989). The autopsies on the neonatal spines have shown that the notochordal tissue associated with the intervertebral disks is not associated with the notochordal remnants within the vertebral bodies. It is therefore only right to assume that the notochordal remnants within the skeleton would be microscopic in size and are most likely located at the spheno-occipital and sacral region.

There have been multiple studies since 1856, showing the presence of notochordal remnants in adults in an extra-osseous location mainly around the spheno-occipital region. They have an approximate autopsy incidence of 2% and appear as small soft tissue nodules, which are soft and gelatinous with physaliferous cells on histological examination. These have been described by various authors as "ecchondrosis physaliphora spheno-occipitalis," "ectopic notochordal rests," and "benign chordoma" (Stewart and Burrow 1923; CONGDON 1952; Lakhani and Martin 2021). They have also been found in the sacrococcygeal location and rarely in the vertebrae where they are called "ecchordosis physaliphora vertebralis" and are very small and microscopic.

Since the advancement in imaging and particularly with the advent of MRI, an increasing number of sporadic cases describing the imaging appearance of asymptomatic notochordal remnants in extra-osseous location started to appear in the radiology literature (Ng et al. 1998). Mehnert et al. identified five cases of retroclival ecchordosis physaliphora, all showing low T1 and high T2 signal with none of them showing any enhancement after administration of contrast (Mehnert et al. 2004). Four of these lesions had signal changes in the adjacent clivus, and a stalk connecting these remnants to the clivus was seen in three cases. Up until 1996, these notochordal remnants were thought to be the precursors of chordomas because of the similar location and distribution in the skeleton. However, the current theory is that these remnants are more likely to be the precursors of benign notochordal cell tumors, and it is the rare malignant transformation of these benign notochordal tumors that in turn results in the development of a chordoma.

3 WHO Classification

The current WHO classification of bone and soft tissue tumors has subdivided notochordal tumors into four subtypes—benign notochordal cell tumors, conventional chordoma, poorly differentiated chordoma, and dedifferentiated chordoma based on their biological behavior and morphological features (Tirabosco et al. 2021). Irrespective of the subtype, these tumors arise from the notochordal tissue and demonstrate expression of cytokeratins and brachyury. Brachyury is a transcription factor encoded by TBXT, which is essential for notochordal development and is the diagnostic hallmark for notochordal tumors. It is the single most important immunohistochemical marker to differentiate notochordal tumors from chondrosarcoma, myoepithelial tumors, metastasis, and meningioma (Tirabosco et al. 2008).

Conventional chordoma is the most common and accounts for 95% of all chordoma cases (Lee et al. 2017). Chondroid chordoma, which was earlier thought to be a distinct variant, is now classified as conventional chondroma in which a large area of the tumor matrix resembles cartilaginous tumors. Dedifferentiated chordoma is characterized by a biphasic appearance, with a mix of conventional chordoma cells, which express brachyury and cells resembling high-grade sarcoma (Choi and Ro 2021). This subtype is rare and is seen in less than 5% of patients. It is more aggressive as suggested by the high-grade sarcomatous component, grows faster, and is more likely to metastasize than the conventional subtype. The poorly differentiated chordoma is a newly described subtype and is characterized by the deletion of the SMARCB1 (INI1) gene (Yeter et al. 2019). It is seen in children and young adults and has a female predominance. It is mostly seen in the skull base followed by the cervical spine and is rarely seen in the sacrococcygeal region.

4 Benign Notochordal Cell Tumors (BNCTs)

In 1996, at the Closed Meeting of the ISS, Cassar-Pullicino and Darby presented an unusual case of a notochordal tumor in the L5 vertebral body, which was treated with vertebrectomy. The plain radiographs and scintigraphy were normal, and this tumor demonstrated faint trabecular sclerosis on the CT without any evidence of bone destruction. MRI demonstrated this lesion to occupy the entire vertebral body and have a low T1 and high T2 signal with no bony destruction or extra-osseous extension. This case was later published in 1999 (Darby et al. 1999), and uncertainty prevailed as to its exact nature as was reflected from the title as well, "Vertebral intra-osseous chordoma or Giant notochordal rest?". There were further reports of vertebral lesions having similar radiological and histological features described by various authors. Mirra and Brien (2001) reported two cases and called them giant notochordal hamartoma of intra-osseous origin. Kyriakos et al. described a lesion confined to the vertebral body with a low T1 and high T2 signal, which was inconspicuous on the plain radiographs, scintigraphy, and CT and called it a giant vertebral notochordal rest (Kyriakos et al. 2003). This tumor lacked the typical histological features of a chordoma but consisted of physaliferous cells. All these papers and publications described a similar novel entity distinct from the known chordoma, confined to the intra-osseous compartment, and all authors struggled at finding the right nomenclature for this new tumoral entity.

The term "benign notochordal cell tumor" was coined by Yamaguchi and his colleagues. They attempted to study the morphological and immunohistochemical characteristic of benign notochordal cell tumors and differentiate them from chordomas and notochordal cell rests. BNCT shows typical physaliferous cells on histology but lacks any necrosis or intercellular myxoid matrix. There was no trabecular destruction; instead, the involved trabeculae were sclerotic. The histological features were distinct from both chordomas and notochordal cell rests. There was an overlap in the immunohistochemistry expression between chordomas and BNCT, but the notochordal vestiges did not demonstrate the expression of cytokeratin 18. As a result, the authors came up with the terminology of benign notochordal cell tumors as they were neither cell rests nor did they fulfill the criteria for hamartomas (Yamaguchi et al. 2004a).

Yamaguchi further examined 100 vertebral columns and 61 clivi dissected from the autopsy specimens and identified 26 benign notochordal cell tumors in 20 cases with a mean age of 63 years and a male:female ratio of 3:1. The respective segment distribution was 11.5% in the clivus, 12% sacrococcygeal segment, 5% cervical, and 2% lumbar vertebrae. This showed that there was a surprisingly high incidence of BNCTs and their anatomical distribution matches that of chordomas, providing supportive evidence that classic chordomas arise from BNCTs (Yamaguchi et al. 2004b).

4.1 Pathology

Histologically, the tumor is characterized by sheets of clear cells interspersed with eosinophilic vacuolated physaliferous cells (Tirabosco et al. 2021; Murphey et al. 2023). The clear cell vacuoles push the nucleus to the side mimicking large clear adipocytes and lipoblasts, which can result in an erroneous diagnosis of fatty marrow or necrotic trabeculae in osteonecrosis. Murakami et al. reported a lesion with low T1 and high T2 signal with no enhancement on contrast administration and sclerosis on CT. Histologically, there was fatty necrosis and vacuolar degeneration, and this was published as a case of vertebral body osteonecrosis without collapse (Murakami et al. 2003). However, subsequently on reviewing the radiological and histological features, they realized that it was typical of what is now described as BNCT. The cells in BNCT are arranged back-to-back with no intervening fibrous septa lacking the lobular architecture, which is typical in chordomas. There is a lack of both intercellular and extracellular myxoid matrix. The cells do not demonstrate any atypia, mitotic figures, necrosis, or hyperchromatism (Iorgulescu et al. 2013). BNCTs interdigitate within the host bone by permeating the marrow around existing bony trabeculae without causing any trabecular destruction and have a sharp demarcation from the surrounding normal marrow. There is no trabecular destruction, and the lesion is well confined to the intra-osseous compartment. Trabecular sclerosis is often seen, which can be due to reactive appositional bone formation (Murphey et al. 2023). Microscopically, BNCT can be difficult to recognize as these lesions resemble fatty marrow, which can also be entrapped within the lesion (Tirabosco et al. 2021).

BNCT shows the same immunohistochemical profile as chordomas, with co-expression of cytokeratins and brachyury (Tirabosco et al. 2021). They have positive immunostaining for cytokeratin 19 differentiating it from notochordal vestiges and fatty marrow lesions. They also show positivity for vimentin, EMA, and S100 like chordomas. It is difficult to differentiate BNCT from early transition to chordoma, and this has given rise to the term "atypical notochordal cell tumor," first suggested by Carter et al., to be used for a subset of notochordal tumors that fail to fulfill the criteria for either BNCT or chordoma (Carter et al. 2017).

4.2 Imaging

BNCTs are usually occult on radiography and do not demonstrate activity on scintigraphy (Carter et al. 2017). The larger lesions can sometime show vertebral sclerosis, most likely in the cervical spine giving rise to ivory vertebrae (Tirabosco et al. 2021).

These lesions show trabecular sclerosis on CT with no evidence of cortical breach or destruction (Fig. 1). On closer inspection, the individual trabeculae are preserved with some thickening of individual trabeculae giving rise to a collective increase in density. This is a very important differentiating feature from other diagnoses such as metastases and chordomas. A large number of BNCTs owe their detection to the advent of MRI as these lesions are often small and asymptomatic and are detected incidentally. These lesions have a reproducible imaging appearance with only slight variations. On MRI, these lesions are sharply marginated and very well demarcated from the surrounding marrow (Fig. 2). These lesions exhibit a low T1 and a high T2 signal and do not enhance after contrast administration (Fig. 3). This correlates with the fact that there is

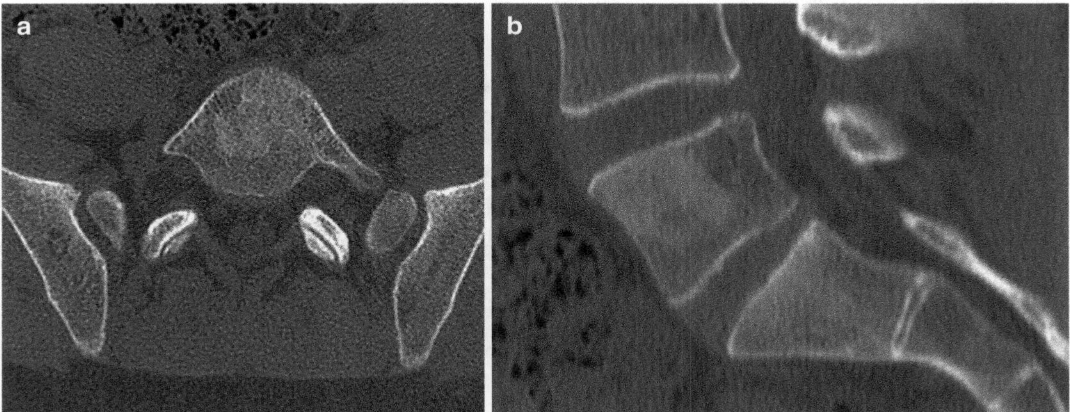

Fig. 1 (**a**) Axial and (**b**) sagittal CT of the lumbosacral spine in a patient with BNCT depicts trabecular sclerosis with no cortical breach or destruction

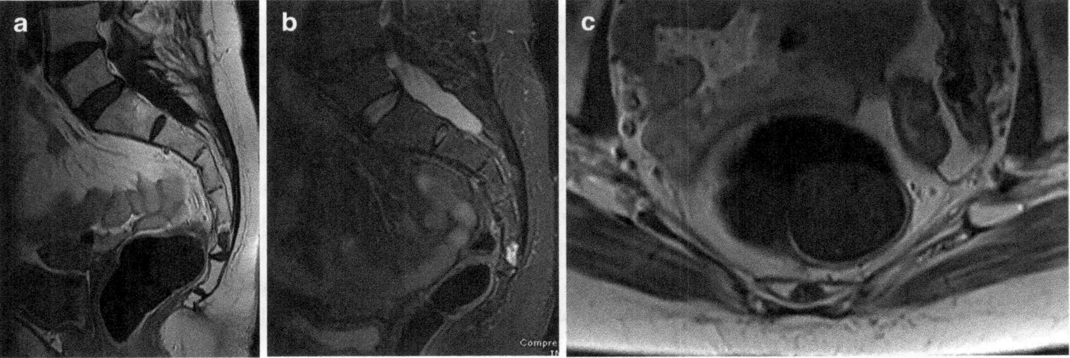

Fig. 2 (**a**) Sagittal T1, (**b**) sagittal STIR, and (**c**) axial T1-weighted MRI shows the BNCT in S5 sacral segment having a low T1 and bright STIR signal. Axial T1 shows the lesion in the midline surrounded by normal fat

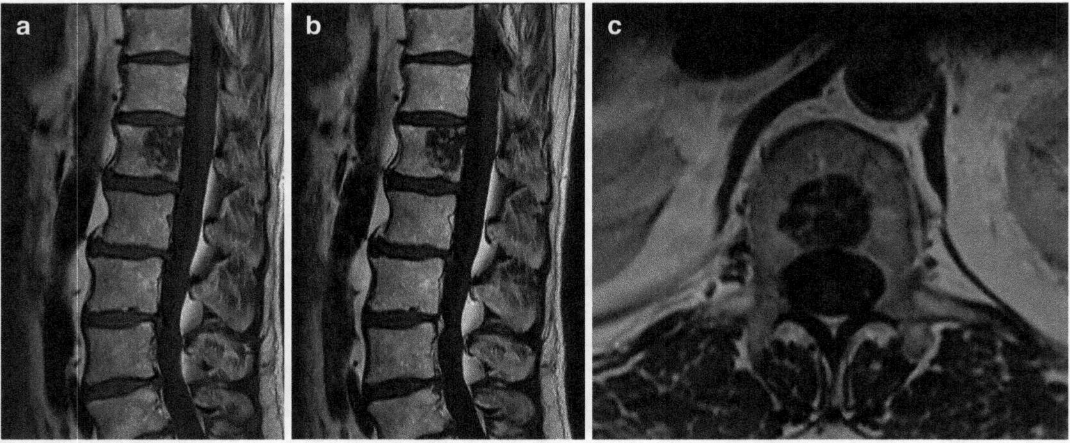

Fig. 3 (**a**) Sagittal T1, (**b**) sagittal postcontrast T1, and (**c**) axial postcontrast T1 MRI depicting a BNCT well confined to the intra-osseous compartment in L1 vertebral body with preserved end plates and posterior vertebral body margin. There are multiple foci of high signal consistent with fat representing areas of trapped normal marrow. On postcontrast administration, there is no enhancement, correlating with the scant vascular network seen histologically in these lesions

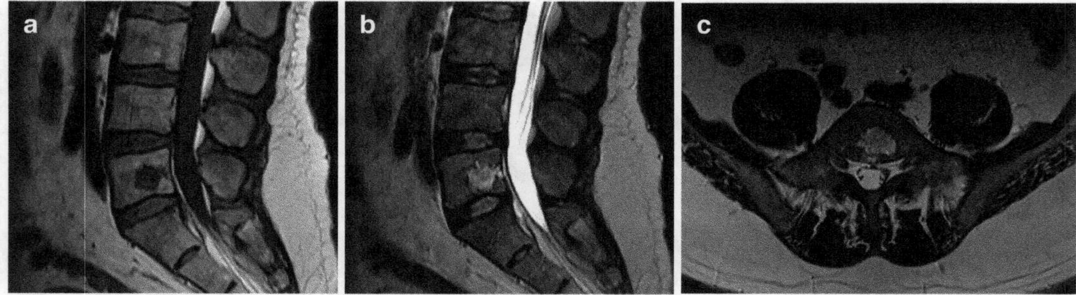

Fig. 4 (**a**) Sagittal T1, (**b**) sagittal T2, and (**c**) axial T2-weighted MRI of a biopsy-proven BNCT demonstrates a T1 hypointense and T2 hyperintense lesion in the L5 vertebral body in the midline confined to the intra-osseous compartment, with no extra-osseous extension

scanty vascular network histologically in these lesions. The lack of enhancement after contrast administration is one of the crucial imaging features to differentiate this from other lesions and chordomas. Areas of entrapped normal marrow can be detected in some of these lesions (Lalam et al. 2012). These lesions are seen in the midline, well confined to the intra-osseous compartment with no extra-osseous extension (Fig. 4). There is evidence of lesions with atypical features, which are difficult to classify having mild enhancement (Yamaguchi et al. 2008) and small extra-osseous component (Carter et al. 2017).

4.3 Differential Diagnosis

The main differential diagnosis is conventional chordoma, and it can be difficult to distinguish BNCT from early transition to chordoma. The most discriminating radiological features are sclerosis with preservation of trabecular pattern and lack of osseous destruction, absence of associated extra-osseous component, and lack of contrast enhancement. Histologically, BNCTs do not have the characteristic lobular morphology with lack of myxoid matrix and absence of necrosis and mitosis.

4.4 Prognosis

BNCT is a benign tumor with excellent prognosis. Some BNCTs can progress to chordomas, but the actual incidence is not known. When presented with a lesion resembling BNCT radiologically, there are two options available for further management, which includes biopsy/histological diagnosis or follow-up imaging. However, increasingly, follow-up imaging without biopsy is being adopted in case of lesions with BNCT-typical MRI and CT radiological appearance. Surveillance imaging is imperative to ensure stability and early detection of a transition to chordoma.

5 Atypical Notochordal Cell Tumors

Yamaguchi et al. proposed the concept of "incipient chordoma" in 2005 for lesions with histological characteristics between that of BNCT and chordoma and proposed a hypothesis that BNCT is the precursor of chordoma (Yamaguchi et al. 2005). They demonstrated two cases characterized by small infiltrative tumors containing less vacuolated cells with mild atypia and a scant amount of intercellular matrix. There was a very fine network of fibrous septa with barely discernible chordoma-specific tumor lobularity. Early in 2002, Yamaguchi demonstrated the first histological confirmed case of transformation of BNCT into chordoma in the coccyx of a 57-year-old. On histology, there was benign notochordal cell tumor adjacent to the chordoma, and two other small benign notochordal cell tumors were seen in the sacrum at a different level (Yamaguchi et al. 2002). Another retrospective histological review by Deshpande et al. suggested a causal link between the BNCT and chordoma based on the identification of coexistent BNCT and chordoma (Deshpande et al. 2007).

The WHO classification divides the notochordal tumors into benign notochordal cell tumors and chordomas with defined radiologic and histologic criteria. The management and treatment of both these lesions are very different. BNCTs are benign and confined to the intraosseous compartment with no cortical destruction or capacity for metastasis. These are generally managed conservatively with serial imaging in order to detect any early transition to chordoma (Fig. 5). Chordomas on the other hand are slow-growing locally destructive lesions with capacity for metastasis. These are treated with en bloc resection along with adjuvant therapy. Being large and bulky and because of their anatomical location, the surgery is often associated with significant morbidity. Therefore, a distinction between BNCT and chordoma is very important, and it is imperative to detect any early transition of BNCT to chordoma. However, Carter et al. found four unusual cases of notochordal tumors that did not fit into the defined criteria for BNCT or chordomas. These tumors had limited extra-osseous extension with minimal cortical permeation. Histologically, all of these resembled BNCT, but two of the lesions had small areas of focal myxoid change. These patients were followed up, two of the lesions showed no growth, one lesion had a slight increase in size of 3.7 mm over a 10-year-old time period, and one underwent sacrectomy (Carter et al. 2017). The authors proposed a designation of atypical notochordal cell tumors for this subset that fails to fulfill the diagnostic criteria for either BNCT or chordomas. They further suggested that these cases should be followed up very closely as they represent a spectrum in between benign BNCT and malignant chordomas. There is growing evidence that BNCT has a potential for malignant transformation into chordoma, and therefore there is consensus that once identified, these lesions should be carefully followed up over a prolonged period of time to detect any early transformation into chordomas (Fig. 6). The frequency of the follow-up has not been universally agreed upon, although intuitively annual MRI surveillance imaging should be done unless there is deterioration of symptoms. Once BNCT is detected, the whole spine should be screened to identify any other coexistent foci.

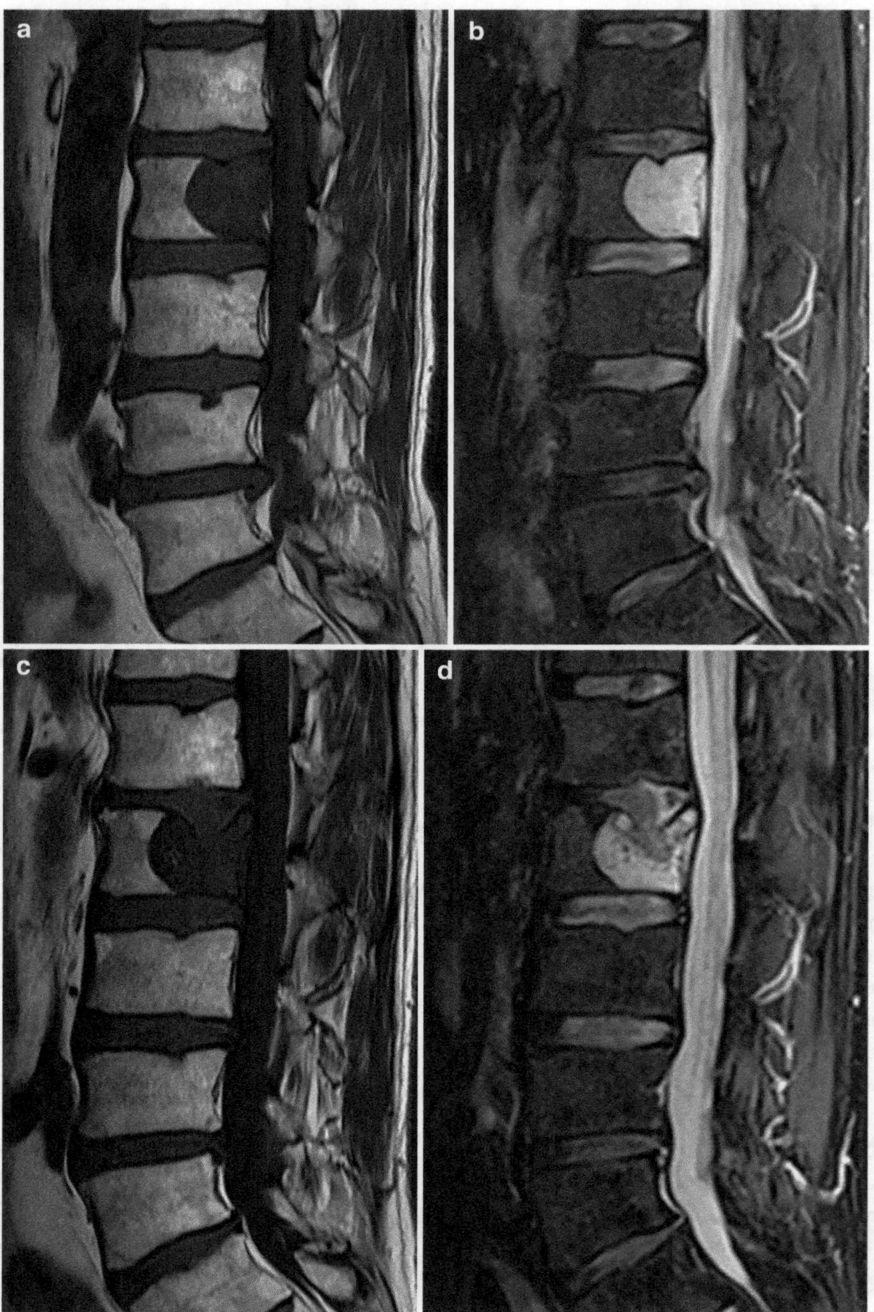

Fig. 5 (**a**) Sagittal T1 and (**b**) STIR MRI lumbosacral spine of a patient demonstrates a lesion well localized to the L2 vertebral body with no bony destruction or extra-osseous extension. The vertebral body end plates were intact. The patient was followed up with serial MRI scans. (**c**) Sagittal T1 and (**d**) STIR images 4 years later demonstrate an increase in size of the lesion with mechanical failure and infraction of the superior end plate. This prompted a CT-guided biopsy, which showed a notochordal tumor demonstrating preservation of the host trabecular bone but displaying features of progression from a "benign notochordal tumor." It was labeled as an atypical notochordal cell tumor/low-grade chordoma. There is increasing evidence that BNCT has a potential for malignant transformation into chordomas and should always be followed up

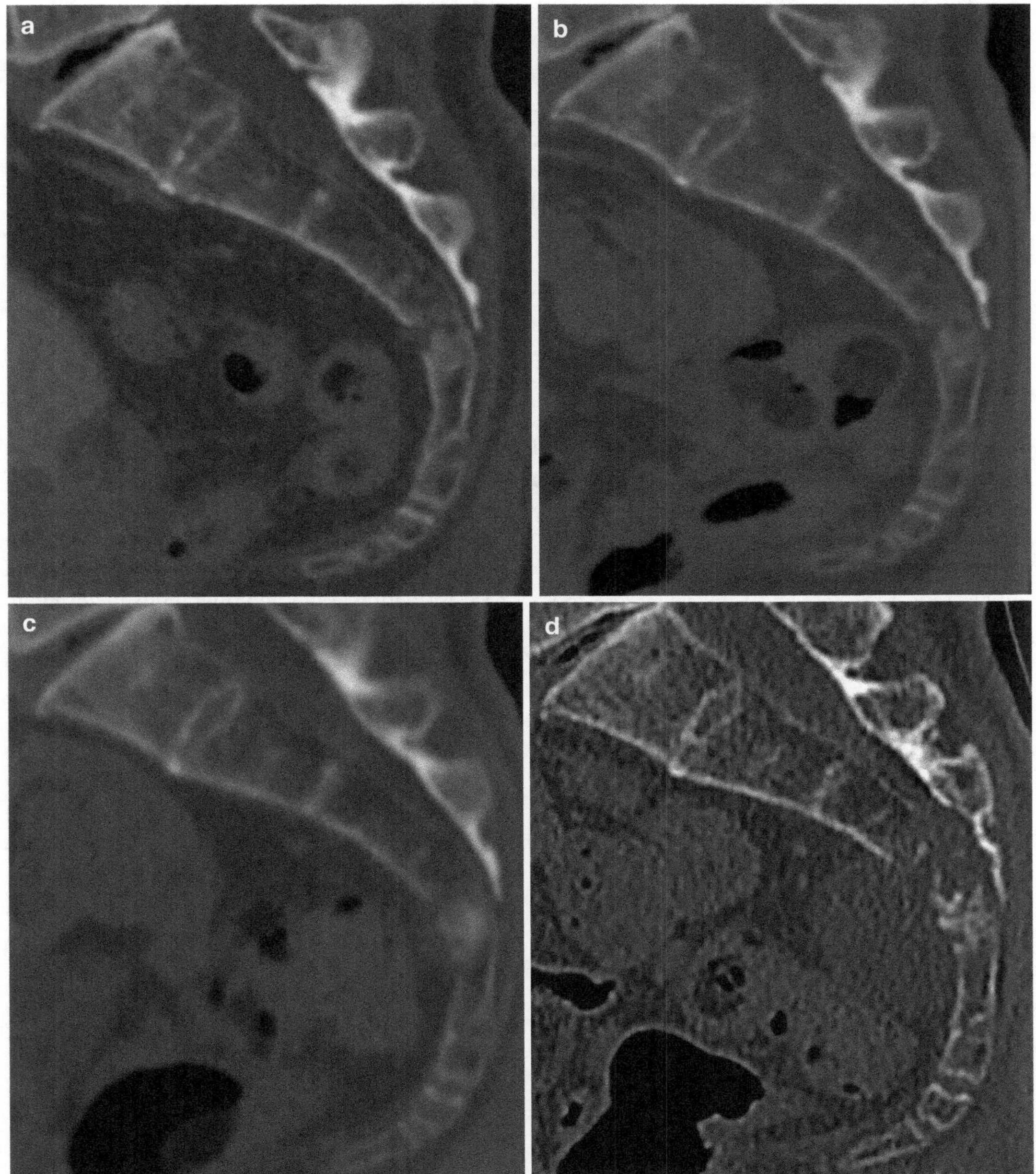

Fig. 6 (**a**) Sagittal reformatted CT in 2009 depicts a small area of anterior cortical breach in S4 spinal segment with no associated extra-osseous soft tissue component. (**b**) Sagittal CT in 2019; 10 years later depicts an increase in the anterior cortical destruction but no soft tissue mass. Further (**c**) CT in 2021 shows a definite anterior soft tissue component with associated cortical breach and trabecular sclerosis in the same spinal segment. (**d**) CT in 2022 demonstrates a large destructive lesion in S4 segment with associated extra-osseous component consistent with that of chordoma. This stresses the fact that chordomas are slow-growing tumors, further demonstrating the conversion or malignant transformation of a presumed BNCT into chordoma

6 Conventional Chordoma

Conventional chordoma is a rare primary bone tumor representing only 1–4% of all primary malignant bone tumors (Smoll et al. 2013; Murphey et al. 2023). It has an annual incidence of 0.08 per 100,000, representing around 300 annual cases in the United States and 450 cases per year in Europe according to the Surveillance, Epidemiology and End Results data from 1973 to 2009 in the United States (Smoll et al. 2013). It is the most common primary bone tumor of the sacrum, constituting of 40% of all sacral tumors and 50% of all malignant sacral tumors. Conventional chordomas can occur at any age but is most prevalent between fifth and seventh decades with a median age at diagnosis being 60 years (Eriksson et al. 1981; Smoll et al. 2013). There is a male predilection with a male-to-female ratio of 1.8:1, and Caucasians are more frequently affected (Bjornsson et al. 1993; Murphey et al. 1996; Tirabosco et al. 2021). It is rare in the Afro-American population and is often solitary.

Historically, it was reported to most commonly involve the sacrococcygeal region followed by the spheno-occipital region and mobile spine (Murphey et al. 2023). However, a more recent study from American registries (SEER program of the National Cancer Institute) found a near-equal distribution with 32% involving base of skull, 33% mobile spine, and 29% sacrococcygeal region (McMaster et al. 2001; Mukherjee et al. 2011). Sacrococcygeal conventional chordoma has a predilection for the lower sacral segments, particularly involving the S4–S5 spinal segment (Eriksson et al. 1981; Murphey et al. 1996). There can be contiguous involvement of the spinal segments or satellite lesions by spreading through the epidural space. It exclusively involves the axial skeleton and tends to be in the midline involving the center of the bone of origin (York et al. 1999).

It is a slow-growing tumor with insidious onset of clinical symptoms, which are nonspecific and location dependent. Sacrococcygeal tumors present with back pain, motor weakness, gradual onset of neuropathy and sensory symptoms, and constipation. When these tumors are large, they typically present with symptoms secondary to mass/pressure effect like bowel or bladder dysfunction, neuropathy, gait disturbance for sacrococcygeal tumors and headaches, diplopia, myelopathy, and cranial nerve dysfunction for clival tumors. Diagnosis is often delayed for months because of the nonspecific symptoms, slow growth, and unfamiliarity with this rare tumor.

6.1 Pathology

Grossly, chordomas appear as multilobulated, solid, gelatinous tumors with a yellow-tan or white-gray appearance associated with significant bone destruction, cortical permeation, and associated extra-osseous invasion. Necrosis and cyst formation containing mucinous material are common. Areas of old and new hemorrhage, sequestered bone fragments, and calcification can be seen. Chordomas are slow-growing tumors and have a low grade of malignancy, often presenting late with advanced destruction in the bone of origin. They are associated with a large extra-osseous component, which compresses and invades the surrounding structures. This includes cranial nerves in the spheno-occipital lesions and sacral plexus, bladder, rectum, and spinal canal in the sacrococcygeal tumors. Tumors in the sacrococcygeal location are often larger at presentation because there is a longer symptom-free interval for the sacrococcygeal lesions because of the anatomic location. On the other hand, symptoms of cranial nerve compression in clival lesions are early to manifest.

Histologically, they are composed of sheets or cords of large vacuolated bubbly physaliferous cells with significant nuclear atypia with pleomorphism and mitosis interspersed with small eosinophilic cells. The cells are arranged in cords and separated by fibrous septa giving the characteristic lobular appearance. There is varying range of myxoid stroma giving rise to pools of mucinous material, which is responsible for the light basophilic appearance. These tumors have a permeative pattern of trabecular destruction,

Table 1 Histological characteristics of BNCT and chordoma

Histological feature	Benign notochordal cell tumor	Chordoma
Gross features	Small intramedullary tumor without any bone expansion or destruction	Multilobulated, solid tumor with bone destruction. Necrotic and cystic areas ++
Microscopy[a]	Adipocyte-like and nonvacuolated cells with eosinophilic cytoplasm	Large epithelioid cells with vacuolated and bubbly cytoplasm-physaliphorous cells
	No intervening septa with tumor cells arranged back-to-back	Lobular architecture with intervening fibrous septa
	No intervening myxoid matrix	Minimal to large pools of mucin
	No mitosis or atypia	Significant atypia and pleomorphism
Immunohistochemistry	Co-expression of brachyury and cytokeratins	Co-expression of brachyury and cytokeratins

[a] Kindly note that BNCT histological features are often seen in cases of proven chordoma

which is often due to recruited osteoclasts. The interface between the lesion and the normal marrow depicts chronically inflamed bone due to the osteoclast recruitment. BNCTs often coexist with chordomas with an incidence of 7.3% in resected specimens of sacrococcygeal chordomas (Deshpande et al. 2007). The histological characteristics of BNCT and chordomas are depicted in Table 1.

In some tumors, the cells are closely packed resembling the pseudo-alveolar pattern seen in renal cell carcinoma. There can be variable atypia with pleomorphism and cellular spindling mimicking myxoid spindle cell sarcoma histologically (Tirabosco et al. 2021). Some tumors have features of hyaline cartilage resembling chondrosarcoma and were known as chondroid chordomas. However, in the recent WHO classification, they are classified as conventional chordoma only.

6.2 Immunohistochemistry

Regardless of the histological subtype, all notochordal tumors are characterized by co-expression of cytokeratins and brachyury. Brachyury is the diagnostic hallmark of the notochordal tumors and is helpful in differentiating these from other malignant tumors like chondrosarcoma, metastatic carcinoma, and meningioma.

An important technical point of note is that decalcification using acids like nitric and formic acid may render the specimen falsely negative for brachyury. So, if chordoma is in the differential diagnosis, specimens should be decalcified using ethylenediaminetetraacetic acid (Tirabosco et al. 2021).

6.3 Imaging Considerations

Chordomas are destructive lytic lesions, and because of the complex anatomy of the sites of involvement, it is often overlooked on plain radiographs (Fig. 7) particularly in the sacrococcygeal area (Firooznia et al. 1976). Osteosclerosis is rare but was reported in 9 out of 14 cases of spinal chordomas by De Bruine and Kroon (1988). However, five out of these nine tumors with sclerosis had no extra-osseous extension or cortical destruction. It is thereby difficult to know whether they represented true chordomas or chordomas arising in sclerotic BNCT. Because of the slow growth of this tumor and a relatively long symptom-free interval, they are often large destructive lesions at presentation associated invariably with a large lobulated extra-osseous component. The presence of mineralization can be due to calcification or entrapped bone fragments. Calcification is seen in 90% of sacral and 15% of vertebral lesions within the tumor along with residual bone fragments (Fig. 8). These tumors can have abundant myxoid matrix with mucinous contents giving rise to lobules of low attenuation on CT (Meyer et al. 1984) returning very low T1 and fluid bright signal on T2-weighted images (Rosenthal et al. 1985). There is often associated hemorrhage and necrosis giving rise to a heterogeneous appearance on MRI with areas of bright T1 signal representing blood products (Fig. 9). On contrast administration, enhancement ranges from minimal in areas of myxoid matrix as these are hypo-vascular to moderate enhancement in the fibrous intervening septa (Fig. 10). There is a prominent crisscrossing pattern secondary to the presence of septa in sacrococcygeal tumors (Sung et al. 2005).

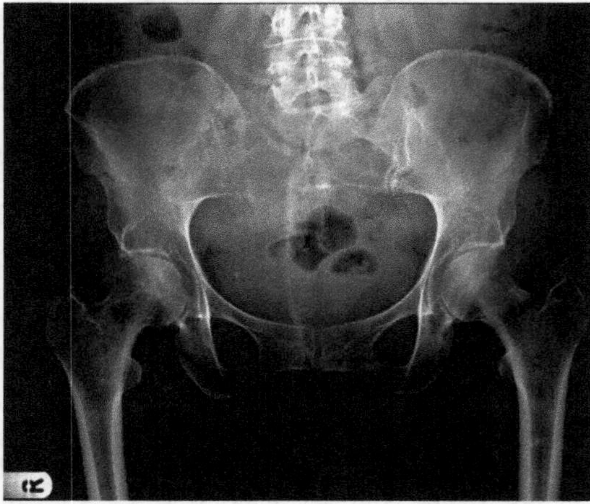

Fig. 7 Conventional AP radiograph of the pelvis demonstrating a large destructive lytic lesion involving the sacrum in a patient with sacral chordoma. It is notoriously difficult to identify chordomas on plain radiograph because of the complex anatomy and superimposition of bowel shadows

Presence of a retropharyngeal mass is common in spheno-occipital lesions, whereas an associated anterior large soft tissue component is often seen in sacrococcygeal tumors. Anterior soft tissue mass was seen in 100% of sacrococcygeal tumors with 77% having evidence of posterior extra-osseous soft tissue extension (Sung et al. 2005).

Vertebral lesions often involve the midline and are also associated with cortical destruction with an associated soft tissue mass. This mass can extend posteriorly into the spinal canal and result in spinal canal compromise (Fig. 11). There is a propensity for contiguous cranio-caudal spread spanning several spinal segments (Fig. 12) characteristically sparing the intervertebral disks till late in the disease (Meyer et al. 1984; Smolders et al. 2003). The intervertebral disks have the same signal intensity and are iso-intense to the tumor tissue; thereby, a very careful evaluation of the end plate on all sequences is important to rule out any disk invasion. The MRI signal characteristic is nonspecific, but chordoma should always be considered whenever there is a destructive lesion of vertebral body with an associated extra-osseous extension and soft tissue component, spanning multiple segments with

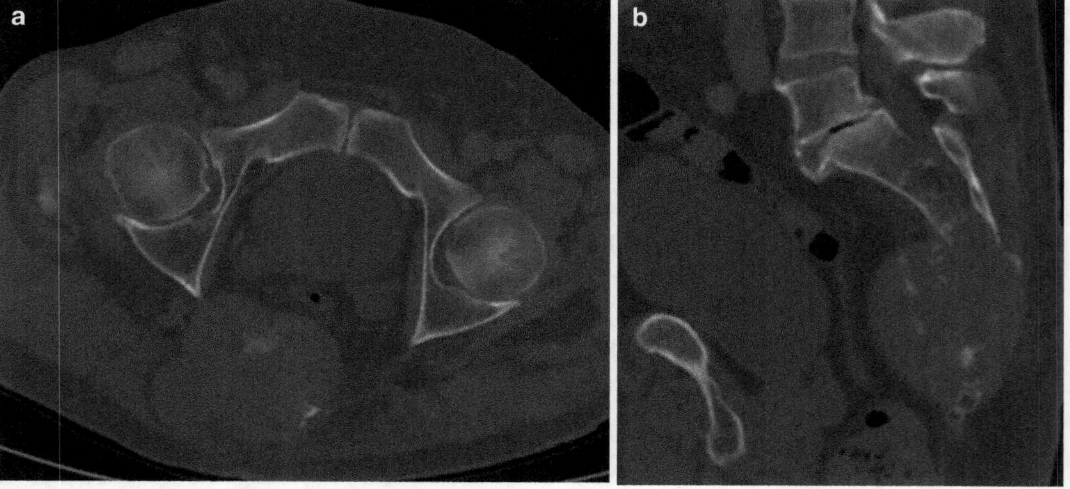

Fig. 8 (**a**) Axial CT pelvis and (**b**) sagittal reformatted CT shows the destructive sacral chordoma with calcification and bone fragments

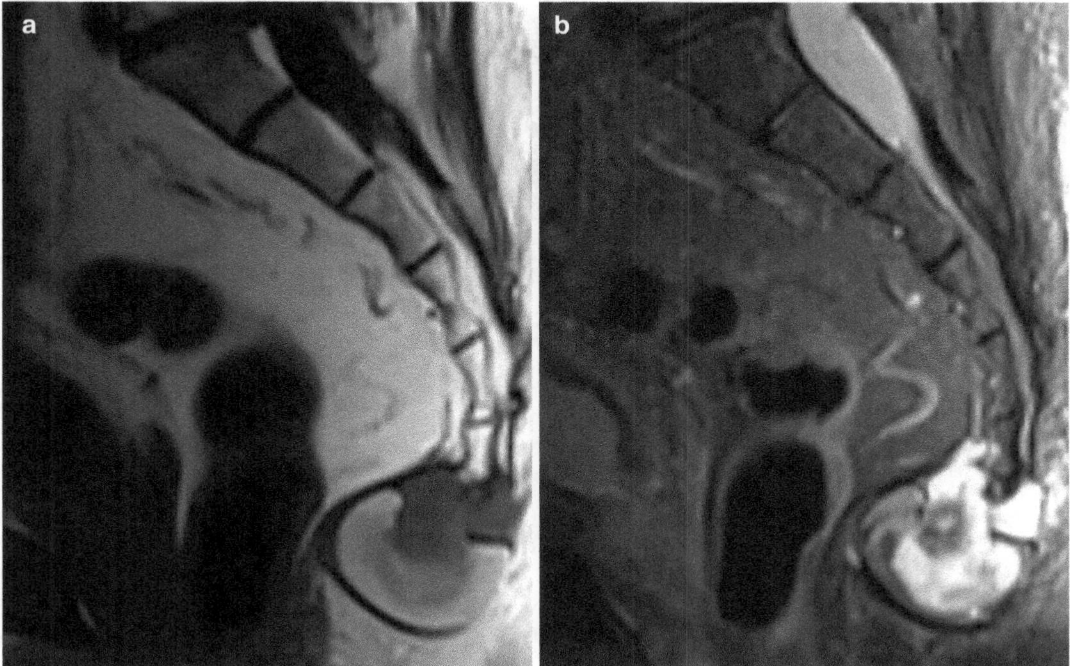

Fig. 9 (**a**) Sagittal T1 and (**b**) sagittal STIR MRI in patient with coccygeal chordoma demonstrates the large lobulated extra-osseous component with a heterogeneous signal on both T1 and STIR sequences, secondary to necrosis and hemorrhage, which is depicted as high signal on the T1-weighted MRI

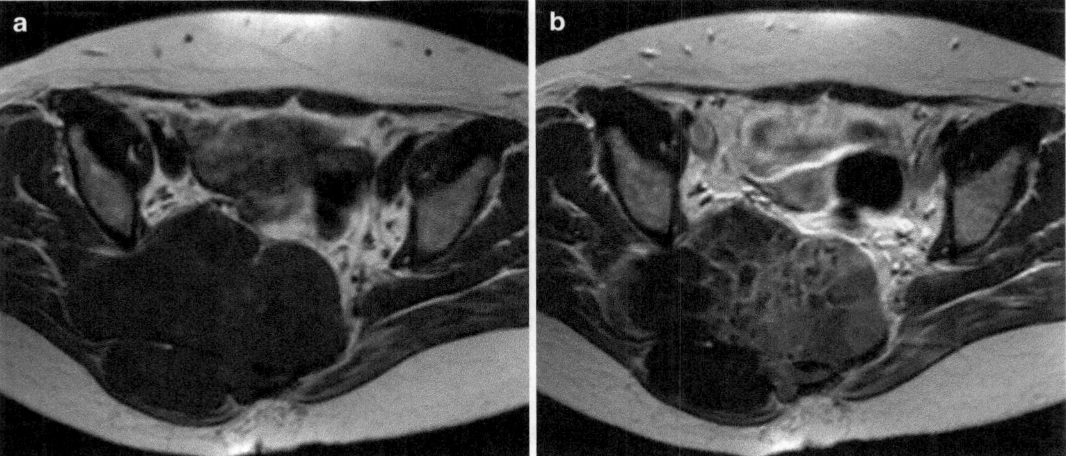

Fig. 10 (**a**) Axial T1 and (**b**) postcontrast axial T1 in a patient with a large biopsy-proven chordoma. There is a heterogeneous pattern of enhancement with areas having minimal to no enhancement, interspersed with moderate-to-avid enhancement of the intervening fibrovascular septa giving rise to the crisscross pattern. The differential diagnosis of the nonenhancing areas includes cystic, necrotic, mucoid, hemorrhagic, and dedifferentiated chordoma. In this case, the nonenhancing areas corresponded to myxoid matrix with mucinous contents

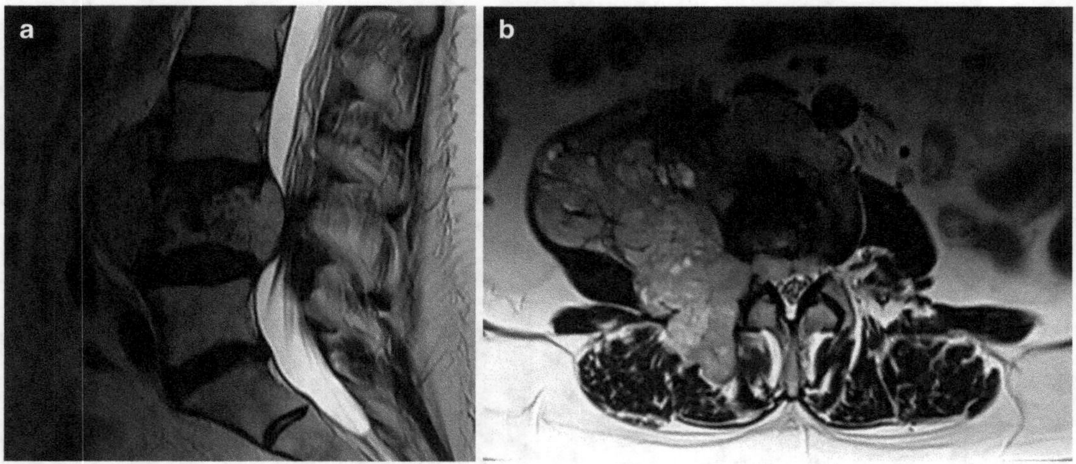

Fig. 11 (**a**) Sagittal T2 and (**b**) axial T2-weighted MRI in a patient with chordoma involving L4 vertebral body. The lesion is seen to involve the entire vertebral body with an associated extra-osseous component both anteriorly and posteriorly. There is soft tissue extending posteriorly in the epidural space encroaching on the spinal canal resulting in canal compromise. There is involvement of the superior end plate with anterior extra-osseous component extending cranially to involve the contiguous L3 segment

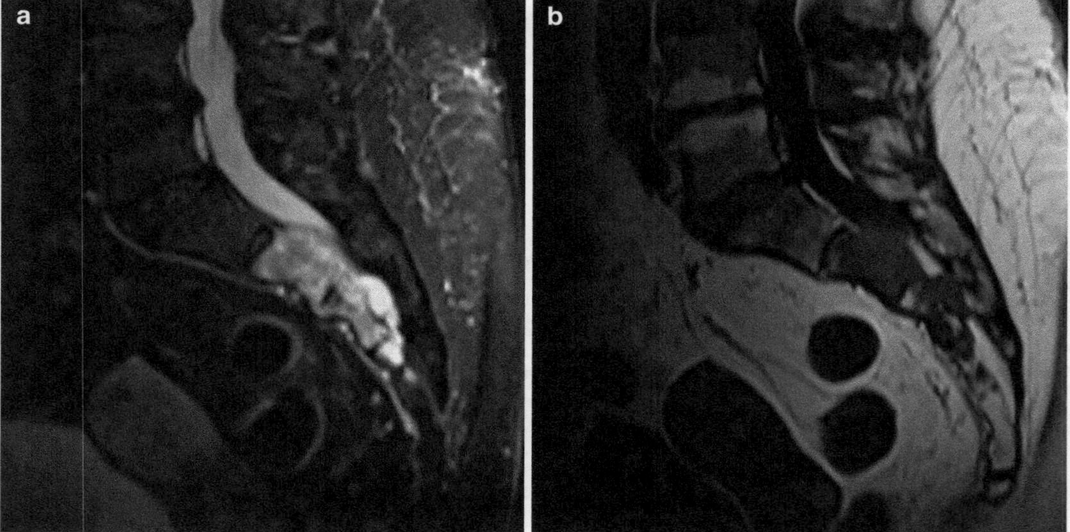

Fig. 12 (**a**) Sagittal STIR and (**b**) sagittal T1 demonstrating the contiguous multisegmental involvement in chordoma, along with posterior extension into the epidural space

sparing of the intervertebral disks. The tumor can extend posteriorly into the epidural space, and once that space is breached, there can be satellite lesions producing cranio-caudal migratory spread. Extension into the epidural space produces the "curtain sign," and if the posterior longitudinal ligament is disrupted, there is enhancement of the "epidural tail sign" (Smolders et al. 2003). There can be extension into the SI joint in 23% of cases at presentation and perineural spread along the sacral nerve roots with formation of pseudopodia in the greater sciatic foramen (Sung et al. 2005). The iliac bone involvement occurs due to the interosseous ligamentous involvement, through the extrasynovial portion of SI joint (Chhaya et al. 2005). Coronal plane is the best imaging plane to detect invasion of the sacral plexus and nerve roots within the foramina. MRI is the best modality to depict the tumor extent, but often the tumor tissue extends beyond the confines seen on the MRI and it is difficult to determine the exact tumor margin. The infiltrative nature of the tumor necessitates a generous en bloc resection with wide margins to reduce the chances of wound contamination and tumor recurrence.

Tumor recurrence is seen on imaging as enhancing soft tissue nodules in the surgical bed. The imaging characteristics are the same as the primary tumor. MRI is the imaging modality of choice to look for any recurrent or residual disease. MRI can also be used to monitor response to adjuvant therapies. There are few studies that have demonstrated the use of PET/CT and SPECT to assess the response and evaluate therapeutic benefit (Zhang et al. 2004; Di Girolamo et al. 2005). It is important to image the entire spine in patients with chordoma as there can be concomitant presence of other notochordal lesions like BNCT. If detected, these lesions can be followed up appropriately, and it avoids any confusion as if not imaged in the first instance, these can be mistaken as metastasis during follow-up.

6.4 Differential Diagnosis

The differential diagnosis for conventional chordoma includes metastasis, chondrosarcoma, myoepithelial tumors, and chordoid meningioma.

Spine involvement is one of the most common sites for metastatic spread, and in many cases, the primary is unknown with a single tumor site in the spine. Histologically, the diagnosis is straightforward; however, metastasis from mucinous adenocarcinoma and renal cell carcinoma is most likely to be confused for chordomas (Tirabosco et al. 2021). In these cases, the brachyury is the single most helpful differentiating specific marker.

A chondroid variety of chordoma was first described in 1973 by Heffelfinger et al., which contained both chondroid and cartilaginous tumor elements indistinguishable from the chondrosarcoma. The cartilaginous tissue can cause diagnostic problems and misinterpretation of these tumors as chondrosarcomas. The postcontrast appearance of chondroid chordomas can also be similar to the classic chondrosarcomas having a ring-and-arc pattern of enhancement. Chondrosarcoma is the second most common primary bone tumor and is in the radiological and histological differential for chordoma. Chondrosarcomas have similar radiological appearance presenting as osteolytic destructive lesions with associated soft tissue components and calcification. Immunohistochemistry is helpful in difficult cases because brachyury and cytokeratin are not expressed by chondrosarcomas. S100 is of no help as it is positive in both chordomas and chondrosarcomas. IDH1/2 mutation is a genetic mutation almost never found in chordomas but present in 70% of chondrosarcomas (Amary et al. 2011a, b; Pansuriya et al. 2011).

Myoepithelial tumors compose of a spectrum of tumors sharing morphological features and immune profile with salivary glands and their cutaneous counterparts. Primary malignant myoepithelial tumor of the bone has been described and often co-expresses cytokeratins and S100 in most cases. Once again, brachyury comes to the diagnostic rescue and is the ultimate distinguishing marker.

Chordoid meningioma is another differential as histologically it is composed of epithelioid cells with variable cytoplasmic vacuolation resembling physaliferous cells. However, it is a rare intracranial tumor with an incidence of 0.32–1% and is in the differential for a clival chordoma. There are areas of more typical meningioma, which help in the diagnosis, and there is strong EMA positivity without exception with no expression of cytokeratin and brachyury (Sangoi et al. 2009).

6.5 Treatment

Despite its low-grade biological behavior and slow growth, conventional chordoma presents numerous challenges for effective control. The tumor is often large at presentation, and proximity to vital structures often precludes complete resection and effective radiation therapy dose. A complete wide en bloc is the cornerstone of treatment and is difficult to achieve (Fig. 13). Negative surgical margin is the most important predictor of survival and local recurrence (Radaelli et al. 2016; Dea et al. 2019). Surgical excision requires resection of at least one sacral segment beyond the area of gross tumor (Fuchs et al. 2005). Subtotal excision of tumor predisposes to increased local recurrence.

Tumors below the SI joint (inferior to S3) are excised using a posterior trans-perineal approach, whereas tumors cranial to S3 need a combined anterior and posterior approach. Achieving wide excision margins unfortunately compromises important osseous and neural structures. Sparing S2 nerves is associated with a higher chance of preserved bladder and bowel function, which is further improved if at least one S3 nerve root is also preserved (Fuchs et al. 2005; Angelini et al. 2015; Radaelli et al. 2016). Complete sacrectomy is associated with extensive morbidity with ambulation difficulties, and sacrifice of bladder and bowel function.

Radiation therapy is largely ineffective in the absence of complete surgical excision. The proximity to important structures like spinal cord, spinal and cranial nerves, and rectum precludes the administration of a higher radiation dose.

Proton beam radiotherapy has better local control of the disease, and a combination of wide en bloc excision and proton beam radiotherapy is the preferred treatment modality (Walcott et al.

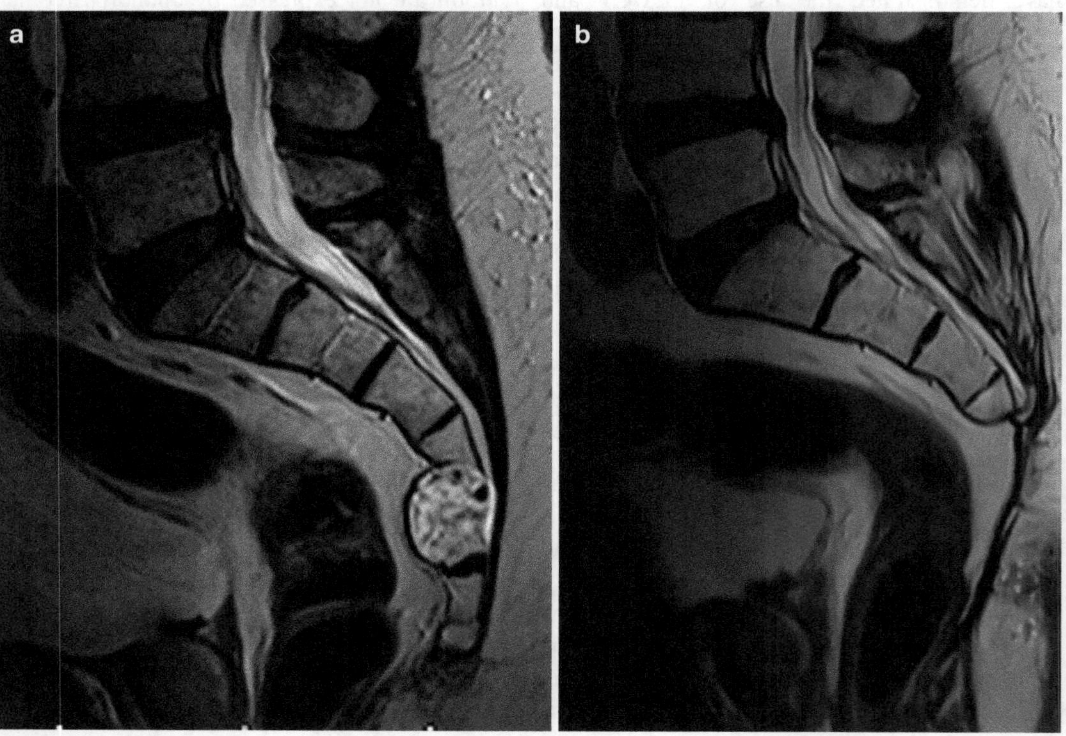

Fig. 13 (**a**) Sagittal T2 MRI depicts a chordoma involving S4/S5 spinal segments. Patient was operated upon and treated with en bloc resection with partial resection of S4. Surveillance imaging 7 years later. (**b**) Sagittal T2 MRI shows no evidence of recurrence

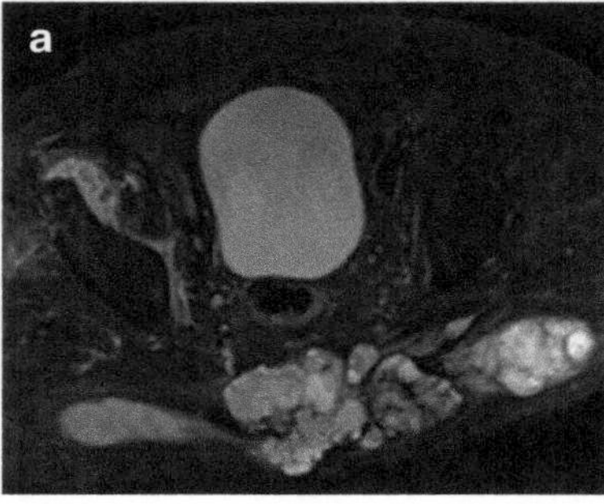
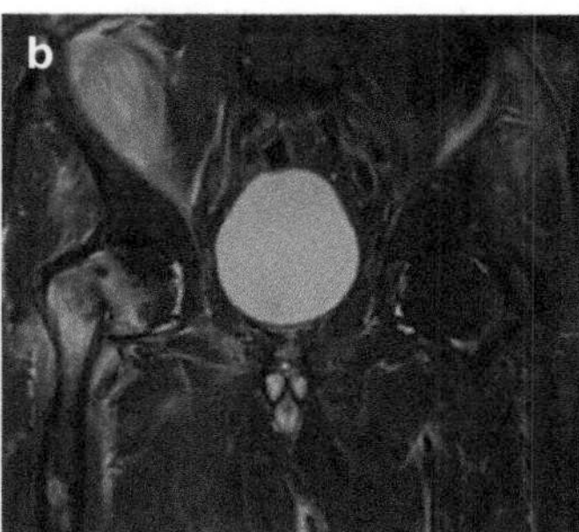
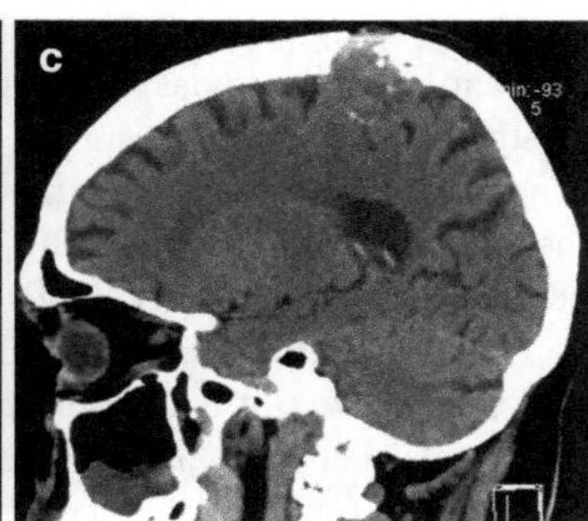

Fig. 14 (**a**) Axial pelvic STIR MRI depicting the extensive extra-osseous spread of chordoma involving posterior epidural space with extension and nodular deposits in gluteal musculature bilaterally. (**b**) Coronal pelvic STIR in the same patient demonstrates a pathological fracture secondary to a metastatic deposit in the right femoral neck. There is another metastatic deposit in the proximal right femoral shaft. (**c**) Sagittal CT skull demonstrates destructive lytic metastatic deposit in the parietal bone

2012; Delaney et al. 2014; Ahmed et al. 2015). Proton beam therapy delivers less radiation to the surrounding tissue, so a high dose of radiation is delivered to the target tumor tissue resulting in better disease control.

6.6 Prognosis

The overall median survival for a conventional chordoma is 7 years (Tirabosco et al. 2021). The prognosis depends on the site of involvement and size at presentation, which in turn governs the likelihood of a complete excision without producing significant morbidity. The median survival is less in patients with spheno-occipital lesions. Although these lesions are slow growing and are not high grade, there is still poor survival attributed to the fact that there is a very high incidence of incomplete surgical excision because of the location and size of the tumor. Tumors above the level of S2 and S3 are associated with a high incidence of local recurrence (Walcott et al. 2012; Smoll et al. 2013).

Local recurrence is frequent owing to intraoperative contamination and positive margins in large tumors in which obtaining negative margins is a challenge because of the invasion of surrounding vital structures. The rates for local recurrence range from 19% to 75% (Smoll et al. 2013; Kayani et al. 2014; Ahmed et al. 2015).

Metastases are rare and usually occur late in the course of disease (Fig. 14). The most common site of metastasis includes lungs, bone, soft tissue, and liver (Walcott et al. 2012; Smoll et al. 2013; Kayani et al. 2014). A chest CT is useful for the diagnosis of lung metastasis and is a part of the diagnostic workup. Metastasis is rare in spheno-occipital tumors as death occurs early because of the invasion of surrounding structures.

7 Poorly Differentiated Chordoma

This type of chordoma is recently added to the WHO classification with only a few cases reported in the literature. It is more commonly seen in the base of the skull and cervical vertebrae. It arises in a younger age group as compared to the conventional chordomas affecting children and young adults with a female-to-male ratio of 2:1 (Renard et al. 2014; Cha et al. 2018; Shih et al. 2018; Tirabosco et al. 2021). Headache, visual disturbances, and site-specific neurology are the most common symptoms.

The imaging appearance overlaps with that of conventional chordomas. There can be a diffuse relatively hypointense signal on the fluid-sensitive sequences and restricted diffusion on the diffusion-weighted imaging suggestive of a cellular tumor (Mobley et al. 2010).

Poorly differentiated chordoma is a solid tumor composed of epithelioid cells with signet ring and rhabdoid appearance and mild-to-moderate pleomorphism. The typical physaliphorous cells are not seen, and there is little or no myxoid stroma. Mitoses are present with substantial tumor necrosis. This type is characterized by loss of SMARCB1 (INI1) expression and by the heterozygous or homozygous deletion of the SMARCB1 gene. The differential diagnosis includes metastatic disease, malignant rhabdoid tumor, and rhabdoid meningioma.

It is very difficult to achieve complete surgical excision because of the complex anatomic location. It is generally treated with a combination of surgery: neoadjuvant or adjuvant radiotherapy and chemotherapy. It is thought to be associated with a worse prognosis than conventional chordoma (Hoch et al. 2006; Owosho et al. 2018; Shih et al. 2018).

8 Dedifferentiated Chordoma

Tumoral differentiation is defined as the emergence of a "histogenetically" distinct (i.e., different differentiation pathway) higher grade tumor in a preexisting tumor. Dedifferentiated chordoma is a biphasic high-grade tumor with a higher growth rate and metastatic potential due to the high-grade sarcomatous component. It can arise de novo or is more commonly reported in recurrences. As chordomas are slow-growing tumors, any sudden increase in size or sudden deterioration should alert the possibility of dedifferentiation. It is a rare tumor which occurs in 2–8% of cases (Hung et al. 2020).

Dedifferentiated chordoma is a high-grade biphasic tumor characterized by the presence of conventional chordoma alongside high-grade sarcomatous component. This tumor also arises in the axial skeleton as in conventional chordoma but most commonly involves the sacrococcygeal region.

The radiological appearance is similar to the conventional chordoma, but it can have a biphasic morphological appearance on MRI. There are lobular high-signal-intensity areas representing the conventional chordoma component interspersed with a demarcated, relatively hypointense mass representing the high-grade sarcoma.

The gross appearance of the tumor also has a biphasic morphology with gross features of conventional chordoma associated with a large fleshy solid tumor with large central necrotic area. Bony destruction and extra-osseous soft tissue extension are common.

On immunohistochemistry, the sarcomatous dedifferentiated component does not express the notochordal immune profile.

The differential diagnosis includes undifferentiated pleomorphic sarcoma of bone, chondrosarcoma, and osteosarcoma. Dedifferentiated chordomas can arise de novo or at the site of previously excised chordoma. A high-grade sarcoma at the site of previous chordoma should be viewed with suspicion. Another tumor to develop at the site of previously excised chordoma is a radiotherapy-induced sarcoma in cases where radiotherapy was delivered to the primary tumor. The time gap between radiation and development of sarcoma can help to differentiate between a dedifferentiated chordoma and a de novo radiation-induced sarcoma.

Dedifferentiated chordoma has a poor prognosis and a survival of less than 2 years (Tirabosco et al. 2021). Surgery is the mainstay of treatment as this tumor is not very chemo- or radiation sensitive.

9 Conclusion

There have been considerable advances in the understanding of these rare tumors over the last 10 years with a clearer role of MRI in the detection and management of these lesions. The emerging concept is that chordomas arise from a very small proportion of BNCTs (through an incipient chordoma phase), which in turn arise from microscopic notochordal remnants. Progression through these recognizable stages to classic chordoma is clearly an extremely rare event. Biopsy identification of chordoid tissue needs to be carefully correlated with MRI and CT appearances to decide if it represents BNCT or chordoma. Currently, the biological triggers of benign and malignant notochordal tumors are unclear. Future advances in molecular genetics and the roles that key molecules (e.g., brachyury) play in notochordal pathophysiology will reduce the gaps in our knowledge and form the basis of future therapeutic advances.

10 Key Points

- Benign notochordal cell tumors are sharply marginated and well demarcated from the surrounding marrow exhibiting a low signal on T1-weighted MRI and bright T2 signal, confined to the intra-osseous compartment with no extra-osseous extension.
- There is no contrast enhancement on postcontrast MRI in these lesions, and this is one of the crucial imaging features to differentiate it from other lesions.
- BNCT does not cause bone destruction and is characterized by trabecular sclerosis of varying degrees.
- There is growing evidence that BNCT has a potential for malignant transformation into chordoma, and therefore there is consensus that once identified, these lesions should be carefully followed up with MRI over a long period of time to detect any early transformation into chordomas.
- Chordomas are destructive lytic lesions having an abundant myxoid matrix giving rise to lobules having low density on CT and returning a low T1 and fluid bright signal on the fluid-sensitive sequences with associated necrosis and hemorrhage.
- Brachyury is the diagnostic hallmark of the notochordal tumors and is helpful in differentiating these from other malignant tumors like chondrosarcoma, metastatic carcinoma, and meningioma.
- A complete en bloc resection with negative surgical margins is the most important predictor of survival and local recurrence in chordomas but is difficult to achieve because of the large size at presentation and proximity to vital structures.
- Metastasis in chordoma is rare and occurs late in the course of disease, with lung, bone, soft tissue, and liver being the most common sites.

References

Ahmed R, Sheybani A, Menezes AH et al (2015) Disease outcomes for skull base and spinal chordomas: a single center experience. Clin Neurol Neurosurg 130:67–73. https://doi.org/10.1016/J.CLINEURO.2014.12.015

Amary MF, Bacsi K, Maggiani F et al (2011a) IDH1 and IDH2 mutations are frequent events in central chondrosarcoma and central and periosteal chondromas but not in other mesenchymal tumours. J Pathol 224:334–343. https://doi.org/10.1002/PATH.2913

Amary MF, Damato S, Halai D et al (2011b) Ollier disease and Maffucci syndrome are caused by somatic mosaic mutations of IDH1 and IDH2. Nat Genet 43(12):1262–1265. https://doi.org/10.1038/ng.994

Angelini A, Pala E, Calabrò T et al (2015) Prognostic factors in surgical resection of sacral chordoma. J Surg Oncol 112:344–351. https://doi.org/10.1002/JSO.23987

Bjornsson J, Wold LE, Ebersold MI, Laws EX (1993) Chordoma of the mobile spine a clinicopathologic analysis of 40 patients. Cancer 71:735–775. https://doi.org/10.1002/1097-0142

Carter JM, Wenger DE, Rose PS, Inwards CY (2017) Atypical notochordal cell tumors. Am J Surg Pathol 41:39–48. https://doi.org/10.1097/PAS.0000000000000766

Cha YJ, Hong CK, Kim DS et al (2018) Poorly differentiated chordoma with loss of SMARCB1/INI1 expression in pediatric patients: a report of two cases and review of the literature. Neuropathology 38:47–53. https://doi.org/10.1111/NEUP.12407

Chhaya S, White LM, Kandel R et al (2005) Transarticular invasion of bone tumours across the sacroiliac joint. Skelet Radiol 34:771–777. https://doi.org/10.1007/S00256-005-0016-X

Choi JH, Ro JY (2021) The 2020 WHO classification of tumors of bone: an updated review. Adv Anat Pathol 28:119–138. https://doi.org/10.1097/PAP.0000000000000293

Congdon CC (1952) Benign and malignant chordomas: a clinico-anatomical study of twenty-two cases. Am J Pathol 28:793

Corallo D, Trapani V, Bonaldo P (2015) The notochord: structure and functions. Cell Mol Life Sci 72:2989–3008. https://doi.org/10.1007/S00018-015-1897-Z

Darby AJ, Cassar-Pullicino VN, McCall IW, Jaffray DC (1999) Vertebral intra-osseous chordoma or giant notochordal rest? Skelet Radiol 28:342–346. https://doi.org/10.1007/S002560050528

De Bruine FT, Kroon HM (1988) Spinal chordoma: radiologic features in 14 cases. AJR Am J Roentgenol 150:861–863. https://doi.org/10.2214/AJR.150.4.861

Dea N, Fisher CG, Reynolds JJ et al (2019) Current treatment strategy for newly diagnosed chordoma of the mobile spine and sacrum: results of an international survey. J Neurosurg Spine 30:119–125. https://doi.org/10.3171/2018.6.SPINE18362

Delaney TF, Liebsch NJ, Pedlow FX et al (2014) Long-term results of phase II study of high dose photon/proton radiotherapy in the management of spine chordomas, chondrosarcomas, and other sarcomas. J Surg Oncol 110:115–122. https://doi.org/10.1002/JSO.23617

Deshpande V, Petur Nielsen G, Rosenthal DI, Rosenberg AE (2007) Intraosseous benign notochord cell tumors (BNCT): further evidence supporting a relationship to chordoma. Am J Surg Pathol 31:1573–1577. https://doi.org/10.1097/PAS.0B013E31805C9967

Di Girolamo S, Ottaviani F, Floris R et al (2005) Indium111 pentetreotide single photon emission computed tomography (In111 pentetreotide SPECT): a new technique to evaluate somatostatin receptors in chordomas. J Laryngol Otol 119:405–408. https://doi.org/10.1258/0022215053945886

Eriksson B, Gunterberg B, Kindblom LG (1981) Chordoma. A clinicopathologic and prognostic study of a Swedish national series. Acta Orthop Scand 52:49–58. https://doi.org/10.3109/17453678108991758

Firooznia H, Pinto RS, Lin JP et al (1976) Chordoma: radiologic evaluation of 20 cases. AJR Am J Roentgenol 127:797–805. https://doi.org/10.2214/AJR.127.5.797

Fuchs B, Dickey ID, Yaszemski MJ et al (2005) Operative management of sacral chordoma. J Bone Joint Surg Am 87:2211–2216. https://doi.org/10.2106/JBJS.D.02693

Hoch BL, Nielsen GP, Liebsch NJ, Rosenberg AE (2006) Base of skull chordomas in children and adolescents: a clinicopathologic study of 73 cases. Am J Surg Pathol 30:811–818. https://doi.org/10.1097/01.PAS.0000209828.39477.AB

Hung YP, Diaz-Perez JA, Cote GM et al (2020) Dedifferentiated chordoma: Clinicopathologic and molecular characteristics with integrative analysis. Am J Surg Pathol 44:1213–1223. https://doi.org/10.1097/PAS.0000000000001501

Iorgulescu JB, Laufer I, Hameed M et al (2013) Benign notochordal cell tumors of the spine: natural history of 8 patients with histologically confirmed lesions. Neurosurgery 73:411–416. https://doi.org/10.1227/01.NEU.0000431476.94783.C6

Kayani B, Hanna SA, Sewell MD et al (2014) A review of the surgical management of sacral chordoma. Eur J Surg Oncol 40:1412–1420. https://doi.org/10.1016/J.EJSO.2014.04.008

Kyriakos M, Totty WG, Lenke LG (2003) Giant vertebral notochordal rest: a lesion distinct from chordoma: discussion of an evolving concept. Am J Surg Pathol 27:396–406. https://doi.org/10.1097/00000478-200303000-00015

Lakhani DA, Martin D (2021) Ecchordosis physaliphora: case report and brief review of the literature. Radiol Case Rep 16:3937–3939. https://doi.org/10.1016/J.RADCR.2021.09.049

Lalam R, Cassar-Pullicino VN, McClure J, Singh J (2012) Entrapped intralesional marrow: a hitherto undescribed imaging feature of benign notochordal cell tumour. Skelet Radiol 41:725–731. https://doi.org/10.1007/S00256-012-1371-Z/METRICS

Lee IJ, Lee RJ, Fahim DK (2017) Prognostic factors and survival outcome in patients with chordoma in the United States: a population-based analysis. World Neurosurg 104:346–355. https://doi.org/10.1016/J.WNEU.2017.04.118

McMaster ML, Goldstein AM, Bromley CM et al (2001) Chordoma: incidence and survival patterns in the United States, 1973-1995. Cancer Causes Control 12:1–11. https://doi.org/10.1023/A:1008947301735/METRICS

Mehnert F, Beschorner R, Küker W et al (2004) Retroclival ecchordosis physaliphora: MR imaging and review of the literature. Am J Neuroradiol 25:1851

Meyer JE, Lepke RA, Lindfors KK et al (1984) Chordomas: their CT appearance in the cervical, thoracic and lumbar spine. Radiology 153:693–696. https://doi.org/10.1148/RADIOLOGY.153.3.6494465

Mirra JM, Brien EW (2001) Giant notochordal hamartoma of intraosseous origin: a newly reported benign entity to be distinguished from chordoma. Report of two cases. Skeletal Radiol 30:698–709. https://doi.org/10.1007/S002560100422

Mobley BC, McKenney JK, Bangs CD et al (2010) Loss of SMARCB1/INI1 expression in poorly differentiated chordomas. Acta Neuropathol 120:745–753. https://doi.org/10.1007/S00401-010-0767-X/METRICS

Mukherjee D, Chaichana K, Gokaslan ZL et al (2011) Survival of patients with malignant primary osseous spinal neoplasms: results from the Surveillance, Epidemiology, and End Results (SEER) database from 1973 to 2003. J Neurosurg Spine 14:143

Murakami H, Kawahara N, Gabata T et al (2003) Vertebral body osteonecrosis without vertebral collapse. Spine (Phila Pa 1976) 28:E323. https://doi.org/10.1097/01.BRS.0000083322.21140.90

Murphey MD, Andrews CL, Flemming DJ et al (1996) From the archives of the AFIP. Primary tumors of the spine: radiologic pathologic correlation. Radiographics 16:1131–1158. https://doi.org/10.1148/RADIOGRAPHICS.16.5.8888395

Murphey MD, Minn MJ, Contreras AL et al (2023) Imaging of spinal chordoma and benign notochordal cell tumor (BNCT) with radiologic pathologic correlation. Skelet Radiol 52:349–363. https://doi.org/10.1007/S00256-022-04158-7

Ng SH, Ko SF, Wan YL et al (1998) Cervical ecchordosis physaliphora: CT and MR features. Br J Radiol 71:329–331. https://doi.org/10.1259/BJR.71.843.9616246

Owosho AA, Zhang L, Rosenblum MK, Antonescu CR (2018) High sensitivity of FISH analysis in detecting homozygous SMARCB1 deletions in poorly differentiated chordoma: a clinicopathologic and molecular study of nine cases. Genes Chromosomes Cancer 57:89–95. https://doi.org/10.1002/GCC.22511

Pandiar D, Thammaiah S (2018) Physaliphorous cells. J Oral Maxillofac Pathol 22:296. https://doi.org/10.4103/JOMFP.JOMFP_265_18

Pansuriya TC, Van Eijk R, D'Adamo P et al (2011) Somatic mosaic IDH1 and IDH2 mutations are associated with enchondroma and spindle cell hemangioma in Ollier disease and Maffucci syndrome. Nat Genet 43(12):1256–1261. https://doi.org/10.1038/ng.1004

Pazzaglia UE, Salisbury JR, Byers PD (1989) Development and involution of the notochord in the human spine. J R Soc Med 82:413

Radaelli S, Stacchiotti S, Ruggieri P et al (2016) Sacral chordoma: long-term outcome of a large series of patients surgically treated at two reference centers. Spine (Phila Pa 1976) 41:1049–1057. https://doi.org/10.1097/BRS.0000000000001604

Renard C, Pissaloux D, Decouvelaere AV et al (2014) Non-rhabdoid pediatric SMARCB1-deficient tumors: overlap between chordomas and malignant rhabdoid tumors? Cancer Genet 207:384–389. https://doi.org/10.1016/J.CANCERGEN.2014.05.005

Rosenthal DI, Scott JA, Mankin HJ et al (1985) Sacrococcygeal chordoma: magnetic resonance imaging and computed tomography. AJR Am J Roentgenol 145:143–147. https://doi.org/10.2214/AJR.145.1.143

Salisbury JR (1993) The pathology of the human notochord. J Pathol 171:253–255. https://doi.org/10.1002/PATH.1711710404

Salisbury JR, Deverell MH, Cookson MJ, Whimster WF (1993) Three-dimensional reconstruction of human embryonic notochords: clue to the pathogenesis of chordoma. J Pathol 171:59–62. https://doi.org/10.1002/PATH.1711710112

Sangoi AR, Dulai MS, Beck AH et al (2009) Distinguishing chordoid meningiomas from their histologic mimics: an immunohistochemical evaluation. Am J Surg Pathol 33:669–681. https://doi.org/10.1097/PAS.0B013E318194C566

Shih AR, Cote GM, Chebib I et al (2018) Clinicopathologic characteristics of poorly differentiated chordoma. Mod Pathol 31:1237–1245. https://doi.org/10.1038/S41379-018-0002-1

Smolders D, Wang X, Drevelengas A et al (2003) Value of MRI in the diagnosis of non-clival, non-sacral chordoma. Skelet Radiol 32:343–350. https://doi.org/10.1007/S00256-003-0633-1

Smoll NR, Gautschi OP, Radovanovic I et al (2013) Incidence and relative survival of chordomas: the standardized mortality ratio and the impact of chordomas on a population. Cancer 119:2029–2037. https://doi.org/10.1002/CNCR.28032

Stewart MJ, Burrow JLEF (1923) Ecchordosis physaliphora spheno-occipitalis. J Neurol Psychopathol 4:218–220. https://doi.org/10.1136/JNNP.S1-4.15.218

Sung MS, Lee GK, Kang HS et al (2005) Sacrococcygeal chordoma: MR imaging in 30 patients. Skelet Radiol 34:87–94. https://doi.org/10.1007/S00256-004-0840-4

Tirabosco R, Mangham DC, Rosenberg AE et al (2008) Brachyury expression in extra-axial skeletal and soft tissue chordomas: a marker that distinguishes chordoma from mixed tumor/myoepithelioma/parachordoma in soft tissue. Am J Surg Pathol 32:572–580. https://doi.org/10.1097/PAS.0B013E31815B693A

Tirabosco R, O'Donnell P, Flanagan AM (2021) Notochordal tumors. Surg Pathol Clin 14:619–643. https://doi.org/10.1016/J.PATH.2021.06.006

Walcott BP, Nahed BV, Mohyeldin A et al (2012) Chordoma: current concepts, management, and future directions. Lancet Oncol 13:e69. https://doi.org/10.1016/S1470-2045(11)70337-0

Yamaguchi T, Iwata J, Sugihara S et al (2008) Distinguishing benign notochordal cell tumors from vertebral chordoma. Skelet Radiol 37:291–299. https://doi.org/10.1007/S00256-007-0435-Y

Yamaguchi T, Suzuki S, Ishiiwa H et al (2004a) Benign notochordal cell tumors: a comparative histological study of benign notochordal cell tumors, classic chordomas, and notochordal vestiges of fetal intervertebral discs. Am J Surg Pathol 28:756–761. https://doi.org/10.1097/01.PAS.0000126058.18669.5D

Yamaguchi T, Suzuki S, Ishiiwa H, Ueda Y (2004b) Intraosseous benign notochordal cell tumours: overlooked precursors of classic chordomas? Histopathology 44:597–602. https://doi.org/10.1111/J.1365-2559.2004.01877.X

Yamaguchi T, Watanabe-Ishiiwa H, Suzuki S et al (2005) Incipient chordoma: a report of two cases of early-stage chordoma arising from benign notochordal cell tumors. Mod Pathol 18:1005–1010. https://doi.org/10.1038/MODPATHOL.3800378

Yamaguchi T, Yamato M, Saotome K (2002) First histologically confirmed case of a classic chordoma arising in a precursor benign notochordal lesion: differential diagnosis of benign and malignant notochordal lesions. Skelet Radiol 31:413–418. https://doi.org/10.1007/S00256-002-0514-Z

Yeter HG, Kosemehmetoglu K, Soylemezoglu F (2019) Poorly differentiated chordoma: review of 53 cases. APMIS 127:607–615. https://doi.org/10.1111/APM.12978

York JE, Kaczaraj A, Abi-Said D et al (1999) Sacral chordoma: 40-year experience at a major cancer center. Neurosurgery 44:74–80. https://doi.org/10.1097/00006123-199901000-00041

Zhang H, Yoshikawa K, Tamura K et al (2004) [(11)C] methionine positron emission tomography and survival in patients with bone and soft tissue sarcomas treated by carbon ion radiotherapy. Clin Cancer Res 10:1764–1772. https://doi.org/10.1158/1078-0432.CCR-0190-3

Langerhans Cell Histiocytosis

Apolline Dufour, Sébastien Aubert, Héloïse Lerisson, Mohamed El Fayoumi, Daniela Rapilat, and Nathalie Boutry

Contents

A. Dufour · H. Lerisson · M. El Fayoumi · D. Rapilat
N. Boutry (✉)
Service d'Imagerie de l'Enfant, Hôpital Jeanne de Flandre, CHRU de Lille, Lille Cedex, France
e-mail: heloise.lerisson@chu-lille.fr; mohamed.elfayoumi@chu-lille.fr; daniela.rapilat@chu-lille.fr; nathalie.boutry@chu-lille.fr

S. Aubert
Service de Pathologie, CHRU de Lille, Lille Cedex, France
e-mail: sebastien.aubert@chu-lille.fr

Med Radiol Diagn Imaging (2023)
https://doi.org/10.1007/174_2023_442,
Published Online: 06 July 2023

Abstract

Langerhans cell histiocytosis (LCH) is a disease of children and young adults that can affect any organ. It leads to a variable infiltration of the organ by cells belonging to the mononuclear phagocytic system. Bone is most often involved (60–80% of cases). Bone involvement in LCH predominates in the axial skeleton, but spinal involvement is rare. It may be unique or more rarely multifocal. In decreasing order of frequency, the thoracic, lumbar, and cervical spines are affected. Involvement of the sacrum is exceptional. On conventional radiography and CT scan, LCH causes nonspecific osteolysis of the vertebral body, which may or may not extend to the posterior arch. The intervertebral disks are preserved. Variable degree of vertebral compression is sometimes associated, sometimes resulting in a *vertebra plana*, which is highly suggestive—although nonspecific—for the LCH in children. MRI is very useful to evaluate tumor extension to the paravertebral soft tissues and especially the epidural and/or foraminal extension, which is generally limited. The final diagnosis is based on histopathological examination of the biopsy specimen from the most accessible site, either osseous or not. Distant staging is based on skeletal radiographs, even if they lack sensitivity. Whole-body MRI (distant staging) and PET-PET/CT (for follow-up and response to treatment) provide useful information but do not necessarily alter treatment management. Since treatment depends largely on the location of the lesions and the potential functional consequences, it varies from watchful waiting to systemic chemotherapy. If the bone involvement is isolated, the prognosis is generally good. It is more reserved in case of multisystemic involvement, especially if the child is very young.

1 Introduction

Langerhans cell histiocytosis (LCH), formerly known as “histiocytosis X,” is a rare disorder characterized by clonal proliferation of cells belonging to the mononuclear phagocyte system and expressing Langerhans markers (CD1a, CD207 also called langerin). By accumulating in the various tissues of the body, Langerhans cells are responsible for focal or more extensive lesions. In decreasing order of frequency, bone, skin, and pituitary gland are most affected (Donadieu et al. 2012; Haupt et al. 2013), but all organs can be involved, including the lung, liver, spleen, hematopoietic system, lymph nodes, central nervous system (other than the pituitary gland), thymus, etc. The clinical spectrum of LCH is therefore very broad, ranging from an isolated, asymptomatic bone lesion to the severe multisystemic involvement that can lead to the death of the patient.

Historically, various clinical entities were initially described:

- The first and most frequent one corresponds to *eosinophilic granuloma*, which is defined as a benign osteolytic lesion, either single or multiple. This is the so-called localized form of the disease. It can occur at any age but most commonly affects children and adolescents. The prognosis is generally good.
- The second form, also called *Hand-Schuller-Christian disease*, is defined by the triad of (1) exophthalmos, (2) diabetes insipidus, and (3) bony lesions of the cranial vault. This represents the so-called chronic relapsing form of the disease. It is most frequent around the age of 2–3 years. The prognosis is variable.
- The third and rarest form is a multisystemic disease called *Letterer-Siwe disease*. This is the so-called fulminant form of the disease, characterized by combined hematological, hepatic, and splenic involvement. It usually occurs before the age of 2 years. The progno-

sis was generally poor before the era of targeted therapies that changed completely the outcome of the disease.
– The last form is very rare and corresponds to an exclusively cutaneous form called *Hashimoto-Pritzker* disease. It is found in newborns. The prognosis is generally excellent because the lesions disappear spontaneously.

Currently, these different clinical entities are grouped under the generic term LCH. Depending on the affected organ and disease extent at initial diagnosis, the Histiocyte Society (2009) now distinguishes patients with monosystemic LCH (SS-LCH) from patients with multisystemic LCH (MS-LCH) (Table 1). Some of these patients present with involvement of the "at-risk" organs such as the hematopoietic system, the spleen, and the liver. In other words, patients with involvement of these organs (OR+) have an increased risk of development of complications compared to patients without involvement of these organs (OR−) (Donadieu et al. 2012). In addition, involvement of some locations requires special attention because of the possible repercussions in terms of prognosis and treatment:

– Patients with involvement of certain anatomical location within the bone and/or critical soft tissue extension: base of the skull, craniofacial involvement (including eye, ear, and oral cavity), odontoid process of C2, vertebral involvement with epidural extension (Donadieu et al. 2012; Grois et al. 2006, 2010; Zhong et al. 2010)
– Patients with neurological damage related to acute pseudotumor lesions (meningeal damage, cerebral pseudotumors) (Grois et al. 2010; Le Guennec et al. 2016)
– Patients with neurocognitive disorders and pseudo-degenerative lesions on MRI (cortical atrophy, hypersignal on T2-weighted images (WI) in the white matter, increased signal in the deep gray matter on T1-WI) (Grois et al. 2010; Le Guennec et al. 2016)

Table 1 Classification of LCH according to the extent of the disease[a]

Monosystemic LCH = SS-LCH Involvement of only one of the following organs: – **Bone** (single piece of bone) – **Skin** – **Pituitary gland** – **Lymph nodes** (except drainage node of another LCH lesion) – **Lungs** – **Central nervous system** – **Other (thymus, thyroid, etc.)**	**Monosystemic LCH = SS-LCH** With **multifocal** bone involvement
	Monosystemic LCH = SS-LCH With involvement of **particular** location
	Monosystemic LCH = SS-LCH Associated with a neurodegenerative risk
Multisystemic LCH = MS-LCH Involvement of **two or more** organs	**Without** involvement of organs at risk = **RO−** (hematopoietic system, spleen, liver)
	With involvement of organs at risk = **RO+** (hematopoietic system, spleen, liver)

[a] Modified from Histiocyte Society (2009)

It should be noted that in monosystemic LCH, patients with isolated pulmonary involvement constitute a separate group requiring specific treatment. It affects predominantly adults, usually smokers (Girschikofsky et al. 2013).

The evolution of LCH at the time of diagnosis is variable and unpredictable, as initial involvement of a single organ can progress in some cases to multisystem involvement (Donadieu et al. 2012; Girschikofsky et al. 2013).

In this chapter, we focus on the involvement of the osseous spine, either isolated (SS-LCH, single involvement), associated with other bone involvement of the axial skeleton and/or the appendicular skeleton (SS-LCH, multifocal involvement), or associated with extra-osseous involvement (MS-LCH).

2 Pathologic Features

Langerhans cells belong to the mononuclear phagocytic system. They originate in the bone marrow and then migrate hematogenously to the skin and the pluristratified epithelia where they organize themselves into networks (Thomas et al. 2007). Described for the first time in 1868 (Langerhans 1868), the Langerhans cell has a characteristic histological appearance. On light optical microscopy, it appears as a dendritic cell containing a kidney-shaped, eccentric nucleus, surrounded by a clear, eosinophilic cytoplasm (Thomas et al. 2007). Its cytoplasm contains specific micro-organelles, also called Birbeck granules, resembling "tennis rackets" on electron microscopy. The Langerhans cell expresses on the surface various phenotypic markers and in particular CD1a antigen, CD207 antigen (langerin), and molecules of the type II major histocompatibility complex (Thomas et al. 2007). Other membrane markers are present but non-specific: protein S100, adenosine triphosphatase (ATPase), and α-D-mannosidase. The Langerhans cell plays an important role in the immune response of the skin as an antigen-presenting cell.

The population of cells found in LCH express the same Langerhans markers (CD1a and CD207) and also contain Birbeck granules. However, they have less antigen-presenting function than Langerhans cells, and they express other membrane markers including peanut agglutinin (PNA), placental alkaline phosphatase (PLAP), and interferon gamma receptor (Thomas et al. 2007). Finally, contrary to the Langerhans cells which are exclusively found in the skin and the pluristratified epithelia, the cells of the LCH can infiltrate one or more organs to form there a tumor resembling histologically an "inflammatory granuloma." This granuloma contains the LCH cells within a polymorphic inflammatory infiltrate made up predominantly of polymorphonuclear eosinophils (hence the old name "eosinophilic granuloma"). Any organ can be affected, but bone is affected in most cases (80%) (Donadieu et al. 2012), in particular, the flat bones of the axial skeleton (cranial vault, ribs, pelvis) and the long bones of the appendicular skeleton (humerus, femur, tibia).

The exact etiology of the condition remains unknown. LCH is currently considered as an inflammatory myeloid neoplasia, similar to Erdheim-Chester disease (non-Langerhans cell histiocytosis) (Haute autorité de Santé 2021; Émile et al. 2016). Various recurrent somatic (non-transmissible) mutations have been identified in these two conditions in approximately ¾ of cases (Héritier et al. 2017), particularly the V600E mutation of the BRAF gene associated with cancers (Girschikofsky et al. 2013; Héritier et al. 2017). This mutation leads to the activation of the RAS-RAF-MEK-ERK signaling pathway of "mitogen activated protein kinases" (MAPKs), proteins involved in various cellular activities (proliferation, differentiation, migration, apoptosis). Its presence is correlated with severe damage in infants and with neurodegenerative damage to LCH (Haute autorité de Santé 2021).

Whatever the etiology may be, LCH leads to clonal proliferation (except for isolated pulmonary LCH (Yousem et al. 2001)) of Langerhans cells, but LCH does not have the characteristics of cancer, as the disease may regress spontaneously, it has no tendency for locoregional extension, and there is absence of distant metastases (Haute autorité de Santé 2021).

3 Epidemiology

LCH is a rare condition with an estimated annual incidence of 2–5 cases/million/year in children and 1–2 cases/million/year in adults (Allen et al. 2018; Reisi et al. 2021). Although it can theoretically occur at any age, most cases (eight out of ten) occur in children and adolescents under 15 years of age (Greenlee et al. 2007). Its peak incidence is between 5 and 15 years of age, with a mean age at diagnosis of 3 years for all clinical forms, 4 years and 6 months for multifocal bone involvement, and 5 years and 6 months for isolated bone involvement (Jha and De Jesus 2022). LCH is extremely rare in the neonatal period and in adults. It is considered exceptional after the age of 50 years (Reisi et al. 2021).

The condition affects predominantly males with a sex ratio of 1.2 to 2:1 (Jha and De Jesus 2022; Zhao et al. 2021). Cases of LCH within the same family have been reported, but the hereditary nature of the disease is not recognized (Jha and De Jesus 2022).

4 Localization

As previously mentioned, LCH lesions can occur anywhere in the body, but the bone is the most frequently affected organ, in 60–80% of cases (Zhao et al. 2021; Angelini et al. 2017). Other organs affected are, in descending order of frequency, skin (33%), pituitary gland (25%), liver (15%), spleen (15%), hematopoietic system (15%), lungs (15%), lymph nodes (5–10%), and central nervous system (2–4%) (Zhao et al. 2021).

Bone involvement predominates in the flat bones of the axial skeleton (skull, ribs, pelvis) and in the metaphysis of the long bones, especially the femur. The skull, ribs, and pelvis alone account for 50% of bone involvement in LCH (Reisi et al. 2021). Furthermore, solitary bone involvement is significantly more common than multifocal involvement, with a ratio of 3 to 4:1 (Reisi et al. 2021). According to Bertram et al., bone involvement is isolated in 79% of cases, multifocal in 7%, and associated with extra-osseous involvement in the remaining 14% of cases (Bertram et al. 2002).

Spinal involvement is rare, occurring in 6.5–25% of LCH with bone involvement (Jiang et al. 2011). It is more often solitary (~30%) than multifocal (~70%), and if multifocal, the involved vertebrae are usually nonadjacent (Vadivelu et al. 2007). When two adjacent vertebrae are involved, the intervertebral disk is preserved. Any segment of the spine may be affected, but the thoracic spine is the most frequently affected (55% of cases), followed by the lumbar spine (35% of cases) and then the cervical spine (10% of cases) (Bertram et al. 2002; Prasad and Divya 2019). Sacral involvement has been very rarely reported (Reisi et al. 2021). LCH preferentially affects the vertebral body; the vertebral end plates are typically spared, at least at the initial stage. Although the posterior arch is typically spared, it is not uncommon that vertebral body involvement extends to the pedicles and, in particular, to the transverse processes at the level of the cervical spine. Although disk involvement by contiguity from the vertebral body and paravertebral soft tissues has been reported in adults (Özdemir et al. 2016), this pattern of extension remains unusual. Finally, isolated involvement of the posterior arch is extremely rare (Jiang et al. 2011; Prasad and Divya 2019).

5 Clinical Presentation

The clinical presentation of spinal LCH is variable, depending on the location, but pain remains the main symptom in about 80% of cases (Thomas et al. 2007). Patients tend to describe pain with an inflammatory pattern (David et al. 1989; Huang et al. 2007). Pain may be associated with limitation of motion, torticollis at the cervical level, or, more rarely, a functional deficit. Swelling may occur if the spinal involvement is accompanied by paravertebral tumor extension (Tyagi et al. 2011). If the soft tissue component extends to the epidural space and/or intervertebral foramina, compression of the spinal cord and/or nerve roots may occur. However, these neurological complications remain rare and are usually of moderate intensity (paresthesia, radiculalgia), although cases of obvious spinal cord (Vadivelu et al. 2007; Tyagi et al. 2011; Villas et al. 1993; Montemurro et al. 2013) or nerve (Bilge et al. 1995) compression have been reported. Neurological complications are more frequent in adults than in children (Huang et al. 2013). In young children, systemic signs such as asthenia and intermittent fever are sometimes present. Other rare symptoms that may reveal LCH include progressive limp (Bodart et al. 1999), atypical painful scoliosis (Huang et al. 2007), or thoracic kyphosis related to one or more vertebral compression fractures.

Overall, the clinical symptomatology of LCH is extremely variable; the spinal signs are not always pronounced, especially if the spinal damage is associated with other bone or extra-osseous involvement. Finally, it should not be forgotten that LCH may be incidentally discovered.

6 Imaging

The key points in imaging are summarized in Table 2.

6.1 Conventional Radiography (CR)

CR of the spine remains the first-line examination for spinal involvement, but it lacks sensitivity in the early stages of the disease, since cortico-medullary destruction must be sufficient (~30–50% at least) to be visible radiographically. In addition, some areas remain difficult to explore radiographically: cervico-occipital junction, upper thoracic spine (due to superimposition of shoulders on lateral views), and lumbar spine (due to superimposition of gas within the gastrointestinal tract on anteroposterior view in children).

Table 2 Spinal involvement in LCH: key points in imaging

- Spinal + extra-spinal bone involvement (axial skeleton +++) > spinal bone involvement alone
- Thoracic spine > lumbar spine > cervical spine (sacrum involvement exceptional)
- Single spinal involvement ≫ multiple spinal involvement
- Vertebral body alone > vertebral body + posterior arch > posterior arch alone
- Mainly osteolysis
- Possible presence of bone sequestration within the osteolysis
- Possible vertebral collapse ± spinal static disorders
- *Vertebra plana* suggestive of the diagnosis in children, but not pathognomonic
- Interest of CT scan to determine the extent of cortico-tabular osteolysis (and to assess the risk of fracture)
- Interest of MRI to judge the possible extension to the spinal canal and intervertebral foramina
- Nonspecific MRI signal but extensive signal anomalies around the bone lesion (bone marrow, soft tissue)
- Extension assessment: skeletal radiographs ± abdominal ultrasound
- Place of CE MRI and PET-PET/CT has to be defined

LCH begins with well-limited osteolysis of the vertebral body, usually respecting the vertebral end plates (Kaplan et al. 1998), the posterior arch, and the overlying and adjacent intervertebral disks. Although the posterior arch is typically preserved on CR, osteolysis may extend to the posterior arch, particularly into one of the pedicles, resulting in a "one-eyed" vertebra on an anteroposterior view (Fig. 1). When the osteolysis progresses further, it may be complicated by vertebral compression (Fig. 2). The collapse may be initially asymmetric on an anteroposterior view before becoming symmetric (Huang et al. 2007). It may or may not be associated with infiltration of the adjacent soft tissues, which is difficult to see on CR. In children, and especially in the thoracolumbar spine, vertebral compression may be complete and results in about 15% of cases in a typical *vertebra plana* (Kaplan et al. 1998) (Fig. 3). This *vertebra plana* is found more rarely in adults (Garg et al. 2006) and at the cervical spine (Dikinson and Farhat 1991). The early onset of symptoms in the case of cervical involvement (pain, torticollis) and the existence of greater compression forces at the thoracolumbar

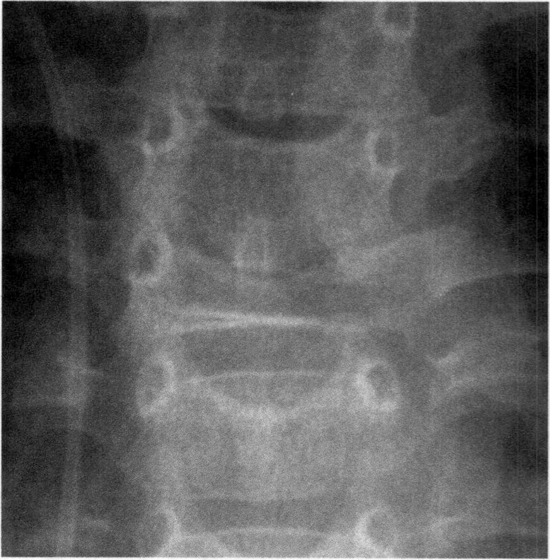

Fig. 1 Note the disappearance of the left pedicle of T5 on the anteroposterior spine radiograph

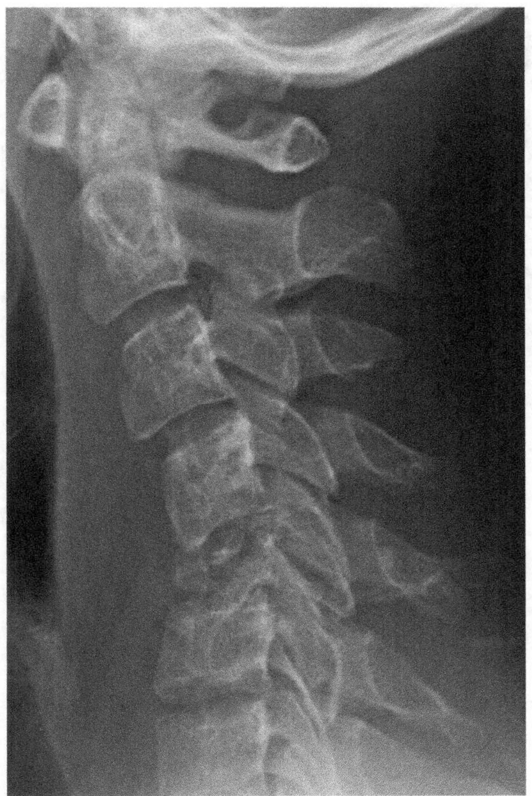

Fig. 2 Presence of an extensive, nonspecific osteolysis of the vertebral body of C5 associated with a kyphotic deformity of the cervical spine on the lateral radiograph

level could explain the greater frequency of *vertebra plana* at the thoracic and lumbar spine (Huang et al. 2007; Dikinson and Farhat 1991). Although not pathognomonic (see differential diagnosis; paragraph 8), *vertebra plana* in children is highly suggestive of LCH.

Exceptionally, osteolysis may involve only the posterior arch (Bodart et al. 1999) or extend to the intervertebral disks (Simnaski et al. 2004).

6.2 Computed Tomography (CT)

If needed, CT may confirm vertebral osteolysis suspected on CR, particularly in anatomically complex areas. CT defines the extent of the cortico-trabecular destruction more accurately in the different planes, thanks to the 2D reconstructions in bone window. CT allows precise assessment whether or not the posterior vertebral wall (Fig. 4) or posterior arch is affected (Fig. 5). The osteolysis is well delineated. It may be associated with subtle intralesional or peripheral sclerosis, particularly in the spine and pelvis.

CT assesses the decrease in height of the vertebral body in case of associated vertebral compression (Fig. 6). In general, it is superior to CR in assessing the fracture risk. It is also superior to CR in demonstrating potential extension into the soft tissues or epidural space, although MRI remains the examination of choice for evaluation of tumor extension to the soft tissues.

CT is the only technique capable of detecting rare intralesional bone sequestration ("button sequestrum") (Fig. 4). Although this does not justify the systematic performance of CT, the presence of a button sequestrum favors the diagnosis of LCH. Apart from the spine, these bone sequestrations can be seen on the skull vault or pelvis as well.

6.3 MRI

6.3.1 Conventional MRI

The signal of a bone lesion is completely nonspecific in LCH: hypo- or isosignal T1-WI and variable hypersignal T2-WI (Rajakulasingam et al. 2021) (Figs. 5 and 7). There is variable enhancement after intravenous injection of gadolinium contrast, ranging from moderate to intense. In case of peripheral enhancement, this may exceptionally simulate an abscess (Özdemir et al. 2016). The precise delineation of the osseous lesion is often difficult to assess on MRI because it is surrounded by inflammatory bone marrow edema. The extent of this edematous reaction is a valuable semiological key feature in the diagnosis of LCH. Inflammatory soft tissue edema adjacent to the bone lesion is typically limited with absence of a mass.

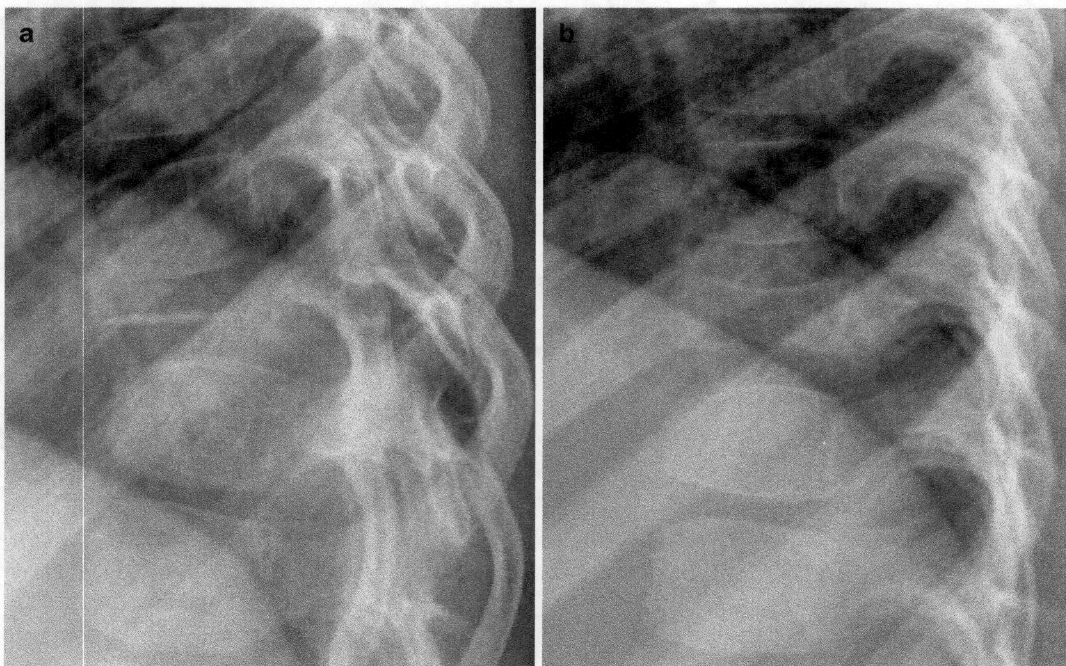

Fig. 3 *Vertebra plana* on CR. (**a**) The vertebral body of T10 is reduced to a bony layer of dense bone extending anteriorly to the adjacent superior and inferior vertebrae. Three years later, the vertebral body of T10 has recovered about half of its original height (**b**)

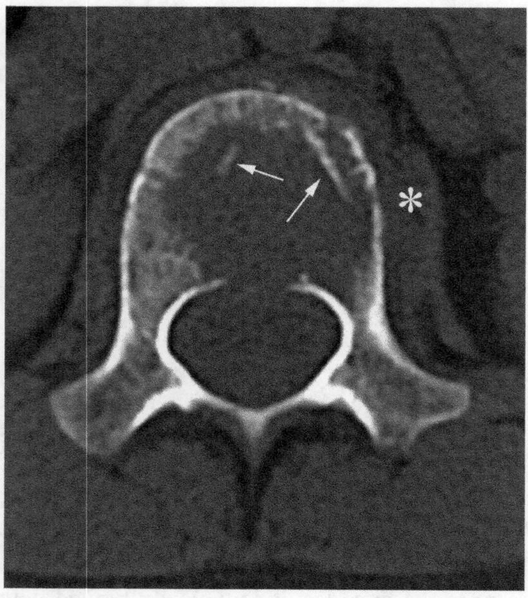

Fig. 4 CT scan of L1 showing osteolysis of the vertebral body extending to the posterior vertebral wall. Note also bone sequestration (arrows). The posterior arch is respected. There is moderate thickening of the left paravertebral soft tissues (asterisk)

MRI is the examination of choice to evaluate lesion extension into the paravertebral soft tissues and especially epidural extension (Fig. 8) and/or the extension to the intervertebral foramina. This epidural and/or foraminal infiltration is usually limited (Figs. 7 and 8), which explains why neurological complications in LCH, at least in children, are rare. In case of *vertebra plana*, the presence of focal and relatively symmetrical soft tissue thickening in the prevertebral as well as in the anterior epidural space is clearly visible on sagittal images following contrast injection and has a characteristic "H" shape (Huang et al. 2013) (Fig. 7). In case of collapse of two adjacent vertebrae, the intervertebral disk may show a decrease in height on T1- and T2-WI and a hyposignal on T2-WI.

In the case of noncontiguous multifocal vertebral involvement (Fig. 9), MRI may be useful in selecting the most suitable vertebra for subsequent biopsy: the vertebra with a T1 hyposignal and T2 hypersignal (representing an "active" lesion) should be preferred, as opposed to a ver-

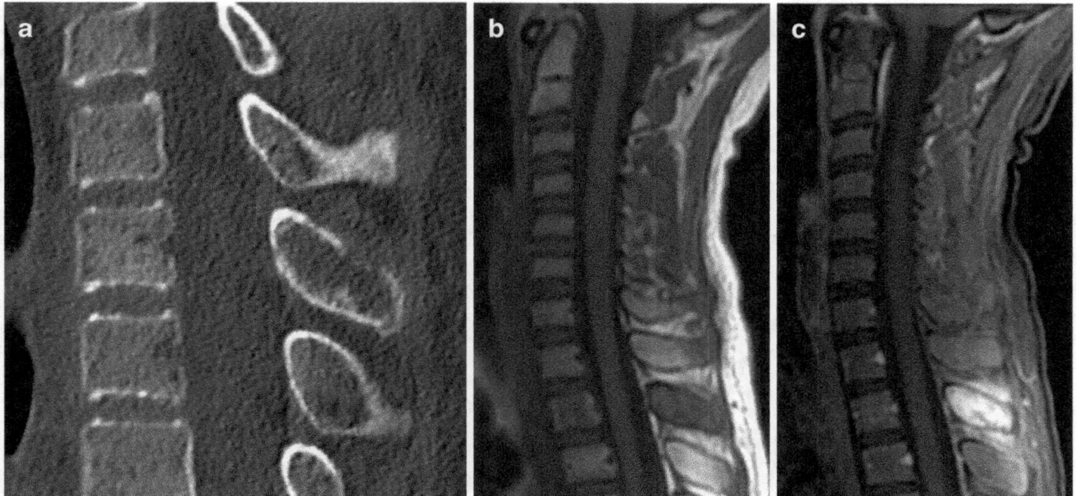

Fig. 5 Isolated posterior arch involvement of T2 on CT. (**a**) Sagittal bone window reformation reveals osteolysis of the spinous process predominantly involving the trabecular bone. (**b**) Corresponding sagittal T1-WI and (**c**) fat-suppressed (FS) T1-WI after IV injection of gadolinium contrast. Note vivid enhancement of spinous process T2

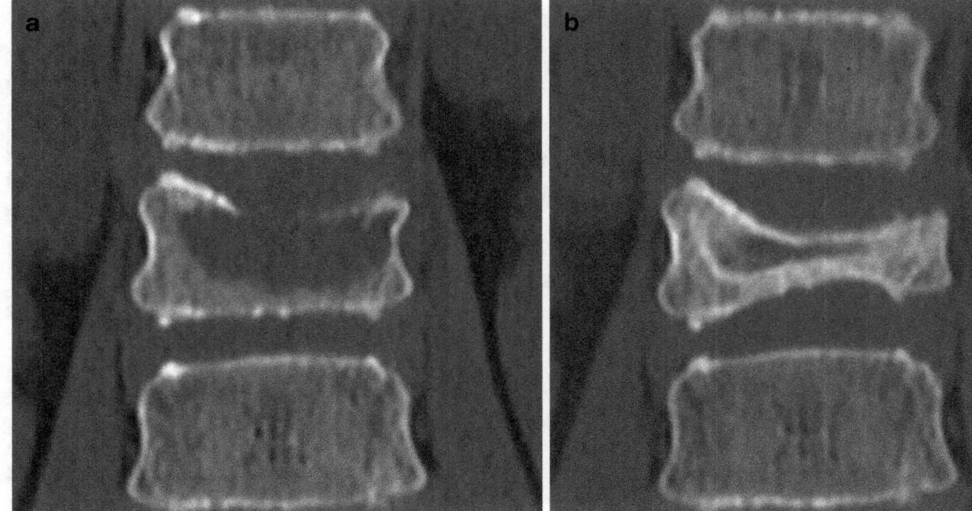

Fig. 6 Vertebral compression fracture of L1 on CT with asymmetric appearance on (**a**) coronal bone window reformat. (**b**) There is decrease of the vertebral height of L1 3 months later but with reappearance of the cortical lining of the upper vertebral plateau and adjacent sclerosis of the bone trabeculae

tebra with a spontaneous T1 hypersignal (representing an "inactive" lesion) (Kaplan et al. 1998). Indeed, the presence of a vertebral compression fracture is not necessarily synonymous with an "active" lesion.

6.3.2 Whole-Body MRI (WBMRI)

WBMRI is superior to radiographs in detecting bone lesions because cortico-medullary osteolysis must be sufficient to be visible on radiography and because certain regions of the axial skeleton

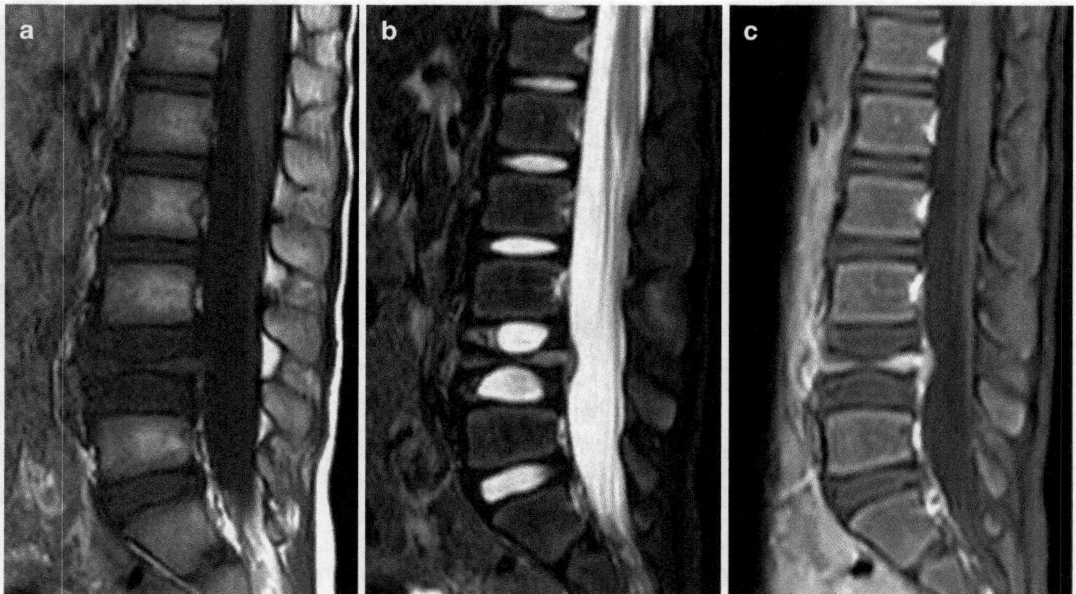

Fig. 7 *Vertebra plana* on MRI. (**a**) Note compression of the entire vertebral body of L4 with nonspecific signal change on T1-WI (**a**), in T2-STIR (**b**), and on FS T1-WI after intravenous injection of gadolinium contrast (**c**). Note also prevertebral soft tissue thickening and moderate anterior epidural extension on contrast-enhanced images

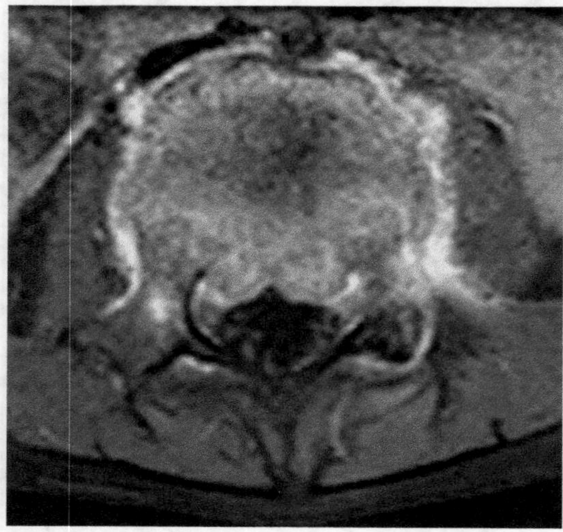

Fig. 8 Paravertebral soft tissue swelling and anterior epidural spread are clearly visible on axial FS T1-WI after intravenous injection of gadolinium contrast. There is no significant compression of the dural sac. The involvement of the vertebral body extends to the pedicles

remain difficult to analyze on radiography because of their anatomical complexity (e.g., the base of the skull) or superimpositions of gastrointestinal gas (e.g., the pelvis). However, even if WBMRI detects more bone lesions than radiographs, this does not always have an impact on the therapeutic management of the patient (Donadieu et al. 2012; Haute autorité de Santé 2021; Rajakulasingam et al. 2021). The potential value of WBMRI lies mainly in its ability to reveal extra-osseous involvement that is not recognized clinically or during imaging workup (see below) such as adenopathy and pulmonary involvement (Perrone et al. 2022; Goo et al. 2006). Indeed, such involvement transforms SS-LCH into MS-LCH and could modify the therapeutic management of the patient. However, the scarce literature data (Perrone et al. 2022; Kim et al. 2019) show that less than 10% of patients are affected. Therefore, the current role of WBMRI in the treatment and follow-up of LCH is not known. In our country, experts recognize the interest of WBMRI but do not recommend its systematic performance before treatment (Haute autorité de Santé 2021), especially since in young children, the examination requires sedation or even general anesthesia. In addition, WBMRI may detect incidental bone lesions without clinical significance in children and

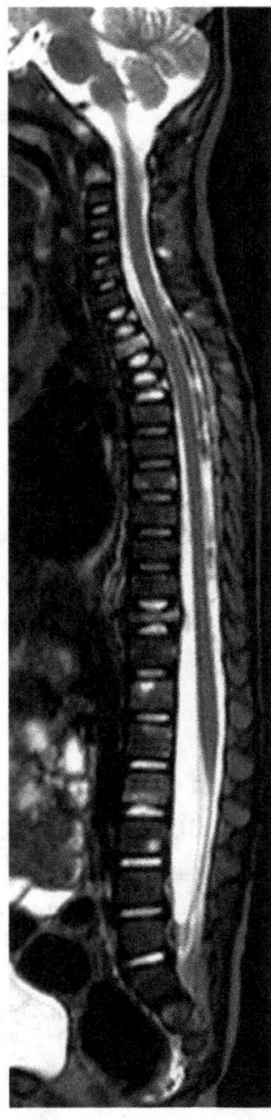

Fig. 9 Multifocal involvement in a 16-month-old child. Sagittal T2-STIR MR image shows diffuse and focal involvement of several vertebrae with *vertebra plana* on multiple levels. The spinal cord is preserved

young adults (in up to 30%), particularly in the lower limbs (Preez et al. 2020).

WBMRI is performed at 1.5 or 3 T, knowing that at 3 T, it should be noted that artifacts are more numerous and the examination time is longer. Ideally, the field of view should cover the skeleton from the vertex to the ankles in order not to miss any bone lesion. The protocol used differs from center to center (T1, T2-STIR, DIXON, diffusion sequences, etc.) (Rajakulasingam et al. 2021; Perrone et al. 2022; Guimarães et al. 2021), but the basic sequences remain coronal T1 and T2-STIR sequences. In case of spinal or cranial involvement, additional axial (cranial) or sagittal (spinal) sequences may be indicated (Rajakulasingam et al. 2021; Perrone et al. 2022; Daldrup-Link et al. 2001). T2-STIR sequences are preferred in children because of high amount of red bone marrow in the axial skeleton. Some authors also perform diffusion sequences (acquisition in the axial plane, reconstructions in the coronal plane according to a "pseudo-scintigraphic" image, also known as *diffusion-weighted* whole-body magnetic resonance *imaging* with background body signal suppression abbreviated as DWIBS) in addition to the T1-WI and T2-STIR sequences or instead of T1-WI, with the latter being performed only in the case of visible T2-STIR or diffusion abnormalities (Perrone et al. 2022). Diffusion sequences are useful but not essential because they increase the examination time. Intravenous injection of gadolinium contrast is generally not indicated (Perrone et al. 2022), except in case of spinal involvement associated with epidural extension. The total duration of a WBMRI varies according to the age of the child and the equipment and the protocol used, but varies generally between 30 min and 1 h. The respective advantages and disadvantages of this technique are shown in Table 3.

Table 3 Whole-body MRI in LCH

Advantages☺	Disadvantages ☹
Nonionizing technique	Sedation or general anesthesia required in small children
Evaluation of osseous and extra-osseous involvement	Long duration
Sensitivity > conventional radiography	Areas of difficult evaluation (calvaria, ribs, lungs)
Sensitivity ≫ bone scintigraphy	Lack of specificity

6.4 Imaging for Monitoring Treatment

LCH may heal either spontaneously, after biopsy, or following treatment. On CR and/or CT, the osteolysis becomes better defined with a peripheral rim of sclerosis or even extensive sclerosis

(Fig. 6) and later complete disappearance of the lesion. On MRI, the perilesional signal abnormalities regress resulting in a better delineated bony lesion, sometimes surrounded by a fatty halo of high T1 signal. With time, the lesion gradually fills with fat (Fig. 10). However, the hyperintense signal on T2-WI and enhancement on contrast-enhanced T1-WI may persist even if the lesion has become inactive on PET (Mueller et al. 2013).

In case of vertebral compression in children, the height of the vertebral body may be restored within a few months or years. This is variable, ranging from 15% to 85% of the initial height (Kaplan et al. 1998; Alarcón-Jaramillo et al. 2022). Restitutio ad integrum of a *vertebra plana* is classically described in LCH, but this is rather exceptional (Fig. 3) (Di Felice et al. 2017; Turgut and Gurçay 1992). The preservation of the vertebral end plates in the initial stage of the disease may explain the restoration of the vertebral height (Kaplan et al. 1998). Formation of a "butterfly" vertebra due to persisting central flattening of the vertebral body with height restoration of the lateral parts is also very rare (Alarcón-Jaramillo et al. 2022).

6.5 PET and PET/CT

6.5.1 Characterization of Bone Lesions

Like MRI, positron emission tomography (PET), alone or in combination with CT (PET/CT), is not able to differentiate LCH from other bone lesions. Indeed, because of its richness in histiocytes, 18FDG uptake in LCH can be very intense, similar to that of an osteosarcoma or a giant cell tumor (Aoki et al. 2001a, b). Therefore, it is not possible to define a standardized uptake value (SUV) indicative of a diagnosis of LCH.

6.5.2 Detection of Bone Lesions

Many studies have highlighted the value of PET/CT for detecting bone lesions in LCH (Fig. 11). False positives are rare (Jessop et al. 2020; Zhou

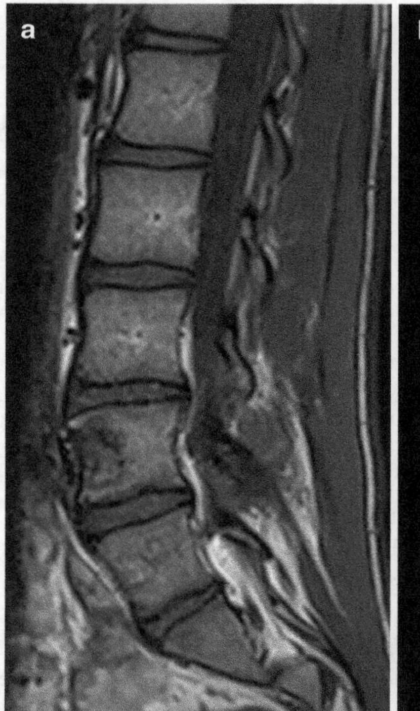

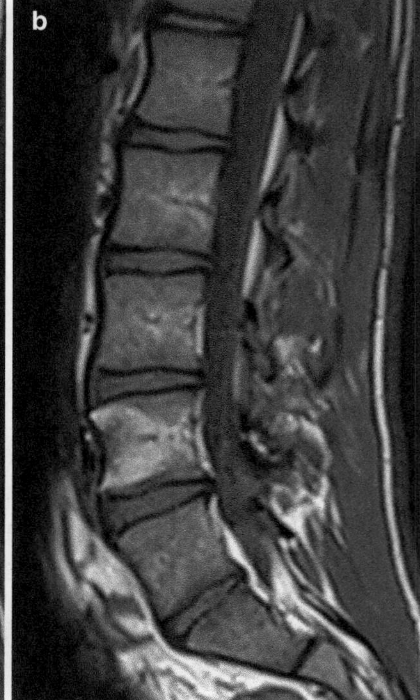

Fig. 10 Follow-up of involvement in L4 (anterior part of the vertebral body and posterior arch). (**a**) Initial sagittal T1-WI. (**b**) Fatty reconversion appeared on the MRI performed 4 months later

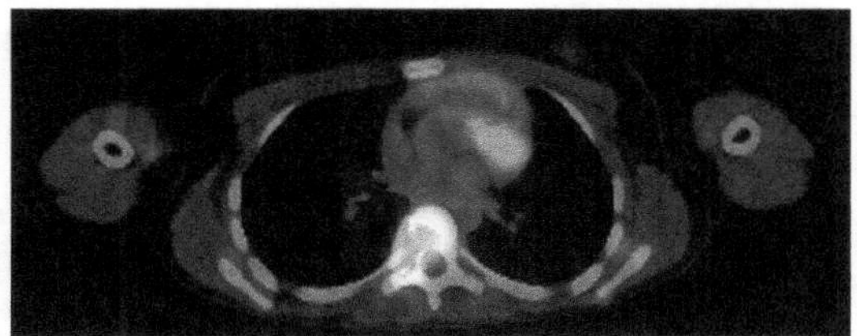

Fig. 11 Intense uptake on PET/CT in T7 resulting in osteolysis of the right posterolateral part of the vertebral body extending to the right posterior arch

et al. 2014). PET/CT undeniably outperforms radiographs or CT scans (Phillips et al. 2009; Kaste et al. 2007; Blum et al. 2002), except for skull lesions because of intense, physiologic uptake of the brain (Phillips et al. 2009; Binkovitz et al. 2003). Several studies (Mueller et al. 2013; Jessop et al. 2020; Zhou et al. 2014; Albano et al. 2017; Lee et al. 2012; Obert et al. 2017; Wu et al. 2020) have compared the performance of PET/CT and WBMRI in the detection of bony lesions of LCH in children and adults, with variable results depending on the methodology used (whether or not extra-osseous involvement was taken into account, PET versus PET/CT): in general, PET/CT was more specific and WBMRI more sensitive. PET would allow better detection of rib lesions (Phillips et al. 2009) but would be less effective in diagnosing subcentimetric bone lesions (Mueller et al. 2013), cranial lesions (Phillips et al. 2009; Binkovitz et al. 2003), and vertebral lesions (Phillips et al. 2009). Like WBMRI, PET may miss small pulmonary nodules (Mueller et al. 2013), but similar to WBMRI, PET assesses soft tissue and reveals possible extra-osseous involvement (Albano et al. 2017).

6.5.3 Monitoring Response to Therapy

PET is the most effective technique for assessing response to therapy and distinguishing metabolically active bone lesions (18FDG uptake) from metabolically inactive bone lesions (no uptake or significant decrease in SUV) (Kaste et al. 2007; Blum et al. 2002; Binkovitz et al. 2003; Lee et al. 2012). Indeed, when the bone lesions begin to regress, radiographic changes (appearance of a peripheral sclerotic border, progressive bone fill-in) and scintigraphic changes (hyperfixation in the periphery of the lesions showing osteoblastic activity) occur late in the healing phase. Moreover, the persistence of hypersignal on T2-WI and contrast enhancement on T1-WI can be seen within a bone lesion when it has become metabolically inactive (Mueller et al. 2013). The specificity of PET is 67% compared with 47% for MRI (Mueller et al. 2013).

Some authors (Mueller et al. 2013) propose to perform PET combined with WBMRI during the initial workup and PET alone during follow-up and evaluation of the response to treatment. However, PET is an ionizing technique and the dose delivered to the gonads during PET (~5–7 mGy) (Phillips et al. 2009; Binkovitz et al. 2003; Huang et al. 2009) is higher than that of radiographs (~1 mGy) (Binkovitz et al. 2003; Huang et al. 2009), which is difficult to justify if the examination must be repeated.

7 Histopathology

The diagnosis of LCH is based on clinical but, more importantly, histological and immunohistochemical evidence (Table 4). It requires prior percutaneous or surgical biopsy, with preference to (1) the most accessible bony site if there is multifocal bone involvement, (2) the most accessible extra-osseous site in case of multisystem involvement (e.g., skin), and (3) a presumably

Table 4 Histological diagnosis of LCH

Presumptive diagnosis	Histological findings under light microscopy
Probable diagnosis	Histological findings by light microscopy and two of the following markers: – Adenosine triphosphatase – S100 protein – α-D-Mannosidase – Peanut agglutinin (PNA)
Definitive diagnosis	Histological findings by light microscopy and at least one of the following two criteria: – Labeling of pathological cells with CD1a antigen – Birbeck granules on electron microscopy

active lesion. In the case of isolated bone lesions, biopsy is systematically done in our institution since LCH has a spontaneous tendency to heal following sampling.

The diagnostic criteria of the Histiocyte Society are summarized in Table 4 (Histiocyte Society 1987). In practice, histological diagnosis is based on the identification of pathologic cells by light microscopy (see pathologic features), together with positive membrane labeling of these cells for S100 protein and CD1a antigen (Fig. 12). Some teams add a positive marking to the CD207 antigen (langerin). The other markers (Table 4) are not widely used. Because the presence of Birbeck granules on electron microscopy correlates with the presence of CD207 antigen (Histiocyte Society 2009; Héritier et al. 2017), and because search for these granules is time-consuming and expensive (Haupt et al. 2013; Thomas et al. 2007), cellular immunostaining is generally preferred to electron microscopy. The anti-BRAFV600E antibody is also sometimes used and will be positive if a mutation is present.

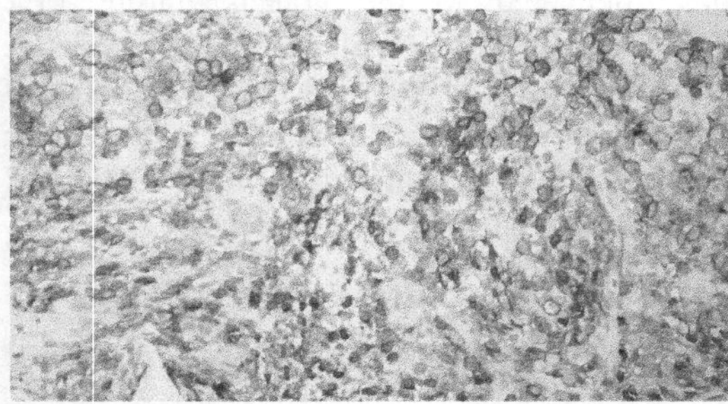

Fig. 12 Histological section at high magnification (×200) showing Langerhans cells with positive membrane marking for CD1a

Exceptionally, biopsy may be deferred in children in specific circumstances such as isolated vertebral bone lesion without adjacent soft tissue involvement (as in *vertebra plana*) in a patient with moderate pain and without alteration of the general condition, under close clinico-radiological surveillance, or in case of isolated vertebral bone lesion that is difficult to access by percutaneous or surgical biopsy (Fig. 13), such as isolated involvement of the odontoid process of C2. Some authors are reluctant to perform a vertebral biopsy in children, citing the risk of iatrogenic injury to the growth plate, but given the sometimes difficult differential diagnosis of LCH on imaging (see below), histological diagnosis is often needed for a final

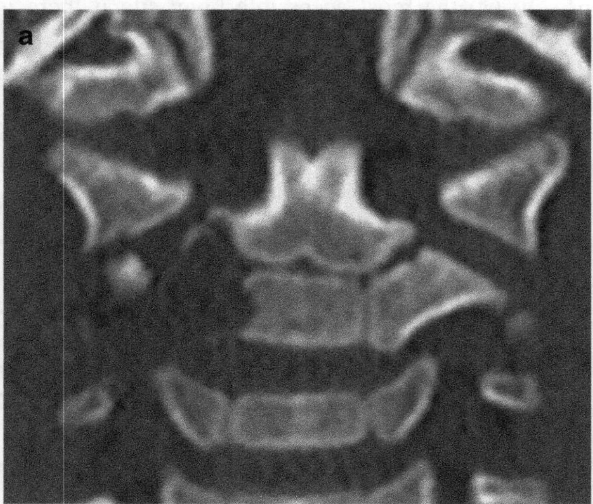

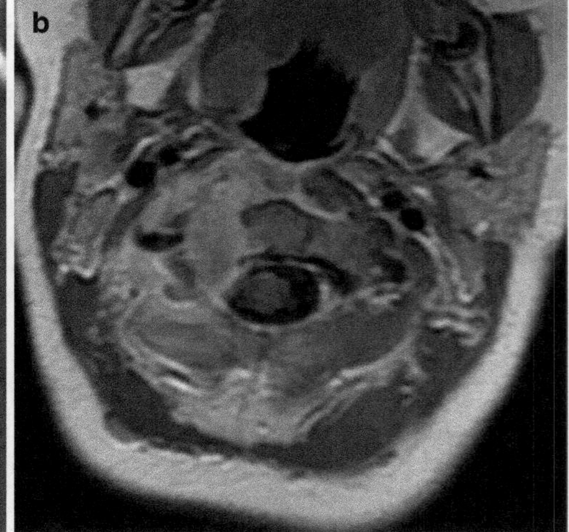

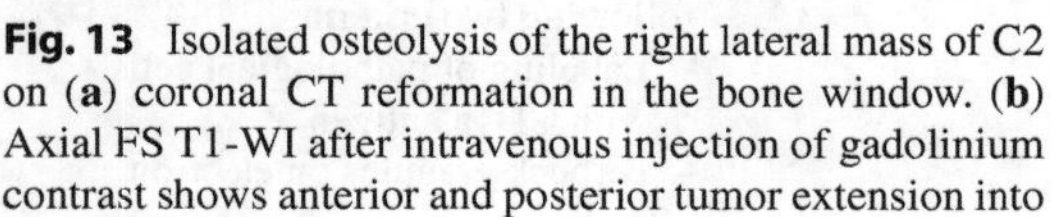

Fig. 13 Isolated osteolysis of the right lateral mass of C2 on (**a**) coronal CT reformation in the bone window. (**b**) Axial FS T1-WI after intravenous injection of gadolinium contrast shows anterior and posterior tumor extension into the adjacent muscles and corresponding intervertebral foramen encompassing the right vertebral artery. There is limited epidural extension

diagnosis. Biopsy is even more essential in case of isolated spinal involvement or when systemic chemotherapy is envisaged.

8 Differential Diagnosis

The main differential diagnoses of LCH in children and adults are summarized in Table 5. The differential diagnosis arises particularly in case of isolated spinal involvement. As intervertebral disk involvement is exceptional in LCH, its presence suggests a possible infectious etiology (in particular with *M. tuberculosis* and atypical mycobacteria) or another primary bone tumor of the spine.

The main differential diagnoses include Ewing's sarcoma, chronic recurrent multifocal osteomyelitis (CRMO), and aneurysmal bone cyst (ABC) in children and lytic metastasis, myeloma, and giant cell tumor (GCT) in adults. In adults, metastasis, myeloma (plasmacytoma), and GCT share a rather similar imaging semiology: aggressive osteolysis on CT (predominantly trabecular bone in plasmacytoma and sometimes GCT); presence of thickened intralesional bone trabeculae (plasmacytoma, GCT); invasion of adjacent soft tissues and epidural infiltration (metastasis, plasmacytoma, GCT); and low T2 signal of the tumor (GCT). Therefore, we will focus on the relevant differential diagnosis in children.

8.1 Main Differential Diagnoses in Children

8.1.1 Ewing's Sarcoma

Ewing's sarcoma primarily involving the spine (10% of cases) is less common than Ewing's sarcoma metastasizing to the spine (Fenoy et al. 2006). The clinical course is more rapid than in LCH, and neurological complications are often present in more than 2/3 of patients (Fenoy et al. 2006). Involvement of the posterior arch is more frequently seen than that of the vertebral body. CT scan reveals an aggressive osteolysis with cortical destruction or sometimes sclerosis. On MRI, a large soft tissue component often exceeding the bone involvement and epidural space invasion (Fig. 14) is usually the rule.

8.1.2 CRMO

Children are usually older than in LCH. CT scan may show mixed sclerosis and osteolysis (Fig. 15) and subtle signs of hyperostosis, but this semiology is inconsistent. WBMRI is useful to search multifocality and lesions with characteristic imaging features (T2 hypersignal of the medial third of the clavicle, the pelvis, and/or the epiphyseal-metaphyseal region of the long bones). In case of a symptomatic isolated vertebral involvement (Fig. 15), a percutaneous/surgical biopsy may be performed at initial presentation (and WBMRI at a later stage when biopsy has formally ruled out LCH).

Table 5 Spinal involvement in LCH: main differential diagnoses on imaging

	Children	Adults
Isolated spinal involvement (± vertebral fracture)	• Ewing's sarcoma • Lymphoproliferative disorder (leukemia, lymphoma) • CRMO • Aneurysmal bone cyst • Osteogenesis imperfecta • Osteoporosis	• Osteosarcoma • Lymphoproliferative disorder (myeloma, lymphoma) • Osteolytic metastasis • (Aggressive) hemangioma • Giant cell tumor • Chordoma • Osteoporosis
Spinal involvement with other bone lesion (± vertebral fracture)	• Leukemia • Lymphoma • Neuroblastoma metastasis • Infection (TB, atypical germs)	• Metastases • Myeloma • Lymphoma

CRMO chronic recurrent multifocal osteomyelitis

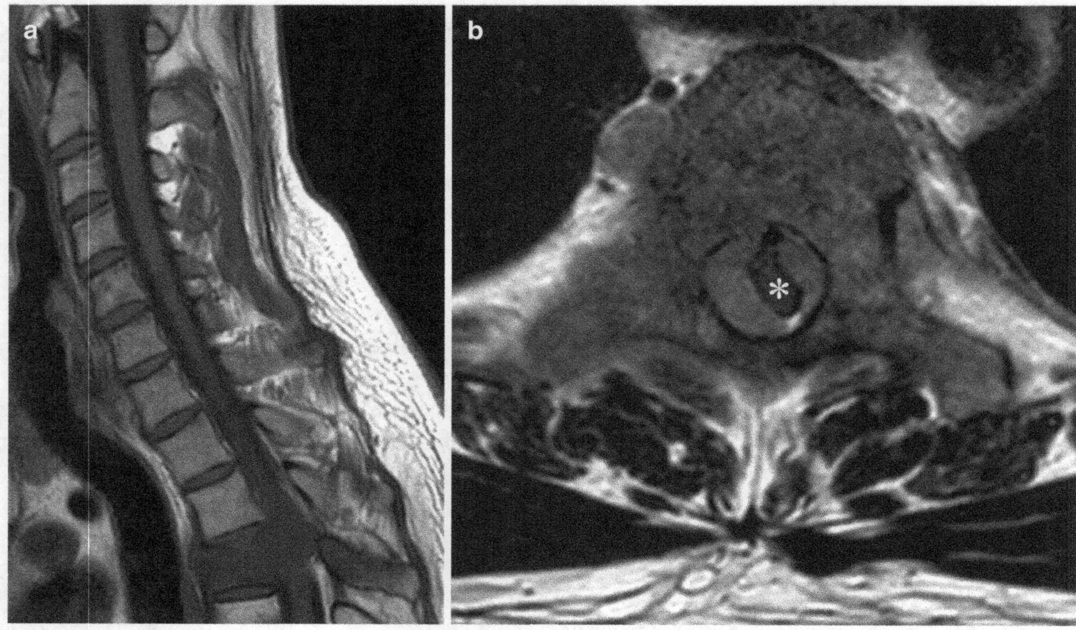

Fig. 14 Ewing's sarcoma T3: (**a**) Sagittal T1-WI and (**b**) axial T2-WI revealing compression of the superior end plate and bone marrow replacement in the vertebral body with extension to the posterior arch. The axial images show significant circumferential epidural extension compressing the spinal cord (asterisk). The patient presented clinically with a motor neurological deficit

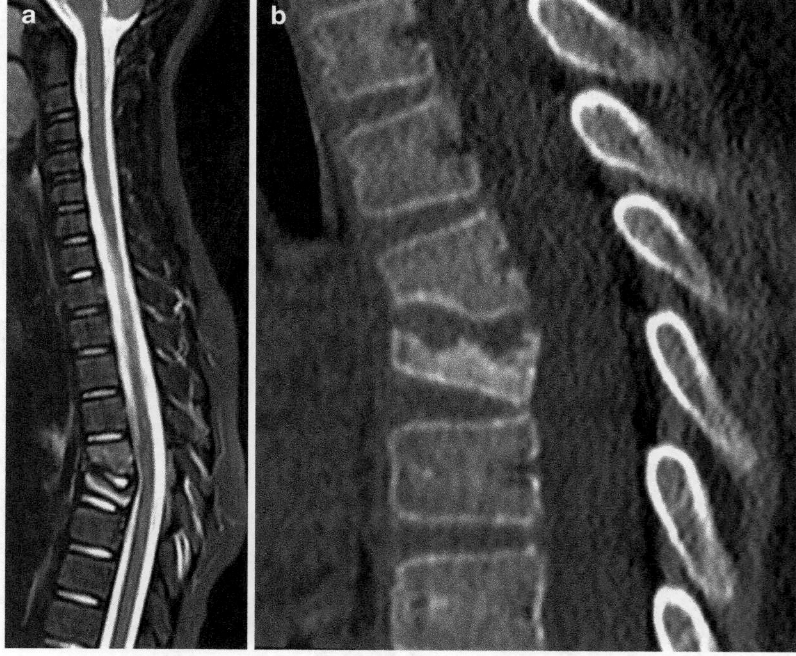

Fig. 15 Chronic recurrent multifocal osteomyelitis (CRMO). (**a**) MRI shows marked vertebral compression of T6 and to a lesser degree of T5, resulting in kyphosis and subtle indentation on the anterior aspect of the spinal cord. (**b**) Corresponding sagittal CT reformat shows marked bone resorption and sclerosis of the trabeculae in T6

Table 6 *Vertebra plana* in children: main etiologies

- Lymphoproliferative disorder (leukemia, lymphoma)
- Ewing's sarcoma
- Neuroblastoma metastasis
- CRMO[a]
- Aneurysmal bone cyst
- Juvenile xanthogranuloma
- Osteoporosis/osteogenesis imperfecta
- Spondylodiscitis (TB, atypical germs)
- Trauma

[a] Chronic recurrent multifocal osteomyelitis

8.1.3 ABC

Vertebral involvement in ABC predominates in the posterior arch, unlike LCH, but may extend to the vertebral body. The osteolysis is usually expansile. CT scans may show a thin peripheral bony shell. On MRI, there may be associated soft tissue signal changes adjacent to an expanding ABC, but there is no mass. Furthermore, MRI shows multiple intralesional cavities with intralesional fluid-fluid levels on T2-WI with peripheral enhancement following gadolinium contrast injection.

8.2 Particular Case of the *Vertebra Plana*

The main etiologies are summarized in Table 6. Underlying neoplasia should always be kept in mind in children (Baky et al. 2020), but true *vertebra plana* consisting of complete loss of height of the vertebral body with only a dense layer of dense bone of a few millimeters thick, extending anteriorly to the adjacent vertebrae (Fig. 3), is the hallmark of LCH. The possibility of CRMO in an older child (Fig. 15) should also be considered but remains a diagnosis of exclusion.

9 Local and Distant Staging

Staging in children (Haupt et al. 2013; Haute autorité de Santé 2021; Satter and High 2008) is better standardized than in adults (Girschikofsky et al. 2013) and is more or less the subject of international consensus.

9.1 Staging in Children (Age Under 18 Years Old)

In our institution, it is based on recommendations from national experts (Haute autorité de Santé 2021) and from European and international experts (Haupt et al. 2013). This workup is mainly aimed at distinguishing SS-LCH from MS-LCH and is based on a complete clinical examination. Each clinical abnormality is subject to appropriate imaging. Clinical examination is completed by (1) blood count, to look for anemia and thrombocytopenia; (2) a liver workup, to look for liver dysfunction and in particular cholestasis; and (3) imaging workup to look for asymptomatic lesions and/or potentially bone lesions at risk related to their location or potential complications: involvement of C2, multiple vertebral involvement with associated epidural extension, craniofacial involvement that may lead to diabetes insipidus, or neurodegenerative involvement (Rajakulasingam et al. 2021).

Initially, the imaging workup includes skeletal surveys and technetium bone scan, which are considered complementary to detect bone lesions (Kumar and Balachandran 1980). However, both techniques lack sensitivity, with figures varying widely depending on the series and the gold standard used (56–100% for radiographs; 22–61% for bone scans) (Rajakulasingam et al. 2021; Kim et al. 2019; Guimarães et al. 2021; Mentzel et al. 2004; Howarth et al. 1996). The efficacy of bone scan is less than CR in the spine and pelvis (Rajakulasingam et al. 2021; Dogan et al. 1996) but higher for detection of osseous lesions in the ribs, facial bones, and mandible (Howarth et al. 1996; Dogan et al. 1996). Bone lesions of the skull are either better (Howarth et al. 1996) or less well seen (Dogan et al. 1996) on scintigraphy than on CR.

On scintigraphy, LCH lesions show either decreased or increased uptake (Schaub et al. 1987), with central decreased uptake surrounded by peripheral increased uptake (Rajakulasingam et al. 2021). Decreased uptake is seen in purely osteolytic lesions or inactive lesions. Increased uptake is seen in case of osteoblastic activity at the periphery of the lesion, indicating healing lesions (Kaplan et al. 1998), which is better seen than on CR (38). The use of skeletal survey is debated in children because of their lack of sensitivity and their ionizing character (~1 mGy delivered to the gonads) (Huang et al. 2009), but they are still relevant (Donadieu et al. 2012; Rajakulasingam et al. 2021; Satter and High 2008). Conversely, technetium bone scintigraphy (~2.4 mGy delivered to the gonads) (Huang et al. 2009) is no longer routinely recommended in the workup of LCH (Donadieu et al. 2012; Broadbent et al. 1989).

Recommendations for initial imaging workup include radiographs of the skull, chest, full spine, and pelvis (Table 7). CR may be supplemented by abdominal ultrasound to look for hepatomegaly, intrahepatic nodular mass, and/or splenomegaly, but its contribution remains limited in the absence of clinical and laboratory abnormalities. Brain MRI is recommended in patients with bony involvement of the skull vault and/or face and in patients with neurological signs or central diabetes insipidus suggestive of pituitary gland involvement (Donadieu et al. 2012). A chest CT scan (high-resolution or low-dose multidetector if available) to study the lung parenchyma is performed in case of abnormal chest radiography.

More recently, techniques such as PET, PET/CT, and WBMRI (see above) have been evaluated in the assessment of the extension of LCH: they provide interesting information (better detection of bony lesions, detection of extra-osseous lesions), but their exact place in the therapeutic algorithm in the follow-up of patients remains to be defined. In our country, these techniques remain optional. Some experts (Haute autorité de Santé 2021) have suggested that the appendicular skeleton should no longer be systematically examined unless there are clinical signs and that the axial skeleton (skull, spine, pelvis) should be systematically examined by MRI, but the relevance of such a workup has to be proven. In addition, the drawbacks of the use of these techniques in young children (such as sedation, general anesthesia) are well known.

Table 7 Radiographic workup for suspected LCH

Systematic assessment of symptomatic anatomical regions	
Skull (AP and lateral view)	Pelvis (AP)
Chest (PA)	Whole spine (AP and lateral view)

AP anteroposterior, *PA* posteroanterior

9.2 Staging in Adults

Staging in adults differs little from staging in children, except that a lateral chest radiograph is recommended in addition to a posteroanterior radiograph, and a low-dose whole-body CT scan may replace a skeletal survey (Girschikofsky et al. 2013). MRI of the skull and PET/CT are optional. PET/CT may replace abdominal ultrasound, low-dose whole-body CT, and chest radiographs (Girschikofsky et al. 2013).

10 Treatment

Schematically, children with single-organ involvement without functional risk require local treatment (e.g., isolated skin involvement) or no treatment at all, unless the evolution is secondarily unfavorable. Other patients will receive systemic chemotherapy (often based on the combination of vinblastine and prednisone) usually for 1 year (Donadieu et al. 2012; Histiocyte Society 2009; Haute autorité de Santé 2021). Infants with OR+ MS require urgent and specialized management and the frequent and necessary use of targeted therapies (see below). In adults, chemotherapy protocols differ (Girschikofsky et al. 2013).

In case of spinal involvement, the therapeutic decision is taken on a case-by-case basis, depending on the location of the lesion, its functional impact, and the acute presentation. In case of a constituted *vertebra plana*, the benefit of treatment is limited. If the spinal injury is isolated, no specific treatment is required, except for symptomatic treatment of pain associated with temporary immobilization until the bone damage heals. In children, this condition requires clinical monitoring to assess the impact on spinal statics, especially if there is vertebral compression. Other therapeutic alternatives have been described many years ago, but they have never really been validated (intralesional injection of corticosteroids) (Egeler et al. 1992) or are currently no longer appropriate in children (low-dose local radiotherapy) (Haute autorité de Santé 2021).

Surgery for vertebral damage has become exceptional, especially in children, because of the possible damage to the vertebral growth plate and its consequences (growth failure, spinal deformities). Various surgical techniques have been described, sometimes radical in adults (Dikinson and Farhat 1991; Chen et al. 2018), but they should be reserved for acute cases of neurological compression, severe instability (Yang et al. 2020), and severe spinal deformity. Indeed, given the self-limiting nature of LCH lesions, the efficacy and good tolerance of conventional chemotherapy, and, more recently, the advent of targeted therapies for forms refractory to chemotherapy, complete surgical removal of a vertebral bone lesion is no longer recommended (Girschikofsky et al. 2013). A few cases of percutaneous vertebroplasty have also been reported (Feng et al. 2013; Tan et al. 2007).

Second-line treatment is intended for patients who are refractory to first-line treatment. In children, 2-CdA (cladribine) and targeted therapy, either BRAF inhibitors or MEK inhibitors, depending on the somatic mutation identified during the diagnostic biopsy, should be emphasized. Finally, a few publications (Elomaa et al. 1989; Kamizono et al. 2002; Farran et al. 2001) have reported the value of bisphosphonates in children and adults in refractory forms to first-line treatment accompanied by disseminated bone involvement.

11 Prognosis

According to the literature, the following factors are associated with a poor prognosis: young age of the child (less than 1–2 years) at the time of diagnosis; the presence or absence of involvement of an organ at risk (hematopoietic system, spleen, liver), which is more frequent at this age; dysfunction of a vital organ (lung, liver, bone marrow); a large number of organs involved (three or more); and a poor initial response to treatment (Donadieu et al. 2012; Thomas et al. 2007; Haute autorité de Santé 2021). Regarding bone involvement, in addition to the anatomical site at risk for complications, the degree of cortico-trabecular destruction and the volume of associated soft tissue involvement are also important parameters. These parameters are more important than the total number of bone lesions (Donadieu et al. 2012). In the future, BRAFV600E molecular status should also be considered in children.

12 Conclusion

LCH is a rare pathology that should be considered in children and young adults. Bone involvement in LCH predominates in the axial skeleton, similar to myeloma in adults. Isolated involvement of the spine is rare. In children, the most characteristic presentation is *vertebra plana*. The appearance on CR and/or CT is that of a nonspecific osteolytic lesion with a predilection for the vertebral body, but associated involvement of the posterior arch is possible. The appearance on MRI is also nonspecific, except for the presence of a significant inflammatory bone marrow reaction in the periphery of the bone lesion. The diagnosis of certainty is therefore made by histopathology after performing a biopsy (either cutaneous, percutaneous imaging-guided, or surgical depending on the most accessible site). Current therapeutic management depends essentially on the location of the lesions and in particular their functional consequences. The contribution of new imaging technologies such as WBMRI (for assessment of extension) and PET-PET/CT (for follow-up and response to treatment) to the management of this condition remains to be proven.

13 Key Points

- Spinal involvement of LCH predominates in the thoracolumbar region and involves the vertebral body more frequently than the posterior arch. The intervertebral disks are typically spared.
- The appearance on CR and CT scan is that of nonspecific osteolysis, associated or not with vertebral compression. Only the *vertebra plana* in children is suggestive of the diagnosis (but remains nonspecific).
- MRI is the key examination to judge the epidural and/or foraminal tumor extension, which is generally limited. Neurological complications are therefore uncommon.
- The final diagnosis is made by histopathological examination after a biopsy of the most accessible site, either osseous or extra-osseous.

Acknowledgments The authors sincerely thank Dr. Sébastien Héritier, MD, PhD, Centre de Référence des Histiocytoses, APHP Sorbonne University, Paris, France, for kindly reviewing and correcting the clinical part of this chapter and Prof. Dr. Filip Vanhoenacker, Belgium, for additional reviewing and editing.

References

Alarcón-Jaramillo J, Moreno-Arango I, Márquez JC (2022) Acquired butterfly vertebra as a sequela of eosinophilic granuloma. Skelet Radiol 52:1243. https://doi.org/10.1007/s00256-022-04249-5

Albano D, Bosio G, Giubbini R et al (2017) Role of ^{18}F-FDG PET/CT in patients affected by Langerhans cell histiocytosis. Jpn J Radiol 35:574–583

Allen CE, Merad M, McClain KL (2018) Langerhans-cell histiocytosis. N Engl J Med 30(379):856–868

Angelini A, Mavrogenis AF, Rimondi E, Rossi G, Ruggieri P (2017) Current concepts for the diagnosis and management of eosinophilic granuloma of bone. J Orthop Traumatol 18:83–90

Aoki J, Watanabe H, Shinozaki T et al (2001a) FDG PET of primary benign and malignant bone tumors: standardized uptake value in 52 lesions. Radiology 219:774–777

Aoki J, Inoue T, Tomiyoshi K et al (2001b) Nuclear imaging of bone tumors: FDG-PET. Semin Musculoskelet Radiol 5:183–187

Baky F, Milbrandt TA, Arndt C et al (2020) Vertebra plana in children may result from etiologies other than eosinophilic granuloma. Clin Orthop Relat Res 478:2367–2374

Bertram C, Madert J, Eggers C (2002) Eosinophilic granuloma of the cervical spine. Spine (Phila Pa 1976) 27:1408–1413

Bilge T, Barut S, Yaymaci Y et al (1995) Solitary eosinophilic granuloma of the lumbar spine in an adult. Case report. Paraplegia 33:485–487

Binkovitz LA, Olshefski RS, Adler BH (2003) Coincidence FDG-PET in the evaluation of Langerhans' cell histiocytosis: preliminary findings. Pediatr Radiol 33:598–602

Blum R, Seymour JF, Hicks RJ (2002) Role of 18FDG-positron emission tomography scanning in the management of histiocytosis. Leuk Lymphoma 43:2155–2157

Bodart E, Nisolle J-F, Maton P et al (1999) Limp as unusual presentation of Langerhans' cell histiocytosis. Eur J Pediatr 158:384–386

Broadbent V, Gadner H, Komp DM et al (1989) Histiocytosis syndromes in children: approach to the clinical and laboratory evaluation of children with Langerhans cell histiocytosis. Med Pediatr Oncol 17:492–495

Chen L, Chen Z, Wang Y (2018) Langerhans cell histiocytosis at L5 vertebra treated with en bloc vertebral resection: a case report. J Surg Oncol 16:96. https://doi.org/10.1186/s12957-018-1399-401

Daldrup-Link HE, Franzius C, Link TM et al (2001) Whole-body MR imaging for detection of bone metastases in children and young adults: comparison with skeletal scintigraphy and FDG PET. AJR 177:229–236

David R, Oria RA, Kumar R et al (1989) Radiologic features of eosinophilic granuloma of bone. Am J Roentgenol 153:1021–1026

Di Felice F, Zaina F, Donzelli S, Negrini S (2017) Spontaneous and complete regeneration of a vertebra plana after surgical curettage of an eosinophilic granuloma. Eur Spine J 26(Suppl 1):225–228

Dikinson LD, Farhat SM (1991) Eosinophilic granuloma of the cervical spine. Surg Neurol 35:57–63

Dogan AS, Conway JJ, Miller JH et al (1996) Detection of bone lesions in Langerhans cell histiocytosis: complementary roles of scintigraphy and conventional radiography. J Pediatr Hematol Oncol 18:51–58

Donadieu J, Chalard F, Jeziorski E (2012) Medical management of Langerhans cell histiocytosis from diagnosis to treatment. Review. Expert Opin Pharmacother 13:1309–1322

Egeler RM, Thompson RC Jr, Voûte PA et al (1992) Intralesional infiltration of corticosteroids in localized Langerhans' cell histiocytosis. J Pediatr Orthop 12:811–814

Elomaa I, Blomqvist C, Porkka L et al (1989) Experiences of clodronate treatment of multifocal eosinophilic granuloma of bone. J Intern Med 225:59–61

Émile JF, Abla O, Fraitag S et al (2016) Revised classification of histiocytoses and neoplasms of the macrophage-dendritic cell lineages. Blood 127:2672–2681

Farran RP, Zaretski E, Egeler RM (2001) Treatment of Langerhans cell histiocytosis with pamidronate. J Pediatr Hematol Oncol 23:54–56

Feng F, Tang H, Chen H et al (2013) Percutaneous vertebroplasty for Langerhans cell histiocytosis of the lumbar spine in an adult: case report and review of the literature. Exp Ther Med 5:128–132

Fenoy AJ, Greenlee JDW, Menezes AH et al (2006) Primary bone tumors of the spine in children. J Neurosurg 105(4 Suppl):252–260

Garg B, Sharma V, Eachempati KK et al (2006) An unusual presentation of eosinophilic granuloma in an adult: a case report. J Orthop Surg (Hong Kong) 14:81–83

Girschikofsky M, Arico M, Castillo D et al (2013) Management of adult patients with Langerhans cell histiocytosis: recommendations from an expert panel on behalf of Euro-Histio-Net. Orphanet J Rare Dis 8:72. https://doi.org/10.1186/1750-1172-8-72

Goo HW, Yang DH, Ra YS et al (2006) Whole-body MRI of Langerhans cell histiocytosis: comparison with radiography and scintigraphy. Pediatr Radiol 36:1019–1031

Greenlee JD, Fenoy AJ, Donovan KA, Menezes AH (2007) Eosinophilic granuloma in the pediatric spine. Pediatr Neurosurg 43:285–292

Grois N, Pötschger U, Prosch H et al (2006) Risk factors for diabetes insipidus in Langerhans cell histiocytosis. Pediatr Blood Cancer 46:228–233

Grois N, Fahrner B, Arceci RJ et al (2010) Central nervous system disease in Langerhans cell histiocytosis. J Pediatr 156:873–881

Guimarães JB, da Cruz IAN, Ahlawat S et al (2021) The role of whole-body MRI in pediatric musculoskeletal oncology: current concepts and clinical applications. J Magn Reson Imaging. https://doi.org/10.1002/jmri.27787. Online ahead of print. Review

Haupt R, Minkov M, Astigarraga I et al (2013) Langerhans cell histiocytosis (LCH): guidelines for diagnosis, clinical work-up, and treatment for patients till the age for 18 years. Pediatr Blood Cancer 60:175–184

Haute autorité de Santé (2021) Protocole national de diagnostic et de soins histiocytose langerhansienne (enfant de moins de 18 ans). https://www.has-sante.fr/jcms/p_3301927/fr/histiocytose-langerhansienne-enfant-de-moins-de-18-ans. Accessed Jan 2023

Héritier S, Donadieu J, Émile JF (2017) Mutations de BRAF et voie des MAP-kinases dans les histiocytoses: détection et intérêt clinique. Correspondances en Onco-Théranostic, vol. VI(2), avril-mai-juin

Histiocyte Society (1987) Histiocytosis syndrome in children. Writing Group of the Histiocyte Society. Lancet 11:1181–1191

Histiocyte Society (2009) Langerhans cell histiocytosis. Evaluation and treatment guidelines. https://www.hematologie-amc.nl/bestanden/hematologie/bijlagennietinDBS/SocietyLCHTreatmentGuidelines.PDF. Accessed Jan 2023

Howarth DM, Mullan BP, Wiseman GA et al (1996) Bone scintigraphy evaluated in diagnosing and staging Langerhans' cell histiocytosis and related disorders. J Nucl Med 37:1456–1460

Huang KY, Lin RM, Yan JJ et al (2007) Langerhans cell histiocytosis as a possible differential diagnosis of painful scoliosis. Joint Bone Spine 74:396–399

Huang B, Law MW, Khong PL (2009) Whole-body PET/CT scanning: estimation of radiation dose and cancer risk. Radiology 251:166–174

Huang WD, Yang XH, Wu ZP et al (2013) Langerhans cell histiocytosis of spine: a comparative study of clinical, imaging features, and diagnosis in children, adolescents, and adults. Spine J 13:1108–1117

Jessop S, Crudgington D, London K et al (2020) FDG PET-CT in pediatric Langerhans cell histiocytosis. Pediatr Blood Cancer 67(1):e28034. https://doi.org/10.1002/pbc.28034. Epub 2019 Oct 10

Jha SK, De Jesus O (2022) Eosinophilic granuloma. In: StatPearls. StatPearls Publishing, Treasure Island, FL

Jiang L, Liu XG, Zhong WQ et al (2011) Langerhans cell histiocytosis with multiple spinal involvement. Eur Spine J 20:1961–1969

Kamizono J, Okada Y, Shirahat A et al (2002) Bisphosphonate induces remission of refractory osteolysis in Langerhans cell histiocytosis. J Bone Miner Res 17:1926–1928

Kaplan GR, Saifuddin A, Pringle JAS et al (1998) Langerhans' cell histiocytosis of the spine: use of MRI in guiding biopsy. Skelet Radiol 27:673–676

Kaste SC, Rodriguez-Galindo C, McCarville ME, Shulkin BL (2007) PET-CT in pediatric Langerhans cell histiocytosis. Pediatr Radiol 37:615–622

Kim JR, Yoon HM, Jung AY et al (2019) Comparison of whole-body MRI, bone scan, and radiographic skeletal survey for lesion detection and risk stratification of Langerhans cell histiocytosis. Sci Rep 9:317. https://doi.org/10.1038/s41598-018-36501-1

Kumar R, Balachandran S (1980) Relative roles of radionuclide scanning and radiographic imaging in eosinophilic granuloma. Clin Nucl Med 5:538–542

Langerhans P (1868) Uber die Nerven der menschlichen Haut. Virchows Arch Path Anat 44:325–337

Le Guennec L, Martin-Duverneuil N, Mokhtari K et al (2016) Neurohistiocytose langerhansienne. Presse Med 46:79. https://doi.org/10.1016/j.lpm.2016.09.014

Lee HJ, Ahn BC, Lee SW et al (2012) The usefulness of F-18 fluorodeoxyglucose positron emission tomography/computed tomography in patients with Langerhans cell histiocytosis. Ann Nucl Med 26:730–737

Mentzel HJ, Kentouche K, Sauner D et al (2004) Comparison of whole-body STIR-MRI and 99mTc-methylene-diphosphonate scintigraphy in children with suspected multifocal bone lesions. Eur Radiol 14:2297–2302

Montemurro N, Perrini P, Vannozzi R (2013) Epidural spinal cord compression in Langerhans cell histiocytosis: a case report. Br J Neurosurg 27:838–839

Mueller WP, Melzer HI, Schmid I et al (2013) The diagnostic value of ^{18}F-FDG PET and MRI in paediatric histiocytosis. Eur J Nucl Med Mol Imaging 40:356–363

Obert J, Vercellino L, Van Der Gucht A et al (2017) 18Ffluorodeoxyglucose positron emission tomography-computed tomography in the management of adult multisystem Langerhans cell histiocytosis. Eur J Nucl Med Mol Imaging 44:598–610

Özdemir ZM, Kahraman AS, Görmeli CA et al (2016) Langerhans cell histiocytosis with atypical intervertebral disc and sacroiliac joint involvement mimicking osteoarticular tuberculosis in an adult. Balkan Med J 33:573–577

Perrone A, Lakatos K, Pegoraro F et al (2022) Whole-body magnetic resonance imaging for staging Langerhans cell histiocytosis in children and young adults. Pediatr Blood Cancer 70:e30064. https://doi.org/10.1002/pbc.30064. Online ahead of print

Phillips M, Allen C, Gerson P et al (2009) Comparison of FDG-PET scans to conventional radiography and bone scans in management of Langerhans cell histiocytosis. Pediatr Blood Cancer 52:97–101

Prasad GL, Divya S (2019) Eosinophilic granuloma of the cervical spine in adults: a review. World Neurosurg 125:301–311

Preez HD, Lasker I, Rajakulasingam R, Saifuddin A (2020) Whole-body magnetic resonance imaging: incidental findings in paediatric and adult populations. Eur J Radiol 130:109156. Published online ahead of print, Jun 30

Rajakulasingam R, Siddiqui M, Michelagnoli M, Saifuddin A (2021) Skeletal staging in Langerhans cell histiocytosis: a multimodality imaging review. Skelet Radiol 50:1081–1093

Reisi N, Raeissi P, Harati Khalilabad T, Moafi A (2021) Unusual sites of bone involvement in Langerhans cell histiocytosis: a systematic review of the literature. Orphanet J Rare Dis 16(1):1

Satter EK, High WA (2008) Langerhans cell histiocytosis: a review of the current recommendations of the Histiocyte Society. Pediatr Dermatol 25:291–295

Schaub T, Ash JM, Gilday DL (1987) Radionuclide imaging in histiocytosis X. Pediatr Radiol 17:397–404

Simnaski C, Bouillon B, Brockmann M et al (2004) The Langerhans' cell histiocytosis (eosinophilic granuloma) of the cervical spine: a rare diagnosis of cervical pain. Magn Reson Imaging 22:589–594

Tan HQ, Li MH, Wu CG et al (2007) Percutaneous vertebroplasty for eosinophilic granuloma of the cervical spine in a child. Pediatr Radiol 37:1053–1057

Thomas C, Émile J-F, Donadieu J (2007) Histiocytose langerhansienne. EMC (Elsevier Masson SAS, Paris), Pédiatrie, 4-082-E-10

Turgut M, Gurçay O (1992) Multi-focal histiocytosis X of bone in two adjacent vertebrae causing paraplegia. Aust N Z J Surg 62:241–244

Tyagi DK, Balasubramaniam S, Savant HV (2011) Langerhans' cell histiocytosis involving posterior elements of the dorsal spine: an unusual cause of extradural spinal mass in an adult. J Craniovertebr Junct Spine 2:93–95

Vadivelu S, Mangano FT, Miller CR et al (2007) Multifocal Langerhans cell histiocytosis of the pediatric spine: a case report and literature review. Childs Nerv Syst 23:127–131

Villas C, Martinez-Peric R, Barrios RH et al (1993) Eosinophilic granuloma of the spine with and without vertebra plana: long-term follow-up of six cases. J Spinal Disord 6:260–268

Wu M, Niu N, Huo L (2020) Clinical utility of 18FDG-PET/CT in adult Langerhans cell histiocytosis: an analysis of 57 patients. J Nucl Med 61:16

Yang IC, Lee GJ, Han MS et al (2020) Langerhans cell histiocytosis involving second cervical vertebra and the hypothalamus and pituitary in an adult. World Neurosurg 142:142–146

Yousem SA, Colby TV, Chen YY et al (2001) Pulmonary Langerhans' cell histiocytosis: molecular analysis of clonality. Am J Surg Pathol 25:630–636

Zhao M, Tang L, Sun S, Cui J, Chen H (2021) Radiologic findings that aid in the reduction of misdiagnoses of Langerhans cell histiocytosis of the bone: a retrospective study. World J Surg Oncol 10(19):146

Zhong WQ, Jiang L, Ma QJ et al (2010) Langerhans cell histiocytosis of the atlas in an adult. Eur Spine J 19:19–22

Zhou W, Wu H, Han Y et al (2014) Preliminary study on the evaluation of Langerhans cell histiocytosis using F-18-fluoro-deoxy-glucose PET/CT. Chin Med J 127:2458–2462

Ewing Sarcoma

Hend Riahi, Emna Labbène, Maher Barsaoui, Mohamed Fethi Ladeb, and Mouna Chelli Bouaziz

Contents

H. Riahi (✉) · E. Labbène · M. F. Ladeb
M. Chelli Bouaziz
Department of Radiology, Institut Mohamed Kassab d'orthopédie, Ksar Said, Tunisia
e-mail: hend.riahi@gmail.com; emnasensei@gmail.com; fethiladeb@hotmail.fr; bouaziz_mouna@yahoo.fr

M. Barsaoui
Department of Orthopedic Surgery, La Rabta, Tunisia
e-mail: barsaoui.maher@yahoo.fr

Abstract

Spinal Ewing sarcoma is an uncommon tumor usually seen in the second decade of life with male predilection. In adolescents, an aggressive solitary osteolytic lesion with a soft tissue mass in the sacrum and less commonly in vertebra should raise suspicion for Ewing sarcoma. Spinal MRI is sensitive in the early detection of Ewing sarcoma and the evaluation of tumor spread to the bone marrow or into adjacent soft tissues. Sacrococcygeal tumors have a poor prognosis. Treatment should be multimodal involving radical surgical excision, radiotherapy, and chemotherapy.

Abbreviations

CT	Computed tomography
EwS	Ewing sarcoma
MRI	Magnetic resonance imaging
WI	Weighted images

1 Introduction

Ewing sarcoma and Ewing-like sarcoma family are highly aggressive round cell mesenchymal neoplasms with various degrees of neuroectodermal differentiation.

It most often occurs in children and young adults. In the 2020 WHO classification, a new

Med Radiol Diagn Imaging (2023)
https://doi.org/10.1007/174_2023_433,
Published Online: 09 June 2023

chapter covering “undifferentiated small round cell sarcomas of bone and soft tissue tumors” has been introduced (de Álava et al. 2020).

The new chapter includes Ewing sarcoma and three main categories showing considerable morphologic overlap (Choi and Ro 2020).

2 Epidemiology

Ewing sarcoma is the second most frequent bone tumor in children and adolescents (Kaatsch 2010).

Metastatic disease to the spine from Ewing tumor at another site is common. However, primary Ewing sarcoma of the spinal column is a relatively rare lesion accounting for approximately 3.5–7% of lesions in two large series of patients with Ewing sarcoma (Whitehouse and Griffiths 1976; Dahlin 1978). Nearly 75% of patients are aged between 5 and 15 years (Boussios et al. 2018).

3 Localization

Ewing sarcoma has been categorized into sacral and non-sacral types based on the differences in the treatment responses and survival rates (Jaiswal et al. 2017).

Sacrum is affected in 55.2% followed by lumbar spine (25%). Cervical spine is the least commonly affected site (3.3% of cases) (Ilaslan et al. 2004).

In non-sacral spine, lesion originates from posterior elements extending to the vertebral body (Patnaik et al. 2016).

4 Pathogenesis

Ewing sarcoma is a model example of solid tumor formation mediated by a specific family of fusion genes. A balanced translocation occurs in the majority of cases between chromosomes 11 and 22, whereas variant rearrangements involving other chromosomes occur less frequently. Specific chimera genes formed between EWSR1 and various fusion partners such as FLI1 (93%), ERG (5%), ETV1, E1AF, FEV, and ZSG (in the remaining cases), all members of the ETS transcription family have been identified (Szuhai et al. 2009).

5 Clinical Presentation

Clinical presentation depends on the affected site and degree of tumor invasion (Grier 1997). Pain is the commonest first symptom. It can be localized, can radiate to the extremities, or both (Qureshi et al. 2007).

Neurologic deficits have been reported in almost two-thirds of patients with vertebral Ewing sarcoma (Barbieri et al. 1998).

Pelvic tumors are mostly deep and are close to other structures that cause vague and insidious presentation. Patients may present late with or without a mass and therefore have higher rate of metastasis (35.6%) (Kadhim et al. 2018).

Systemic manifestations such as fever and anemia have been described.

6 Imaging

6.1 Radiographs

Radiographic abnormalities may be subtle and difficult to detect, especially in the sacral spine of young patients. Thus, radiographic analysis of bone and soft tissues must be very accurate, and subsequent imaging (MRI, CT) must be performed promptly in doubtful cases or when radiographs are considered normal.

Radiographs show variable degrees of osteolysis or sclerosis with partial (Fig. 1) or complete vertebral collapse (Fig. 2). Osteosclerotic Ewing sarcoma is a rare but well-known phenomenon in the appendicular skeleton and histologically corresponds to necrotic and reactive bone formation (Ilaslan et al. 2004). Vertebra plana has also been reported as a presentation. Extension into adjacent vertebral bodies may be observed (Flemming et al. 2000). Disc space narrowing or rarely widening may be seen. Bony expansion and radiographically evident calcification within Ewing sarcoma is rare (Weinstein et al. 1984).

6.2 Computed Tomography

CT allows a very clear evaluation of density and cortical integrity. It demonstrates the aggressive growth of the lesions and the soft tissue extension (Figs. 3 and 4). Moth eaten and permeative patterns are usual. CT-guided needle biopsy of vertebral or paravertebral lesions can be accomplished with accuracy and relative ease.

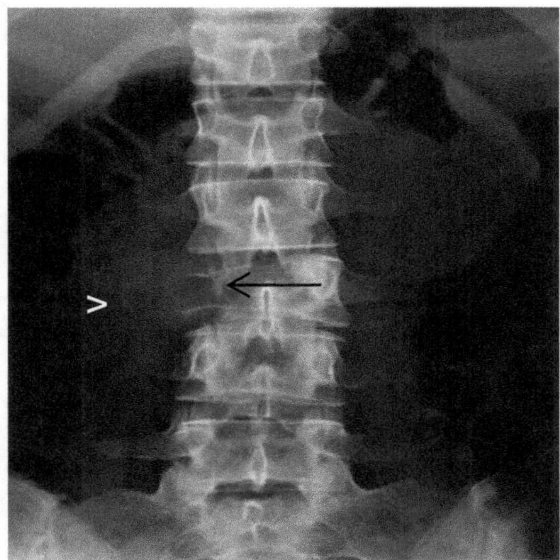

Fig. 1 Ewing sarcoma of L3: anteroposterior radiograph of lumbar spine shows lytic lesion within the right lateral aspect of the L3 vertebral body and the right pedicle and transverse apophysis (arrow). An associated heterogeneous soft tissue mass extends from this lesion into the right (arrowhead)

6.3 Magnetic Resonance Imaging

MRI is very sensitive in the early detection of Ewing sarcoma in the spine.

After scout views in three orthogonal planes, we perform mostly T1-weighted images (WI), T2-WI images in a sagittal and axial plane.

For sacral tumors, slices are acquired in three planes, but the most important plane is the coronal oblique plane, parallel to the long axis of the sacrum (Leclère et al. 2007).

STIR may be reliable for determining the extension into the soft tissues, encasement of the neurovascular bundle, and visualizing intratumoral necrosis.

T1-WI after intravenous injection of Gadolinium is performed in the same imaging plane as that of the precontrast series and in the axial plane (Vanhoenacker et al. 2010).

Anatomic T1-WI and T2-WI or STIR MR images provide relevant information for diagnosis, staging, and surgical planning.

MRI of the spine is superior for visualizing epidural extension and tumor spread to the bone marrow or extension into adjacent soft tissues.

Fig. 2 Ewing sarcoma of C5: radiograph anteroposterior and lateral view showing C5 vertebra plana (arrowhead)

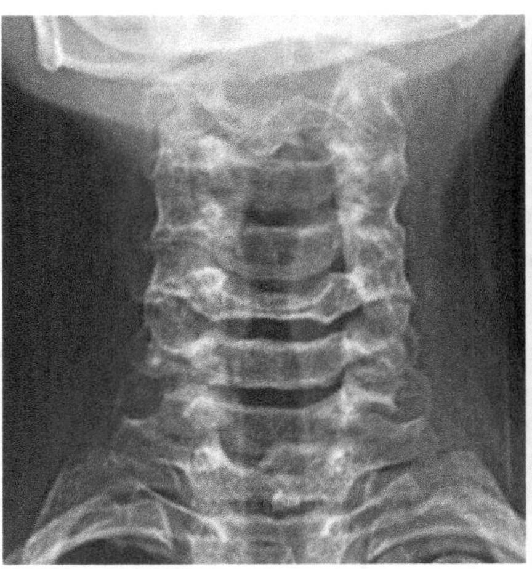

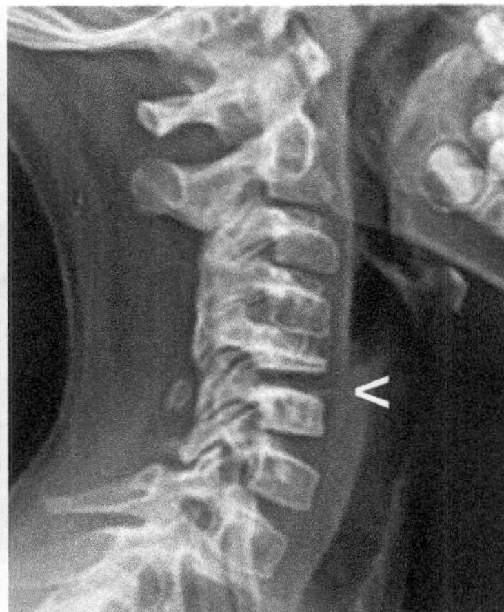

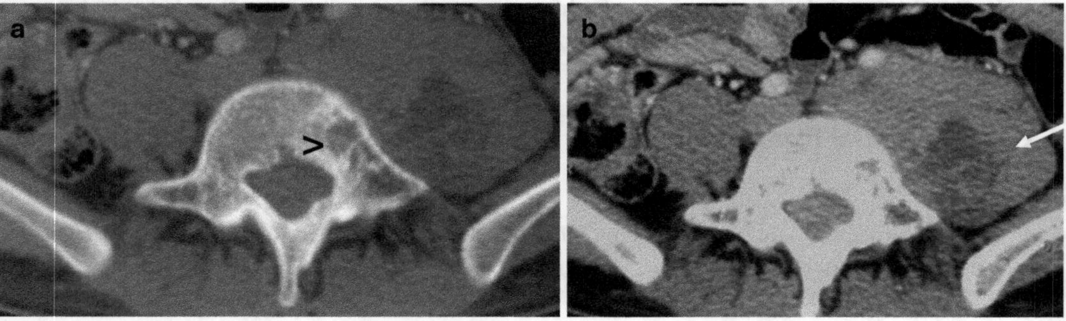

Fig. 3 Ewing sarcoma of L4: axial CT shows mixed lucency and sclerosis (**a**, bone window) of L4 vertebral body and transverse process with hypodense soft tissue mass (**b**, soft tissue window)

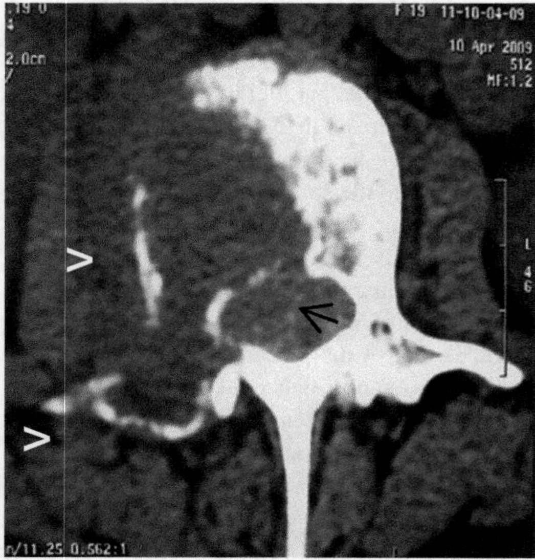

Fig. 4 Ewing sarcoma of L3. Axial CT scan shows a unilateral posterolateral lytic lesion within the right vertebral body of L3 with lateral soft tissue extension (arrowhead) and extension into the spinal canal (arrow)

The relationship of tumor to adjacent vessels can also be determined.

MRI is superior to CT for the delineation of the soft tissue mass, which is often a prominent feature. The presence and size of a soft tissue mass are useful MRI signs to distinguish Ewing sarcoma from differential diagnosis such as osteomyelitis (Kasalak et al. 2019).

The MR imaging appearance is nonspecific, with lesions having intermediate signal intensity on T1-WI and intermediate to high signal intensity on T2-WI (Garcia et al. 2017) (Fig. 5).

Ewing sarcoma shows a wide intramedullary transition between the tumor and the normal bone marrow (Kaste 2011).

It typically shows inhomogeneous contrast enhancement caused by the presence of internal necrosis or hemorrhage, which, depending on its time of evolution, may appear hyper-, iso-, or hypointense to muscle (Clemente et al. 2022).

There is no relevant literature to support the use of whole-body MRI without and with IV contrast in the initial staging for extrapulmonary metastasis of Ewing sarcoma (Stanborough et al. 2022).

6.4 Nuclear Medicine Imaging

In the Euro Ewing study protocol, 18F-FDG PET-CT should be performed three times: at staging, at early response assessment, and at late response assessment. Pre-therapeutic 18F-FDG PET-CT of patients with Ewing sarcoma improves detection of metastases compared to conventional imaging. False FDG positive lesions are quite common, and supplementary imaging or biopsies is often necessary (Johnsen et al. 2018).

For the American College of Radiology, FDG-PET/CT whole body is usually appropriate in the evaluation of extrapulmonary metastases for the initial staging. Although the panel did not agree on recommending fluoride PET/CT whole body, because there is insufficient medical literature to conclude whether these patients would benefit from the procedure, its use may be appropriate (Stanborough et al. 2022).

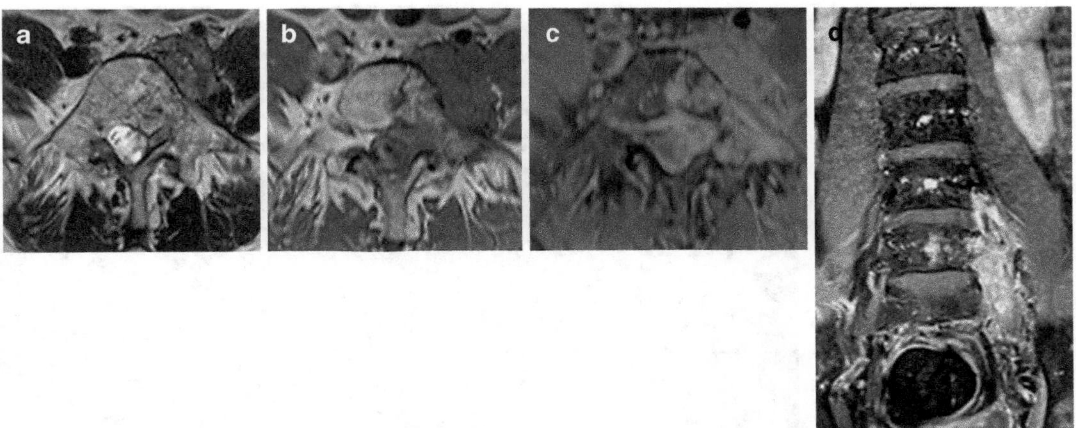

Fig. 5 Ewing sarcoma of L4. Axial T2-WI (**a**), T1-WI (**b**), T1-WI postcontrast (**c**), and coronal T1-WI postcontrast (**d**), MR imaging demonstrating tumor mass arising from left pedicle, transverse process, and vertebral body of L4 invading spinal canal and left psoas muscle

7 Histopathology

In gross examination, the cut surface of untreated EwS is gray-white, soft and frequently includes areas of hemorrhage and necrosis. Histologically, EwS has a solid pattern of growth, and is composed of monomorphic small cells with round nuclei. CD99 is a cell surface glycoprotein and a very sensitive but poorly specific diagnostic marker for Ewing sarcoma (Marcilla et al. 2021).

Currently, the diagnosis of Ewing sarcoma can only be confirmed by molecular pathology. FISH-based detection of EWSR1 rearrangements and/or RT-PCR detection of FET–ETS gene fusions specific for Ewing sarcoma have been used (Sorensen et al. 1993).

8 Differential Diagnosis

Differential diagnosis consists in this age-group of an eosinophilic granuloma (EG) (Fig. 6). If a Ewing sarcoma does not show the sclerotic pattern, imaging features are quite similar. However, paravertebral soft tissue component and isolated posterior element involvement are uncommon in EG (Prasad and Divya 2019).

In sclerotic appearing Ewing sarcoma, the differential diagnosis is osteosarcoma. Mineralization of the soft tissue mass is the hallmark for an osteosarcoma (Erlemann 2006).

Lymphoma should be considered in the differential diagnosis of any sclerotic vertebral lesion (Mechri et al. 2018).

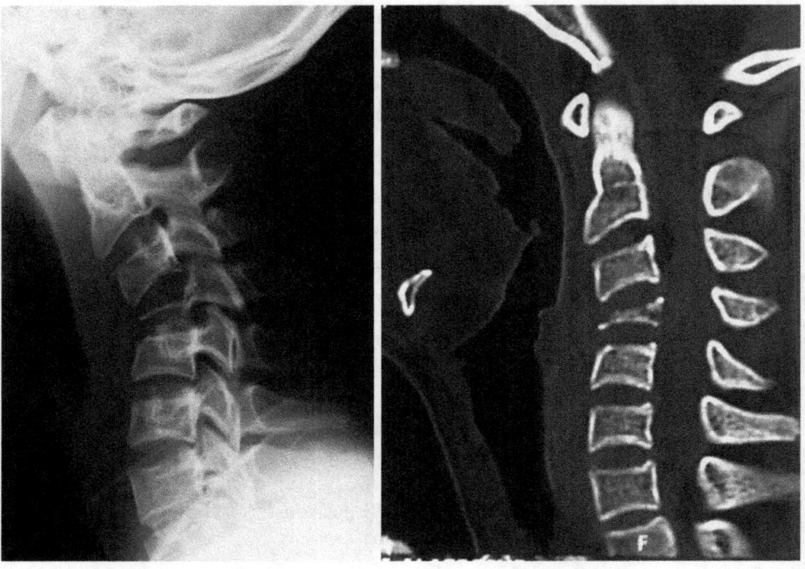

Fig. 6 Eosinophilic granuloma: radiograph lateral view and sagittal CT showing C4 vertebra plana

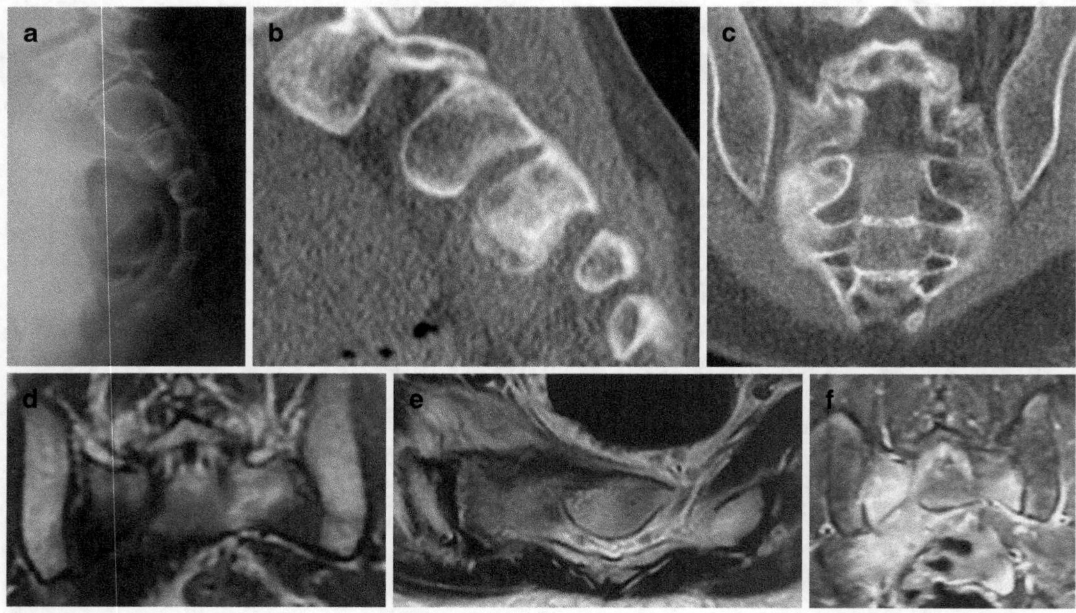

Fig. 7 Chronic multifocal osteomyelitis: lateral view of sacral radiograph (**a**), sagittal (**b**), and coronal oblique (**c**) CT, coronal T1-WI (**d**), axial T2-WI (**e**), and coronal T1-WI postcontrast MR (**f**) imaging showing sclerotic lesion of S2 and S3 of low T1 and T2 signal and extensive enhancement after intravenous Gadolinium contrast injection

Spinal involvement of chronic multifocal osteomyelitis although less common than in the long tubular bones has been reported. Radiologic findings include partial or complete loss of height of the vertebral body, lytic lesion with surrounding sclerosis, or a purely sclerosis appearance (Fig. 7).

9 Local and Distant Staging

Imaging guidelines for patients with EwS have been proposed (Meyer et al. 2008).

MRI is the method of choice for visualizing the local extent of the tumor. The native T1 sequence is best suited for determining the resection height. The protocol must be completed with T2-WI TSE and the T1-WI TSE sequence with contrast media and fat saturation, to address extraosseous tumor infiltration of adjacent vascular/nerve bundles or joint compartments as these findings impact the extent and technique of local therapy.

18F-FDG-PET/CT with chest CT, and either 18F-FDG-PET/MRI or whole-body MRI, each combined with a chest CT, are reliable diagnostics in staging of Ewing sarcoma patients (Zöllner et al. 2021).

10 Treatment

Treatment consists of a combination of an aggressive chemotherapy followed by radiation therapy. Surgical resection is often not feasible because of the lesion location and the large size of the soft tissue components (Orguc and Remide 2014).

Subtotal or partial resection should be avoided; en-bloc resection with negative tumor margins should be the surgical goal (Boussios et al. 2018).

For tumors that invade the vertebral body and entrap the spinal cord from its anterior side, decompressive laminectomy is not considered. Extensive tumor resection could lead to loss of stability of the spine, which is a major concern. This risk has been minimized by the anterior interbody fusion with or without instrumentation (Alfonso and Burgos 2012).

For localized pelvic EwS surgery is indicated if clear margins can be achieved, but in all other cases, the role of RT in single or combinatorial modalities for local control plays a greater role. Tumors which cross the midline in the sacrum or sacral tumors involving the S1 nerve route are not considered resectable because of the morbidity associated with surgery (Gerrand et al. 2020).

11 Prognosis

Nearly total local control and a long-term survival of more than 70% for patients with non-sacral tumors can be achieved. Sacrococcygeal tumors have a poor prognosis, with about 60% local control and about 25% long-term survival. This is due to the larger tumor size at diagnosis. It has been clearly shown that prognosis, particularly long-term survival, is related to tumor size at presentation (Erlemann 2006).

12 Key Messages

- Ewing sarcoma is most commonly seen in children and young adults, with a peak incidence in the second decade of life.
- The spine is usually involved in metastatic disease, primary vertebral Ewing sarcoma (PVES) is uncommon with a reported incidence of 3.5%.
- The sacrum is the most frequent site of involvement followed by the lumbar spine and the cervical spine.
- Radiograph and CT usually show lytic pattern, osteosclerotic Ewing sarcoma is rare and it corresponds to necrotic and reactive bone formation.
- MRI is more sensitive in detecting the tumor, delineating soft tissue extension and spinal cord compression.

References

Alfonso M, Burgos J (2012) Ewing's sarcoma of the spine with initial myeloradicular involvement in children and adolescents. Eur Orthop Traumatol 3:189–194

Barbieri E, Chiaulon G, Bunkeila F et al (1998) Radiotherapy in vertebral tumors. Indications and limits; a report on 28 cases of Ewing's sarcoma of the spine. Chir Organi Mov 83:105–111

Boussios S, Hayward C, Cooke D, Zakynthinakis-Kyriakou N, Tsiouris AK, Chatziantoniou AA, Kanellos FS, Karathanasi A (2018) Spinal Ewing sarcoma debuting with cord compression: have we discovered the thread of Ariadne? Anticancer Res 38(10):5589–5597. https://doi.org/10.21873/anticanres.12893. PMID: 30275176

Choi JH, Ro JY (2020) The 2020 WHO classification of tumors of soft tissue: selected changes and new entities. Adv Anat Pathol 28(1):44–58. https://doi.org/10.1097/pap.0000000000000284

Clemente EJI, Navarro OM, Navallas M, Ladera E, Torner F, Sunol M, Barber I (2022) Multiparametric MRI evaluation of bone sarcomas in children. Insights Imaging 13(1):1–18

Dahlin DC (1978) Ewing's tumor. In: Bone tumors, 3rd edn. Thomas, Springfield, p 274

De Álava E, Lessnick SL, Stamenkovic I, The WHO Classification of Tumours Editorial Board (2020) Ewing sarcoma WHO classification of tumours soft tissue and bone tumours, 5th edn. IARC Press, Lyon, pp 323–325

Erlemann R (2006) Imaging and differential diagnosis of primary bone tumors and tumor-like lesions of the spine. Eur J Radiol 58(1):48–67

Flemming DJ, Murphey MD, Carmichael BB, Bernard SA (2000) Primary tumors of the spine. Semin Musculoskelet Radiol 4(3):0299–0320

Garcia DAV, Aivazoglou LU, Garcia LAL et al (2017) Diagnostic imaging of primary bone tumors of the spine. Curr Radiol Rep 5:30. https://doi.org/10.1007/s40134-017-0220-1

Gerrand C, Bate J, Seddon B, Dirksen U, Randall RL, van de Sande M, O'Donnell P, Tuckett J, Peake D, Jeys L et al (2020) Seeking international consensus on approaches to primary tumour treatment in Ewing sarcoma. Clin Sarcoma Res 10:21

Grier HE (1997) The Ewing family of tumors: Ewing sarcoma and primitive neuroectodermal tumors. Pediatr Clin North Am 44(4):991–1004

Ilaslan H, Sundaram M, Unni KK, Dekutoski MB (2004) Primary Ewing's sarcoma of the vertebral column. Skeletal Radiol 33(9):506–513. https://doi.org/10.1007/s00256-004-0810-x. Epub 2004 Jun 30. PMID: 15232658

Jaiswal S et al (2017) Primary Ewing's sarcoma of spine, its management & outcome: a retrospective analysis. Int J Neurol Neurosurg 9(1):33. https://doi.org/10.21088/ijnns.0975.0223.9117.5

Johnsen B, Fasmer KE, Boye K et al (2018) Added value of 18F-FDG PET-CT in staging of Ewing sarcoma in children and young adults. Eur J Hybrid Imaging 2:13

Kaatsch P (2010) Epidemiology of childhood cancer. Cancer Treat Rev 36(4):277–285. https://doi.org/10.1016/j.ctrv.2010.02.003. Epub 2010 Mar 15. PMID: 20231056

Kadhim M, Oyoun NA, Womer RB, Dormans JP (2018) Clinical and radiographic presentation of pelvic sarcoma in children. SICOT J 4:44. https://doi.org/10.1051/sicotj/2018040. Epub 2018 Oct 19. PMID: 30339522; PMCID: PMC6195345

Kasalak Ö, Overbosch J, Adams HJ et al (2019) Diagnostic value of MRI signs in differentiating Ewing sarcoma from osteomyelitis. Acta Radiol 60(2):204–212. https://doi.org/10.1177/0284185118774953

Kaste SC (2011) Imaging pediatric bone sarcomas. Radiol Clin North Am 49:749–765

Leclère J, Vanel D, Missenard G, Brisse H, Neuenschwander S (2007) Imaging of sacral tumours. Skeletal Radiol 37(4):277–289. https://doi.org/10.1007/s00256-007-0413-4

Marcilla D, Machado I, Grunewald TGP, Llombart-Bosch A, de Alava E (2021) (Immuno)histological analysis of Ewing sarcoma. Methods Mol Biol 2226:49–64. https://doi.org/10.1007/978-1-0716-1020-6_5

Mechri M, Riahi H, Sboui I, Bouaziz M, Vanhoenacker F, Ladeb M (2018) Imaging of malignant primitive tumors of the spine. J Belg Soc Radiol 102(1):56. https://doi.org/10.5334/jbsr.1410. PMID: 30915424; PMCID: PMC6425224

Meyer JS, Nadel HR, Marina N, Womer RB, Brown KL, Eary JF, Gorlick R, Grier HE, Randall RL, Lawlor ER et al (2008) Imaging guidelines for children with Ewing sarcoma and osteosarcoma: a report from the Children's Oncology Group Bone Tumor Committee. Pediatr Blood Cancer 51:163–170. https://doi.org/10.1002/pbc.21596

Orguc S, Remide A (2014) Primary tumors of the spine. Semin Musculoskelet Radiol 18:280–299

Patnaik S, Jyotsnarani Y, Uppin SG, Susarla R (2016) Imaging features of primary tumors of the spine: a pictorial essay. Indian J Radiol Imaging 26:279–289

Prasad GL, Divya S (2019) Eosinophilic granuloma of the cervical spine in adults: a review. World Neurosurg 125:301

Qureshi AA, Qureshi GA, Hassan M (2007) A case of Ewing sarcoma involving cervical spine. Am Euras J Sci Res 2(1):57–59

Sorensen PH, Liu XF, Delattre O, Rowland JM, Biggs CA, Thomas G, Triche TJ (1993) Reverse transcriptase PCR amplification of EWS/FLI-1 fusion transcripts as a diagnostic test for peripheral primitive neuroectodermal tumors of childhood. Diagn Mol Pathol 2:147–157. https://doi.org/10.1097/00019606-199309000-00002

Stanborough R, Demertzis JL, Wessell DE, Lenchik L, Ahlawat S, Baker JC, Banks J, Caracciolo JT, Garner HW, Hentz C, Lewis VO, Lu Y, Maynard JR, Pierce JL, Scott JA, Sharma A, Beaman FD (2022) ACR appropriateness criteria® malignant or aggressive primary musculoskeletal tumor-staging and surveillance: 2022 update. J Am Coll Radiol 19(11S):S374–S389. https://doi.org/10.1016/j.jacr.2022.09.015. PMID: 36436964

Szuhai K, Ijszenga M, de Jong D, Karseladze A, Tanke HJ, Hogendoorn PC (2009) The NFATc2 gene is involved in a novel cloned translocation in a Ewing sarcoma variant that couples its function in immunology to oncology. Clin Cancer Res 15(7):2259–2268. https://doi.org/10.1158/1078-0432.CCR-08-2184. Epub 2009 Mar 24. PMID: 19318479

Vanhoenacker FM, Van Dyck P, Gielen J, De Schepper AM, Parizel PM (2010) Musculoskeletal system. In: Reimer P et al (eds) Clinical MR imaging. Springer, pp 265–355

Weinstein JB, Siegel MJ, Griffith RC (1984) Spinal Ewing sarcoma: misleading appearances. Skeletal Radiol 11:262–265. https://doi.org/10.1007/BF00351350

Whitehouse GH, Griffiths GJ (1976) Roentgenologic aspects of spinal involvement by primary and metastatic Ewing's tumor. J Can Assoc Radiol 27:290

Zöllner SK et al (2021) Ewing sarcoma—diagnosis, treatment, clinical challenges and future perspectives. J Clin Med 10(8):1685

Spinal Bone Lymphoma

Mohamed Chaabouni, Mouna Chelli Bouaziz, and Mohamed Fethi Ladeb

Contents

Abstract

Bone lymphoma is a heterogeneous set of distinct clinicopathological entities with different disease stages and prognoses. It can be categorized into primary solitary lymphoma of bone, primary multifocal or polyostotic lymphoma of bone, and disseminated lymphoma with bone involvement. Primary lymphoma of bone is rare, and secondary bone lymphoma is more frequent. Spinal location is not uncommon and has the particularity of proximity to the central nervous system. Clinical presentation and imaging features are nonspecific. Open surgery biopsy is preferred for histological and immunohistochemical examination. MRI is the imaging modality of choice for local staging. ^{18}F-FDG-PET/CT is the gold standard for distant staging. Whole-body MRI with diffusion-WI is an interesting alternative. Treatment is based on chemotherapy and radiotherapy. Surgical treatment is reserved for neurological complications and spinal instability. Primary lymphoma of bone has the best prognosis, whereas polyostotic and disseminated lymphomas have more variable reserved prognosis. The spinal location is associated with a worse outcome compared to the appendicular skeleton location.

M. Chaabouni (✉) · M. Chelli Bouaziz · M. F. Ladeb
Department of Radiology, MT Kassab Institute of Orthopaedics, Ksar Said, Tunisia

Faculty of Medicine of Tunis, Tunis-El Manar University, Tunis, Tunisia

Med Radiol Diagn Imaging (2023)
https://doi.org/10.1007/174_2023_467,
Published Online: 06 December 2023

1 Introduction

Lymphoma is a heterogeneous group of malignancies that arise from the clonal proliferation of lymphocytes (mostly in lymph nodes), representing approximately 5% of all cancers. Lymphoma is broadly classified into Hodgkin's lymphoma (HL) (10%) and non-Hodgkin's lymphoma (NHL) (90%) (Jamil and Mukkamalla 2023).

Lymphoma of bone accounts for 5% of extranodal lymphomas and can be categorized into primary lymphoma of bone (PLB), multifocal PLB, or disseminated lymphoma with secondary osseous involvement (Messina et al. 2015).

PLB is defined by the 2020 World Health Organization (WHO) classification of soft tissue and bone tumors as a neoplasm composed of malignant lymphoid cells, producing one or more lesions within bone with no (supraregional) lymph node or other extranodal lesion involvement (Cleven and Ferry 2020). By convention, an interval of 6 months between the skeletal manifestation and the development of extraskeletal disease is also required for the tumor to be considered as PLB (Saifuddin 2021).

PLB is a rare disease that constitutes approximately 7% of all malignant bone tumors and less than 1% of all malignant lymphomas (Saifuddin 2021).

Secondary bone lymphoma is more common and occurs in the setting of hematogenous spread or direct extension from surrounding involved lymph nodes or soft tissues, implying stage IV disease (Saifuddin 2021).

Age range is wide, commonly between 45 and 60 years with slight male predominance.

Spinal bone lymphoma presents almost always with pain, and neurologic impairment is frequent, due to spinal canal invasion.

Imaging features are suggestive but nonspecific of bone lymphoma.

We herein review the histopathology, epidemiology, imaging features, up-to-date staging methods, treatment, and prognosis of spinal bone lymphoma.

2 Pathogenesis

More than 80% of PLBs are diffuse large B-cell lymphomas (DLBCLs).

Other rare subtypes include follicular, marginal zone, lymphoblastic, ALK-positive and ALK-negative anaplastic large cell, NK/T-cell, Burkitt, indolent, and HL (Cleven and Ferry 2020).

Primary bone DLBCL probably arises from centrocytes that originate from naive B cells in the germinal center light zone of lymphoid follicles as part of an inflammatory or immunological response. Alternatively, the centrocytes may derive from extra-osseous lymphoid tissue, migrate to the bone, and give rise to lymphoma (Cleven and Ferry 2020).

3 Epidemiology

PLB is uncommon, accounting for about 7% of all malignant bone tumors, less than 1% of all malignant lymphomas, and 4–5% of all extranodal lymphomas (Saifuddin 2021).

Spinal location accounts for about 30% of all PLBs (Ramadan et al. 2007; Liu et al. 2020).

Median age at diagnosis is 45–60 years, but the age range is wide (15–99 years). Pediatric cases were also reported (Messina et al. 2015).

Most reports suggest a slight male prevalence.

PLB typically arises sporadically. PLB has rarely arisen on a background of HIV-positive patients, patients with long-standing osteomyelitis, or Paget's disease of bone (Cleven and Ferry 2020).

Secondary bone lymphoma is more common, occurring in 16% of disseminated lymphomas. The prevalence is higher in children, accounting for 25% of cases. The most frequent sites of bone metastases are the spine, pelvis, and skull (Malloy et al. 1992).

4 Localization

Thoracic spine is the most involved segment (57%) followed by the lumbar spine (27%), whereas 15% of spinal lymphomas involve junction zones (Barz et al. 2021).

Sacral lymphoma is rare (1%), with few case reports (Mavrogenis et al. 2017; Barz et al. 2021).

In most cases, lymphoma involves the anterior vertebral column, whereas posterior involvement is rare (Mechri et al. 2018).

5 Clinical Presentation

Most patients present with insidious and intermittent bone pain in the involved spinal segment. Other symptoms include local swelling and a palpable mass (Vannata and Zucca 2015).

Systemic symptoms such as fever, weight loss, or night sweats are rare at presentation (Cleven and Ferry 2020).

Hypercalcemia may be observed, but related symptoms such as constipation, lethargy, and somnolence are uncommon (Messina et al. 2015).

Clinical presentation is nonspecific, and the reported delay between symptoms' onset and diagnosis is 6–8 months (Vannata and Zucca 2015).

Up to 50% of patients present with neurologic impairment due to spinal cord compression (Ramadan et al. 2007).

Vertebral collapse is present at presentation in 38% of cases (Messina et al. 2015).

6 Imaging

6.1 Radiographs

Radiographic findings are nonspecific and underestimate the true extent of the osseous infiltration. Radiographs may be normal. Paravertebral masses may precede radiographic evidence of bone involvement.

Osteolysis is the most common pattern and may be permeative, moth eaten, geographic poorly, or well defined, with or without cortical disruption (Fyllos et al. 2021). Osteolytic and mixed lytic-sclerotic lesions account for almost 90% of cases (Saifuddin 2021).

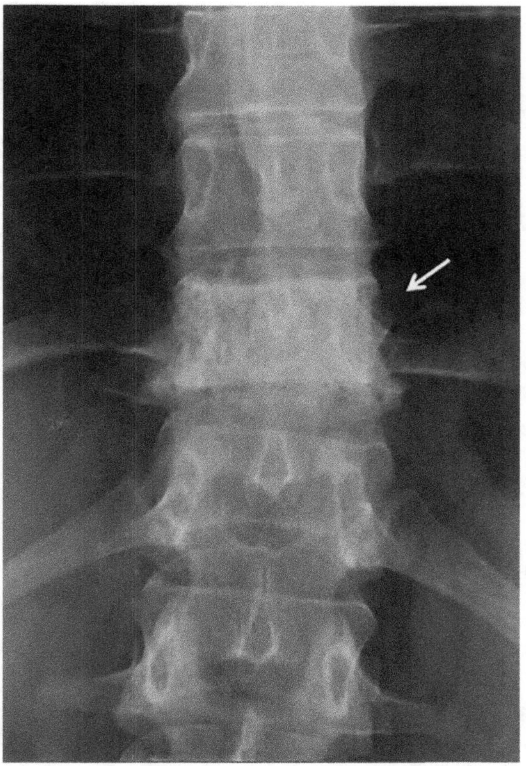

Fig. 1 Bone lymphoma of T11 vertebra: frontal view radiograph: diffuse osteosclerosis of the vertebral body giving it the appearance of "ivory vertebra"

Vertebral collapse occurs early with lytic lesions, occasionally producing vertebra plana (Saifuddin 2021).

Purely osteosclerotic pattern is very rare and is seen more commonly in HL. A vertebral body with diffuse osteosclerosis, known as "ivory vertebra" (Fig. 1), is a characteristic but not pathognomonic sign of spinal bone lymphoma (Lim and Ong 2013).

6.2 CT

Computed tomography (CT) is more sensitive than radiography for detecting spinal bone lesions and identifying the vertebral segment(s) involved (Fig. 2). It is also superior in analyzing cortical

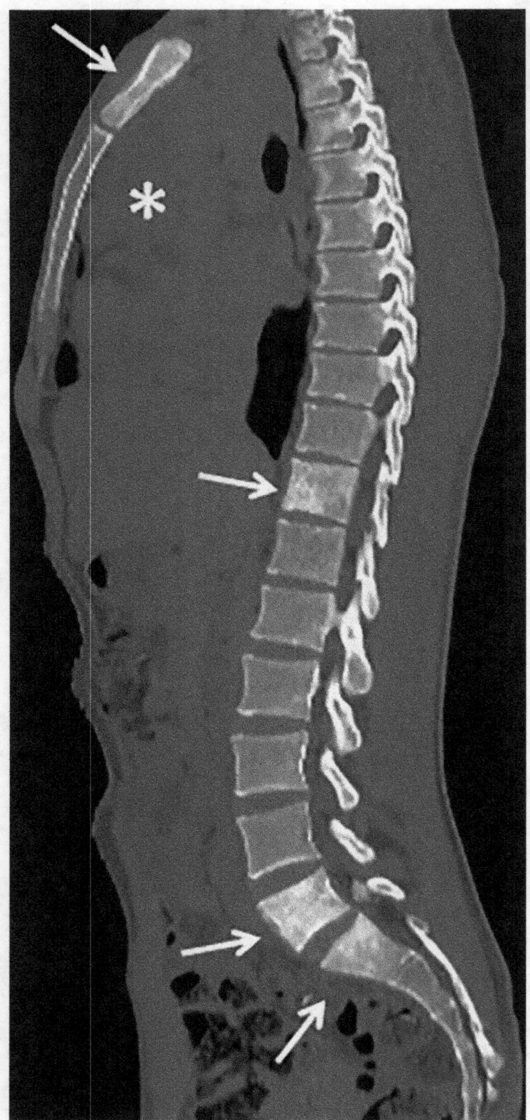

Fig. 2 Disseminated nodal lymphoma with multifocal bone involvement: thoraco-abdominopelvic CT, sagittal reconstruction in bone window: osteosclerotic lesions of the vertebral bodies of T11, L5, S1 and the sternal manubrium (arrows). Note the bulky mediastinal disease (asterisk)

disruption and potential soft tissue paravertebral and epidural extension (Fig. 3) (Fyllos et al. 2021; Saifuddin 2021).

Bone sequestra, a recognized feature of bone lymphoma, is better seen on CT (Fig. 3) (Mechri et al. 2018).

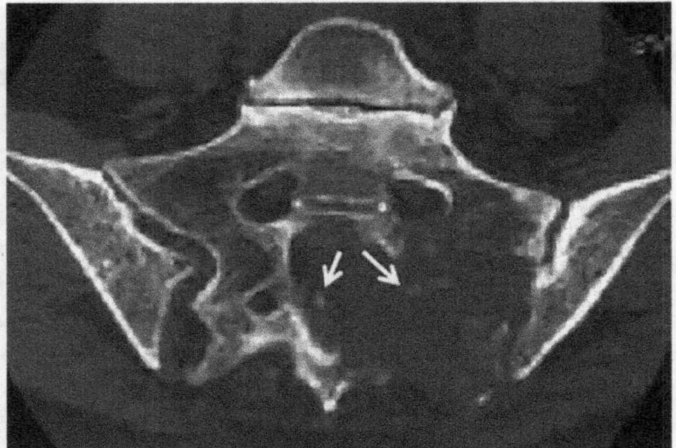

Fig. 3 Lymphoma of the sacrum: CT oblique axial image with bone window: a destructive osteolytic lesion of sacrum extending to the left sacral foramina and sacroiliac joint. Note the bone sequestra (arrows)

Contrast-enhanced CT may be performed for disease staging, ideally during a single visit in combination with positron emission tomography (PET). It allows an accurate measurement of the nodal localizations, characterizes focal parenchymal lesions, distinguishes between viscera and lymphadenopathy, and evaluates thrombosis or great thoracic vessel compression (Barrington et al. 2014).

Lymphoma is the most common malignancy that results in nondiagnostic CT-guided needle biopsy: 22% of bone lymphoma's and 17% of soft tissue lymphoma's CT-guided needle biopsies are nondiagnostic (Chang et al. 2015).

The accuracy of image-guided bone biopsy is lower than that of soft tissue biopsy (Wang et al. 2019).

In case of nondiagnostic image-guided needle biopsy, with high suspicion of lymphoma, it may be more appropriate to refer the patient for open surgical biopsy rather than for repeat image-guided biopsy. If a repeated biopsy is decided, variations in technique and an increased number of needle passes may increase diagnostic yield. The previous biopsy images should be reviewed and, if possible, sampling a different portion of the lesion should be attempted (Meek et al. 2020).

Diagnosis of lymphoma is often aided by using flow cytometry, in which biopsy samples are placed in saline solution instead of formalin (Meek et al. 2020).

6.3 PET and PET/CT

^{18}F-fluorodeoxyglucose-PET (^{18}F-FDG PET) is a functional imaging modality that explores the whole body and identifies tumor lesions with high glucose metabolism (Fig. 4a).

PET/CT is a hybrid imaging technique that simultaneously provides functional and anatomical information (Fig. 4).

94% of all lymphomas are avid for FDG, such as HL, DLBCL, and follicular lymphoma (Saifuddin 2021).

PET/CT has a better diagnostic performance than CT with 97% sensitivity and 100% specificity, especially for normal-sized lymph nodes and extranodal sites (including bone marrow), as it detects diffuse or focal metabolic uptake where no significant abnormalities are noted on CT (Fig. 4). This led to frequent disease upstage and treatment modification (Wang 2015).

PET/CT also provides a better evaluation of bone marrow involvement compared to bone marrow biopsy, which evaluates a very limited sample, whereas PET/CT may identify focal involvement in the whole body. The sensitivity and specificity of PET/CT in detecting bone marrow involvement are 84% and 100%, respectively (Kaddu-Mulindwa et al. 2021).

This renders bone marrow biopsy no longer indicated for the routine staging of FDG-avid lymphoma if a PET/CT is performed (Cheson et al. 2014).

PET/CT is widely used for staging and response assessment in FDG-avid lymphoma. Response assessment PET/CT studies are performed during and after treatment (Cheson et al. 2014).

The parameter most commonly used in response assessment is the standardized uptake value (SUV) at sites of disease, compared to

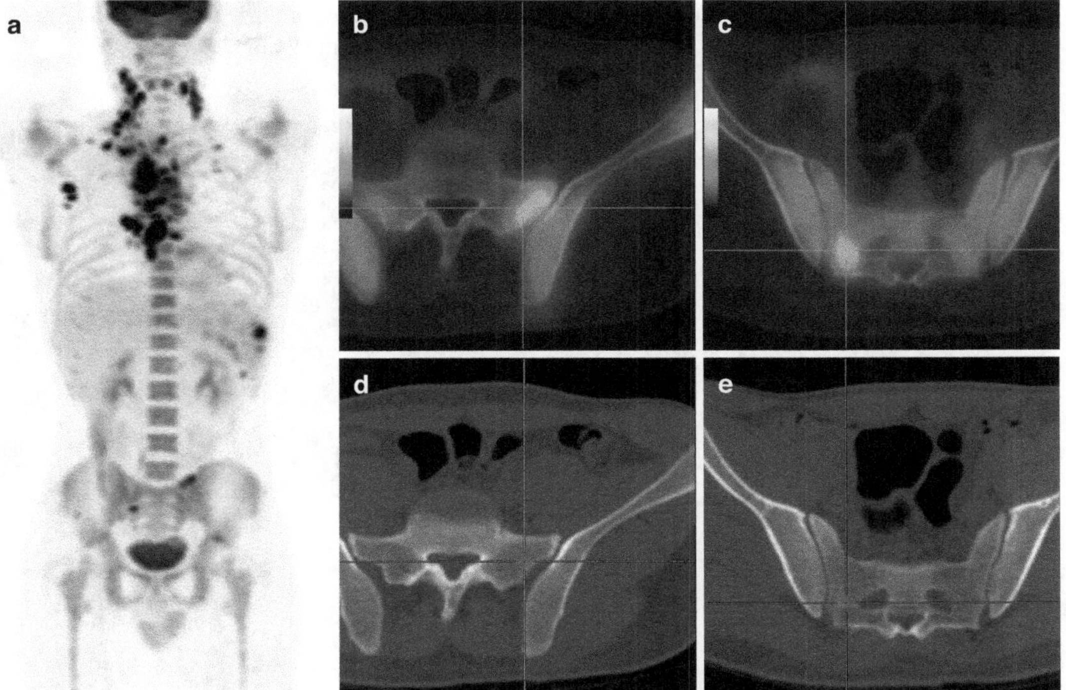

Fig. 4 Disseminated lymphoma with bone involvement: ^{18}F-FDG PET/CT: (**a**) PET shows high FDG uptake foci and makes an exhaustive disease extent assessment: cervical, mediastinal, and right axillary lymph nodes; nodular splenic lesion; and bone marrow focal involvement in the sacrum and right acetabular roof. Bone marrow biopsy of the right iliac crest was negative. CT component provides precise anatomical location of the areas with increased uptake (**b**, **c**). Note the normal appearance of these areas on CT (**d**, **e**)

physiological activity in reference areas (mediastinum and liver) and reported using the 5-point Deauville scale (Barrington et al. 2014).

PET/CT-derived quantitative parameters, such as metabolic tumor volume, total lesion glycolysis, and textural and shape analysis (radiomics), may predict prognosis or treatment outcome (Frood et al. 2021).

6.4 MRI

With its high sensitivity, MRI is the imaging modality of choice for assessing bone marrow replacement and lesion extent to the surrounding soft tissue, especially epidural, nerve, and spinal cord involvement (Patnaik et al. 2016).

Bone marrow replacement may be focal or diffuse. Signal intensity characteristics are nonspecific, commonly low on T1-weighted images (WI) and high and heterogeneous on T2-WI. Fibrosis within the tumor may appear hypointense on T2-WI. Short tau inversion recovery (STIR) sequences are also helpful in the detection of hyperintense lesions on a background of a hypointense fatty marrow. These lesions enhance following contrast medium administration (Fig. 5) (Mikhaeel 2012; Lim and Ong 2013).

The presence of a large soft tissue paravertebral and/or epidural mass with maintenance of the cortical outline of the vertebral body is highly suggestive of lymphoma (Fig. 5) (Saifuddin 2021). This feature may be explained by cytokine-mediated neoplastic action causing increased local bone resorption and formation of penetrating channels through the cortex, allowing the tumor cells to leave the intramedullary space and spread to the surrounding soft tissues without overt cortical destruction (Hicks et al. 1995).

Contiguous vertebral bodies' involvement can occur (Patnaik et al. 2016).

Because of the intense physiologic FDG uptake in the central nervous system (CNS), detection of lymphomatous involvement (especially leptomeningeal infiltration) is difficult with PET/CT. MRI is preferred to assess suspected CNS involvement (Wang 2015).

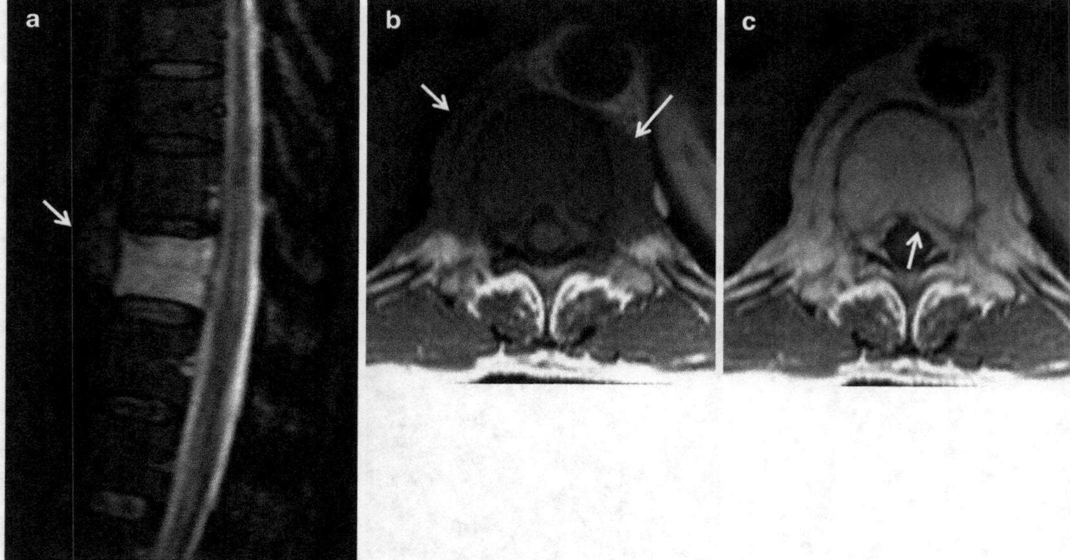

Fig. 5 DLBC lymphoma of bone in the thoracic spine: MRI: sagittal STIR-WI (**a**), axial T1-WI before (**b**) and after (**c**) gadolinium administration: lesion affecting the vertebral body, hypointense on T1-WI, hyperintense on STIR-WI with post-gadolinium enhancement. Extension to the paravertebral soft tissues and epidural space with little cortical changes (arrows)

Malignant lymphoma of bone and soft tissue has characteristically high signal intensity on diffusion-WI (DWI) with lower apparent diffusion coefficient (ADC) values than other malignant musculoskeletal tumors due to high cellularity and nucleocytoplasmic ratio (Rao et al. 2019).

An increased posttreatment ADC value correlates with higher tumor necrosis, suggesting tumor response, and is usually consistent with decreased FDG uptake on PET/CT (Messina et al. 2015).

Recent studies show an excellent agreement between PET/CT and whole-body MRI with DWI (WB-DWI MRI) in the detection of nodal and extranodal locations of disease (Maccioni et al. 2023).

Moreover, unlike the FDG avidity which varies substantially according to histology and aggressiveness of lymphoma, the morphological and functional parameters obtained with MRI, especially DWI, seem to be influenced only by its cellularity (Balbo-Mussetto et al. 2017).

WB-DWI MRI is a radiation-free alternative to the standard staging and follow-up PET/CT and CT, which increase cancer risk in patients with lymphoma by about one excess cancer per 100 patients during both the first year after diagnosis and a follow-up period of 5 years (Fabritius et al. 2016).

The strengths and shortcomings of each imaging modality in lymphoma tumor burden assessment are summarized in Table 1.

Table 1 Advantages and disadvantages of the main imaging modalities in patients with lymphoma (Albano et al. 2021)

Imaging modality	Advantages	Disadvantages
Contrast-enhanced CT	Wide availability	Radiation exposure
	High spatial resolution	Contrast medium injection
	Short acquisition time	No functional/metabolic evaluation
^{18}F-FDG PET/CT	Metabolic evaluation	Radiation exposure
	Bone marrow evaluation	Low performance in the central nervous system locations
	Standard protocol	Variable/low FDG avidity of some lymphomas
	Recognized SUV_{max} 2.5 cutoff	Long examination time
	Standard response assessment reporting (Deauville score)	
WB-DWI MRI	Morphologic and functional evaluation	No clear ADC cutoff values
	Less histology dependent	Lower performance in hilar mediastinal and lung locations
	High contrast resolution in soft tissue and bone marrow	Long examination time (generally lower than that of PET/CT)
	Bone marrow evaluation	Contraindications (pacemaker, claustrophobia, etc.)
	Best performance for central nervous system locations	
	No radiation exposure	
	Contrast medium not necessary	
	Feasible in pregnancy	

7 Histopathology

7.1 Macroscopic Appearance

Gross specimens of PLB are rarely obtained because diagnosis is made on biopsy material and surgery is not routinely performed. If available, macroscopy shows a greyish-white and fleshy tumor with frequent areas of necrosis (Cleven and Ferry 2020).

7.2 Microscopic Appearance

HL's hallmark is the presence of Hodgkin and Reed–Sternberg cells in an inflammatory background. These pathognomonic malignant cells are multinucleate giant cells or large mononuclear cells (Shanbhag and Ambinder 2018).

DLBCL is characterized by a diffuse growth of large atypical lymphoid cells filling the marrow space, sometimes with prominent fibrosis. These cells have large, round, or irregular nuclei, with often cleaved or multilobulated appearance and variably prominent nucleoli. Cytoplasm is not abundant and may be amphophilic. Areas of nonneoplastic lymphocytes and histiocytes are also found (Cleven and Ferry 2020).

The crush artifact is common, occurring due to tissue compression and distortion while sampling or sample cutting, resulting in tissue morphologic changes and chromatin squeezed out of nuclei (Chatterjee 2014). This finding should raise the possibility of lymphoma. The crush artifact, reactive cells, and bone may obscure the neoplastic population, sometimes requiring a second biopsy to obtain diagnostic tissue (Cleven and Ferry 2020).

7.3 Immunohistochemistry

A panel of immunohistochemical markers are used for the diagnostic workup of PLB including CD20, PAX5, CD3, CD5, CD10, BCL6, BCL2, IRF4 (MUM1), MYC, and Ki-67, as well as in situ hybridization for Epstein-Barr virus using EBV-encoded small RNA (EBER). Most PLBs are DLBCLs that express CD20, PAX5, and CD79a (Cleven and Hogendoorn 2017).

The Hans algorithm is applied to further classify tumors as germinal center B-cell (GCB) type and non-GCB type: CD10+ or CD10−, BCL6+, IRF4 (MUM1)− supports GCB type, whereas CD10−, BCL6− or CD10−, BCL6+, IRF4 (MUM1)+ supports non-GCB type. Non-GCB type has a worse prognosis (Abdulla et al. 2020).

Available data on primary bone T-cell lymphomas are sparse. Most reported cases of primary bone T-cell lymphomas are anaplastic large cell lymphoma (ALCL) diffusely positive for CD30 and usually positive for at least one pan-T-cell marker such as CD3, CD2, CD4, or CD5. In cases with an *ALK* translocation, expression of ALK protein is observed (ALK-positive ALCL) (Cleven and Ferry 2020).

8 Differential Diagnosis

The differential diagnosis of spinal bone lymphoma includes other primary malignant and benign bone tumors, hematological neoplasms, metastases, and spinal osteomyelitis.

Due to marrow infiltration, bone lymphoma shows discrepancy between normal or subtle findings on radiographs and florid appearance on MRI or PET/CT. This feature is also found in other small round cell neoplasms such as Ewing sarcoma, leukemia, and multiple myeloma (Lim and Ong 2013).

Bone sequestra have been described in patients with Langerhans' cell histiocytosis, chronic osteomyelitis, fibrosarcoma, malignant fibrous histiocytoma, and desmoplastic fibroma (Mulligan et al. 1999).

Infection, especially granulomatous such as tuberculous spondylitis, may mimic spinal bone lymphoma (Khor et al. 2012). Moreover, spinal lymphoma may be rarely superinfected (Liu et al. 2012).

The etiological suspicion should be strongly oriented by patients' age, physical examination, and biological survey. Histology establishes the definitive diagnosis.

9 Local and Distant Staging

Staging of bone lymphoma begins with precise medical history and complete physical examination.

Blood tests include full blood count, alkaline phosphatase, lactate dehydrogenase, erythrocyte sedimentation rate, C-reactive protein, beta-2 microglobulin, and protein electrophoresis (Messina et al. 2015).

Anatomical MRI is the imaging modality of choice for local staging of spinal PLB.

PET/CT is currently the gold standard for disease distant staging and response assessment in FDG-avid lymphomas and may obviate the need for bone marrow biopsy in FDG-avid lymphoma (Cheson et al. 2014; Vitolo et al. 2016).

Contrast-enhanced CT of the neck, chest, abdomen, and pelvis is recommended for lymphomas with variable or low FDG avidity (Cheson et al. 2014; Vitolo et al. 2016). Frontal chest radiography is no longer systematic since it has been replaced by chest CT.

The osseous spine (along the skull) location is of risk of CNS involvement or relapse due to the anatomic close apposition. Gadolinium-enhanced brain MRI and cerebrospinal fluid flow cytometry can be recommended in this location (Vitolo et al. 2016).

To date, WB-DWI MRI is not considered in the international guidelines for staging or response assessment in patients with nodal and extranodal lymphoma (Cheson et al. 2014; Vitolo et al. 2016).

The standard Ann Arbor/Lugano staging system was intended for lymphomas with primary nodal involvement, although applicable to primary extranodal lymphoma (Cheson et al. 2014). An adapted staging system for bone lymphoma has been proposed (Table 2) (Messina et al. 2015; Vitolo et al. 2016).

The WHO definition of PLB implies a stage IE or IIE disease (E standing for extranodal). Disseminated lymphoma with bone involvement is a stage IV disease. A particular subcategory of stage IV is multifocal or polyostotic PLB (stage IVE) (Table 2).

Table 2 Adapted Ann Arbor/Lugano staging system for lymphoma of bone (Messina et al. 2015; Vitolo et al. 2016)

Stage	Disease extent
IE	Single bone lesion without regional nodal involvement
IIE	Single bone lesion with regional nodal involvement
IVE (polyostotic lymphoma)	Multifocal lesions in a single bone without nodal or other extranodal involvement/lesions in multiple bones without nodal or other extranodal involvement
IV	Disseminated lymphoma with at least one bone lesion

10 Treatment

Treatment of spinal PLB is based on systemic therapy, and the current modalities include chemotherapy or immunochemotherapy with or without radiotherapy.

Anthracycline-based multi-agent chemotherapy comprising cyclophosphamide, doxorubicin, vincristine, and prednisone (CHOP) with or without the addition of rituximab (R-CHOP) is the preferred modality. The choice of chemotherapy regimen is based on the histology of PLB. R-CHOP is preferred when the PLB is of B-cell origin and CHOP when of T-cell origin. If anthracyclines are contraindicated, etoposide or gemcitabine can be used instead (Kanavos et al. 2023).

Chemotherapy and radiotherapy are usually combined, since a combined modality has a significantly superior outcome than single-modality therapy, achieving a 5-year overall survival (OS) rate of 80–90% (Kanavos et al. 2023).

In case of neurological impairment without spinal instability, radiotherapy is still the first line of treatment. Rapid neurologic deterioration requires urgent operative decompression. Surgical stabilization is also needed in case of spinal instability. Additionally, surgery enables open biopsy for diagnosis (Barz et al. 2021).

11 Prognosis

Of all primary bone malignancies, PLB is associated with the best prognosis (DiCaprio 2017).

The 5-year survival rate exceeds 70% (Yang et al. 2022).

The prognosis is significantly related to the stage of disease: 5-year OS of bone DLBCL varies from 82% for patients with stage IE disease to 38% for patients with stage IV disease (Messina et al. 2015).

Multifocal PLB (stage IVE) exhibits a significantly better prognosis than disseminated lymphoma with bone involvement (stage IV) with 5-year OS rate of 74% versus 36% (Messina et al. 2014).

OS and cancer-specific survival are significantly lower for tumors in the spine compared to the appendicular skeleton, which may be related to the spinal cord and nerve compression with subsequent complications, and the potential CNS involvement and relapse (Liu et al. 2020; Yang et al. 2022).

Age older than 61 years is another poor prognosis factor (Wang et al. 2020).

The prognostic significance of the phenotypic and genetic characteristics of primary bone DLBCL has been studied. GCB phenotype and related molecular features are associated with favorable outcome in primary bone DLBCL, whereas non-GCB type and related features have worse outcome (Abdulla et al. 2020).

Prognosis is poorer in primary bone T-cell lymphomas than in primary bone B-cell lymphomas (Messina et al. 2015).

12 Key Points

- Spinal bone lymphoma occurs frequently in the setting of a disseminated disease with secondary bone infiltration, and rarely as primary single or multiple lymphomas of bone.
- Suggestive but not pathognomonic imaging features of bone lymphoma include:
  - Marked abnormality on PET/CT or MR imaging with normal or nearly normal findings on radiographs
  - Focal marrow replacement and a surrounding soft tissue mass with surprisingly little cortical destruction
  - Bone sequestra
- Open surgery biopsy is preferred for diagnosis. If an image-guided biopsy is planned, soft tissue components should be targeted rather than bone lesions.
- ^{18}F-FDG PET/CT is currently the gold standard for disease distant staging and response assessment in FDG-avid lymphomas
- WB-DWI MRI has similar sensitivity and specificity to PET/CT for detection of FDG-avid lymphomas and outperforms PET/CT in lymphomas with variable/low FDG avidity. This promising technique is yet to be validated by further studies and upcoming recommendations.
- Primary lymphoma of bone is a disease with a good prognosis, but the spinal location is associated with a worse outcome compared to the appendicular skeleton location.

References

Abdulla M, Hollander P, Pandzic T et al (2020) Cell-of-origin determined by both gene expression profiling and immunohistochemistry is the strongest predictor of survival in patients with diffuse large B-cell lymphoma. Am J Hematol 95(1):57–67

Albano D, Micci G, Patti C et al (2021) Whole-body magnetic resonance imaging: current role in patients with lymphoma. Diagnostics (Basel) 11(6):1007

Balbo-Mussetto A, Saviolo C, Fornari A et al (2017) Whole body MRI with qualitative and quantitative analysis of DWI for assessment of bone marrow involvement in lymphoma. Radiol Med 122:623–632

Barrington SF, Mikhaeel NG, Kostakoglu L et al (2014) Role of imaging in the staging and response assessment of lymphoma: consensus of the International Conference on Malignant Lymphomas Imaging Working Group. J Clin Oncol 32(27):3048–3058

Barz M, Aftahy K, Janssen I et al (2021) Spinal manifestation of malignant primary (PLB) and secondary bone lymphoma (SLB). Curr Oncol 28(5):3891–3899

Chang CY, Huang AJ, Bredella MA et al (2015) Percutaneous CT-guided needle biopsies of musculoskeletal tumors: a 5-year analysis of non-diagnostic biopsies. Skelet Radiol 44(12):1795–1803

Chatterjee S (2014) Artefacts in histopathology. J Oral Maxillofac Pathol 18(Suppl 1):S111–S116

Cheson BD, Fisher RI, Barrington SF et al (2014) Recommendations for initial evaluation, staging, and response assessment of Hodgkin and non-Hodgkin lymphoma: the Lugano classification. J Clin Oncol 32(27):3059–3068

Cleven AHG, Ferry JA (2020) Primary non-Hodgkin lymphoma of bone. In: WHO Classification of Tumours Editorial Board (ed) WHO classification of soft tissue and bone tumours, 5th edn. IARC Press, Lyon, pp 488–491

Cleven AHG, Hogendoorn PCW (2017) Hematopoietic tumors primarily presenting in bone. Surg Pathol Clin 10(3):675–691

DiCaprio MR (2017) Malignant tumors of bone and soft tissue. In: Grauer JN (ed) Orthopaedic knowledge update, 12th edn. American Academy of Orthopaedic Surgeons, Rosemont, IL, pp 259–273

Fabritius G, Brix G, Nekolla E et al (2016) Cumulative radiation exposure from imaging procedures and associated lifetime cancer risk for patients with lymphoma. Sci Rep 6:35181

Frood R, Burton C, Tsoumpas C et al (2021) Baseline PET/CT imaging parameters for prediction of treatment outcome in Hodgkin and diffuse large B cell lymphoma: a systematic review. Eur J Nucl Med Mol Imaging 48(10):3198–3220

Fyllos A, Zibis A, Markou A et al (2021) Clinical and imaging features of primary bone lymphoma: a pictorial essay. Hellenic J Radiol 6(2):32–43

Hicks DG, Gokan T, O'Keefe RJ et al (1995) Primary lymphoma of bone. Correlation of magnetic resonance imaging features with cytokine production by tumor cells. Cancer 75(4):973–980

Jamil A, Mukkamalla SKR (2023) Lymphoma. In: StatPearls. StatPearls Publishing, Treasure Island, FL. Available from: https://www.ncbi.nlm.nih.gov/books/NBK560826/

Kaddu-Mulindwa D, Altmann B, Held G et al (2021) FDG PET/CT to detect bone marrow involvement in the initial staging of patients with aggressive non-Hodgkin lymphoma: results from the prospective, multicenter PETAL and OPTIMAL>60 trials. Eur J Nucl Med Mol Imaging 48(11):3550–3559

Kanavos T, Birbas E, Papoudou-Bai A et al (2023) Primary bone lymphoma: a review of the literature with emphasis on histopathology and histogenesis. Diseases 11(1):42

Khor LK, Wang S, Lu SJ (2012) Anaplastic large cell lymphoma of the vertebra masquerading as tuberculous spondylitis: potential pitfalls of conventional imaging. Intern Emerg Med 7:573–577

Lim CY, Ong KO (2013) Imaging of musculoskeletal lymphoma. Cancer Imaging 13(4):448–457

Liu CW, Tsai TY, Li YF et al (2012) Infected primary non-Hodgkin lymphoma of spine. Indian J Orthop 46(4):479–482

Liu CX, Xu TQ, Xu L et al (2020) Primary lymphoma of bone: a population-based study of 2558 patients. Ther Adv Hematol 11:2040620720958538

Maccioni F, Alfieri G, Assanto GM et al (2023) Whole body MRI with diffusion weighted imaging versus 18F-fluorodeoxyglucose-PET/CT in the staging of lymphomas. Radiol Med 128(5):556–564

Malloy PC, Fishman EK, Magid D (1992) Lymphoma of bone, muscle, and skin: CT findings. AJR Am J Roentgenol 159(4):805–809

Mavrogenis AF, Panagopoulos GN, Angelini A et al (2017) Lymphoma and myeloma of the sacrum. In: Ruggieri P, Angelini A, Vanel D, Picci P (eds) Tumors of the sacrum. Springer, Cham, pp 227–235

Mechri M, Riahi H, Sboui I et al (2018) Imaging of malignant primitive tumors of the spine. J Belg Soc Radiol 102(1):56

Meek RD, Mills MK, Hanrahan CJ et al (2020) Pearls and pitfalls for soft-tissue and bone biopsies: a cross-institutional review. Radiographics 40(1):266–290

Messina C, Ferreri AJ, Govi S et al (2014) Clinical features, management and prognosis of multifocal primary bone lymphoma: a retrospective study of the international extranodal lymphoma study group (the IELSG 14 study). Br J Haematol 164(6):834–840

Messina C, Christie D, Zucca E et al (2015) Primary and secondary bone lymphomas. Cancer Treat Rev 41(3):235–246

Mikhaeel NG (2012) Primary bone lymphoma. Clin Oncol (R Coll Radiol) 24(5):366–370

Mulligan ME, McRae GA, Murphey MD (1999) Imaging features of primary lymphoma of bone. AJR Am J Roentgenol 173(6):1691–1697

Patnaik S, Jyotsnarani Y, Uppin SG et al (2016) Imaging features of primary tumors of the spine: a pictorial essay. Indian J Radiol Imaging 26(2):279–289

Ramadan KM, Shenkier T, Sehn LH et al (2007) A clinicopathological retrospective study of 131 patients with primary bone lymphoma: a population-based study of successively treated cohorts from the British Columbia Cancer Agency. Ann Oncol 18:129–135

Rao A, Sharma C, Parampalli R (2019) Role of diffusion-weighted MRI in differentiating benign from malignant bone tumors. BJR Open 1(1):20180048

Saifuddin A (2021) Bone marrow disorders: haematological neoplasms. In: Adam A et al (eds) Grainger & Allison's diagnostic radiology, vol 65, 7th edn. Elsevier Ltd, pp 1703–1723

Shanbhag S, Ambinder RF (2018) Hodgkin lymphoma: a review and update on recent progress. CA Cancer J Clin 68(2):116–132

Vannata B, Zucca E (2015) Primary extranodal B-cell lymphoma: current concepts and treatment strategies. Chin Clin Oncol 4(1):10

Vitolo U, Seymour JF, Martelli M et al (2016) Extranodal diffuse large B-cell lymphoma (DLBCL) and primary mediastinal B-cell lymphoma: ESMO Clinical Practice Guidelines for diagnosis, treatment and follow-up. Ann Oncol 27(Suppl 5):v91–v102

Wang X (2015) PET/CT: appropriate application in lymphoma. Chin Clin Oncol 4(1):4

Wang Z, Shi H, Zhang X et al (2019) Value of CT-guided percutaneous needle biopsy of bone in the diagnosis of lymphomas based on PET/CT results. Cancer Imaging 19(1):42

Wang HH, Dai KN, Li AB (2020) A nomogram predicting overall and cancer-specific survival of patients with primary bone lymphoma: a large population-based study. Biomed Res Int 2020:4235939

Yang XY, He X, Zhao Y (2022) Nomogram-based prediction of overall and cancer-specific survival in patients with primary bone diffuse large B-cell lymphoma: a population-based study. Evid Based Complement Alternat Med 2022:1566441

Plasmacytoma

Thomas Van Den Berghe, Denim Brack, Alexander De Clercq, Jo Van Dorpe, Julie Dutoit, Filip M. Vanhoenacker, and Koenraad L. Verstraete

Contents

T. Van Den Berghe (✉) · K. L. Verstraete
Department of Diagnostic Sciences, Faculty of Medicine and Health Sciences, Ghent University, Ghent, Belgium

Department of Radiology and Medical Imaging, Ghent University Hospital, Ghent, Belgium
e-mail: thovdnbe.vandenberghe@ugent.be; koenraad.verstraete@ugent.be

D. Brack · A. De Clercq
Department of Diagnostic Sciences, Faculty of Medicine and Health Sciences, Ghent University, Ghent, Belgium
e-mail: denim.brack@ugent.be; alexander.declercq@ugent.be

J. Van Dorpe
Department of Diagnostic Sciences, Faculty of Medicine and Health Sciences, Ghent University, Ghent, Belgium

Department of Pathology, Ghent University Hospital, Ghent, Belgium

Cancer Research Institute (CRIG), Ghent University Hospital, Ghent, Belgium
e-mail: jo.vandorpe@ugent.be

J. Dutoit
Department of Diagnostic Sciences, Faculty of Medicine and Health Sciences, Ghent University, Ghent, Belgium

Department of Radiology and Medical Imaging, General Hospital Groeninge—Campus Kennedylaan, Kortrijk, Belgium

F. M. Vanhoenacker
Department of Diagnostic Sciences, Faculty of Medicine and Health Sciences, Ghent University, Ghent, Belgium

Department of Radiology and Medical Imaging, General Hospital Sint-Maarten Mechelen, Mechelen, Belgium

Department of Radiology and Medical Imaging, University Hospital Antwerp, Edegem, Belgium

Faculty of Medicine and Health Sciences, University of Antwerp, Antwerp, Belgium

Faculty of Medicine and Health Sciences, KU Leuven, Leuven, Belgium
e-mail: filip.vanhoenacker@telenet.be

Med Radiol Diagn Imaging (2023)
https://doi.org/10.1007/174_2023_452,
Published Online: 15 October 2023

Abstract

Solitary plasmacytoma of bone is one of many existing types of bone tumors and is part of the plasma cell disorder spectrum. It is a local clonal plasma cell proliferation without evidence of symptomatic multiple myeloma. It occurs slightly more frequently in males with a median age at diagnosis of 55 years. The thoracic vertebrae are most frequently involved. The exact etiology is unknown, although a role for acquired B-cell defects is suggested. In children and young adults, preceding trauma might play a role in the development of solitary plasmacytoma of bone. Compared to extramedullary plasmacytoma, solitary plasmacytoma of bone has a significantly worse prognosis, progressing to symptomatic multiple myeloma in over 50% of cases. The survival rates are significantly worse in case of abnormal serum immunoglobulin free light chain ratio, in patients diagnosed after the age of 60 years and in female patients.

In one-third of presumed "solitary" plasmacytomas, an additional lesion is characterized with subsequent diagnostic imaging, marking the importance of further investigations when an apparent solitary plasmacytoma of bone is encountered. Conventional radiography plays a distinct role in the imaging and detection of solitary plasmacytoma of bone, mostly in the presence of clear clinical symptoms. It may show a "punched-out" lesion appearance with generally clear margins and normal surrounding bone. More advanced cases may be paired with marked erosion and cortical bone destruction, creating a "soap bubble" appearance. On CT, solitary plasmacytoma of bone presents as a uni- or multilocular lesion, causing focal trabecular destruction. A characteristic "mini brain" appearance may be observed. On conventional MRI, a plasmacytoma is iso- to hypointense on T1-weighted images and hyperintense on (fat-saturated) T2-weighted images compared to muscle and enhances homogeneously after gadolinium contrast administration. Specialized MRI techniques such as dynamic contrast-enhanced MRI and diffusion-weighted imaging also play an important role, especially in assessing disease extent and differentiation with multiple myeloma, where a focal solitary plasmacytoma of bone is accompanied by surrounding or distant bone marrow invasion. ^{18}F-FDG PET/CT is useful in the evaluation and has a prognostic value both at diagnosis and in the evaluation of treatment.

Abbreviations

ADC	Apparent diffusion coefficient
BM	Bone marrow
BMI	Body mass index
b-Value	Diffusion-sensitizing gradient
CRAB	Calcemia, renal failure, anemia, bone lesions
DCE-MRI	Dynamic contrast-enhanced MRI
DD	Differential diagnosis
DWI(BS)	Diffusion-weighted whole-body imaging with background body signal suppression
EBV	Epstein-Barr virus
EMP	Extramedullary plasmacytoma
FDG	Fluorodeoxyglucose
FLC	Free light chain
Gd	Gadolinium
Hb	Hemoglobin
HE	Hematoxylin and eosin
(i)AUC	Initial-area-under-curve
Ig	Immunoglobulin
IMWG	International Myeloma Working Group
MDE	Myeloma-defining events
MGUS	Monoclonal gammopathy of undetermined significance
MM	Multiple myeloma
M-protein	Monoclonal protein
MRD	Minimal residual disease
MVD	Microvessel density
MYRADS	Myeloma response assessment and diagnosis system
OS	Overall survival
PC(D)	Plasma cell (disorder)
PET	Positron emission tomography
PFS	Progression-free survival
ROI	Region-of-interest
(s)FLC	(serum) Free light chain
SI	Signal intensity
SLIM	Sixty, light chains, MRI
SMM	Smoldering multiple myeloma
SNR	Signal-to-noise ratio
SP(B)	Solitary plasmacytoma (of bone)
STIR	Short tau inversion recovery
SUV	Standardized uptake value
T1-WI	T1-weighted imaging
T2FS-WI	Fat-saturated T2-weighted imaging
TCC	Time-concentration curve
TIC	Time-intensity curve
TTP	Time-to-peak
WBLDCT	Whole-body low dose computed tomography
WBMRI	Whole-body magnetic resonance imaging
WBXR	Whole-body conventional radiography

1 Introduction

1.1 Definitions and Criteria

Solitary plasmacytoma (SP) is a rare and early-stage plasma cell dyscrasia accounting for about 3–5% of all plasma cell disorders (PCDs) (Dimopoulos et al. 2000). In SP, a solitary localized mass with a proliferation of monoclonal plasma cells (PCs) without radiological evidence for other skeletal lesions exists. Examination of the surrounding bone marrow (BM) shows a normal morphology, although a PC percentage of <10% is possible in SP with minimal BM involvement (Table 1). When an apparent SP is associated with ≥10% clonal surrounding BM PC, it is considered to be multiple myeloma (MM). Two

Table 1 International Myeloma Working Group (IMWG) 2014 diagnostic criteria for solitary plasmacytoma without and with minimal surrounding bone marrow involvement

	SP	SP with minimal surrounding bone marrow involvement
Biopsy-proven solitary lesion of bone or soft tissue with evidence of clonal plasma cells	Yes *AND*	Yes *AND*
Surrounding bone marrow	Normal bone marrow without evidence of clonal plasma cells *AND*	Clonal bone marrow plasma cells <10% *AND*
Normal skeletal MRI or CT of spine and pelvic region except for the solitary lesion	Yes *AND*	Yes *AND*
Absence of end-organ damage (no CRAB features) that can be attributed to a proliferative plasma cell disorder	Yes	Yes

Table modified from Van Den Berghe et al. (2022)—Review of diffusion-weighted imaging and dynamic contrast-enhanced MRI for multiple myeloma and its precursors (monoclonal gammopathy of undetermined significance and smoldering myeloma). Available from Van Den Berghe et al. (2022) Skeletal Radiology
CRAB calcemia, renal failure, anemia, bone lesions, *SP* solitary plasmacytoma
CRAB (criteria for end-organ damage in multiple myeloma and related disorders): hypercalcemia (serum calcium >0.25 mmol/L (>1 mg/dL) higher than the upper limit of normal or >2.75 mmol/L (>11 mg/dL)), renal insufficiency (creatinine clearance <40 mL/min/1.73 m^2 or serum creatinine >177 µmol/L (>2 mg/dL)), anemia (hemoglobin (Hb) >2 g/dL below the lower limit of normal, or Hb <10 g/dL), one or more osteolytic lesions on skeletal radiography, CT or ^{18}F-FDG PET/CT

Table 2 International Myeloma Working Group (IMWG) 2014 diagnostic criteria for multiple myeloma and related plasma cell disorders

	MGUS	SMM	MM
M-protein	<30 g/L (serum) *AND*	≥30 g/L (serum) OR ≥500 mg/24 h (urine) *AND/OR*	≥30 g/L (serum) OR ≥500 mg/24 h (urine) *AND/OR*
Monoclonal plasma cells	<10% *AND*	10–60% *AND*	≥10%[a] *AND*
SLIM-CRAB	No	No	Yes

Table modified from Van Den Berghe et al. (2022)—Review of diffusion-weighted imaging and dynamic contrast-enhanced MRI for multiple myeloma and its precursors (monoclonal gammopathy of undetermined significance and smoldering myeloma). Available from Van Den Berghe et al. (2022) Skeletal Radiology
MGUS monoclonal gammopathy of undetermined significance, *MM* multiple myeloma, *M-protein* monoclonal protein, *SLIM-CRAB* criteria for myeloma-defining events (MDEs) (SLIM) and end-organ damage in multiple myeloma (CRAB), *SLIM* clonal bone marrow plasma cells ≥60%, involved/uninvolved serum free light chain (FLC) ratio ≥100 (involved free light chain must be ≥100 mg/L), >1 focal lesion on MRI studies (≥5 mm), *CRAB* calcemia, renal failure, anemia, bone lesions, *CRAB* (criteria for end-organ damage in multiple myeloma and related disorders) hypercalcemia (serum calcium >0.25 mmol/L (>1 mg/dL) higher than the upper limit of normal or >2.75 mmol/L (>11 mg/dL)), renal insufficiency (creatinine clearance <40 mL/min/1.73 m^2 or serum creatinine >177 µmol/L (>2 mg/dL)), anemia (hemoglobin (Hb) >2 g/dL below the lower limit of normal, or Hb <10 g/dL), one or more osteolytic lesions on skeletal radiography, CT, or ^{18}F-FDG PET/CT, *SMM* smoldering multiple myeloma
[a] Or biopsy-proven bone or extramedullary plasmacytoma

types of SP exist: solitary plasmacytoma of bone (SPB) and solitary extramedullary plasmacytoma (EMP), depending on whether the lesion occurs in the bones or soft tissues, respectively. The focus of this chapter is on primary spinal SPB.

SP is situated together with monoclonal gammopathy of undetermined significance (MGUS) and smoldering myeloma (SMM) before MM on the PCD spectrum (Table 2) (Rajkumar 2016a). It is thought to be a precursor of MM with about

50–70% of SP cases progressing to MM within two years post-treatment (Dimopoulos et al. 2000; de Waal et al. 2016).

1.2 Disease Course and Risk Factors

The prognosis of SPB is significantly worse compared to EMP, with some studies showing as high as 57% of SPB cases progressing to MM with a median progression time of 2.5 years (Reed et al. 2011; Finsinger et al. 2016). About 10% of all SP cases progress to MM within three years, compared to 20–60% of SP cases with minimal BM involvement, highlighting the importance of the correct and detailed characterization of BM infiltration on imaging (Rajkumar 2016b). Moreover, in SPB, the extent of BM plasmacytosis and infiltration is prognostic for progression-free survival (PFS) (Warsame et al. 2012). Also, the subtype of M-protein has an effect on prognosis. Patients with immunoglobulin G (IgG) M-protein show better MM-free survival compared to patients with IgA and IgM proteins (Suh et al. 2012). Complete disappearance of the monoclonal protein following therapy, on the other hand, is associated with lower risk of relapse and progression to MM (Wilder et al. 2002). Patients diagnosed at age >60 years have a significantly worse 5-year overall survival (OS) compared to younger patients. Female sex is also associated with worse survival (Jawad and Scully 2009; Shen et al. 2021).

2 Pathologic Features

The exact etiology of SPB is unknown. There are very rare familial cases, but it is considered to be an acquired disorder. It is proposed that genetic B-cell defects make these cells more susceptible for environmental toxins. These genetic defects can cause subclinical MGUS or SPB, which can be present for years before a change of the environment triggers the evolution to a full-blown MM. Commonly accepted environmental triggers are ionizing radiation and occupational exposure to metals and pesticides (Pingali et al. 2012). The presence of Epstein-Barr virus (EBV) has also been described as a possible trigger for the development of PCD in general in organ-transplant patients (Dharnidharka 2018).

Neoplastic PCs arise from post-germinal center B-cells, after somatic hypermutation and after homing of the clonal PC to the BM. There, the clonal PC and the extracellular matrix interact. Via cell-surface adhesion molecules, the PCs adhere to the stromal cells. In turn, these cell-surface adhesion molecules also encourage PC proliferation, indicating a great importance of the interaction between the proliferating tumoral cells and the microenvironment, leading to the characteristic bone destruction (receptor activator of nuclear factor kappa B ligand stimulates osteoclasts, initiating osteolysis) and increased vascularization (vascular endothelial growth factor stimulates neoangiogenesis) (Pingali et al. 2012).

3 Epidemiology

SPB features a slight male predominance, with male-to-female ratios ranging from 1.18:1 to 1.5:1. The median age at diagnosis is 55 years (Dimopoulos et al. 2000; Finsinger et al. 2016).

In children and young adults, SPB is extremely rare, suggesting that in such young individuals, trauma plays a role in the development of SPB. A 2012 study reviewing 13 cases of SPB in individuals between 14 and 29 years of age found a history of preceding trauma in eight of these patients (Pasch et al. 2012).

4 Localization

SPB can occur in any bone but most often affects the axial skeleton, especially the vertebrae (50% of patients), with a predilection to the thoracic spine (Dimopoulos et al. 2000; Finsinger et al. 2016; Pinter et al. 2016). It is the most common primary vertebral tumor and accounts for about 26% of primary vertebral tumors (Kelley et al. 2007). The vertebral body is the most commonly involved site due to the red BM content, although there is often extension to the pedicles (Rodallec et al. 2008). As plasmacytomas preferentially replace the cancellous bone, the result is most often a hollow vertebral body or pedicle (Rodallec et al. 2008). With vertebral involvement, pathological fractures of the vertebral end plates are often observed (Rodallec et al. 2008). In about 8% of cases, SPB may involve the cervical spine. These patients might present with neck pain and instability in the neck/head region (Yurac et al. 2021).

In one-third of presumed "solitary" plasmacytomas, an additional lesion is characterized with subsequent diagnostic imaging, marking the importance of further investigations when an apparent SP is detected (Pinter et al. 2016).

5 Clinical Presentation

Patients with SP are often asymptomatic and do not present with the signs and symptoms associated with MM. The most common symptom is pain, caused by bone destruction. When the vertebrae are involved, pathological compression fractures associated with spinal cord or nerve root compression symptoms may be present (Dimopoulos et al. 2000; Peker et al. 2019).

When patients with SPB also present with signs of demyelinating polyneuropathy, the syndrome of polyneuropathy, organomegaly, endocrinopathy, M-protein, and skin changes (POEMS) should be excluded (Dimopoulos et al. 2000).

6 Imaging

Conventional radiography plays a limited role in the imaging of bone tumors and is more of a complementary technique to CT and MRI imaging (Patnaik et al. 2016). CT and MRI are both necessary to evaluate the tumor itself as well as possible soft tissue involvement. In cervical spinal tumors, the relationship to the supra-aortic trunks is important, whereas in lumbar tumors, the relationship with the retroperitoneum should be evaluated (Patnaik et al. 2016). CT is the preferred method to evaluate the degree of osseous involvement and bone destruction, while MRI is optimal for the evaluation of the epidural space and neural structures (Table 3).

6.1 Conventional Radiography (CR)

Radiographically, SPB presents as an osteolytic lesion with a "punched-out" appearance (similar to MM but solitary). Most often, a clear margin with normal surrounding bone/BM is present, and purely sclerotic plasmacytomas are rare (Dimopoulos et al. 2000; Pinter et al. 2016; Hansford et al. 2020). The tumor preferentially replaces the cancellous bone, whereas the cortical bone is partly preserved or even sclerotic, resulting in a hollow vertebral body or pedicle. In this way, the vertebral compression can be less pronounced despite severe bone destruction. More advanced SPB can present with marked erosion, expansion and destruction of the bone cortex, sometimes with thick ridging around the periphery, creating a "soap bubble" appearance (Fig. 1, Table 3). The sensitivity of classic radiographs is low for the detection of osteolytic lesions, as more than 30% of trabecular bone loss needs to be present for lytic lesions to become visible. The European Myeloma Network advises to replace whole-body radiography by whole-body low-dose CT (WBLDCT) as the standard imaging modality in patients with MM, and this could also be applied to patients with SPB (Terpos et al. 2016). Nevertheless, conventional radiography plays a distinct role in the imaging and detection of solitary plasmacytoma of bone, mostly in the presence of clear clinical symptoms. It may show a "punched-out" lesion appearance with generally clear margins and normal surrounding bone.

6.2 Computed Tomography (CT)

On CT images, SPB presents as a solitary osteolytic uni- or multilocular lesion, or as one that completely destroys and replaces the bone (Hansford et al. 2020). A characteristic "mini brain" appearance, caused by cortical preservation/thickening and lytic vertebral body lesions, may be observed on spinal axial CT images (Rodallec et al. 2008) (Figs. 2a and 3) (Table 3). Focal end-plate fractures are frequently observed in patients with SPB. CT can also be used as ana-

Table 3 Typical features of solitary plasmacytoma of bone on different imaging modalities

Imaging modality	Imaging characteristics of solitary plasmacytoma of bone
Conventional radiography	Solitary "punched-out" or osteolytic lesion (rarely sclerotic) Clear margin with normal surrounding bone (marrow) *Expansion and cortical destruction with "soap bubble" appearance* *Extra-osseous soft tissue involvement*
CT	Solitary osteolytic uni- or multilocular lesion or complete destruction and replacement of bone Clear margin with normal surrounding bone (marrow) *"Mini brain" appearance*[a] *Soft tissue involvement*
MRI	**Conventional anatomical MRI** – T1-weighted iso- to hypointense SI compared to muscle – (Fat-saturated) T2-weighted hyperintense SI compared to muscle – Homogeneous gadolinium contrast enhancement on fat-saturated T1-weighted images – Clear margin with normal surrounding bone (marrow) – *"Mini brain" appearance* – *Soft tissue involvement* **DWI** – Diffusion restrictive focal lesion (high SI on high *b*-value images + low ADC) – Normal surrounding bone marrow (low SI on high *b*-value images + normal ADC) **DCE-MRI** – Highly vascularized focal lesion (type IV TIC + malignant (semi)quantitative parameters) – Normally vascularized surrounding bone marrow (type I/II TIC + normal (semi) quantitative parameters)
^{18}F-FDG PET/CT	CT characteristics as described above PET: solitary lesion with high ^{18}F-FDG uptake (high SUV) and normal surrounding bone marrow
Bone scintigraphy	No enhancement (no osteoblastic or sclerotic reaction), except in concomitant fracture and/or surrounding invasion

Characteristics in italic can be present but are not necessary for the diagnosis of solitary plasmacytoma of bone
^{18}F-FDG PET 18-fluorodeoxyglucose positron emission tomography, *ADC* apparent diffusion coefficient, *b-value* diffusion-sensitizing gradient, *DCE* dynamic contrast-enhanced, *DWI* diffusion-weighted imaging, *SI* signal intensity, *SUV* standardized uptake value, *TIC* time-intensity curve
[a] Caused by cortical preservation/thickening and lytic vertebral body lesions

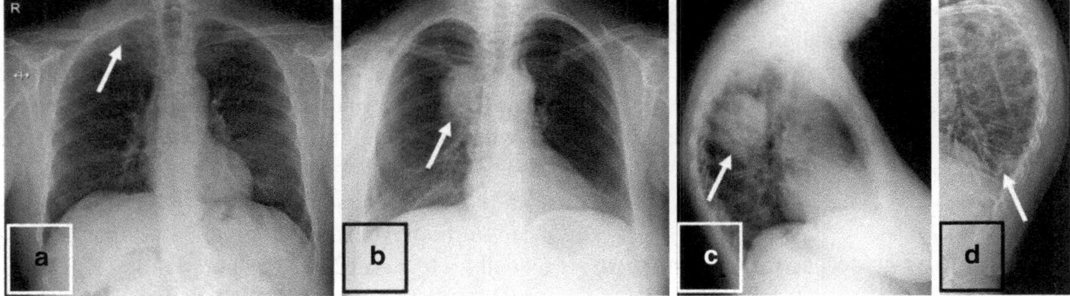

Fig. 1 Conventional radiography appearance of solitary plasmacytomas of bone. (**a**) Male, 69 years old. Clear osteolytic lesion (white arrow) of the middle and sternal end of the right clavicle with cortical destruction but without sclerosis. (**b**, **c**) Female, 58 years old. Thoracic plasmacytoma (white arrow) without sclerosis in the fifth, sixth and seventh thoracic vertebral body. Cortical destruction and extra-osseous expansion of the lesion with "soap bubble" multi-loculated appearance in the surrounding soft tissues can be observed. The largest extra-osseous component is located on the right side of the spine. (**d**) Female, 73 years old. Plasmacytoma of the tenth thoracic vertebral body and tenth rib (white arow). As a plasmacytoma tends to initially only replace cancellous bone with the cortical bone being partly preserved, only a (partly) "hollow vertebral body" appearance can be observed. Moreover, >30% bone loss needs to be present for lytic lesions to become visible. In this way, the vertebral compression is less pronounced despite severe bone destruction. Here, a 30% (8 mm, grade II, moderate fracture) anterior height loss of the vertebral body can be observed

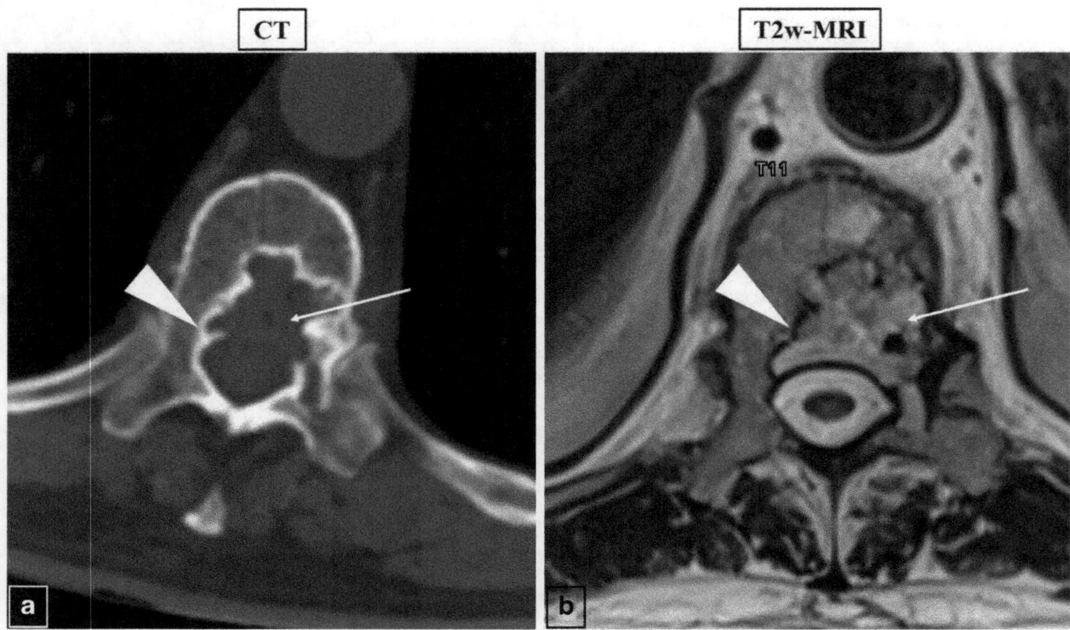

Fig. 2 "Mini brain" appearance of a plasmacytoma of bone in the 11th thoracic vertebral body as observed on CT (**a**) and T2-weighted MRI (**b**) images in a 79-year-old patient (white arrow). A solitary osteolytic multilocular lesion with complete destruction and replacement of trabecular bone and a clear partly sclerotic margin (white arrowhead, high density (**a**) on CT image and low signal intensity (**b**) on T2-weighted MRI image) is observed. The typical "mini brain" appearance occurs due to a large lytic vertebral body lesion in combination with a thickened and preserved cortex. *T2w-MRI* T2-weighted MRI image

tomical guidance for vertebral SPB biopsies. WBLDCT is superior for the detection of osteolytic lesions compared to standard radiography. The lesions may sometimes be very subtle on CT images, making them imperceivable on radiographic images. Some authors therefore endorse replacing radiography with WBLDCT in the workup of patients with MM and this could also be the case for SPB (Terpos et al. 2016; Mena et al. 2022).

6.3 Magnetic Resonance Imaging (MRI)

6.3.1 Conventional Spin-Echo MRI

6.3.1.1 Principles of Spin-Echo MRI in the Evaluation of Normal Bone Marrow

Both T1- and T2-weighted sequences are used for the evaluation of BM. T1-weighted images (WI) are more suited for this due to the high BM fat content, appearing hyperintense compared to surrounding structures (muscle, intervertebral disks) (Dutoit and Verstraete 2017). Indeed, yellow (fatty) BM will appear more hyperintense on T1-WI compared to red BM. On T2-WI, BM appears iso- to hypointense compared to subcutaneous fat and hyperintense compared to muscle and intervertebral disks (Lecouvet 2016). Images with gadolinium (Gd) contrast agent can be accentuated by the application of fat suppression. Short tau inversion recovery (STIR) produces more homogeneous fat suppression than chemically selective T2-WI fat suppression (T2FS-WI) (Dutoit and Verstraete 2017).

6.3.1.2 MRI Findings in Solitary Plasmacytoma of Bone

Relative to muscle, SPB presents as an iso- to hypointense signal intensity (SI) lesion on T1-WI and a hyperintense SI lesion on T2-WI (Figs. 4 and 5). The previously mentioned "mini brain" appearance of SPB can also be appreciated on MRI images (Fig. 2b). Compression of neural

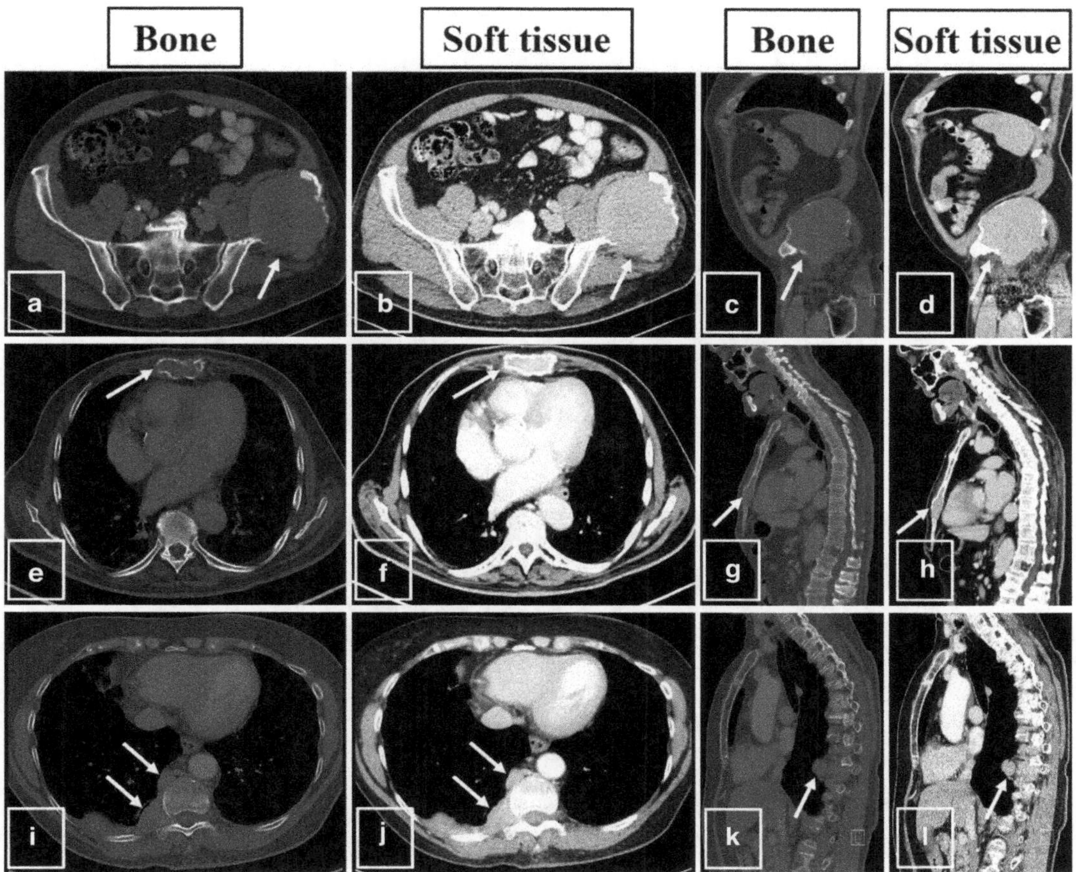

Fig. 3 CT appearance of solitary plasmacytomas of bone. Axial and sagittal bone and soft tissue window CT images of solitary plasmacytomas of bone in the left iliac wing of a 66-year-old male patient (**a–d**), the sternal body in an 87-year-old male patient (**e–h**) and the tenth thoracic vertebral body and tenth rib in a 74-year-old female patient (**i–l**) (white arrows) show solitary uni- or multilocular osteolytic lesions with (complete) destruction and replacement of bone and clear margins with normal bone (marrow). Cortical destruction and soft tissue involvement can be observed (white arrows in **a–d**, **i–l**)

structures by an extra-osseous component may be more accurately observed on MRI images. Administration of Gd contrast agent causes lesion enhancement on T1-WI, which is best evaluated on fat-saturated T1-WI. Postcontrast T1-WI is also useful to demonstrate epidural extension and subligamentous extension to the neighboring vertebral body. However, contrast-enhanced nonfat-saturated T1-WI remains valuable, as inhomogeneous suppression of the fat signal can impair image quality because of motion artifacts (Rodallec et al. 2008) (Table 3).

Although MRI of the spine and pelvic region is not necessary for the diagnosis of SPB according to the IMWG diagnostic criteria of SPB (Tables 1 and 2) and although CT is a valid alternative, MRI shows the extent of SPB more clearly than CT and certainly than radiography. Therefore, some authors endorse the use of MRI on all patients with SPB to detect occult widespread disease, by which it may upstage the SPB to MM and thus influence therapy (Terpos et al. 2016). While whole-body MRI (WBMRI) imaging is preferred for the diagnosis of MM, the IMWG has acknowledged that axial spinal and pelvic MRI is an acceptable alternative in cases where WBMRI is not available (Mena et al. 2022).

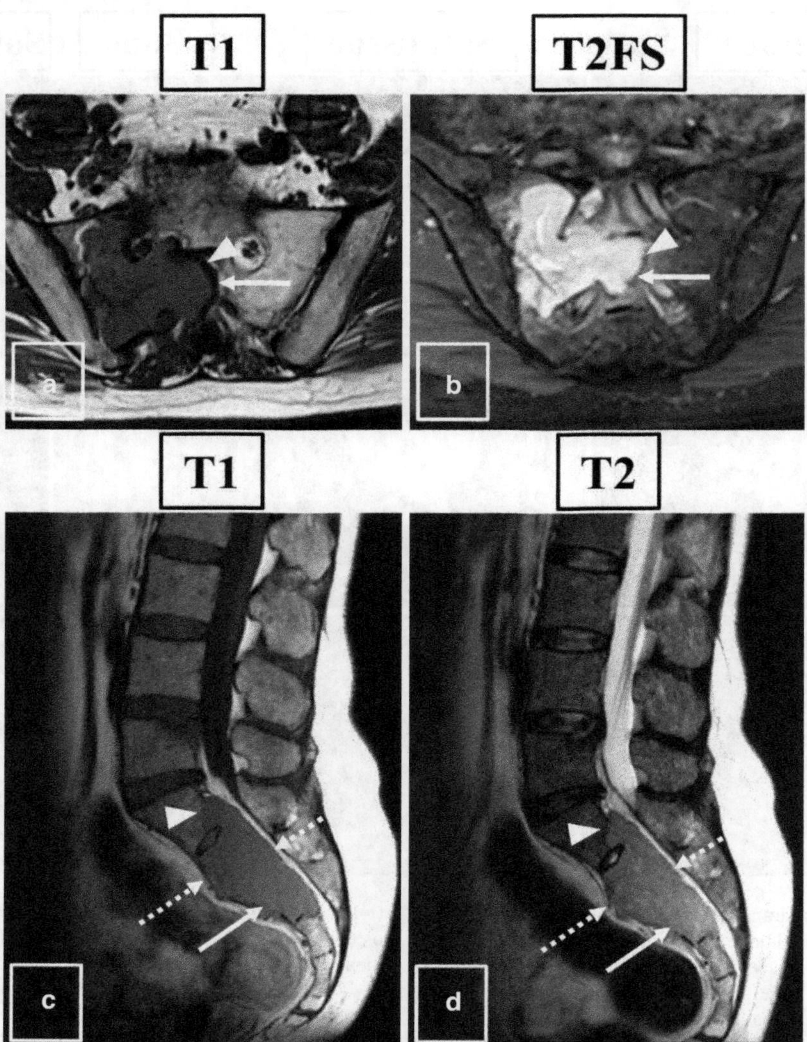

Fig. 4 MRI appearance of solitary plasmacytomas of bone. A solitary plasmacytoma of bone is observed in the right hemi-sacrum of a 77-year-old male patient (**a**, **b**) and in the S1–S4 vertebral bodies of a 64-year-old female patient (**c**, **d**) (white arrows), presenting as iso- to hypointense lesions on T1-weighted imaging as compared to muscle (**a**, **c**) and slightly to highly hyperintense lesions on (fat-saturated) T2-weighted images (**b**, **d**) as compared to muscle. Clear margins with the normal surrounding bone (marrow) can be observed (white arrowheads). Cortical breakthrough, subligamentous extension from one to a neighboring vertebral body and soft tissue extension with compression of neurological structures in the vertebral canal (dotted arrows in **c**, **d**) can be observed. *T1* T1-weighted image, *T2(FS)* (fat-saturated) T2-weighted image

6.3.1.3 MRI Findings in Plasma Cell Disorders

Bone Marrow Infiltration Patterns and Focal Lesions

Apart from detection of focal lesions and SPB, WBMRI allows for differentiation of four other BM infiltration patterns in PCD, which is important for the differentiation of SPB versus other PCDs: normal BM, salt-and-pepper pattern, diffuse pattern and combined diffuse and focal pattern (Dimopoulos et al. 2015; Martí-Bonmatí et al. 2015; Lee et al. 2019; Biffar et al. 2010b). A diffuse pattern is more predominant in SMM,

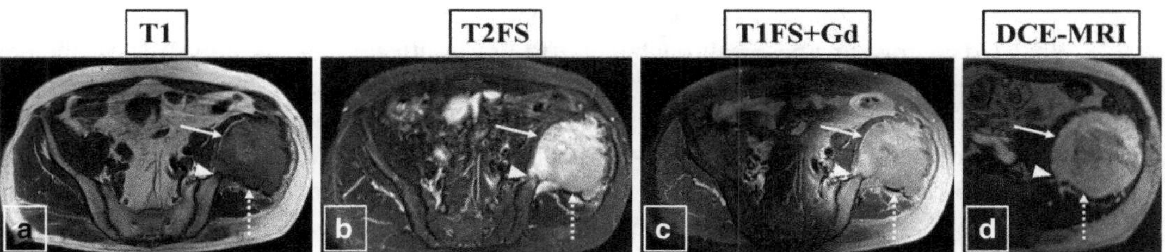

Fig. 5 MRI appearance of solitary plasmacytomas of bone. A solitary plasmacytoma of bone is observed in the left iliac wing (white arrows) in a 66-year-old male patient as an iso- to hypointense lesion on the T1-weighted image as compared to muscle (**a**), a highly hyperintense lesion on the fat-saturated T2-weighted image (**b**) as compared to muscle and with homogeneous gadolinium contrast enhancement on the fat-saturated T1-weighted image. A clear margin with the normal surrounding bone (marrow) is observed (white arrowheads). Cortical breakthrough and soft tissue extension can be observed (dashed arrows). On DCE-MRI, the lesion was highly vascularized (type IV time-intensity curve focal lesion) with normally vascularized surrounding bone marrow (type I/II time-intensity curve) as can be observed on the dynamic T1-weighted image with gadolinium contrast enhancement (**d**). *DCE-MRI* dynamic contrast-enhanced MRI, *T1* T1-weighted image, *T1FS+Gd* fat-saturated T1-weighted image with gadolinium contrast enhancement, *T2FS* fat-saturated T2-weighted image

whereas focal infiltration is more prevalent in MM. These findings suggest that, despite high PC counts, PCs are more scattered and diffuse in the preclinical stages of MM, therefore being undetectable by anatomical MRI imaging. The presence of such diffuse BM infiltration is prognostic for progression from MGUS/SMM/SPB to MM (Hillengass et al. 2010, 2014; Merz et al. 2014). As for focal lesions, the presence of more than one focal lesion on MRI is the cutoff as a prognostic parameter for MGUS and asymptomatic myeloma (Hillengass et al. 2010, 2014). In accordance with these findings, the IMWG recommends that patients with SMM with more than one focal lesion >5 mm should be considered to have symptomatic myeloma that requires treatment (Dutoit and Verstraete 2017). Patients with MGUS and focal lesions are also at an increased risk, but MRI is not yet recommended for the routine workup in these patients, unless high suspicion is present (Dutoit and Verstraete 2017).

Multiple Myeloma Lesions

Lesions in MM appear hypointense on T1-WI as compared to muscle, because the fat content is lowered. They appear rather hyperintense on T2FS-WI/STIR images as compared to muscle due to the higher water content and cellularity (Silva et al. 2013). The predilection sites for MM lesions are the axial skeleton, shoulders and proximal femora, stressing the importance of WBMRI for the adequate assessment of the extent of disease and differentiation from SPB (Dutoit et al. 2013; Schmidt et al. 2007).

6.3.1.4 Solitary Plasmacytoma of Bone in the Plasma Cell Disorder Spectrum

Because SP(B) is part of the PCD spectrum and often progresses to MM (in 50–70% of cases within two years), it is important to understand the more advanced imaging modalities that can help in the prognosis and differentiation of the multiple types of PCD in the earliest of its stages. Diffusion-weighted imaging (DWI-MRI) and dynamic contrast-enhanced MRI (DCE-MRI) are of particular value (Van Den Berghe et al. 2022) (Table 3).

6.3.2 Dynamic Contrast-Enhanced MRI

6.3.2.1 Principles of Dynamic Contrast-Enhanced MRI

DCE-MRI allows for the noninvasive evaluation of BM microcirculation, by collecting a time series of images after intravenous injection of Gd contrast agent. Multiple biological characteristics can be evaluated, such as tissue vascularization, perfusion, capillary resistance, permeability and volume of and bulk water flow in the interstitial space (Merz et al. 2015; Van Den Berghe et al. 2022). When Gd contrast first passes through the capillaries, fast diffusion into tissues occurs due to a high concentration gradient between the intravascular and interstitial space (*wash-in*). Approximately 50% of the contrast agent diffuses from blood to the interstitial space in healthy tissues. After this initial first pass, the concentration gradient drops, causing the diffusion rate to drop (Dutoit and Verstraete 2017). When equilibrium is achieved, meaning an equal concentration of contrast intravascular and interstitial, the contrast medium is washed out from the interstitium (*washout*). In highly vascularized lesions with a small interstitial space, early washout (this is within the first few minutes post-contrast injection) occurs (Verstraete et al. 1996). The analysis of dynamic images can be performed in four manners: the native review method, qualitatively, semiquantitatively or quantitively (Cuenod and Balvay 2013; García-Figueiras et al. 2015; Koutoulidis et al. 2018). The native review method is the only one of the four methods that does not require post-processing of the images. The post-processing consists of manually placing regions-of-interest (ROIs) in affected and healthy tissues, thereby acquiring time-intensity curves (TIC) that plot the SI against time points, reflecting the passage of Gd contrast from the intravascular space to the interstitial space (Van Den Berghe et al. 2022).

6.3.2.2 Methods of Analysis in Dynamic Contrast-Enhanced MRI

The *native review method* comprises the visual evaluation of a series of images at different points in time after the administration of Gd contrast agent to detect differences in contrast enhancement over time (Fig. 6a). *Qualitative analysis* of DCE-MRI images consists of visually scoring the TIC type of the ROI (I–V) based on enhancement patterns (Fig. 6b, Table 4). *Semiquantitative analysis* is based on the calculation of descriptive parameters of the TICs (SIs with corresponding time points, absolute and relative enhancement of a vertebra or lesion compared to muscle, slope wash-in, slope washout, area under curve (AUC), maximum (relative) enhancement, amplitude wash-in/washout, time to peak (TTP), arrival time (AT)) (Fig. 6c) (Cuenod and Balvay 2013;

Fig. 6 Different methods for the evaluation of dynamic contrast-enhanced MRI images. (**a**) Native review method showing a lesion in the L2 vertebral body (white arrow), increasingly enhancing from 45–55 s after gadolinium contrast injection and decreasing enhancement after 75 s. *Gd* gadolinium, *s* seconds. (**b**) Qualitative method showing time-intensity curve types. Higher curve types are indicative of higher disease stage, progression, therapy failure or relapse. Lower curve types indicate lower disease stage or therapy response. Curve types I and II have low wash-in (low tissue vascularization, perfusion and capillary permeability) and are "inactive curve types." Type I: very low/no enhancement. Type II: slow sustained enhancement. Curve types III, IV and V have a steep wash-in (indicating high tissue vascularization, perfusion and capillary permeability) and are "active curve types." Type III: plateau. Type IV: rapid washout (small interstitial space, high cellularity). Type V: continuous wash-in (large interstitial space). *A.U.* arbitrary units, *s* seconds, *SI* signal intensity. (**c**) Semiquantitative method showing descriptive parameters of the time-intensity curves. *AT* arrival time, *A.U.* arbitrary units, *AUC* area-under-the-curve, *s* seconds, *SI* signal intensity, *T* time, *TTP* time-to-peak. (**d**) Quantitative method with a two-compartment tissue model reflecting bidirectional transport of gadolinium contrast agent between plasma and extravascular extracellular space. *AIF* arterial input function, *DCE* dynamic contrast-enhanced, *EES* extravascular extracellular space, *Gd* gadolinium, *ROI* region-of-interest, *T1* T1-weighted images. Blue rectangles represent cells in tissue. (Reproduced from Van Den Berghe et al. (2022)—Review of diffusion-weighted imaging and dynamic contrast-enhanced MRI for multiple myeloma and its precursors (monoclonal gammopathy of undetermined significance and smoldering myeloma). Available from Van Den Berghe et al. (2022) Skeletal Radiology; Reproduced from Lecouvet et al. (2022)—Imaging of treatment response and minimal residual disease in multiple myeloma: state of the art WB-MRI and PET/CT. Available from Lecouvet et al. (2022) Skeletal Radiology)

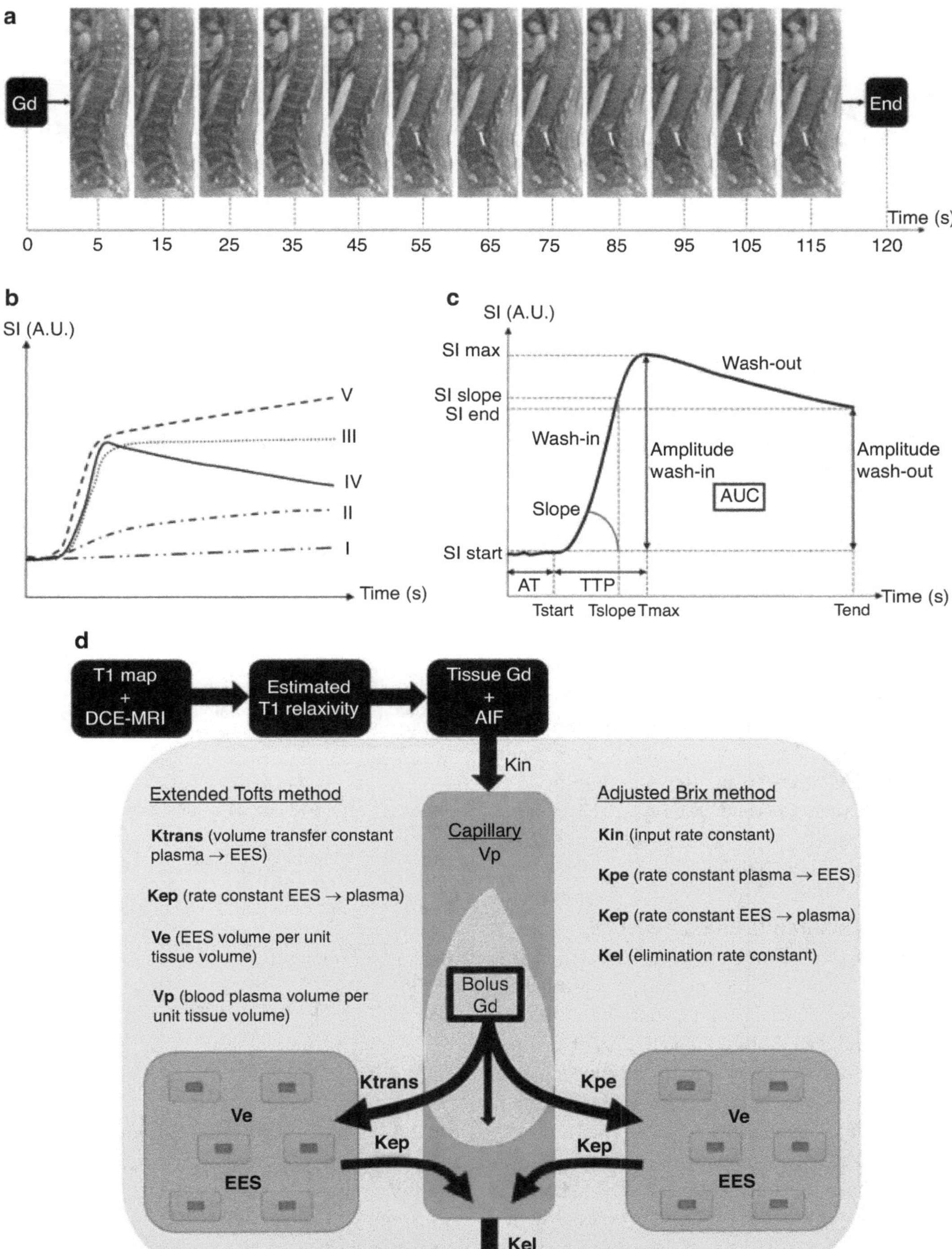
a
Gd
End
Time (s)
0
5
15
25
35
45
55
65
75
85
95
105
115
120
b
SI (A.U.)
V
III
IV
II
I
Time (s)
c
SI (A.U.)
SI max
SI slope
SI end
Wash-out
Wash-in
Amplitude wash-in
Amplitude wash-out
AUC
Slope
SI start
AT
TTP
Tstart
Tslope
Tmax
Tend
Time (s)
d
T1 map + DCE-MRI
Estimated T1 relaxivity
Tissue Gd + AIF
Kin
Extended Tofts method
Ktrans (volume transfer constant plasma → EES)
Kep (rate constant EES → plasma)
Ve (EES volume per unit tissue volume)
Vp (blood plasma volume per unit tissue volume)
Capillary
Vp
Bolus Gd
Adjusted Brix method
Kin (input rate constant)
Kpe (rate constant plasma → EES)
Kep (rate constant EES → plasma)
Kel (elimination rate constant)
Ktrans
Kep
Kpe
Kep
Ve
EES
Ve
EES
Kel

Table 4 Possible dynamic contrast-enhanced MRI curve types for qualitative analysis with curve description and accompanying physiological properties such as tissue vascularization, tissue perfusion and capillary permeability

DCE-MRI curve type	Curve description	Tissue vascularization, tissue perfusion and capillary permeability	Associated plasma cell disorder
I	Very low or no enhancement Low wash-in and first pass	Low	Healthy/MGUS
II	Slow and sustained enhancement	Low	Healthy/MGUS
III	Steep wash-in followed by plateau	High	SMM MM (rare)
IV	Steep wash-in followed by rapid washout	High (small interstitial space, high cellularity)	MM SMM (rare) SPB/EMP
V	Steep wash-in followed by sustained wash-in	High (large interstitial space)	MM/SPB/EMP in early therapy response (evolution from type IV)

DCE dynamic contrast-enhanced, *EMP* extramedullary plasmacytoma, *MGUS* monoclonal gammopathy of undetermined significance, *MM* multiple myeloma, *SMM* smoldering myeloma, *SPB* solitary plasmacytoma of bone

Koutoulidis et al. 2018; Dutoit et al. 2013, 2016; Lavini et al. 2007). For the *quantitative analysis*, pharmacokinetic models (extended Tofts/adjusted Brix) are applied, thereby deriving a time-concentration curve (TCC). This curve is then interpreted quantitatively by distribution parameters over the vascular/cellular/interstitial compartments with corresponding parametric maps (Ktrans, Kep, Ve, Vp, initial area under curve (iAUC), Kpe, Kin, Kel and amplitude *A*) (Fig. 6d) (Cuenod and Balvay 2013; García-Figueiras et al. 2015; Koutoulidis et al. 2018; Dutoit et al. 2013, 2016) (Table 5).

6.3.2.3 Qualitative Characteristics

Lower curve types indicate lower disease stage or therapy response. Higher curve types are indicative of higher disease stage, progression, therapy failure or relapse (Tables 1 and 2, Fig. 6b). Type I and II curves with very low or absent enhancement are seen in both healthy patients and in MGUS (Dutoit et al. 2013, 2016). Type III curves, characterized by a steep wash-in followed by a plateau phase, are most common in SMM but can also be present in MM. Type IV curves, with a steep wash-in followed by a rapid washout, reflect the small interstitial space and high cellularity of the tissues and are most common in patients with MM and SPB (Koutoulidis et al. 2018; Dutoit et al. 2016).

Table 5 Quantitative dynamic contrast-enhanced parameters in the extended Tofts and adjusted Brix models

Parameter	Description
Ktrans (eTofts)	Volume transfer constant from intravascular to tumoral interstitium (~wash-in)
Kep (eTofts, aBrix)	Rate constant reverse transport of contrast medium from interstitium to intravascular space (~washout)
Ve (eTofts)	Extravascular extracellular space volume per unit of tissue volume
Vp (eTofts)	Blood plasma volume per unit of tissue volume
Kin (aBrix)	Input rate constant
Kpe (aBrix)	Rate constant from intravascular to tumoral interstitium
Kel (aBrix)	Elimination rate constant
AUC	Total contrast medium inflow

aBrix adjusted Brix model, *AUC* area-under-the-curve, *eTofts* extended Tofts model

6.3.2.4 Semiquantitative Characteristics

In patients with MGUS, no difference with healthy controls can be made based on curve types nor TIC parameters. This indicates that (neo)vascularization has not yet started in MGUS (Dutoit et al. 2013). There is a positive correlation between the maximal enhancement/wash-in slope and BM histological infiltration grade. TTP is inversely correlated to both BM histological infiltration grade and R-ISS stage. So, low TTP is associated with bad prognosis, shorter PFS and worse OS. The highest TTP is seen in MGUS/healthy subjects, intermediate TTP in SMM and low TTP in MM and SPB (Terpos et al. 2017; Lin et al. 2009; Zha et al. 2010) (Table 2).

6.3.2.5 Quantitative Characteristics

Amplitude *A* is correlated positively with both BM plasmacytosis and microvessel density (MVD) (Nosàs-Garcia et al. 2005). However, it appears that amplitude *A* has a prognostic effect in patients with SMM and asymptomatic MM but not in patients with MGUS. For example, SMM patients that show an amplitude *A* of ≥0.89 have an 80% risk of progression to symptomatic disease within two years (Hillengass et al. 2016; Merz et al. 2016). In plasmacytoma, the Kep appears to be significantly higher than in metastasis, which might be useful in the differential diagnosis between the two (in one study 0.78 ± 0.17 vs. 0.61 ± 0.18, $p = 0.02$) (Zhang et al. 2020). The application of other quantitative characteristics in diagnosis of PCD appears to be insufficiently studied and further research is warranted (Table 5).

6.3.2.6 Added Value of Dynamic Contrast-Enhanced MRI in the Diagnosis of Plasma Cell Disorders

Studies show that high-grade angiogenesis (measured in MVD) in SPB is associated with a higher risk of progression to MM as well as a shorter PFS compared to SPB with low-grade angiogenesis. In SPB, the MVD in the surrounding BM does not appear to be increased, supporting the theory that the BM is not (or very minimally, plasmacytosis <10%) affected in strict SPB (Kumar et al. 2003). The same theory holds for MGUS, which also does not show increased BM perfusion (Hillengass et al. 2009). In SMM, however, diffuse microcirculation patterns corresponding with high-grade angiogenesis of the BM are linked with a poor prognosis (Rajkumar et al. 2000; Hillengass et al. 2009). These changes in MVD occur before morphological changes appear (Rana et al. 2010; Mena et al. 2011). Following the principle of angiogenic switch from early to advanced stages of disease, the added value of DCE-MRI lies in the early detection of such increased vascularization and detection of lesions that would otherwise be missed on anatomical MRI sequences. This can upstage the disease (both SPB and MGUS/SMM) and have an impact on therapy and therefore on patient outcomes (Dutoit and Verstraete 2017; Van Den Berghe et al. 2022) (e.g., Fig. 7).

6.3.2.7 Pitfalls and Conclusion of Dynamic Contrast-Enhanced MRI in Imaging of Plasma Cell Disorders

Firstly, there is a lack of clinical validation concerning the use of DCE-MRI in PCD. Also, vascularization is dependent on various factors such as age, sex, BMI and anatomical level of BM and a high inter-patient variability exists (Dutoit and Verstraete 2017). Moreover, it is important to note that an overlap between hypercellular BM of healthy young individuals and hypercellular BM after administration of BM-stimulating factors with neoplastic BM exists (Dutoit et al. 2013). In such cases, it may be more difficult to differentiate between normal hypercellular and neoplastic BM or SPB. Furthermore, the evaluation of the BM involvement type (normal, diffuse, focal, salt-and-pepper) and the placement of the ROI are subjective in nature. These highly observer-dependent factors result in a poor reproducibility of this technique (Dutoit et al. 2016). Also, since BM in MGUS does not appear to show increased levels of vascularization, DCE-MRI does not offer prognostic value in these patients (Hillengass et al. 2016). It does however in patients with SMM, asymptomatic MM and SPB.

6.3.3 Diffusion-Weighted Imaging

6.3.3.1 Principles of Diffusion-Weighted Imaging

DWI provides information on tissue cellularity, extracellular space viscosity and integrity of cellular membranes by measuring the random

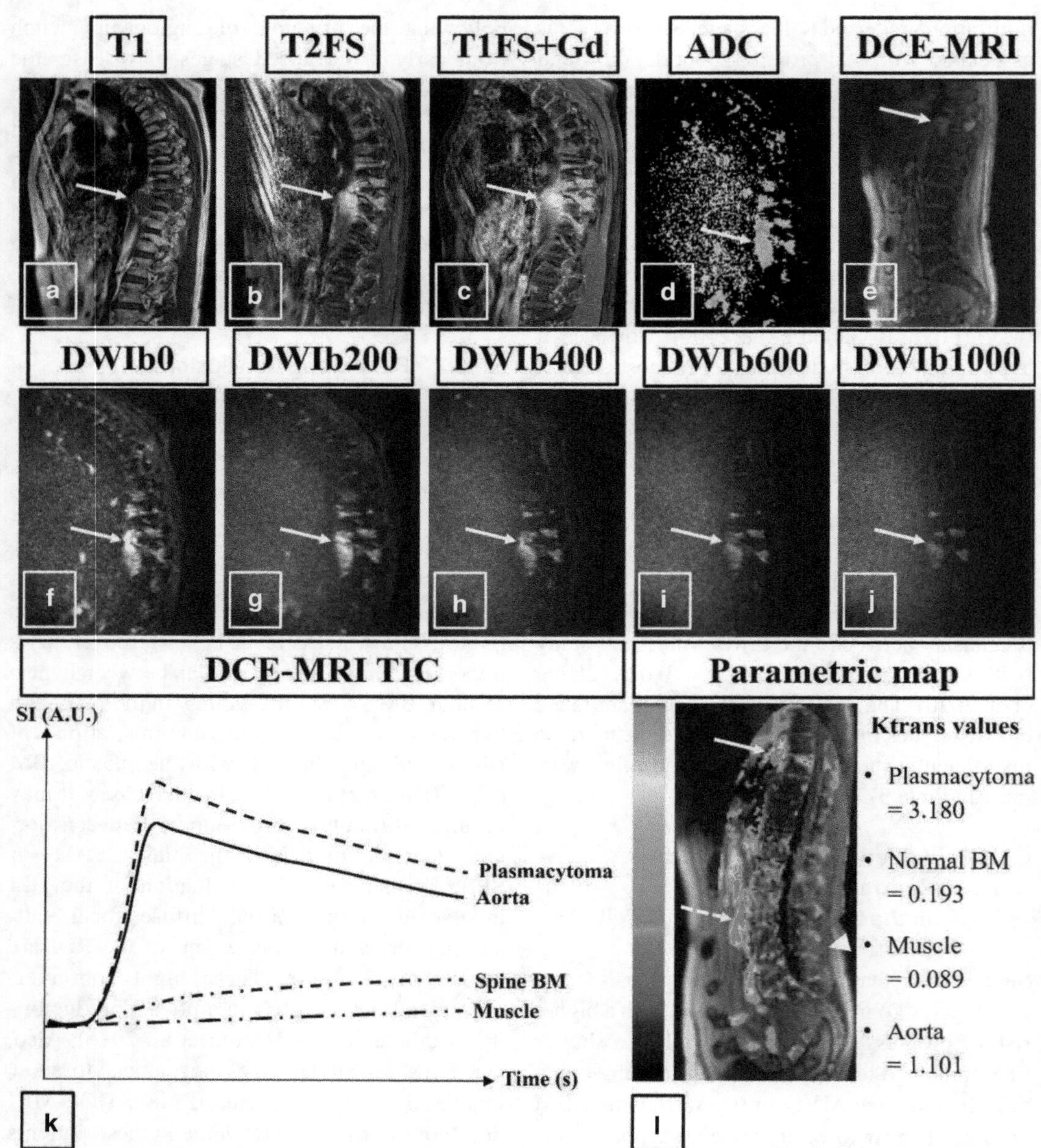
T1
T2FS
T1FS+Gd
ADC
DCE-MRI
a
b
c
d
e
DWIb0
DWIb200
DWIb400
DWIb600
DWIb1000
f
g
h
i
j
DCE-MRI TIC
Parametric map
SI (A.U.)
Plasmacytoma
Aorta
Spine BM
Muscle
Time (s)
k
Ktrans values
• Plasmacytoma = 3.180
• Normal BM = 0.193
• Muscle = 0.089
• Aorta = 1.101
l

Fig. 7 MRI appearance of solitary plasmacytomas of bone with emphasis on diffusion-weighted imaging and dynamic contrast-enhanced MRI. A solitary plasmacytoma of bone with extensive cortical destruction and soft tissue extension is observed in a 74-year-old female patient in the tenth rib and in the vertebral body of the tenth thoracic vertebra (white arrows). The lesion has an iso- to hypointense signal intensity as compared to muscle on T1-weighted imaging (**a**), a hyperintense signal intensity as compared to muscle on fat-saturated T2-weighted imaging (**b**) and a homogeneous gadolinium contrast enhancement on fat-saturated T1-weighted imaging (**c**). On conventional anatomical MRI sequences, a clear margin with normal surrounding bone (marrow) can be observed (**a**–**c**). On diffusion-weighted imaging, the lesion presents as a diffusion restrictive focal lesion with high signal intensity on high *b*-value images (**j**, $b = 1000$ s/mm^2) and low ADC (**d**). On the different *b*-value images (**f**, $b = 0$ s/mm^2; **g**, $b = 200$ s/mm^2; **h**, $b = 400$ s/mm^2; **i**, $b = 600$ s/mm^2; **j**, $b = 1000$ s/mm^2), the high signal intensity as present on the *b*0 images (**f**) is only retained in the solitary plasmacytoma of bone on the *b*1000 images (**j**), indicating diffusion restriction in the focal lesion and normal surrounding bone (marrow) without diffusion restriction. On the dynamic contrast-enhanced MRI (**e**, dynamic T1-weighted sequence after gadolinium contrast enhancement, 34 s after contrast injection), the solitary plasmacytoma of bone presents as an early and intensely enhancing focal lesion, surrounded by nonenhancing normal bone (marrow). On the time-intensity curve (**k**), the solitary plasmacytoma of bone presents with a high vascularization (type IV curve with high first pass, rapid wash-in, high maximal enhancement and rapid washout), which is comparable to the vascularization of the aorta. The surrounding bone (marrow) and muscles show normal vascularization (type I/II curve with low first pass, slow wash-in and no further or slow sustained enhancement). As an example, the dynamic contrast-enhanced MRI Ktrans parametric map is calculated, showing very high Ktrans (volume transfer constant) values in the solitary plasmacytoma of bone (white arrow) as compared to the normal surrounding spinal bone marrow and the paravertebral muscles (white arrowhead) and aorta (dashed white arrow) as reference tissues (**l**). *ADC* apparent diffusion coefficient, *A.U.* arbitrary unit, *BM* bone marrow, *DCE-MRI (TIC)* dynamic contrast-enhanced MRI (time-intensity curve), *DWIb0–DWIb1000* diffusion-weighted imaging with different diffusion sensitizing gradients (0–1000 s/mm^2), *Ktrans* volume transfer constant, *s* second, *SI* signal intensity, *T1* T1-weighted image, *T1FS+Gd* fat-saturated T1-weighted image with gadolinium contrast enhancement, *T2FS* fat-saturated T2-weighted image

Brownian motion of water molecules (Biffar et al. 2010a; Dutoit and Verstraete 2017; Koutoulidis et al. 2018). The diffusion sensitizing gradient or *b*-value (s/mm^2) of the applied pulse sequence is an important parameter in DWI imaging. Lower *b*-values render a higher signal-to-noise ratio (SNR) but are influenced by perfusion effects, while higher *b*-values are better at highlighting the differences in diffusion restriction independently from perfusion effects but have a lower SNR (Gariani et al. 2018). Generally, a maximal *b*-value of 1000 s/mm^2 is used (Sommer et al. 2011). The Myeloma Response Assessment and Diagnosis System (MYRADS) recommends the use of two *b*-values for clinical protocols to avoid long acquisition times and three *b*-values for research. For better evaluation of potential malignancies, diffusion-weighted whole-body imaging with background body signal suppression (DWIBS) can be performed. This necessitates relatively high diffusion weightings and excellent fat suppression (Van Den Berghe et al. 2022).

6.3.3.2 Qualitative Interpretation

Qualitative evaluation of DWI images is performed by visually assessing different *b*-value images ranging from *b*0 to *b*1000 to compare the SI of ROIs with those of adjacent reference tissues (Dutoit et al. 2014). Loss of SI over time on the different images indicates movement of water molecules and no diffusion restriction, while retained high SI indicates the presence of diffusion restriction. The use of a *b*-value of $\geq$800 s/mm^2 results in signal suppression of normal tissues, allowing for the identification of high SI foci with restricted diffusion (Martí-Bonmatí et al. 2015). However, the interpretation of SI on high *b*-value images is subjective and therefore susceptible to inter- and intraobserver variability.

6.3.3.3 Quantitative Interpretation

For quantitative assessment, apparent diffusion coefficient (ADC) values and ADC maps are calculated using a minimum of two different *b*-values per pixel in the image (Biffar et al. 2010a; Messiou and Kaiser 2015; Horger et al. 2011;

Paternain et al. 2020). ADC maps are created by plotting the ADC values in that way that dark voxels represent a low ADC and vice versa (Van Den Berghe et al. 2022). With increasing *b*-values, the contrast between tissues with different ADCs increases. However, this process is limited by the SNR, as overall SI decreases with increasing *b*-values. At a certain point, the tissue SI will reach the noise level of the image, biasing the determined ADC (Sommer et al. 2011; Messiou and Kaiser 2015; Dutoit et al. 2014; Dietrich et al. 2010). Low ADC values are indicative of diffusion restriction. ADC values and ADC maps should always be interpreted together with the *b*-value images (e.g., Fig. 7).

6.3.3.4 Physiological Changes in Bone Marrow with Age and Location and the Effects on Diffusion-Weighted Imaging

With increasing age, the BM transitions from red (high cellularity and water content) to yellow (low cellularity and water content). The high cellular and water content in younger BM will contribute to high ADC values and a higher SI on high *b*-value images. In older patients, the lower cellular and water content as well as the hydrophobic nature of fat will contribute to low ADC values and a low SI on high *b*-value images (Biffar et al. 2010a, b; Herrmann et al. 2012). The lumbar spine contains significantly less water and more fat compared to the thoracic spine, making for physiologically lower ADC values and *b*-value image SIs at the lumbar level (Dutoit and Verstraete 2017; Van Den Berghe et al. 2022).

6.3.3.5 Added Value of Diffusion-Weighted Imaging in the Diagnosis, Staging and Follow-Up of Plasma Cell Disorders

When a presumed focal lesion is identified on anatomical MRI (focal MM lesion or SPB), the detection of diffusion restriction is a sign of malignancy. In the case of SPB, which presents as a solitary diffusion restrictive lesion, there might not be any other visible abnormality on anatomical WBMRI sequences, but DWI images and ADC values and corresponding ADC maps may be able to visualize diffusion restriction in other parts of the body, indicating progression of the disease to MM (Tables 1, 2, and 3). DWI images and ADC values can thus aid in better detection and characterization of lesions that would otherwise be missed or misdiagnosed (Van Den Berghe et al. 2022). It can help in the timely upstaging of patients and can therefore have an impact on therapy and patient outcomes. DWI images and ADC values may also be of value in the absence of focal lesions on anatomical MRI sequences, but when diffuse signal abnormalities are observed (e.g., low SI on T1-WI), diffusion restriction may be demonstrated, thus giving a clue that an underlying malignant process might be present in a diffuse distribution pattern.

The correlation of ADC with the cellularity of BM appears to follow a biphasic pattern. Initially, higher ADC values are noted, possibly due to increased water content and because smaller PCs cause less restriction of water diffusion compared to larger fat cells. After this initial increase in ADC values, they drop due to the replacement of fat cells by abundant monoclonal PCs, which massively produce Ig, thus increasing the interstitial viscosity. This increased cellularity results in diffusion restriction and thus lower ADC values (Koutoulidis et al. 2018; Padhani et al. 2013; Khoo et al. 2011). Lower ADC values also correlate with higher levels of monoclonal protein, indicative of higher BM plasmacytosis and interstitial viscosity (Sommer et al. 2011).

6.3.3.6 Role of Diffusion-Weighted Imaging in Vertebral Fractures

Although morphological features on anatomical sequences are often enough to differentiate between benign and malignant fractures (e.g., diffuse low T1-WI SI, convex vertebral bodies, and pedicle involvement are more frequent in malignant fractures), DWI with ADC can be used in vertebral fractures to help differentiate between benign and malignant fractures caused by SPB or MM focal lesions. In benign (osteoporotic) fractures, there will be a low SI on high *b*-value images and a high ADC value, both indicating no diffusion restriction. Increased BM edema and free water flow through the osteoporotic bone are observed. In malignant fractures in SPB or MM focal lesions, there will be a high SI on high *b*-value images and a low ADC value, indicating diffusion restriction due to closely packed tumor cells and increased interstitial viscosity (Biffar et al. 2010b; Dietrich et al. 2017; Suh et al. 2018; Messiou and Kaiser 2015).

6.3.3.7 Potential Pitfalls of Diffusion-Weighted Imaging

With aging, the red BM is gradually replaced by fatty yellow BM. High *b*-value DWI can be used for tumor detection in patients with higher adiposity BM, as SI differences between yellow BM and SPB do not overlap. In young patients, patients with BM reconversion (obesity, anemia, physical activity) or reactive hyperplasia (chemotherapy, erythropoietin), the overall BM SI will increase on high *b*-value images, making the detection of BM malignancies more difficult, rendering DWI for tumor detection less useful (Messiou and Kaiser 2015; Dutoit et al. 2014; Padhani et al. 2013). In these cases, correlation with the ADC values can help to differentiate with malignancy. They will be higher in red BM/BM reconversion/reactive hyperplasia and lower in MM focal lesions and SPB.

A second pitfall is the T2 shine-through phenomenon. As DWI reflects both cellular and water content of tissues, it can cause high SI on high *b*-value images even if there is no diffusion restriction. Here again, correlation with the ADC values can provide information that may be able to confirm the presence of T2 shine-through (generally evident from a high SI on high *b*-value images and corresponding high ADC) (Messiou and Kaiser 2015; Sommer et al. 2011; Khoo et al. 2011).

6.4 Positron Emission Tomography With or Without CT

^{18}F-fluorodeoxyglucose (^{18}F-FDG) PET/CT is an imaging modality that has a place in the diagnosis of many types of cancers. The most significant advantage it has over other imaging techniques is the ability to assess the burden of disease with good accuracy and to distinguish between metabolically active and inactive lesions. The field of view of ^{18}F-FDG PET/CT should include at least the skull, upper limbs, and femurs in the diagnostic workup of SPB to detect additional lesions or diffuse surrounding bone marrow invasion, thus upstaging SPB to MM (Cavo et al. 2017) (Fig. 8). The maximum standardized uptake value (SUV) based on body weight is a semiquantitative parameter that can be used for image interpretation (Cavo et al. 2017). When evaluating ^{18}F-FDG PET/CT images, it is important to realize that there might be false-positive cases due to infection, inflammation and hyperglycemia, among others. False-negative scans are associated with hyperglycemia, recent use of high-dose steroid therapy and genetic defects hampering tumoral glucose uptake (Terpos et al. 2016; Cavo et al. 2017). ^{18}F-FDG PET/CT has been able to discover additional plasmacytoma lesions that were not visible on other imaging modalities, thereby upstaging the extent of the disease. It can therefore have a major impact on the diagnosis and treatment of SPB, especially in cases where the presumed SPB is a local manifestation of an underlying MM (Salaun et al. 2008; Schirrmeister et al. 2003; Nanni et al. 2008; Cavo et al. 2017). The IMWG released a consensus statement recommending the use of ^{18}F-FDG PET/CT to confirm the diagnosis of SPB when WBMRI is unavailable. Also, according to the IMWG, patients with focal lesions on ^{18}F-FDG PET but without lytic lesions on the CT part of ^{18}F-FDG PET/CT are at a high risk of progression to active MM (Cavo et al. 2017). However, it must be noted that there is at least one case in the literature where ^{18}F-FDG PET/CT has missed a known plasmacytoma of bone (Schirrmeister et al. 2003). ^{18}F-FDG PET/CT is therefore not an ideal substitution for conventional imaging modalities, but it can be a useful technique to help distinguish SPB from SPB with minimal BM involvement or even MM, especially in cases with an atypical presentation (Warsame et al. 2012) (Tables 1, 2, and 3).

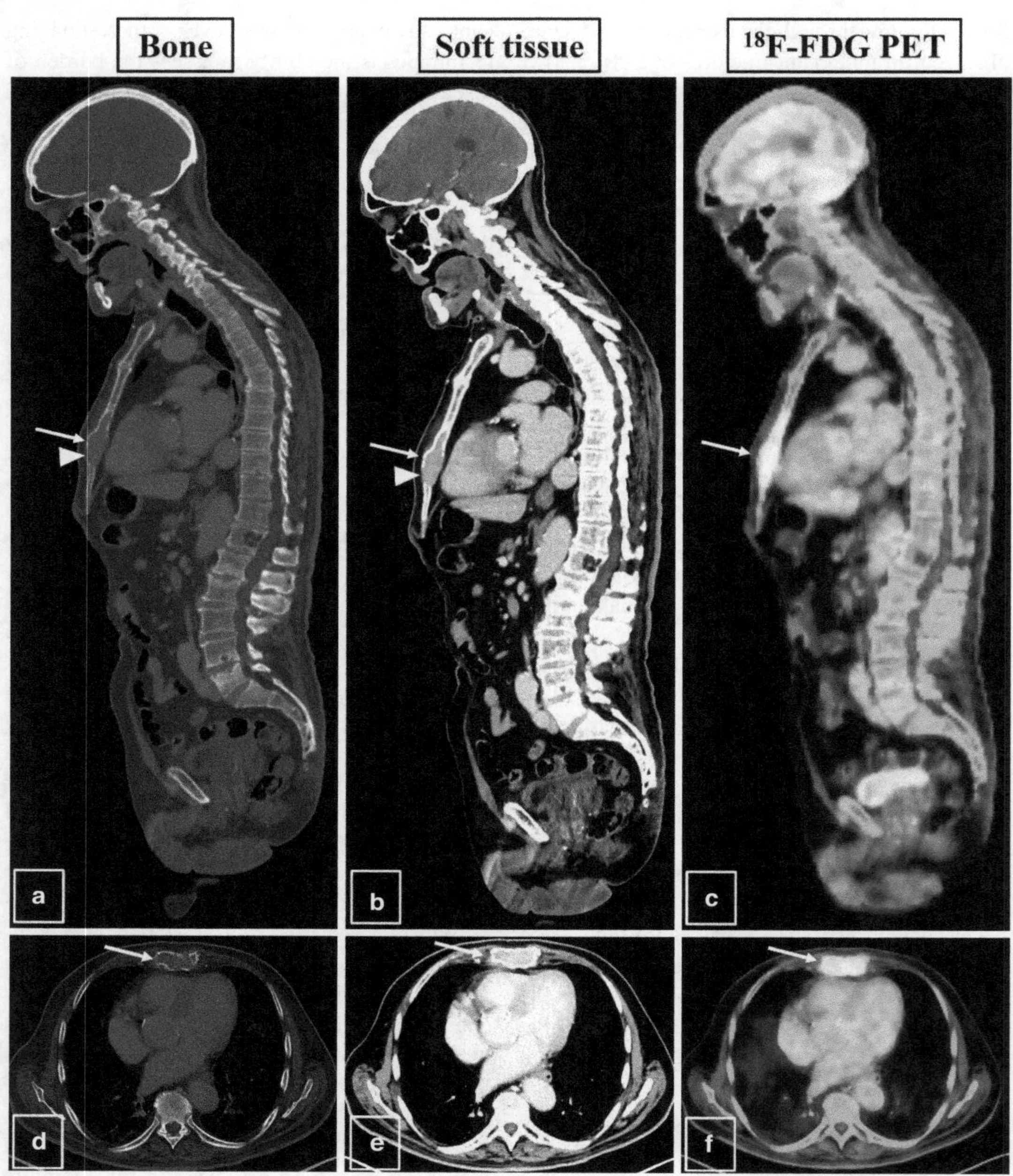

Fig. 8 ^{18}F-FDG PET/CT appearance of a solitary plasmacytoma of bone. A solitary plasmacytoma of bone is observed in an 87-year-old male patient as a solitary osteolytic unilocular lesion with complete destruction and replacement of normal bone and clear margins in the sternal body on the axial and sagittal bone and soft tissue CT images (white arrows in **a**, **b** and **d**, **e**). Cortical destruction without soft tissue involvement is observed (white arrowhead in **a**, **b**). On ^{18}F-FDG PET images, a solitary lesion with high ^{18}F-FDG uptake (white arrows in **c**, **f**) with normal surrounding bone marrow in the sternum, mandible, skull, ribs, scapulae and entire spine is observed. This differentiates a solitary plasmacytoma of bone from other plasma cell disorders like (smoldering) multiple myeloma, in which higher ^{18}F-FDG uptake is expected. Total administered activity: 303 MBq. SUVmax plasmacytoma: 14.4. *^{18}F-FDG PET* 18-fluorodeoxyglucose positron emission tomography

In MM, ^{18}F-FDG PET/CT is considered as the best imaging modality for evaluation of therapy response. Metabolic changes assessed by ^{18}F-FDG PET/CT provide an earlier evaluation of response compared with MRI and allow for better evaluation of minimal residual disease (MRD) (Jamet et al. 2019; Terpos et al. 2016; Cavo et al. 2017; Mena et al. 2022). In patients with plasmacytoma, ^{18}F-FDG PET/CT has value for staging and planning of radiotherapy and potentially also in response assessment of radiotherapy (Kim et al. 2009). It can help exclude unsuspected sites of disease that may define active MM (Ulaner and Landgren 2020). To conclude, ^{18}F-FDG PET/CT is useful in the evaluation of SPB and has a prognostic value both at the moment of diagnosis and in the evaluation of treatment response.

6.5 Bone Scintigraphy

There is usually no increased uptake, because osteoblastic reaction is absent, except in cases of concomitant fracture and/or surrounding invasion. Scintigraphy is therefore not a reliable imaging modality for staging or monitoring of SPB and plays little to no role in SPB (Table 3).

A general overview of advantages and disadvantages of different imaging modalities in SPB is presented in Table 6.

Table 6 Advantages and disadvantages of different imaging modalities in solitary plasmacytoma of bone

	Advantages	Disadvantages
WBXR	– Low cost – Availability – Time-efficient	– Limited sensitivity – Low detection rate – >30% bone destruction necessary – Patient discomfort (repositioning, multiple films) – No bone marrow assessment – No differentiation between benign and malignant fractures – No treatment response assessment
WBLDCT	– More sensitive and specific – Time-efficient – Bone marrow involvement can be visible – Evaluation of extramedullary disease	– Higher radiation exposure – More expensive than WBXR – Unclear prognostic significance of lesion number
MRI	– No radiation – DCE-MRI and DWI techniques – Evaluation of neurological structures and soft tissues – Bone marrow assessment with differentiation from MGUS, SMM and MM – Assessment of number of focal lesions with prognostic significance – Evaluation of extramedullary disease	– High costs – Long acquisition times – Claustrophobia – Contraindicated for certain medical devices or implants – Relatively limited availability
^{18}F-FDG PET/CT	– Prognostic value pre- and post-treatment – Best assessment of response and minimal residual disease – Evaluation of extramedullary disease	– High costs – Limited availability – False positive in infection, inflammation – False negative in hyperglycemia, high-dose steroid use, glucose transport genetic defects – Poor resolution unless combined with CT

Modified from Terpos et al. (2016)—The Role of Imaging in the Treatment of Patients With Multiple Myeloma in 2016. Am Soc Clin Oncol Educ Book. 2016;35:e407–17. https://doi.org/10.1200/EDBK_159074. Available from ASCO Educational Book 2016

^{18}F-FDG PET 18-fluorodeoxyglucose positron emission tomography, *DCE* dynamic contrast-enhanced, *DWI* diffusion-weighted imaging, *MGUS* monoclonal gammopathy of undetermined significance, *MM* multiple myeloma, *SMM* smoldering multiple myeloma, *WBLDCT* whole-body low-dose CT, *WBXR* whole-body radiography

7 Histopathology

SP is a rare solitary tumor characterized by a local clonal PC proliferation without evidence of multiple myeloma. As discussed earlier, it can be present either in bone (SPB) or in extra-osseous tissue (EMP). These SPB cells are identical to PC in MM, both cytologically and immunophenotypically (Jawad and Scully 2009).

Histological analysis of tissue shows infiltration of PC without a significant lymphoid component. Using immunohistochemistry, in situ hybridization or flow cytometry, clonality of PC can be determined based on kappa or lambda light chain restriction. Confirmation of PC clonality can be performed by detection of heavy- and light-chain gene rearrangement via polymerase chain reaction (Peker et al. 2019). High-grade angiogenesis, measured in MVD in SPB, is associated with a higher risk of progression to MM as well as a shorter PFS compared to SPB with low-grade angiogenesis. In SPB, the MVD in the surrounding BM does not appear to be increased, supporting the theory that the BM is not (or very minimally, plasmacytosis <10%) affected in strict SPB (Kumar et al. 2003). The MVD does not appear to be linked to tumor location nor other prognostic factors such as age or monoclonal protein levels (Kumar et al. 2003). These findings are closely linked to the ones in MM, where high-grade angiogenesis of the BM is linked with a poor prognosis of MM (Rajkumar et al. 2000). After hematoxylin-eosin staining of biopsied SPB tissue, intracytoplasmic crystals may be identified in a significant proportion of cells, representing crystallized Ig. These crystals are eosinophilic and can be either needle-shaped or elongated rhomboid-shaped (Chan 2014) (Figs. 9 and 10).

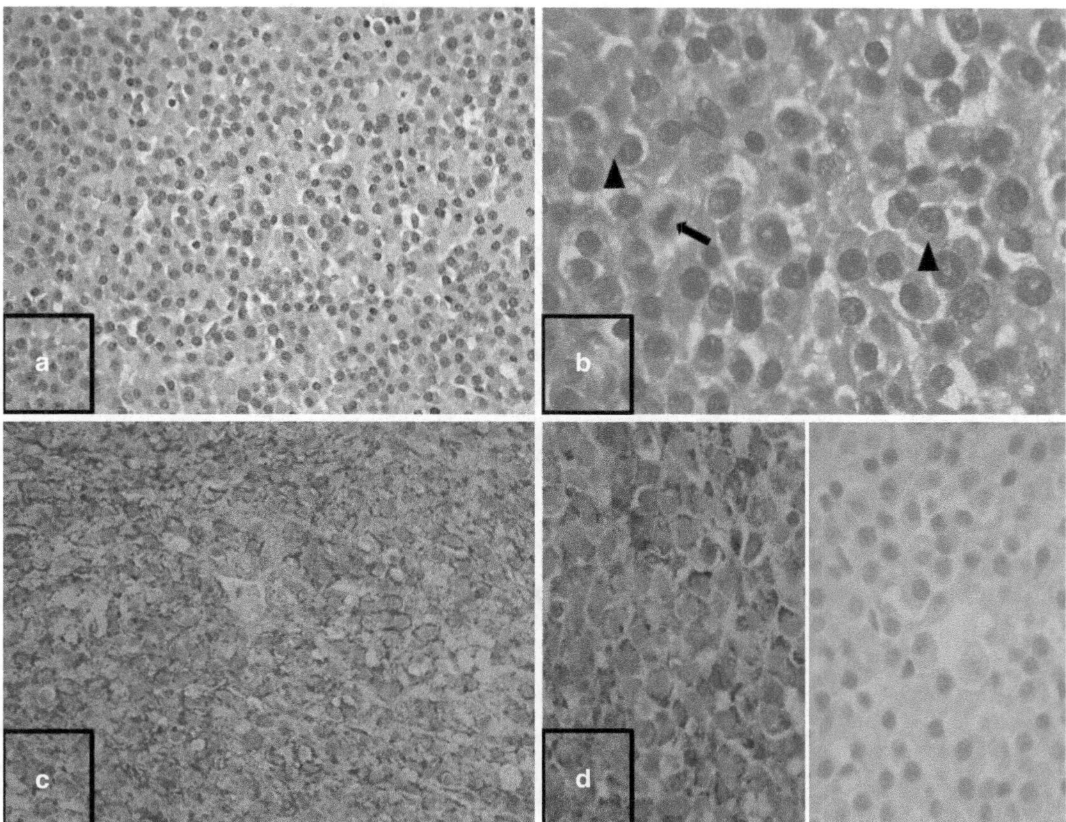

Fig. 9 Histological assessment of a solitary plasmacytoma of bone. (**a**) Solitary plasmacytoma of bone completely replacing normal bone marrow (hematoxylin and eosin staining, ×20 magnification). (**b**) High magnification of the same lesion as in (**a**) showing neoplastic plasma cells, containing abundant cytoplasm with a prominent Golgi apparatus (arrowheads) and an eccentrically placed nucleus. Compared to nuclei of normal plasma cells, cell nuclei of these neoplastic plasma cells are slightly larger and irregular. The typical spoke-wheel or clock-face chromatin of normal plasma cells is no longer visible in this neoplasm. A mitotic figure is indicated by an arrow (hematoxylin and eosin staining, ×100 magnification). (**c**) Immunohistochemistry for the general plasma cell marker CD138, confirming the plasma cell origin of this neoplastic lesion (×20 magnification). (**d**) Immunohistochemistry demonstrating strong cytoplasmic positivity for kappa light chain (left), but not for lambda light chain (right), confirming the monoclonal aspect of these plasma cells (×40 magnification)

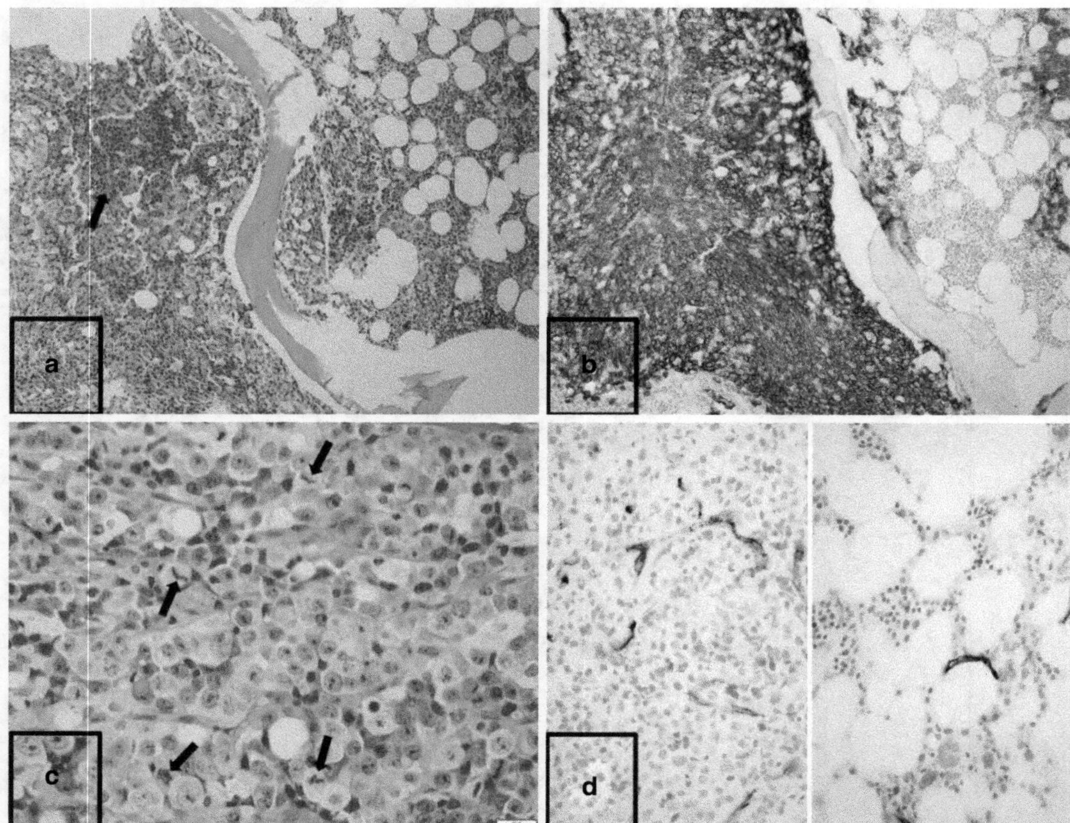

Fig. 10 Histological assessment of solitary plasmacytoma of bone. (**a**) Trephine biopsy showing a plasma neoplasm (black arrow) with an immature morphology (hematoxylin and eosin staining, ×20 magnification). (**b**) The neoplastic plasma cell focus becomes easily visible after immunohistochemical staining for CD138 (×20 magnification). (**c**) Hematoxylin and eosin staining demonstrating plasma cells with an immature morphology, containing irregular and enlarged nuclei with a "blastic" aspect (resembling the nuclei of immunoblasts or plasmablasts). Nucleoli in these cell nuclei are prominent. Several mitoses are indicated by arrows (×40 magnification). (**d**) Immunohistochemistry staining for CD34 (brown) comparing a dense neoplastic cell focus showing an increased microvascular density (left) and an area of unaffected bone marrow from the same patient (right) (×40 magnification)

8 Differential Diagnosis

In the broad differential diagnosis of SPB, all tumors involving bone and BM should be included, especially the osteolytic lesions. An overview of the imaging characteristics differentiating SPB from alternative diagnoses is described in Table 7.

First, around one-third of presumed "solitary" plasmacytomas are in fact not SPB but one of multiple other lesions found in the context of MM and other PCD. Further imaging is important to differentiate SPB from MM and other diseases (Choi et al. 2014). MGUS is situated before SPB on the PCD spectrum (Rajkumar 2016b). SMM is a PCD that falls in between MGUS and MM (Choi et al. 2014).

Second, other cancers that affect the BM, such as lymphoma and leukemia, should also be considered. Patients with lymphoma involving the

Table 7 Plasmacytoma differential diagnosis and imaging characteristics to distinguish between plasmacytoma and alternative diagnoses (according to Choi et al. 2014, Dammacco et al. 2015, Nguyen et al. 2020, Delorme and Baur-Melnyk 2011, Patnaik et al. 2016, Zhang et al. 2009, Morales et al. 2018, Hwang et al. 2021)

Differential diagnosis	SPB	Alternative diagnosis
Plasma cell dyscrasias—monoclonal gammopathy of undetermined significance	*WBMRI*: large focal lesion *[18]F-FDG PET/CT*: large focal lesion positive	*WBMRI*: small focal lesion(s) are rare *[18]F-FDG PET/CT*: small focal lesion(s) positive but rare
Plasma cell dyscrasias—smoldering myeloma	*WBMRI*: focal lesion only *DWI*: no diffusion restriction in surrounding BM *DCE-MRI*: normal vascularization in surrounding BM (TIC type I/II) *[18]F-FDG PET/CT*: focal lesion positive	*WBMRI*: focal lesion and/or diffuse BM infiltration *DWI*: diffuse diffusion restriction in surrounding BM in diffuse disease *DCE-MRI*: high vascularization in surrounding BM (TIC type III/IV) in diffuse disease *[18]F-FDG PET/CT*: diffuse mostly negative but a single focal lesion can be positive
Plasma cell dyscrasias—multiple myeloma	Single focal lesion No diffuse BM infiltration	Single or multiple focal lesions Diffuse BM infiltration can be present
Lymphoma/leukemia	*WBMRI*: no diffuse BM infiltration *[18]F-FDG PET/CT*: only positive in focal lesion	*WBMRI*: diffuse BM infiltration *[18]F-FDG PET/CT*: positive in entire axial skeleton
Bone marrow metastasis	No diffuse invasion, only focal lesion *MRI T1-WI*: less hypointense to muscle *MRI T2(FS)-WI*: less hyperintense compared to muscle *MRI T2(FS)-WI*: less peritumoral edema *MRI T2-WI and T1-WI+Gd*: homogeneous signal *DWI*: lower ADC (mean 760 μm²/s) *[18]F-FDG PET/CT*: only positive in focal lesion	Diffuse invasion by multiple metastases possible *MRI T1-WI*: hypointense compared to muscle *MRI T2(FS)-WI*: hyperintense compared to muscle *MRI T2(FS)-WI*: intense peritumoral edema *MRI T2-WI and T1-WI+Gd*: heterogeneous signal *DWI*: higher ADC (mean 1214 μm²/s) *[18]F-FDG PET/CT*: positive in multiple metastases
Hemangioma of bone	*Conventional radiography*: mini brain sign *Axial CT*: mini brain sign *MRI T1-WI and T2(FS)-WI*: iso- to hypointense compared to muscle on T1-WI and hyperintense compared to muscle on T2(FS)-WI *[18]F-FDG PET/CT*: positive single focal lesion *DCE-MRI*: higher semiquantitative TIC parameters, Vp, Ktrans	*Conventional radiography*: vertical orientation (corduroy) *Axial CT*: polka dot sign *MRI T1-WI and T2(FS)-WI*: hyperintense compared to muscle *[18]F-FDG PET/CT*: negative (cold) or positive (hot) lesions *DCE-MRI*: lower semiquantitative TIC parameters, Vp, Ktrans

(continued)

Table 7 (continued)

Differential diagnosis	SPB	Alternative diagnosis
Aneurysmal bone cyst	Primarily in vertebral body	Primarily in posterior spinal elements (e.g., lamina) with anterior spread into vertebral body
	CT: no cortical thinning	*CT*: cortical thinning (eggshell thin cortex)
	No fluid-fluid levels	Fluid-fluid levels
	Conventional radiography: purely lytic lesion	*Conventional radiography*: lytic with bone remodeling
	MRI: solid-like appearance	*MRI:* cyst-like appearance, varying signal intensity (blood products at various stages)
	MRI T1-WI and T2-WI: no surrounding rim of low signal intensity	*MRI T1-WI and T2-WI*: surrounding rim of low signal intensity
	MRI T1-WI+Gd: no peripheral and septal enhancement pattern, less bone marrow edema and soft tissue edema	*MRI T1-WI+Gd*: peripheral and septal enhancement pattern with bone marrow edema and soft tissue edema
Giant cell tumor of bone	Most common in spine	Most common in upper sacrum, 7% in spine
	No cystic regions	Cystic regions
	No hemorrhagic foci	Hemorrhagic foci
	No fluid-fluid levels	Fluid-fluid levels
	Homogeneous lesion	Heterogeneous lesion
	MRI T1-WI: hypointense to muscle without hyperintense hemorrhagic zones	*MRI T1-WI*: hypointense to muscle with hyperintense hemorrhagic zones
	MRI T2-WI: high signal intensity	*MRI T2-WI*: low to intermediate signal intensity (hemosiderin and high collagen content)

μm^2 square micrometer, *[18]F-FDG PET/CT* 18-fluorodeoxyglucose positron emission tomography CT, *ADC* apparent diffusion coefficient, *BM* bone marrow, *DCE-MRI* dynamic contrast-enhanced MRI, *DWI* diffusion-weighted imaging, *Ktrans* volume transfer constant, *s* second, *SPB* solitary plasmacytoma of bone, *T1-WI(+Gd)* T1-weighted imaging on MRI (+gadolinium contrast enhancement), *T2(FS)-WI* (fat-saturated) T2-weighted imaging on MRI, *TIC* time-intensity curve, *Vp* blood plasma volume per unit tissue volume, *WBMRI* whole-body MRI

BM can benefit from ^{18}F-FDG PET/CT since it is accurate and sensitive and has a strong negative predictive value. In acute myeloid leukemia, imaging techniques only have a supporting function, as opposed to malignant lymphoma, such as for the management of infections or the detection of unusual presentation sites (Choi et al. 2014). Lymphoma is further discussed in Part III, chapter "Lymphoma."

Third, the spine is the third most frequent location for metastatic disease. Spinal metastases are the most frequent type of spinal tumors. In comparison to CT, MRI is more effective at detecting osseous metastases.

Fourth, hemangioma of bone is another differential diagnosis of SPB. According to the dominant vessel type, this benign vascular malformation can be categorized as capillary cavernous or venous. Hemangioma is further discussed in Part III, chapter "Vertebral Hemangioma and Angiomatous Neoplasms."

Fifth, aneurysmal bone cysts can easily be mistaken for more aggressive lesions. They are believed to result from underlying neoplasms or trauma and commonly occur in patients under 20 years of age. Typical radiographic findings include a lytic extended bone remodeling lesion, which may also affect the nearby soft tissues. Aneurysmal bone cyst is further discussed in Part III, chapter "Aneurysmal Bone Cyst and Other Cystic Lesions."

Lastly, a giant cell tumor may mimic SPB. Giant cell tumor is further discussed in Part III, chapter "Giant Cell Tumor."

9 Local and Distant Staging

SPBs are considered stage I myeloma in accordance with the Durie and Salmon staging criteria. As a result, stage I myeloma meets all the following requirements: hemoglobin >10 g/dL, normal serum calcium level, normal bone structure or SPB exclusively and low M-component (IgG <5 g/dL, IgA <3 g/dL, urine light chains <4 g/24 h) (Kilciksiz et al. 2012).

In the Fourth Edition of the WHO Classification of Tumors of Hematopoietic and Lymphoid Tissues, SPB is described as having two subtypes. The first one is an SPB lacking clonal BM PC remote from the plasmacytoma itself. Therefore, it discloses a normal surrounding BM. In 10% of cases, this subtype progresses to MM in three years. The second subtype exhibits minimal (<10%) clonal BM PC. It has a more pronounced progression rate of SPB to MM, namely 60% in three years. The IMWG conclusions do not adopt the clear distinction as outlined in the WHO update. The two isolated plasmacytoma types in this report are combined to form a single SP that is labeled as "not otherwise specified" (SP-NOS). This is thought to be a single-type lesion made up of clonal PC with varying degrees of differentiation, either in soft tissue or bone. At the time of diagnosis, these patients' iliac crest BM has no clonal PC. When excluding the isolated primary tumor, MRI or CT scans of the spine and pelvis reveal only normal bones. Moreover, there is no obvious end-organ damage that is directly linked to the PCD. Within three years, 10% of these patients could progress to MM. The IMWG further separates SP with low (<10%) clonal BM PC at diagnosis from the SP-NOS. Only one characteristic distinguishes this subtype from the so-called SP-NOS: evidence of <10% clonal BM PC upon diagnosis. Yet, this subset's trajectory differs noticeably from the SP-NOS group because 60% of individuals with this subtype SPB will progress to MM within three years. The EMP of this subset, however, will only proceed to MM in 20% of patients after three years (Table 8) (Ohana et al. 2018).

Table 8 Definition and course of solitary plasmacytoma according to the International Myeloma Working Group

Type	Features
SP-NOS	– Solitary disorder of bone or soft tissue, composed of monoclonal PC (by biopsy) – Bone marrow biopsy, remote from the plasmacytoma, is normal – MRI or CT shows normal skeleton, except for the plasmacytoma – No evidence of CRAB – Progression to MM in 10% of cases in three years
SP with <10% of bone marrow involvement	– Same criteria as SP-NOS with additional monoclonal BM PC <10% in a sporadic bone marrow biopsy – 60% of SPB will develop into MM in three years – 20% of EMP will transform into MM in three years

Modified from Ohana et al. (2018)—Classification of Solitary Plasmacytoma, Is it more Intricate than Presently Suggested? A Commentary. J Cancer. 2018 Oct 10;9(21):3894–3897. https://doi.org/10.7150/jca.26854. Available from: Ohana et al. (2018) J Cancer

BM bone marrow, *CRAB* calcemia, renal failure, anemia, bone lesions, *EMP* extramedullary plasmacytoma, *MM* multiple myeloma, *NOS* not otherwise specified, *PC* plasma cells, *SP(B)* solitary plasmacytoma (of bone)

10 Treatment

10.1 Radiotherapy

Clonal PCs are very radiation sensitive and initial clinical trials support high response rates of SP to radiation therapy (local control in >90%), making it the treatment of choice for SPB (Caers et al. 2018). Although no clear relationship between radiotherapy dose and response has been documented to date, the consensus is a dose of 40–50 Gy over a period of four weeks with a daily dosage of 1.8–2.0 Gy per fraction (Dimopoulos et al. 2000; Reed et al. 2011; Caers et al. 2018). Because microscopic extension surrounding the lesion increases disease recurrence risk, both the imaging-identified affected tissues and a margin of healthy tissue of at least 2 cm should be included in the treatment area (Caers et al. 2018). For spinal lesions, including one normal vertebra above and below the affected vertebra in the treatment field is recommended (Dimopoulos et al. 2000, Reed et al. 2011, Caers et al. 2018). Following local radiotherapy, radiographs may show sclerosis and bone remineralization in up to 50% of patients. MRI images may still show BM abnormalities, even after successful treatment of SPB (Dimopoulos et al. 2000) (Fig. 11).

10.2 Surgery

Surgery is not indicated as a routine therapeutic procedure in patients with SPB and should be reserved for specific cases. However, newer studies have observed an improvement in overall survival when complementary surgery was performed by reducing the tumor burden, thereby eradicating clones that are potentially resistant to radiotherapy (Shen et al. 2021; Kilciksiz et al. 2008; Jawad and Scully 2009; Xie et al. 2020). An argument against the use of complementary surgery is that it causes a delay of radiotherapy, hereby potentially limiting its efficacy (Li et al. 2015). For spinal lesions, laminectomy may be indicated before starting radiotherapy when the patient presents with rapidly developing neurological impairments (Dimopoulos et al. 2000).

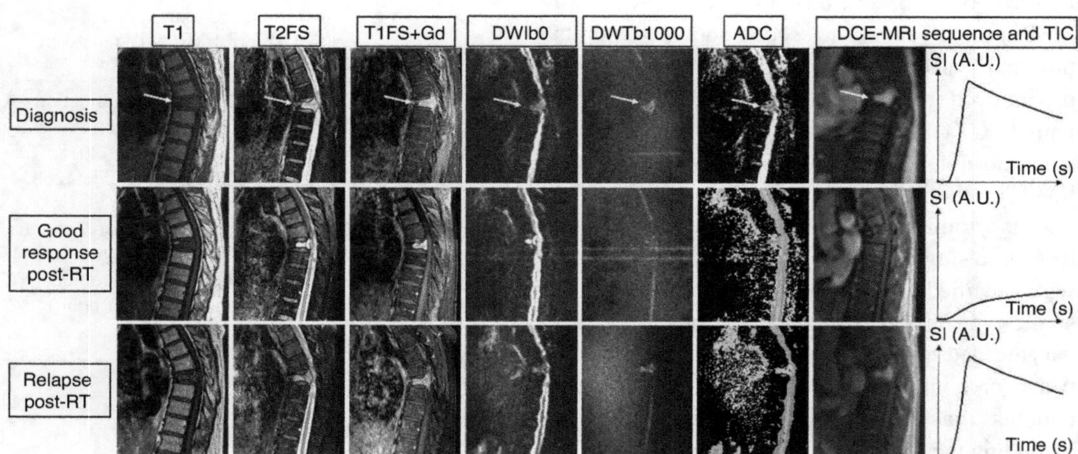

Fig. 11 MRI treatment response assessment. Multiparametric conventional MRI, diffusion-weighted MRI and dynamic contrast-enhanced MRI evaluation of a solitary plasmacytoma of bone in the seventh thoracic vertebral body at diagnosis (**upper row**, 69-year-old male patient) at the time of good response to local radiotherapy (**middle row**, 71-year-old male patient) and at the time of relapse after initial good response to local radiotherapy (**lower row**, 75-year-old male patient). At diagnosis, the lesion causes a grade III vertebral collapse with posterior cortical breakthrough, vertebral canal stenosis and subsequent neurological compression (white arrows). The lesion is iso- to hypointense to muscle on T1-weighted imaging and hyperintense to muscle on fat-saturated T2-weighted imaging, shows homogeneous intense contrast enhancement on fat-saturated T1-weighted imaging after gadolinium contrast enhancement, is diffusion restrictive and has a type IV time-intensity curve, indicating high vascularization and perfusion. At the time of good response to local radiotherapy, the lesion shows higher signal intensity on fat-saturated T2-weighted images (gelatinous transformation) with central necrosis, absent diffusion restriction and normal vascularization (type II time-intensity curve). At relapse, the initial imaging characteristics as at the time of diagnosis reappear. *ADC* apparent diffusion coefficient, *A.U.* arbitrary unit, *DCE-MRI (TIC)* dynamic contrast-enhanced MRI (time-intensity curve), *DWIb0/b1000* diffusion-weighted imaging with a diffusion sensitizing gradient of 0/1000 s/mm^2, *RT* radiotherapy, *s* second, *SI* signal intensity, *T1* T1-weighted image, *T1FS+Gd* fat-saturated T1-weighted image after gadolinium contrast administration, *T2FS* fat-saturated T2-weighted image

10.3 Chemotherapy

Despite the general consensus that adjuvant chemotherapy does not have a significant impact on the progression of SPB to MM or on OS/PFS, some recent studies find a tendency towards better event-free survival (Finsinger et al. 2016; Suh et al. 2012). Some authors suggest that, because of the high probability of developing MM in patients with SPB (even after local radiotherapy), adding systemic treatment with novel agents, such as proteasome inhibitors, might be beneficial for the outcome in these patients (de Waal et al. 2016). Bortezomib, a proteasome inhibitor used in MM, has shown possible efficacy in SPB in multiple case reports (Shen et al. 2021).

11 Prognosis

There are three failure patterns in SPB after therapy: emergence of evolving MM, local recurrence and emergence of new bone lesions free of MM (Kilciksiz et al. 2012). While radiotherapy can provide good local control for SPB, progression to MM is the main problem in these patients. The prognosis is rather poor, with more than 50–70% of patients developing MM within two years after radiotherapy (Dimopoulos et al. 2000; de Waal et al. 2016). The median OS in patients with treated SPB lies around 70–90 months, with a 10-year OS of 50% (Dingli et al. 2006; Shen et al. 2021). The role of surgery in the treatment of SPB remains debatable in respect to OS. Improvement in the survival of patients diagnosed in 2008–2016 as compared to 1976–2007 is possibly attributed to the use of novel agents such as proteasome inhibitors and immunomodulators (Shen et al. 2021).

A minimum lesion size of 5 cm, age (e.g., patients 40 years and older), spine lesions, radiotherapy dose, high M-protein levels, presence of light chains and persistence of M-protein after treatment have all been found to affect patient outcomes in some series and may indicate the presence of higher risks of progression to MM. With radiotherapy treatment, M-protein is dramatically reduced in the majority of SPB patients. M-protein disappearance is even observed in 20–50% of the patients. A poor prognostic indicator is post-treatment persisting M-protein levels (Kilciksiz et al. 2012).

The advances in imaging techniques are however also relevant and might play a role in the amelioration of survival outcomes. Further work needs to be performed, however. For instance, there are currently no high-quality data available about the potential contribution of qualitative and semiquantitative ^{18}F-FDG PET/CT characteristics to the prediction of the transformation to MM in SPB. The findings in the literature are not conclusive. Therefore, more research is required (Albano et al. 2020).

12 Key Points

- Solitary plasmacytoma of bone is a part of the plasma cell disorder spectrum and can evolve to symptomatic full-blown multiple myeloma.
- The prognosis of solitary plasmacytoma of bone is rather poor with 50–70% of patients developing symptomatic full-blown multiple myeloma.
- Solitary plasmacytoma of bone should be included in the differential diagnosis of spinal bone tumors and should ideally be excluded with further imaging when a solitary bone lesion is observed on imaging.
- Multiple imaging modalities have their place in the evaluation of solitary plasmacytoma of bone and other plasma cell disorders.
- The mainstay of solitary plasmacytoma of bone treatment remains high-dose focused radiotherapy.

References

Albano D, Tomasini D, Bonù M, Giubbini R, Bertagna F (2020) (18)F-FDG PET or PET/CT role in plasmacytoma: a systematic review. Rev Esp Med Nucl Imagen Mol (Engl Ed) 39(4):220–224

Biffar A, Baur-Melnyk A, Schmidt GP, Reiser MF, Dietrich O (2010a) Multiparameter MRI assessment of normal-appearing and diseased vertebral bone marrow. Eur Radiol 20(11):2679–2689

Biffar A, Dietrich O, Sourbron S, Duerr HR, Reiser MF, Baur-Melnyk A (2010b) Diffusion and perfusion imaging of bone marrow. Eur J Radiol 76(3):323–328

Caers J, Paiva B, Zamagni E, Leleu X, Bladé J, Kristinsson SY et al (2018) Diagnosis, treatment, and response assessment in solitary plasmacytoma: updated recommendations from a European Expert Panel. J Hematol Oncol 11(1):10

Cavo M, Terpos E, Nanni C, Moreau P, Lentzsch S, Zweegman S et al (2017) Role of (18)F-FDG PET/CT in the diagnosis and management of multiple myeloma and other plasma cell disorders: a consensus statement by the International Myeloma Working Group. Lancet Oncol 18(4):e206–e217

Chan JK (2014) The wonderful colors of the hematoxylin-eosin stain in diagnostic surgical pathology. Int J Surg Pathol 22(1):12–32

Choi YY, Kim JY, Yang SO (2014) PET/CT in benign and malignant musculoskeletal tumors and tumor-like conditions. Semin Musculoskelet Radiol 18(2):133–148

Cuenod CA, Balvay D (2013) Perfusion and vascular permeability: basic concepts and measurement in DCE-CT and DCE-MRI. Diagn Interv Imaging 94(12):1187–1204

Dammacco F, Rubini G, Ferrari C, Vacca A, Racanelli V (2015) ^{18}F-FDG PET/CT: a review of diagnostic and prognostic features in multiple myeloma and related disorders. Clin Exp Med 15(1):1–18

de Waal EG, Leene M, Veeger N, Vos HJ, Ong F, Smit WG et al (2016) Progression of a solitary plasmacytoma to multiple myeloma. A population-based registry of the northern Netherlands. Br J Haematol 175(4):661–667

Delorme S, Baur-Melnyk A (2011) Imaging in multiple myeloma. Recent Results Cancer Res 183:133–147

Dharnidharka VR (2018) Comprehensive review of post-organ transplant hematologic cancers. Am J Transplant 18(3):537–549

Dietrich O, Biffar A, Baur-Melnyk A, Reiser MF (2010) Technical aspects of MR diffusion imaging of the body. Eur J Radiol 76(3):314–322

Dietrich O, Geith T, Reiser MF, Baur-Melnyk A (2017) Diffusion imaging of the vertebral bone marrow. NMR Biomed 30(3). https://doi.org/10.1002/nbm.3333

Dimopoulos MA, Moulopoulos LA, Maniatis A, Alexanian R (2000) Solitary plasmacytoma of bone and asymptomatic multiple myeloma. Blood 96(6):2037–2044

Dimopoulos MA, Hillengass J, Usmani S, Zamagni E, Lentzsch S, Davies FE et al (2015) Role of magnetic resonance imaging in the management of patients with multiple myeloma: a consensus statement. J Clin Oncol 33(6):657–664

Dingli D, Kyle RA, Rajkumar SV, Nowakowski GS, Larson DR, Bida JP et al (2006) Immunoglobulin free light chains and solitary plasmacytoma of bone. Blood 108(6):1979–1983

Dutoit JC, Verstraete KL (2017) Whole-body MRI, dynamic contrast-enhanced MRI, and diffusion-weighted imaging for the staging of multiple myeloma. Skelet Radiol 46(6):733–750

Dutoit JC, Vanderkerken MA, Verstraete KL (2013) Value of whole body MRI and dynamic contrast enhanced MRI in the diagnosis, follow-up and evaluation of disease activity and extent in multiple myeloma. Eur J Radiol 82(9):1444–1452

Dutoit JC, Vanderkerken MA, Anthonissen J, Dochy F, Verstraete KL (2014) The diagnostic value of SE MRI and DWI of the spine in patients with monoclonal gammopathy of undetermined significance, smouldering myeloma and multiple myeloma. Eur Radiol 24(11):2754–2765

Dutoit JC, Claus E, Offner F, Noens L, Delanghe J, Verstraete KL (2016) Combined evaluation of conventional MRI, dynamic contrast-enhanced MRI and diffusion weighted imaging for response evaluation of patients with multiple myeloma. Eur J Radiol 85(2):373–382

Finsinger P, Grammatico S, Chisini M, Piciocchi A, Foà R, Petrucci MT (2016) Clinical features and prognostic factors in solitary plasmacytoma. Br J Haematol 172(4):554–560

García-Figueiras R, Padhani AR, Beer AJ, Baleato-González S, Vilanova JC, Luna A et al (2015) Imaging of tumor angiogenesis for radiologists—part 1: biological and technical basis. Curr Probl Diagn Radiol 44(5):407–424

Gariani J, Westerland O, Natas S, Verma H, Cook G, Goh V (2018) Comparison of whole body magnetic resonance imaging (WBMRI) to whole body computed tomography (WBCT) or (18)F-fluorodeoxyglucose positron emission tomography/CT ((18)F-FDG PET/CT) in patients with myeloma: systematic review of diagnostic performance. Crit Rev Oncol Hematol 124:66–72

Hansford BG, Hanrahan CJ, Girard N, Silbermann R, Morag Y (2020) Untreated plasmacytoma of bone containing macroscopic intralesional fat and mimicking intraosseous lipoma: a case report and review of the literature. Clin Imaging 64:18–23

Herrmann J, Krstin N, Schoennagel BP, Sornsakrin M, Derlin T, Busch JD et al (2012) Age-related distribution of vertebral bone-marrow diffusivity. Eur J Radiol 81(12):4046–4049

Hillengass J, Zechmann C, Bäuerle T, Wagner-Gund B, Heiss C, Benner A et al (2009) Dynamic contrast-enhanced magnetic resonance imaging identifies a subgroup of patients with asymptomatic monoclonal plasma cell disease and pathologic microcirculation. Clin Cancer Res 15(9):3118–3125

Hillengass J, Fechtner K, Weber MA, Bäuerle T, Ayyaz S, Heiss C et al (2010) Prognostic significance of focal lesions in whole-body magnetic resonance imaging in patients with asymptomatic multiple myeloma. J Clin Oncol 28(9):1606–1610

Hillengass J, Weber MA, Kilk K, Listl K, Wagner-Gund B, Hillengass M et al (2014) Prognostic significance of whole-body MRI in patients with monoclonal gammopathy of undetermined significance. Leukemia 28(1):174–178

Hillengass J, Ritsch J, Merz M, Wagner B, Kunz C, Hielscher T et al (2016) Increased microcirculation detected by dynamic contrast-enhanced magnetic resonance imaging is of prognostic significance in asymptomatic myeloma. Br J Haematol 174(1):127–135

Horger M, Weisel K, Horger W, Mroue A, Fenchel M, Lichy M (2011) Whole-body diffusion-weighted MRI with apparent diffusion coefficient mapping for early response monitoring in multiple myeloma: preliminary results. AJR Am J Roentgenol 196(6):W790–W795

Hwang H, Lee SK, Kim JY (2021) Comparison of conventional magnetic resonance imaging and diffusion-weighted imaging in the differentiation of bone plasmacytoma from bone metastasis in the extremities. Diagn Interv Imaging 102(10):611–618

Jamet B, Bailly C, Carlier T, Touzeau C, Nanni C, Zamagni E et al (2019) Interest of pet imaging in multiple myeloma. Front Med 6:69

Jawad MU, Scully SP (2009) Skeletal plasmacytoma: progression of disease and impact of local treatment; an analysis of SEER database. J Hematol Oncol 2:41

Kelley SP, Ashford RU, Rao AS, Dickson RA (2007) Primary bone tumours of the spine: a 42-year survey from the Leeds Regional Bone Tumour Registry. Eur Spine J 16(3):405–409

Khoo MM, Tyler PA, Saifuddin A, Padhani AR (2011) Diffusion-weighted imaging (DWI) in musculoskeletal MRI: a critical review. Skelet Radiol 40(6):665–681

Kilciksiz S, Celik OK, Pak Y, Demiral AN, Pehlivan M, Orhan O et al (2008) Clinical and prognostic features of plasmacytomas: a multicenter study of Turkish Oncology Group-Sarcoma Working Party. Am J Hematol 83(9):702–707

Kilciksiz S, Karakoyun-Celik O, Agaoglu FY, Haydaroglu A (2012) A review for solitary plasmacytoma of bone and extramedullary plasmacytoma. ScientificWorldJournal 2012:895765

Kim PJ, Hicks RJ, Wirth A, Ryan G, Seymour JF, Prince HM et al (2009) Impact of 18F-fluorodeoxyglucose positron emission tomography before and after definitive radiation therapy in patients with apparently solitary plasmacytoma. Int J Radiat Oncol Biol Phys 74(3):740–746

Koutoulidis V, Papanikolaou N, Moulopoulos LA (2018) Functional and molecular MRI of the bone marrow in multiple myeloma. Br J Radiol 91(1088):20170389

Kumar S, Fonseca R, Dispenzieri A, Lacy MQ, Lust JA, Wellik L et al (2003) Prognostic value of angiogenesis in solitary bone plasmacytoma. Blood 101(5):1715–1717

Lavini C, de Jonge MC, van de Sande MG, Tak PP, Nederveen AJ, Maas M (2007) Pixel-by-pixel analysis of DCE MRI curve patterns and an illustration of its application to the imaging of the musculoskeletal system. Magn Reson Imaging 25(5):604–612

Lecouvet FE (2016) Whole-body MR imaging: musculoskeletal applications. Radiology 279(2):345–365

Lecouvet FE, Vekemans MC, Van Den Berghe T, Verstraete K, Kirchgesner T et al (2022) Imaging of treatment response and minimal residual disease in multiple myeloma: state of the art WB-MRI and PET/CT. Skeletal Radiol. 51(1):59–80. Published online 2021 Aug 7. https://doi.org/10.1007/s00256-021-03841-5. PMCID: PMC8626399. PMID: 34363522.

Lee K, Park HY, Kim KW, Lee AJ, Yoon MA, Chae EJ et al (2019) Advances in whole body MRI for musculoskeletal imaging: diffusion-weighted imaging. J Clin Orthop Trauma 10(4):680–686

Li QW, Niu SQ, Wang HY, Wen G, Li YY, Xia YF et al (2015) Radiotherapy alone is associated with improved outcomes over surgery in the management of solitary plasmacytoma. Asian Pac J Cancer Prev 16(9):3741–3745

Lin C, Luciani A, Belhadj K, Maison P, Vignaud A, Deux JF et al (2009) Patients with plasma cell disorders examined at whole-body dynamic contrast-enhanced MR imaging: initial experience. Radiology 250(3):905–915

Martí-Bonmatí L, Ramirez-Fuentes C, Alberich-Bayarri Á, Ruiz-Llorca C (2015) State-of-the-art of bone marrow imaging in multiple myeloma. Curr Opin Oncol 27(6):540–550

Mena E, Choyke P, Tan E, Landgren O, Kurdziel K (2011) Molecular imaging in myeloma precursor disease. Semin Hematol 48(1):22–31

Mena E, Turkbey EB, Lindenberg L (2022) Modern radiographic imaging in multiple myeloma, what is the minimum requirement? Semin Oncol 49(1):86–93

Merz M, Hielscher T, Wagner B, Sauer S, Shah S, Raab MS et al (2014) Predictive value of longitudinal whole-body magnetic resonance imaging in patients with smoldering multiple myeloma. Leukemia 28(9):1902–1908

Merz M, Ritsch J, Kunz C, Wagner B, Sauer S, Hose D et al (2015) Dynamic contrast-enhanced magnetic resonance imaging for assessment of antiangiogenic treatment effects in multiple myeloma. Clin Cancer Res 21(1):106–112

Merz M, Moehler TM, Ritsch J, Bäuerle T, Zechmann CM, Wagner B et al (2016) Prognostic significance of increased bone marrow microcirculation in newly diagnosed multiple myeloma: results of a prospective DCE-MRI study. Eur Radiol 26(5):1404–1411

Messiou C, Kaiser M (2015) Whole body diffusion weighted MRI—a new view of myeloma. Br J Haematol 171(1):29–37

Morales KA, Arevalo-Perez J, Peck KK, Holodny AI, Lis E, Karimi S (2018) Differentiating atypical hemangiomas and metastatic vertebral lesions: the role of T1-weighted dynamic contrast-enhanced MRI. AJNR Am J Neuroradiol 39(5):968–973

Nanni C, Rubello D, Zamagni E, Castellucci P, Ambrosini V, Montini G et al (2008) 18F-FDG PET/CT in myeloma with presumed solitary plasmacytoma of bone. In Vivo 22(4):513–517

Nguyen TT, Thelen JC, Bhatt AA (2020) Bone up on spinal osseous lesions: a case review series. Insights Imaging 11(1):80

Nosàs-Garcia S, Moehler T, Wasser K, Kiessling F, Bartl R, Zuna I et al (2005) Dynamic contrast-enhanced MRI for assessing the disease activity of multiple myeloma: a comparative study with histology and clinical markers. J Magn Reson Imaging 22(1):154–162

Ohana N, Rouvio O, Nalbandyan K, Sheinis D, Benharroch D (2018) Classification of solitary plasmacytoma, is it more intricate than presently suggested? A commentary. J Cancer 9(21):3894–3897

Padhani AR, van Ree K, Collins DJ, D'Sa S, Makris A (2013) Assessing the relation between bone marrow signal intensity and apparent diffusion coefficient in diffusion-weighted MRI. AJR Am J Roentgenol 200(1):163–170

Pasch W, Zhao X, Rezk SA (2012) Solitary plasmacytoma of the bone involving young individuals, is there a role for preceding trauma? Int J Clin Exp Pathol 5(5):463–467

Paternain A, García-Velloso MJ, Rosales JJ, Ezponda A, Soriano I, Elorz M et al (2020) The utility of ADC value in diffusion-weighted whole-body MRI in the follow-up of patients with multiple myeloma. Correlation study with (18)F-FDG PET-CT. Eur J Radiol 133:109403

Patnaik S, Jyotsnarani Y, Uppin SG, Susarla R (2016) Imaging features of primary tumors of the spine: a pictorial essay. Indian J Radiol Imaging 26(2):279–289

Peker D, Wei S, Siegal GP (2019) Bone pathology for hematopathologists. Surg Pathol Clin 12(3):831–847

Pingali SR, Haddad RY, Saad A (2012) Current concepts of clinical management of multiple myeloma. Dis Mon 58(4):195–207

Pinter NK, Pfiffner TJ, Mechtler LL (2016) Neuroimaging of spine tumors. Handb Clin Neurol 136:689–706

Rajkumar SV (2016a) Updated diagnostic criteria and staging system for multiple myeloma. Am Soc Clin Oncol Educ Book 35:e418–e423

Rajkumar SV (2016b) Myeloma today: disease definitions and treatment advances. Am J Hematol 91(1):90–100

Rajkumar SV, Leong T, Roche PC, Fonseca R, Dispenzieri A, Lacy MQ et al (2000) Prognostic value of bone marrow angiogenesis in multiple myeloma. Clin Cancer Res 6(8):3111–3116

Rana C, Sharma S, Agrawal V, Singh U (2010) Bone marrow angiogenesis in multiple myeloma and its correlation with clinicopathological factors. Ann Hematol 89(8):789–794

Reed V, Shah J, Medeiros LJ, Ha CS, Mazloom A, Weber DM et al (2011) Solitary plasmacytomas: outcome and prognostic factors after definitive radiation therapy. Cancer 117(19):4468–4474

Rodallec MH, Feydy A, Larousserie F, Anract P, Campagna R, Babinet A et al (2008) Diagnostic imaging of solitary tumors of the spine: what to do and say. Radiographics 28(4):1019–1041

Salaun PY, Gastinne T, Frampas E, Bodet-Milin C, Moreau P, Bodéré-Kraeber F (2008) FDG-positron-emission tomography for staging and therapeutic assessment in patients with plasmacytoma. Haematologica 93(8):1269–1271

Schirrmeister H, Buck AK, Bergmann L, Reske SN, Bommer M (2003) Positron emission tomography (PET) for staging of solitary plasmacytoma. Cancer Biother Radiopharm 18(5):841–845

Schmidt GP, Reiser MF, Baur-Melnyk A (2007) Whole-body imaging of the musculoskeletal system: the value of MR imaging. Skelet Radiol 36(12):1109–1119

Shen X, Liu S, Wu C, Wang J, Li J, Chen L (2021) Survival trends and prognostic factors in patients with solitary plasmacytoma of bone: a population-based study. Cancer Med 10(2):462–470

Silva JR Jr, Hayashi D, Yonenaga T, Fukuda K, Genant HK, Lin C et al (2013) MRI of bone marrow abnormalities in hematological malignancies. Diagn Interv Radiol 19(5):393–399

Sommer G, Klarhöfer M, Lenz C, Scheffler K, Bongartz G, Winter L (2011) Signal characteristics of focal bone marrow lesions in patients with multiple myeloma using whole body T1w-TSE, T2w-STIR and diffusion-weighted imaging with background suppression. Eur Radiol 21(4):857–862

Suh YG, Suh CO, Kim JS, Kim SJ, Pyun HO, Cho J (2012) Radiotherapy for solitary plasmacytoma of bone and soft tissue: outcomes and prognostic factors. Ann Hematol 91(11):1785–1793

Suh CH, Yun SJ, Jin W, Lee SH, Park SY, Ryu CW (2018) ADC as a useful diagnostic tool for differentiating benign and malignant vertebral bone marrow lesions and compression fractures: a systematic review and meta-analysis. Eur Radiol 28(7):2890–2902

Terpos E, Dimopoulos MA, Moulopoulos LA (2016) The role of imaging in the treatment of patients with multiple myeloma in 2016. Am Soc Clin Oncol Educ Book 35:e407–e417

Terpos E, Matsaridis D, Koutoulidis V, Zagouri F, Christoulas D, Fontara S et al (2017) Dynamic contrast-enhanced magnetic resonance imaging parameters correlate with advanced revised-ISS and angiopoietin-1/angiopoietin-2 ratio in patients with multiple myeloma. Ann Hematol 96(10):1707–1714

Ulaner GA, Landgren CO (2020) Current and potential applications of positron emission tomography for multiple myeloma and plasma cell disorders. Best Pract Res Clin Haematol 33(1):101148

Van Den Berghe T, Verstraete KL, Lecouvet FE, Lejoly M, Dutoit J (2022) Review of diffusion-weighted imaging and dynamic contrast-enhanced MRI for multiple myeloma and its precursors (monoclonal gammopathy of undetermined significance and smouldering myeloma). Skelet Radiol 51(1):101–122

Verstraete KL, Van der Woude HJ, Hogendoorn PC, De-Deene Y, Kunnen M, Bloem JL (1996) Dynamic contrast-enhanced MR imaging of musculoskeletal tumors: basic principles and clinical applications. J Magn Reson Imaging 6(2):311–321

Warsame R, Gertz MA, Lacy MQ, Kyle RA, Buadi F, Dingli D et al (2012) Trends and outcomes of modern staging of solitary plasmacytoma of bone. Am J Hematol 87(7):647–651

Wilder RB, Ha CS, Cox JD, Weber D, Delasalle K, Alexanian R (2002) Persistence of myeloma protein for more than one year after radiotherapy is an adverse prognostic factor in solitary plasmacytoma of bone. Cancer 94(5):1532–1537

Xie L, Wang H, Jiang J (2020) Does radiotherapy with surgery improve survival and decrease progression to multiple myeloma in patients with solitary Plasmacytoma of bone of the spine? World Neurosurg 134:e790–e798

Yurac R, Silva A, Delgado M, Nuñez M, Lopez J, Marre B (2021) Pathological axis fracture secondary to a solitary bone plasmacytoma: two cases and a literature review. Surg Neurol Int 12:165

Zha Y, Li M, Yang J (2010) Dynamic contrast enhanced magnetic resonance imaging of diffuse spinal bone marrow infiltration in patients with hematological malignancies. Korean J Radiol 11(2):187–194

Zhang Z, Meng Q, Gao Z, Ma L (2009) MR imaging features of solitary plasmacytoma of the spine. Clin Oncol Cancer Res 6:241–244

Zhang J, Chen Y, Zhang Y, Zhang E, Yu HJ, Yuan H et al (2020) Diagnosis of spinal lesions using perfusion parameters measured by DCE-MRI and metabolism parameters measured by PET/CT. Eur Spine J 29(5):1061–1070

Lipogenic Tumors

Maarten J. Steyvers and Valerie S. Van Ballaer

Contents

M. J. Steyvers (✉) · V. S. Van Ballaer
Department of Radiology, University Hospitals Leuven, Leuven, Belgium
e-mail: maarten.steyvers@uzleuven.be; valerie.vanballaer@uzleuven.be

Med Radiol Diagn Imaging (2023)

https://doi.org/10.1007/174_2023_439,
Published Online: 28 June 2023

Abstract

Apart from the very common vertebral hemangioma, lipogenic tumors of the osseous spine are very rare and usually benign. Nevertheless, diagnosing these lesions correctly is necessary to exclude an infrequent malignancy (e.g., liposarcoma) or to avoid overdiagnosis. This chapter reviews the most common lipogenic benign tumors of the osseous spine (lipoma, hibernoma, osteolipoma), malignant lesions (liposarcoma), and pseudotumoral fat-containing lesions (fatty island, fatty corner, and fatty reconversion). The purpose is to provide an up-to-date overview of the sometimes scarce literature about some of these tumors. Emphasis is put on the prevalent imaging findings and the differential diagnosis.

1 Introduction

Lipogenic tumors of the spinal column are generally rare tumors that arise from adipose tissue in the vertebrae. They are usually benign, slow-growing tumors that nevertheless may require surgical intervention in selected cases. If symptomatic, they can present with a variety of symptoms including back pain, weakness, and sensory disturbances. The diagnosis requires a combination of imaging studies, such as computed tomography (CT), magnetic resonance imaging (MRI), positron emission tomography (PET)/CT, PET/MRI, as well as biopsy in selected cases. Despite being rare, lipogenic tumors of the spine are important to recognize and diagnose correctly, especially in case of benignity to avoid unnecessary additional (invasive) investigations and therapeutic interventions.

This chapter does not discuss intraspinal non-osseous or neurogenic fat-containing lesions (e.g., intraspinal lipoma-liposarcoma, neurofibroma, myxopapillary ependymoma, and intraspinal metastases). Also, vertebral hemangioma will be discussed in a separate chapter.

2 Intra-osseous Vertebral Lipoma

2.1 Introduction

Vertebral lipomas are rare benign primary tumors that arise almost exclusively within the medulla of the vertebral bones (WHO classification 2020). Lipomas of the bone are however the most common lipogenic osseous tumors (Murphey et al. 2004). They are composed of mature white adipocytes without interspersed bony trabeculae or hematopoietic tissue (Davies et al. 2009; Sen et al. 2015).

2.2 Epidemiology

The exact prevalence is not well known. However, they are estimated to represent less than 1% of all primary bone tumors and less than 2% of all benign spinal tumors (Propeck et al. 2000). Vertebral lipomas can occur at any age but are most commonly reported in middle-aged individuals (fourth and fifth decades), and are somewhat more common in males (1.3:1) (Campbell et al. 2003; WHO classification 2020). The etiology is not well understood, but some studies suggest that it may be related to genetic factors, endocrine-metabolic disorders (obesity), and certain medications.

2.3 Localization

Most intra-osseous lipomas occur in the lower limb, with the most common site of presentation being the calcaneum, followed by the femoral subtrochanteric region and proximal tibia. They also have been reported in the upper limb, spine, skull, sinonasal cavities, mandible, pelvis, and ribs (Sen et al. 2015). In the vertebrae, intra-osseous lipomas can occur in the body or any of the posterior elements, such as the spinous and transverse processes (Fig. 1). Sometimes, it may present in adjacent vertebral bodies (e.g., Pande et al. 1988; Yang et al. 2015).

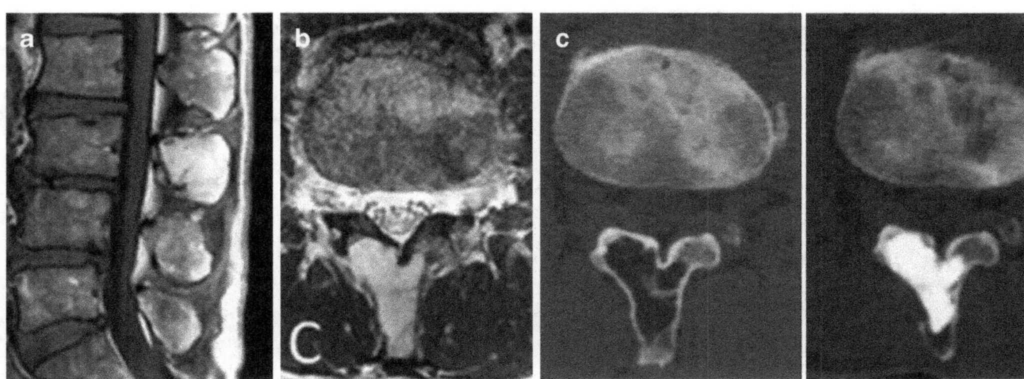

Fig. 1 Intra-osseous lipoma of the third lumbar spine. A 54-year-old man presented with a 3-month history of low-back pain. (**a**) Sagittal T1-weighted image, (**b**) axial T2-weighted image, (**c**) axial CT image before and after intervention, respectively. MRI revealed a homogenous fat-containing lesion in the L3 vertebral arch and spinous process. CT demonstrated a well-defined osteolytic lesion with a thin sclerotic rim and mild cortical bulging. The image on the far right shows the CT result after curettage and filling the defect with hydroxyapatite bone. Patient recovered without any rest symptoms and without recurrence 3 years postoperatively. (Adapted from Teekhasaenee et al. 2015)

2.4 Clinical Presentation

Vertebral lipomas can be asymptomatic, although in up to 70% of intra-osseous lipomas, aching pain is reported (Campbell et al. 2003). The etiology is most likely due to expansile bone remodeling or coexistent ischemic changes. Symptoms depend on their location and size. Specifically for vertebral intra-osseous lipomas, biomechanical stress due to end plate cortical thinning may be a predisposition for backache. Pathologic fractures are rare.

2.5 Imaging

Vertebral lipomas are mainly detected as incidentalomas. The fat components of intra-osseous lipomas may show different amounts of involution and necrosis. Milgram (1988) subdivided intra-osseous lipomas into three categories based on their histological findings (section "Histopathology", see below). The radiological findings parallel the histopathological stage.

On plain radiography, Milgram stage I lesions are well-circumscribed, lucent intramedullary lesions occasionally associated with mild focal cortex expansion and a thin sclerotic rim. There is no evidence of cortical disruption or periosteal reaction. If vertebral intra-osseous lipoma is suspected based on radiographic findings, further imaging studies such as CT or MRI may be necessary to confirm the diagnosis and assess the extent of the lesion. On CT, the intralesional fat is clearly demonstrated, with occasionally a thin rim of sclerosis and expansile remodeling of the intramedullary canal. On MRI, the intralesional fat has the same intensity as the subcutaneous fat and shows similar suppression on fat-saturated sequences.

Milgram stage II or III lesions appear as lucent lesions on radiography and CT, with internal ring-like calcifications or ossifications. CT is superior in delineating intralesional fat and bone surface changes. MRI, however, is considered the imaging modality of choice and is superior in distinguishing complex fatty lesions. Focal areas of fat necrosis are seen as zones of low signal on T1-weighted images (WI) and high signal on T2-WI. Internal cystic components are of low signal on T1-WI and high signal on T2-WI and show peripheral enhancement after administration of gadolinium contrast. Calcifications are apparent as regions of signal voids. Expansile remodeling of bone and rounded margins are additional characteristics.

PET/CT imaging is not typically used, as vertebral lipomas do not exhibit increased metabolic activity.

2.6 Histopathology

Based on histological findings, an intra-osseous lipoma can be subdivided by Milgram into three stages. Stage I consists of a lesion composed of mature adipocytes without abnormal cytological features, with a surrounding fibrous capsule. The cells are well differentiated, and there is no evidence of mitotic activity or cellular atypia. Stage II refers to predominantly fatty lesions with areas of fat necrosis, hemorrhage, and dystrophic calcifications or ossifications. These areas typically contain cholesterol crystals or hemosiderin deposits. Stage III consists of lesions with extensive fat necrosis, calcification, and cyst formation (Milgram 1988). In case of significant necrosis, biopsy may be required to exclude malignancy.

2.7 Differential Diagnosis

Differential diagnosis of vertebral lipoma includes other benign bone lesions, malignant bone tumors, as well as non-tumoral conditions.

Benign lesions that need to be considered include bone cyst, osteochondroma, osteoid osteoma, and enchondroma. Intra-osseous vertebral lipomas may occasionally mimic hemangioma and osteoporotic bone with increased fatty marrow.

Malignant bone tumors to be excluded include plasmocytoma, osteosarcoma, chondrosarcoma, and metastases.

Osteomyelitis is a non-tumoral differential to be considered. Obviously, aggressive characteristics indicate a malignant or infectious etiology. In case of symptomatic vertebral lipomas, the more common causes of back pain (e.g., disk herniation, spinal canal stenosis) need to be excluded.

2.8 Treatment and Prognosis

Asymptomatic and stable lesions do not require any treatment. Symptomatic cases or those with imminent fractures are treated surgically with curettage and bone grafting or vertebroplasty/kyphoplasty (Teekhasaenee et al. 2015). The risk of recurrence after surgical excision is very low. Reports of malignant transformation have been rarely described (Milgram 1990; Campbell et al. 2003).

3 Intra-osseous Hibernoma

3.1 Introduction

Hibernoma is a rare benign adipocytic tumor of brown fat cells, which typically occurs in soft tissues, usually in middle-aged adults. Discovered in 1906 by Merkel as "pseudolipoma", they were renamed as "hibernoma" in 1914 because of their similarity to the brown fat of hibernating animals (Bonar et al. 2014). In mammals, brown fat gradually disappears with age and becomes white fat (Gesta et al. 2007).

3.2 Epidemiology

Hibernomas in humans are usually observed in soft tissues (Furlong et al. 2001).

Intra-osseous hibernomas are rare and are reported to present as isolated sclerotic lesions in adults aged 40–85 years, with a female predominance (Bonar et al. 2014; Hafeez et al. 2015; Ringe et al. 2013; Song et al. 2017). Most reported intra-osseous hibernomas are located in the axial skeleton (predominantly the pelvis), with only a number of case reports of spinal hibernomas that have been described (e.g., Bonar et al. 2014; Hafeez et al. 2015; Song et al. 2017; Um et al. 2020).

3.3 Localization

Soft tissue hibernomas are most common in the thigh, followed by shoulder, back, neck, chest, arm, and abdominal cavity (Furlong et al. 2001). Intra-osseous hibernomas have been reported in the femur, pelvis (sacrum, ileum), thoracic spine, and lumbar spine (e.g., Hafeez et al. 2015; Kumar et al. 2011; Reyes et al. 2008).

3.4 Clinical Presentation

Most lesions are detected in asymptomatic patients, but some patients may present with nonspecific (musculoskeletal) pain, necessitating further investigation (Hafeez et al. 2015; Song et al. 2017).

3.5 Imaging

Intra-osseous hibernomas are often incidentalomas and are discovered incidentally during the workup for other indications. On plain radiographs and CT, hibernomas characteristically present as a densely sclerotic lesion with trabecular thickening and variable delineation.

MRI shows variable T1 hypointense (sometimes with internal hyperintense foci) and T2/STIR heterogenous hyperintense or intermediate signal, with (incomplete) fat suppression and moderate contrast enhancement (Botchu et al. 2013; Hafeez et al. 2015; Ko et al. 2020; Song et al. 2017) (Fig. 2).

Brown fat cells of hibernomas are rich in mitochondria, resulting in glucose hypermetabolism and mildly increased 18F-FDG uptake on PET/CT scans, although normal uptake has been reported (Um et al. 2020). As a consequence of

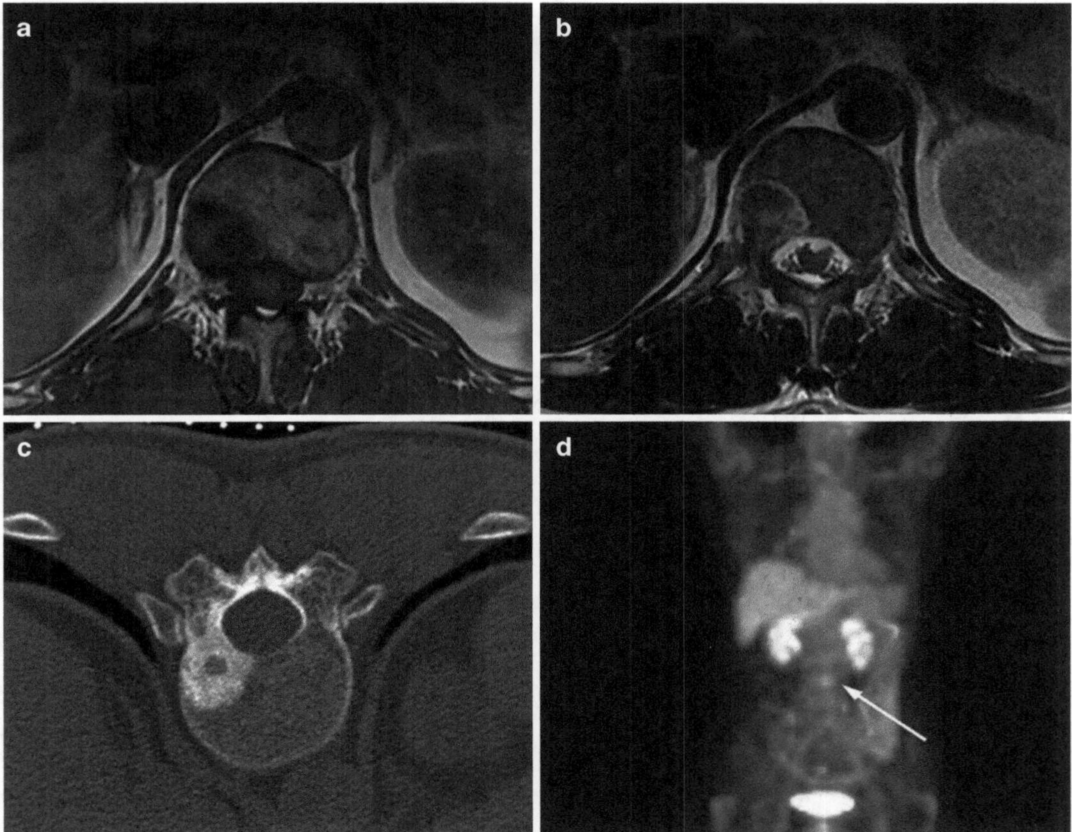

Fig. 2 Intra-osseous vertebral hibernoma. Characteristic imaging features with low signal intensity on T1-weighted imaging (WI) (**a**), heterogeneous intermediate and high signal intensity on T2-WI (**b**), densely sclerotic on CT (**c**), and mild hypermetabolism on PET (arrow) (**d**). (Image adapted from Song et al. 2017)

the combined imaging findings, lesions are commonly (mis)interpreted for a malignancy (metastasis) and biopsy is warranted (Ko et al. 2020).

3.6 Histopathology

Microscopically, the bone marrow space is replaced by sheets and clusters of brown fat cells with voluminous multivacuolated (as opposed to the mononuclear adipocytes in lipomas) cytoplasm and centrally located small nuclei with no or minimal nuclear atypia (Furlong et al. 2001; Hafeez et al. 2015). Bony trabeculae are kept intact as intra-osseous hibernomas infiltrate in between them, unlike intra-osseous lipomas. Immunohistological staining is positive for S100 and negative for CD68, epithelial membrane antigen, and AE1/AE3 (Hafeez et al. 2015; Song et al. 2017). Their heterogeneous nature suggests etiologies of (1) reactive secondary sclerosis and (2) upregulation of brown fat adipogenesis and bone formation (Bai et al. 2013; Song et al. 2017).

3.7 Differential Diagnosis

Due to their rarity and suspicious imaging findings (T1 hypointense and enhancing), intra-osseous hibernomas are often mistaken for malignancy (e.g., metastasis, lymphoma, liposarcoma, chordoma) or osteomyelitis. Other differential considerations are dense bone island, lipoma, hemangioma, and notochordal rest (Hafeez et al. 2015; Kumar et al. 2011; Ko et al. 2020).

3.8 Treatment and Prognosis

In general, intra-osseous hibernomas require no further follow-up. In case of symptomatic lesions, successful treatment with radiofrequency ablation and kyphoplasty is reported (Ringe et al. 2013; Ko et al. 2020). Malignant transformation has not been reported.

4 Osteolipoma

4.1 Introduction

Lipomas can contain other mesenchymal components such as fibrous tissue (fibrolipoma) and cartilage (chondrolipoma). An osteolipoma is defined as a lesion with mature adipose tissue and randomly distributed trabeculae of laminated bone (Obermann et al. 1999). Osteolipoma (ossifying lipoma, osseous lipoma) is an extremely rare benign variant of lipoma, constituting only 1% of all lipomas. If the fatty component predominates, the term ossifying lipoma is used, whereas those lesions without a dominant fatty component are referred to as osteolipoma (Obermann et al. 1999). Although lipomas originating in the bony tissues are common, isolated osteolipomas are extremely rare.

Most osteolipomas are reported in the oral cavity, brain (tuber cinereum, hypothalamus, suprasellar region), and soft tissues of the head and neck (Castilho et al. 2004; Sinson et al. 1998). They are scarcely reported in the extremities (Heffernan et al. 2008; Val-Bernal et al. 2007) and intraspinal area (see below).

Its etiology is believed to be related to repeated microtrauma or ischemia (to induce ossification), metaplasia of fibroblast to osteoblasts, and chondro-ossification of multipotent mesenchymal cells. Translocations involving the 12q13-15 chromosome have been observed (Fritchie et al. 2012).

4.2 Clinical Presentation

As far as we are aware, only five cases of intraspinal (or intraspinally extending) osteolipomas have been reported (Lin et al. 2001; Aiyer et al. 2016; Dilip Chand Raja et al. 2018; Jain et al. 2019; Brones et al. 2010). Symptoms are dependent on many factors, including location. Patients can be asymptomatic or present with features of compressive myelopathy/radiculopathy.

Lin et al. reported a cervical intraspinal extradural ossifying lipoma in a 20-year-old woman.

She presented with slowly progressive paraparesis and dysesthesia in both legs. Laminectomy was performed with amelioration of symptoms (Lin et al. 2001).

An intraspinal adipose lesion may also be associated with spinal dysraphism (Jaiswal et al. 2005; Brones et al. 2010). Jaiswal et al. (2005) reported an intradural lipoma in an 8-year-old, neurologically intact girl who presented with an enlarging swelling over the lumbar region. Imaging revealed an intradural lipoma connected with a large subcutaneous lipoma, together with a prominent island of bone and a dermal sinus. The lesion was excised by laminotomy without postoperative neurological defects (Jaiswal et al. 2005). A somewhat similar case was published by Brones et al. (2010), discussing the case of a 21-month-old neurologically intact girl with a posterior cervical subcutaneous osteolipoma that was attached to the spinal cord.

Aiyer et al. (2016) reported the case of a 61-year-old male with dorsal column symptoms due to an intraspinal extradural osteolipoma in the cervical spinal canal (arising at the posterior spinolaminar line at C5) causing myelum compression. Surgical excision resulted in complete resolution of symptoms (Aiyer et al. 2016).

Finally, Dilip Chand Raja et al. discussed a 36-year-old male with a lumbar intraspinal dural based osteolipoma (attached to the L2 inferior articular process) presenting as a cauda equina syndrome. Again, laminectomy resulted in recovery without recurrence (Dilip Chand Raja et al. 2018).

4.3 Imaging

Radiographs can demonstrate a lobulated mass with fat density and trabecular bone. In case of intraspinal osteolipoma, CT and MRI can visualize a well-defined fat-containing (intraspinal) mass, possibly expansile (Jaiswal et al. 2005). On MRI, heterogeneous T1 and T2 hyperintense signal within the lesion would raise the suspicion for both fat and osseous tissue. Enhancement characteristics are these of a plain lipoma. CT can be done for further confirmation. It would show an ossified (intraspinal) lipomatous lesion and would potentially further aid in preoperative planning for surgical decompression (Dilip Chand Raja et al. 2018).

4.4 Histopathology

Osteolipomas consist of well-capsulated mature adipose tissue with interspersed islands of osteoid matrix and mature trabeculae of lamellar or woven bone, surrounded by fibrous tissue bands and without connection to the neighboring bone (Demiralp et al. 2009).

4.5 Differential Diagnosis

The differential diagnosis of spinal osteolipomas is broad and includes fat-containing lesions with ossification, such as calcified synovial cyst, dermoid, teratoma, hemangioma, (well-differentiated) liposarcoma, tumoral calcinosis, extra-osseous osteochondroma, myositis ossificans, and ossifying fibroma. Another mimicker of an intraspinal osteolipoma is ossification of the ligamentum flavum or posterior longitudinal ligament (Aiyer et al. 2016).

4.6 Treatment and Prognosis

Surgical excision is the recommended treatment in symptomatic patients or when malignancy is suspected. No recurrence has been reported (Cheng et al. 2012). The overall prognosis is favorable, similar to plain lipomas (Jaiswal et al. 2005).

5 Primary Liposarcoma of the Spine

5.1 Introduction

Liposarcoma is a malignant soft tissue tumor that originates from primitive mesenchymal cells. They are the most frequent type of sarcomas in adults, but primary liposarcoma of bone is a very rare type of tumor (Torok et al. 1983). Primary vertebral involvement is even rarer, with only a limited number of cases described.

5.2 Epidemiology

The WHO classifies liposarcoma into four different histologic subtypes: well differentiated/dedifferentiated, myxoid/round cell, pleiomorphic, and mixed. To the best of our knowledge, no cases of primary well-differentiated or dedifferentiated liposarcoma of the spine have been reported, but sporadic case reports of myxoid and pleiomorphic primary liposarcoma involving the spine have been published. Myxoid liposarcoma is the second most common liposarcoma subtype, occurring more frequently in the fourth and fifth decades, with a male-to-female predominance (6:1) (Schwab et al. 2007a; Zhao et al. 2016). Pleomorphic liposarcoma is the rarest and most aggressive of all subtypes and has the highest prevalence in the sixth and seventh decades, with an equal sex distribution (Dei Tos 2001; Oliveira and Nascimento 2001). However, epidemiological features are not clear because of the lack of large number of series with long-term follow-up (Zhao et al. 2016).

5.3 Localization

Myxoid spinal liposarcoma has been described in the cervical, thoracic, and lumbar spine, as well as the sacrum (Zhao et al. 2016). Localizations of primary spinal liposarcomas that have been described in literature are vertebrae T7–T8 (Hamlat et al. 2005), L1–L3 (Morales-Codina et al. 2016), L4 (de Moraes et al. 2015), and L4–L5 (Lmejjati et al. 2008).

5.4 Clinical Presentation

The most common symptoms are neck pain, backache, or unilateral of bilateral lumbo-ischialgia (Zhao et al. 2016). Secondary neurological symptoms such as gait abnormality and motor or sensory deficit can be present.

5.5 Imaging

Patients' symptoms instigate additional imaging including radiography, CT, MRI, and nuclear imaging. As compared to FDG-PET, MRI has superior diagnostic accuracy to detect spinal liposarcoma (especially for the myxoid subtype), and whole-spine MRI is the imaging modality of choice (Schwab et al. 2007a, b). In case of a primary spinal liposarcoma, it may show vertebral body infiltration with edema (being hypointense on T1-weighted images and hyperintense on T2-weighted images), with prevertebral epidural extension (Fig. 3). A pathological fracture may be seen. CT of the chest, abdomen, and pelvis may show evidence of metastatic disease.

5.6 Histopathology

Liposarcomas can be subdivided into five types (see above). Only the myxoid and pleomorphic types have been described as primary tumors of the spine. Pleomorphic liposarcoma can be hard to discern as being lipomatous in origin, with a composition of atypical mesenchymal cells with multiple mitoses and necrosis. Myxoid liposarcoma consists of abundant mucin deposition and a plexiform capillary network (Fletcher et al. 2002).

5.7 Differential Diagnosis

Primary tumors of the spine are relatively infrequent compared with metastatic disease, multiple myeloma, and lymphoma. Other considerations are (tuberculous) spondylitis, malignant fibrous histiocytoma, and high-grade pleomorphic sarcoma (Turanli et al. 2000). Although rare, liposarcoma should be considered in the differential diagnosis of spinal/vertebral tumors.

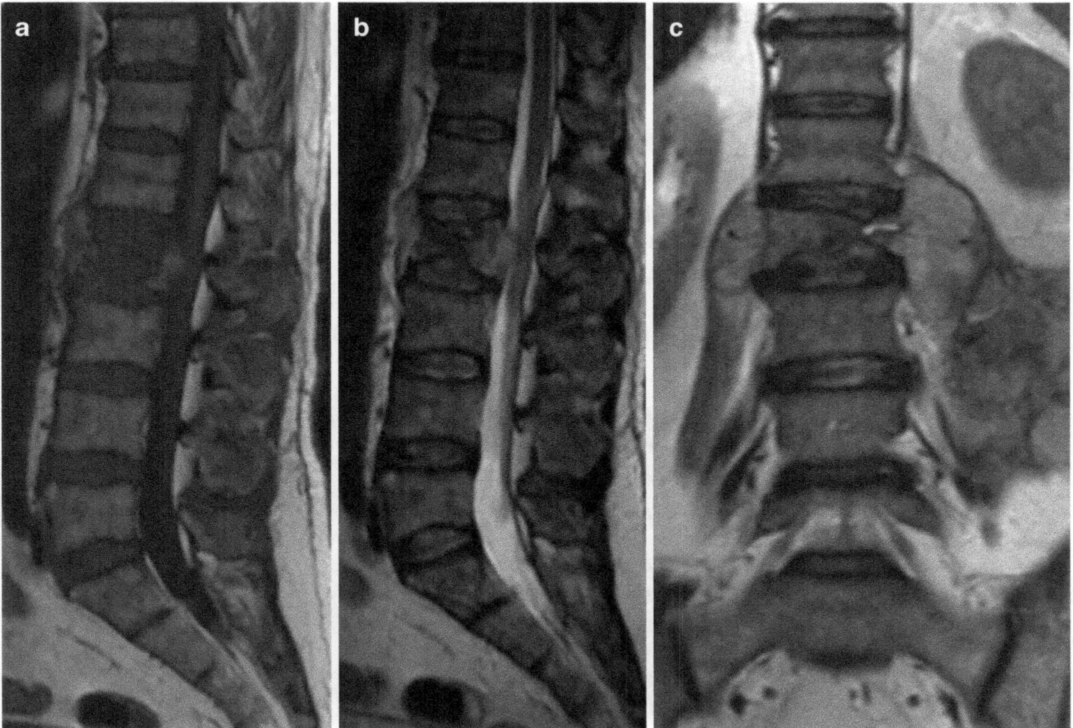

Fig. 3 Primary liposarcoma of the spine. Sagittal T1-WI (left, **a**) and T2-WI (middle, **b**) show a diffusely infiltrated body of L2, fracture, prevertebral extension, and anterior epidural component (left). A coronal T2-WI (right, **c**) better illustrates the paravertebral extension. Histology showed a pleomorphic liposarcoma. (From Morales-Codina et al. 2016)

5.8 Treatment and Prognosis

Surgical resection is the treatment of choice for liposarcoma, but local control is not always possible in spinal liposarcoma given the size and the complex anatomical structures. In a series of seven patients presented by Zhao et al. (2016), the spinal cord and/or nerve roots were always involved in tumor extension. Total en bloc spondylectomy is recommended for solitary spinal lesions, but for the majority of liposarcoma patients, only marginal resection is feasible, and surgical treatment is combined with (intraoperative) chemotherapy and adjuvant radiotherapy. Adjuvant radiotherapy is assumed to reduce the risk of local recurrence of lesions in the extremities; however, there are no data justifying this treatment in other locations. Concerning adjuvant chemotherapy, sensitivity profiles for each subtype of liposarcoma still need to be determined (Borghei-Razavi et al. 2015; Morales-Codina et al. 2016).

Prognosis is generally poor and depends on the tumor size and location, neurological status when diagnosed, local recurrence, and metastases. In case of irresectability and/or distant metastasis, effective treatment options are currently limited (Zhao et al. 2016). As far as we know, no data concerning the 5-year survival rate for primary spinal liposarcomas are available to date.

6 Spinal Metastases of Liposarcoma

Most soft tissue liposarcomas arise in the deep soft tissues of extremities or the retroperitoneum, and the most common site of metastasis is the lungs. Myxoid liposarcoma has the propensity to metastasize to extrapulmonary sites, such as soft tissue, retroperitoneum, mediastinum, chest wall, peritoneal surfaces, and spine (Fig. 4). Nevertheless, the spine remains an unusual location, even as a metastasis. Bone scan and FDG-PET lack sensitivity to detect spinal metastases in myxoid liposarcoma, and instead total spine MRI is advocated when screening for metastases in this population (Ishii et al. 2003; Schwab et al. 2007a, b). Turanli et al. (2000), Ogose et al. (2001), and Borghei-Razavi et al. (2015) present patients with metastatic myxoid liposarcoma to the epidural space, and Cho et al. (2010) describe a patient with multicentric myxoid liposarcoma with intradural involvement.

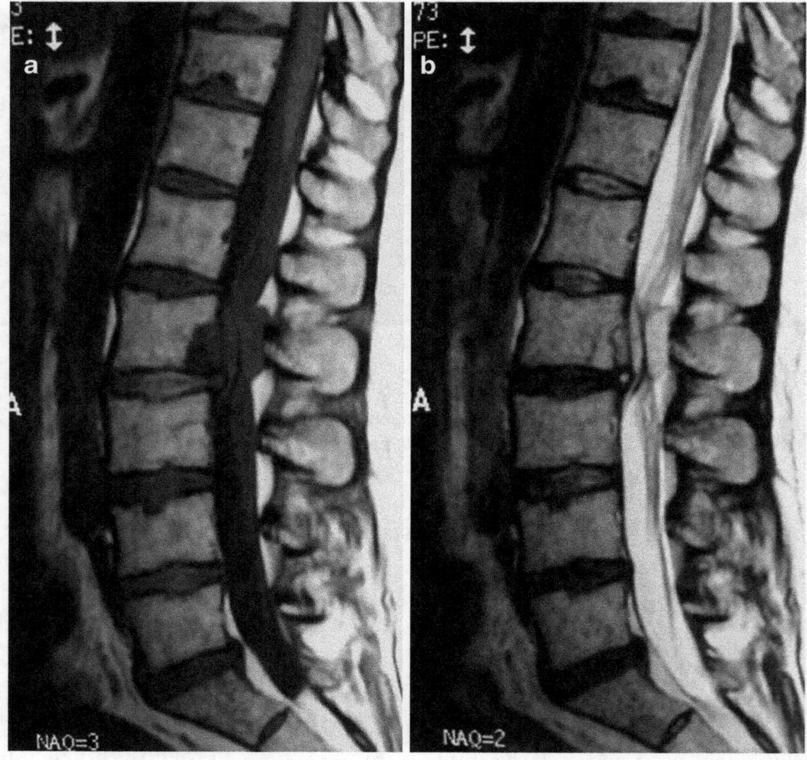

Fig. 4 Spinal metastasis from myxoid liposarcoma. T1-WI without fat saturation (left, **a**) of the lower thoracic and lumbar spine shows an area of abnormal low signal intensity in the posteroinferior corner of the L2 vertebral body with epidural invasion. T2-WI (right, **b**) shows an almost similar signal as normal vertebral bone marrow in the corresponding area, with epidural invasion. The lesion proved to be a metastasis from myxoid liposarcoma. (From Ishii et al. 2003)

7 Benign Notochordal Cell Tumor

Benign notochordal cell tumors are vertebral lesions usually discovered incidentally. Notochordal cell tumors are extremely common and are most likely underreported. The majority are asymptomatic, but a limited number of patients can present with chronic back pain (Amer and Hameed 2010). They are most commonly located in the clivus, but can occur also in the vertebrae, sacrum, and coccyx.

On imaging, they appear as well-defined lesions, with on CT preserved trabeculae, sclerosis, and without cortical destruction. On MRI, T1 hyperintense punctiform foci may be seen within the lesion, due to entrapped fat lobules. There is no soft tissue extension, no diffusion restriction, and usually no enhancement following intravenous contrast. The lack of metabolic activity most often shows no uptake in nuclear imaging.

Benign notochordal cell tumors should be differentiated from malignant chordomas. Chordomas are aggressive vertebral lesions, characterized by osseous destruction and extraosseous extension. PET/MR imaging provides detailed anatomic evaluation of benign notochordal cell tumor, and the lack of aggressiveness and metabolic activity distinguishes it from chordoma (Gupta 2018).

For further discussion of benign notochordal cell tumor, see chapter "Notochordal Tumors."

8 Focal Pseudotumoral Lesions Containing Fat

8.1 Focal Fatty Island in Bone Marrow

Focal fatty deposits ("marrow islands") are well-defined fat islands in the bone marrow of the spine or other parts of the axial skeleton (Frühwald et al. 1988). Focal fatty deposits are characterized by a localized replacement of normal hematopoietic bone marrow by a higher percentage of adipocytes. This is a normal variant and might be associated with degenerative changes or chronic inflammatory conditions such as spondylosis, scoliosis, or axial spondylarthritis. On CT, the focal fatty islands are typically more hypodense than normal marrow. MRI however is the imaging modality of choice, showing a well-defined vertebral lesion, T1 and T2 hyperintense, with low signal on fat-saturated sequences (Fig. 5). This benign entity should not be confused with melanoma metastases, focal hemorrhage, intra-osseous lipoma, hemangioma, or degenerative end plate changes, Modic type 2.

8.2 Reactive

8.2.1 Fatty Corner Lesion

A fatty corner lesion is a well-demarcated fat infiltration in the corner of a vertebral body, visible on T1-weighted MRI (Chung et al. 2019) (Fig. 6). Initially suggested as a diagnostic aid for spondyloarthropathy (SpA) by Bennett et al. (2010), the study by Chung et al. (2019) confirmed that the presence of at least three anterior thoracic fatty corner lesions or five whole-spine lesions suggests a diagnosis of SpA in patients with clinical features without additional MRI of the SI joints.

8.2.2 Fatty Reconversion After Radiotherapy

Radiation therapy is known to alter the signal intensity of bone marrow. In the acute phase, an increase in signal intensity on STIR/T2-WI may be visible due to early bone marrow edema. After around 10–14 days, the bone marrow starts to undergo fatty replacement in the radiation field, visible as hyperintense areas on T1-WI and dark on fat-suppressed sequences (Daldrup-Link et al.

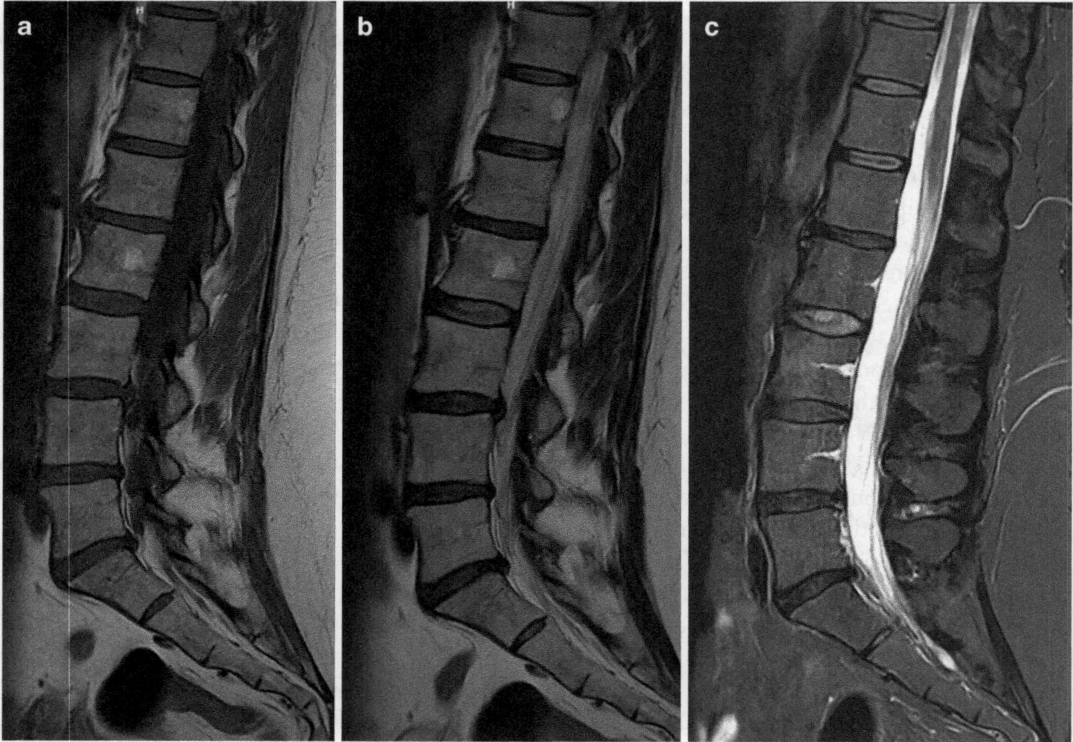

Fig. 5 Focal fatty islands in the thoracolumbar spine in a 53-year-old woman with ischialgia. (**a**) Sagittal T1-weighted image, (**b**) sagittal T2-weighted image, and (**c**) sagittal T2-weighted image with fat saturation. MRI of the thoracolumbar spine revealed a right-sided subarticular/foraminal hernia level L3–L4 as well as central posterior bulging of the disk L4–L5 and L5–S1. Focal fatty islands were incidentally detected in Th12 en L2, showing as hyperintense rounded lesions on both T1- and T2-weighted images, with nulling of the signal after fat saturation. (Case courtesy: Prof. Dr. F. Vanhoenacker)

2007). This fatty replacement may be homogeneous or band-like. In some cases, the edema may persist for weeks and fatty reconversion may become visible only months after radiation. Fatty replacement of the bone marrow is reversible with cumulative radiation doses of up to 30–40 Gy and irreversible after an irradiation with more than 40 Gy (Daldrup-Link et al. 2007; Ollivier et al. 2015).

Additionally, bone marrow outside the irradiation field may also show these changes, but to a much lower degree, most likely due to scattering of the radiation beam (Daldrup-Link et al. 2007; Ollivier et al. 2015).

8.2.3 Chronic Fracture and Bone Marrow Hemorrhage

In vertebral fracture, edema and hemorrhage initially present as areas of T1 hypointensity on MRI. As the edema disappears and the blood products mature, the methemoglobin in vertebral marrow hemorrhage may present as increased T1 signal, resulting in variable T1 signal with areas of T1 hyperintensity and hypointensity. Additionally, evolving bone marrow necrosis may contain blood and proteinaceous debris within the hyperemic marrow, which may result in areas of T1 and T2 hyperintensity (Hanrahan and Shah 2011).

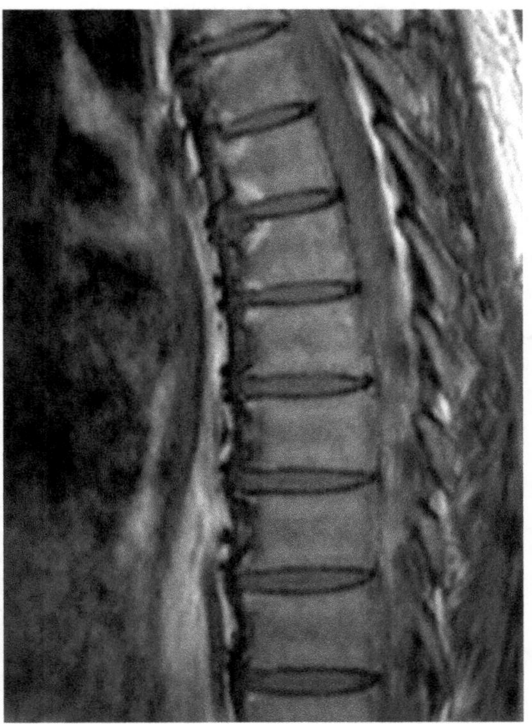

Fig. 6 Fatty corner lesions. T1-WI shows well-demarcated triangular hyperintense lesions in the (anterior) corners of multiple thoracic vertebrae. (Without modifications from Chung et al. 2019 (http://creativecommons.org/licenses/by/4.0/))

8.3 Fatty Hemangioma

Vertebral hemangiomas are benign venous malformations within the vertebrae. They are usually intra-osseous but may have an epidural component. They are classically asymptomatic and incidentally detected. Rarely, vertebral hemangiomas can be locally aggressive (Riahi et al. 2018). For the discussion of vertebral hemangiomas, see chapter "Vertebral Hemangioma and Angiomatous Neoplasms."

9 Key Points

- Vertebral hemangioma is the most common fat-containing vertebral lesion. Increased usage of medical imaging will raise the detection of other (rare) lipomatous lesions.
- Intra-osseous hibernoma can mimic a solitary vertebral malignancy (metastasis).
- Intraspinal osteolipoma is a very rare benign lesion that may present with acute neurological symptoms.
- (Primary) spinal liposarcoma is rare. MRI has better sensitivity as compared to FDG-PET, particularly in myxoid liposarcoma.

References

Aiyer SN, Shetty AP, Kanna R et al (2016) Isolated dorsal column dysfunction due to an intraspinal Osteolipoma - case report and review of literature. J Clin Orthop Trauma 7(Suppl 1):2–4

Amer HZ, Hameed M (2010) Intraosseous benign notochordal cell tumor. Arch Pathol Lab Med 134(2):283–288

Bai S, Mies C, Stephenson J et al (2013) Intraosseous hibernoma: a potential mimic of metastatic carcinoma. Ann Diagn Pathol 17:204–206

Bennett AN, Rehman A, Hensor EM et al (2010) The fatty Romanus lesion: a non-inflammatory spinal MRI lesion specific for axial spondyloarthropathy. Ann Rheum Dis 69(5):891–894

Bonar SF, Watson G, Gragnaniello C et al (2014) Intraosseous hibernoma: characterization of five cases and literature review. Skeletal Radiol 43(7):939–946

Borghei-Razavi H, Daabak K-M, Bakhti S et al (2015) Primary epidural liposarcoma of the cervical spine: technical case report and review of the literature. Interdiscip Neurosurg 2(1):1–5

Botchu R, Puls F, Hock YL et al (2013) Intraosseous hibernoma: a case report and review of the literature. Skeletal Radiol 42:1003–1005

Brones A, Mengshol S, Wilkinson CC (2010) Ossifying lipoma of the cervical spine. Case report. J Neurosurg Pediatr 5(3):283–284

Campbell RSD, Grainger AJ, Mangham DC et al (2003) Intraosseous lipoma: report of 35 new cases and a review of the literature. Skeletal Radiol 32(4):209–222

Castilho RM, Squarize CH, Nunes FD et al (2004) Osteolipoma: a rare lesion in the oral cavity. Br J Oral Maxillofac Surg 42(4):363–364

Cheng S, Lu SC, Zhang B et al (2012) Rare massive osteolipoma in the upper part of the knee in a young adult. Orthopedics 35(9):e1434–e1437

Cho SH, Rhim SC, Hyun SJ, Bae CW et al (2010) Intradural involvement of multicentric myxoid liposarcoma. J Korean Neurosurg Soc 48(3):276–280

Chung HY, Yiu RSW, Chan SCW et al (2019) Fatty corner lesions in T1-weighted magnetic resonance imaging as an alternative to sacroiliitis for diagnosis of axial spondyloarthritis. BMC Rheumatol 3:17

Daldrup-Link HE, Henning T, Link TM (2007) MR imaging of therapy-induced changes of bone marrow. Eur Radiol 17:743–761

Davies AM, Sundaram M, James SJ (2009) Imaging of bone tumors and tumor-like lesions. Springer. ISBN: 9783540779827

de Moraes FB, Cardoso AL, Tristão NA et al (2015) Primary liposarcoma of the lumbar spine: case report. Rev Bras Ortop 47(1):124–129

Dei Tos AP (2001) Lipomatous tumor. Curr Diagn Pathol 7:8–16

Demiralp B, Alderete JF, Kose O et al (2009) Osteolipoma independent of bone tissue: a case report. Cases J 2:8711

Dilip Chand Raja S, Kanna RM et al (2018) Lumbar intraspinal osteolipoma presenting as cauda equina syndrome: a case report and review of literature. Case Rep Orthop 2018:1945149

Fletcher CDM, Unni KK, Mertens F (2002) Pathology and genetics of tumors of soft tissue and bone. World Health Organization

Fritchie KJ, Renner JB, Rao KW et al (2012) Osteolipoma: radiological, pathological, and cytogenetic analysis of three cases. Skeletal Radiol 41(2):237–244

Frühwald F, Frühwald S, Hajek PC et al (1988) Focal fatty deposits in spinal bone marrow—MR findings. MRI of focal fatty deposits. Rofo 148(1):75–78

Furlong MA, Fanburg-Smith J, Miettinen M (2001) The morphologic spectrum of hibernoma: a clinicopathologic study of 170 cases. Am J Surg Pathol 25:809–814

Gesta S, Tseng YH, Kahn CR (2007) Developmental origin of fat: tracking obesity to its source. Cell 131:242–256

Gupta R (2018) Benign notochordal remnant. In: PET/MR imaging. Springer, Cham

Hafeez I, Shankman S, Michnovicz J et al (2015) Intraosseous hibernoma: a case report and review of the literature. Spine 40(9):E558–E561

Hamlat A, Saikali S, Gueye EM et al (2005) Primary liposarcoma of the thoracic spine: case report. Eur Spine J 14(6):613–618

Hanrahan CJ, Shah LM (2011) MRI of spinal bone marrow: Part 2, T1-weighted imaging-based differential diagnosis. AJR Am J Roentgenol 197(6):1309–1321

Heffernan EJ, Lefaivre K, Munk PL et al (2008) Ossifying lipoma of the thigh. Br J Radiol 81(968):e207–e210

Ishii T, Ueda T, Myoui A et al (2003) Unusual skeletal metastases from myxoid liposarcoma only detectable by MR imaging. Eur Radiol 13:L185–L191

Jain R, Raj S, Sandhu GS, Bhatia VPM (2019) Intraspinal osteolipoma: a rare case. Indian J Musculoskelet 1(2):108–110

Jaiswal AK, Garg A, Mahapatra AK (2005) Spinal ossifying lipoma. J Clin Neurosci 12(6):714–717

Ko A, Rowell CC, Vogler JB (2020) Intraosseous hibernoma: a metastatic mimicker to consider on the differential. Radiol Case Rep 15:2677–2680

Kumar R, Deaver MT, Czerniak BA et al (2011) Intraosseous hibernoma. Skeletal Radiol 40:641–645

Lin YC, Huang CC, Chen HJ (2001) Intraspinal osteolipoma. Case report. J Neurosurg 94(1 Suppl):126–128

Lmejjati M, Loqa C, Haddi M et al (2008) Primary liposarcoma of the lumbar spine. Joint Bone Spine 75(4):482–485

Milgram JW (1988) Intraosseous lipomas. A clinicopathologic study of 66 cases. Clin Orthop Relat Res 231:277–302

Milgram JW (1990) Malignant transformation in bone lipomas. Skeletal Radiol 19(5):347–352

Morales-Codina AM, Martín-Benlloch JA, Corbellas Aparicio M (2016) Primary pleomorphic liposarcoma of the spine. Case report and review of the literature. Int J Surg Case Rep 25:114–119

Murphey M, Carroll J, Flemming D et al (2004) From the archives of the AFIP: benign musculoskeletal lipomatous lesions. Radiographics 24(5):1433–1466

Obermann EC, Bele S, Brawanski A et al (1999) Ossifying lipoma. Virchows Arch 434(2):181–183

Ogose A, Hotta T, Inoue Y et al (2001) Myxoid liposarcoma metastatic to the thoracic epidural space without bone involvement: report of two cases. Jpn J Clin Oncol 31(9):447–449

Oliveira AM, Nascimento AG (2001) Pleiomorphic liposarcoma. Semin Diagn Pathol 18:274–285

Ollivier L, Brisse H, Leclère J (2015) Bone marrow imaging: follow-up after treatment in cancer patients. Cancer Imaging 2(2):90–92

Pande KC, Ceccherini AF, Webb JK et al (1988) Intraosseous lipomata of adjacent vertebral bodies. Eur Spine J 7(4):344–347

Propeck T, Bullard MA, Lin J et al (2000) Radiologic-pathologic correlation of intraosseous lipomas. AJR Am J Roentgenol 175(3):673–678

Reyes AR, Irwin R, Wilson JD et al (2008) Intraosseous hibernoma of the femur: an unusual case with a review of the literature (poster #20). In: Paper presented at: Annual College of American Pathologists Meeting, San Diego, CA, vol 132, p 3

Riahi H, Mechri M, Barsaoui M et al (2018) Imaging of benign tumors of the osseous spine. J Belg Soc Radiol 102(1):13

Ringe KI, Rosenthal H, Langer F et al (2013) Radiofrequency ablation of a rare case of an intraosseous hibernoma causing therapy-refractory pain. J Vasc Interv Radiol 24(11):1754–1756

Schwab JH, Boland PJ, Antonescu C et al (2007a) Spinal metastases from myxoid liposarcoma warrant screening with magnetic resonance imaging. Cancer 110(8):1815–1822

Schwab JH, Boland P, Guo T et al (2007b) Skeletal metastases in myxoid liposarcoma: an unusual pattern of distant spread. Ann Surg Oncol 14(4):1507–1514

Sen D, Satija L, Chatterji S et al (2015) Vertebral intraosseous lipoma. Med J Armed Forces India 71(3):293–296

Sinson G, Gennarelli TA, Wells GB (1998) Suprasellar osteolipoma: case report. Surg Neurol 50(5):457–460

Song B, Ryu HJ, Lee C et al (2017) Intraosseous hibernoma: a rare and unique intraosseous lesion. J Pathol Transl Med 51(5):499–504

Teekhasaenee C, Kita K, Takegami K et al (2015) Intraosseous lipoma of the third lumbar spine: a case report. J Med Case Rep 9:52

Torok G, Meller Y, Maor E (1983) Primary liposarcoma of bone. Case report and review of the literature. Bull Hosp Jt Dis Orthop Inst 43(1):28–37

Turanli S, Ozer H, Ozyürekoglu T et al (2000) Liposarcoma in the epidural space. Spine 25:1733–1735

Um MK, Lee E, Lee JW et al (2020) Spinal intraosseous hibernoma: a case report and review of literature. Taehan Yongsang Uihakhoe Chi 81(4):965–971

Val-Bernal JF, Val D, Garijo MF et al (2007) Subcutaneous ossifying lipoma: case report and review of the literature. J Cutan Pathol 34(10):788–792

WHO Classification of Tumours Editorial Board (2020) WHO classification of tumours editorial. Soft tissue and bone tumours. WHO. ISBN: 9789283245025

Yang J-S, Chu L, Li X et al (2015) Multiple intraosseous vertebral lipomas with chronic back pain. Spine J 15(7):1676–1677

Zhao C, Han Z, Xiao H et al (2016) Surgical management of spinal liposarcoma: a case series of 7 patients and literature review. Eur Spine J 25(12):4088–4093

Paget's Disease of the Spine

Sinan Al-Qassab, Radhesh Lalam, and Victor N. Cassar-Pullicino

Contents

Abstract

Paget's disease of bone (PDB) is a chronic metabolic disease due to the disturbance in the normal homeostasis of bone remodeling. The spine is the second most commonly affected part in the body. There is strong evidence that the prevalence of the disease is declining as is its extent and severity as well as increasing age at time of diagnosis. Patients can be asymptomatic, and the disease may be incidentally discovered while other patients may have symptoms from the disease itself or as a result of its complications. Spinal changes due to PDB can be very difficult to depict on radiography and very subtle on MRI and may present a diagnostic dilemma. In fact, PDB may mimic other pathologies including neoplasia and may be incorrectly diagnosed as such. This is particularly important given that PDB usually affects elderly population in whom the risk of malignancy is already high. In this chapter, we discuss the epidemiological and pathological background of the disease and describe important practical radiological principles and imaging features that will assist in achieving a sound and confident diagnosis. The chapter also goes into details of potential complications in the spine.

S. Al-Qassab · R. Lalam (✉) · V. N. Cassar-Pullicino
Department of Radiology, The Robert Jones and Agnes Hunt Orthopaedic Hospital,
Oswestry, Shropshire, UK
e-mail: radhesh.lalam@nhs.net

Med Radiol Diagn Imaging (2023)
https://doi.org/10.1007/174_2023_454,
Published Online: 24 September 2023

1 Introduction

In 1877, Sir James Paget described a bone disorder of unknown etiology in five patients, remarkably without the aid of radiographs, characterized by osteolysis and excessive attempts of repair resulting in expansion and deformity of the affected bones, and termed it "osteitis deformans" (Paget 1877). Currently, this is commonly referred to as Paget's disease of bone (PDB).

2 Epidemiology

Paget's disease of bone (PDB) is the second most common metabolic bone disease following osteoporosis (Whitehouse 2002). It is most prevalent in the Northwest of England, with Lancashire being the focus in the United Kingdom with a prevalence of 7% in the population over 55 years (Barker et al. 1980). The disease is most common in people of British descent in the United Kingdom, Australia, New Zealand, South Africa, and North America (Altman 2002). It is rare in Scandinavia, the Middle East, Africa, India, and the Far East (Whitehouse 2002). In fact, it has been hypothesized that the disease originated in Britain and from there spread to the rest of the world by migration and admixture of the British populations. This has been proven by Mays when he reviewed the literature of Paget's disease of bone (PDB) in archeological specimens published between 1889 and 2010, which fulfilled the radiological and/or histological criteria of PDB. He identified 109 cases dating back to the first century AD Roman Empire, where all the cases came from Western Europe, 94% of which were from England (Mays 2010). Interestingly, no credible evidence of PDB is available from the archeological remains of the great civilizations of Mesopotamia, Egypt, Far East, and South America, further supporting this hypothesis (Mays 2010). Analysis of Beethoven's skeletal appearances suggests that he might have had PDB, which contributed to his hearing loss (Naiken 1971).

The disease is rare before 50 years of age (Nebot Valenzuela and Pietschmann 2017). The overall prevalence is 3–5% above this age, increasing to 10% by the age of 90 years. The disease is more common in men with a male-to-female ratio of 1.6:1 (Schmorl 1932; Altman 2002; Lalam et al. 2016). Recent studies show significant change in the epidemiology. The prevalence of the disease is reducing with increasing age at the time of onset. There is also evidence that the severity and extent of the disease are reducing with higher incidence of monostotic disease (Cundy 2007; Dell'Atti et al. 2007; Lalam et al. 2016). Bastin et al. looked at 3350 abdominal radiographs of people older than 54 years of age in New Zealand between 2005 and 2006. They found Paget's disease in 2.6% of the study sample in which the cases were older patients who demonstrated milder disease compared to previously (Bastin et al. 2009).

3 Etiology

The exact etiology behind PDB is not clearly understood. Infectious, inflammatory, autoimmune, and tumoral pathologies have been suggested. The currently accepted etiology is thought to be due to a combination of environmental factors on the background of genetic predisposition. Genetic susceptibility is supported by cases reported in identical twins. 15–40% of patients with PDB have affected first-degree relatives (Lucas et al. 2008). Linkage analysis has identified several potential loci for susceptibility to PD, but the most important of these is the PDB3 locus on chromosome 5q35, particularly mutations affecting sequestosome 1 (SQSTM1) gene. Mutations of this gene were found in 20–50% of familial cases and 5–10% of sporadic cases of PDB (Layfield 2007).

The environmental factors that have been suggested are viruses, reduced dietary calcium intake, increased mechanical loading, and exposure to toxins (Lalam et al. 2016). Members of the myxovirus and paramyxovirus families have been suspected including measles. The reduction in the incidence of the disease could be linked to the reduction in theses viral infections secondary to universal immunization. However, despite experimental evidence of the effect of paramyxoviruses on osteoclast activity, studies have failed to isolate live viruses or viral RNA from affected specimens (Mee et al. 1998; Friedrichs et al. 2002; Matthews et al. 2008).

4 Pathology

In normal bones, the osteoblastic and osteoclastic activity is orderly maintained. In PDB, there is disruption to this normal homeostasis resulting in increased bone turnover and remodeling. This is the basis of the clinical, pathological, as well as radiological features of this disease with pathomechanical changes contributing to the subsequent potential complications.

Hyperosteoclastosis from increased multinucleated giant cell osteoclasts results in bone resorption and associated fibrosis. Biochemically, this is reflected as an increase in alkaline phosphatase (ALP). Meanwhile, hyperosteoblastosis will result in increased bone deposition in a chaotic fashion of "mosaic" woven bone, which is mechanically weak with alternating heavily calcified and fibrotic areas. There is varying degree of vascularity and marrow fibrosis (Al-Rashid et al. 2015; Nebot Valenzuela and Pietschmann 2017). These changes constitute the basis of the clinically and pathologically recognized three phases of PDB, where the initial phase represents the osteoclastic activity, the late phase represents the osteoblastic activity, and the intermediate mixed phase represents a combination of both. A fourth "inactive sclerotic" phase has been described where there is chronic quiescent sclerosis with normal or reduced bone activity (Dell'Atti et al. 2007; Lalam et al. 2016). Radiologically, these background changes may give similar appearances to other diseases including neoplasia, and hence PDB is a great mimicker of other pathologies.

Four different patterns of bone remodeling at the periosteal/endosteal interface have been described as a result of the various combinations of periosteal and endosteal new bone formation due to osteoblastic activity termed apposition and endosteal bone resorption due to abnormal osteoclastic activity termed resorption. These patterns are periosteal and endosteal apposition (Fig. 1), periosteal apposition and endosteal resorption (Fig. 1), periosteal apposition with normal endosteum, and focal periosteal apposition "pumice stone" appearance. There may be a combination of these patterns in the same vertebra, but usually one

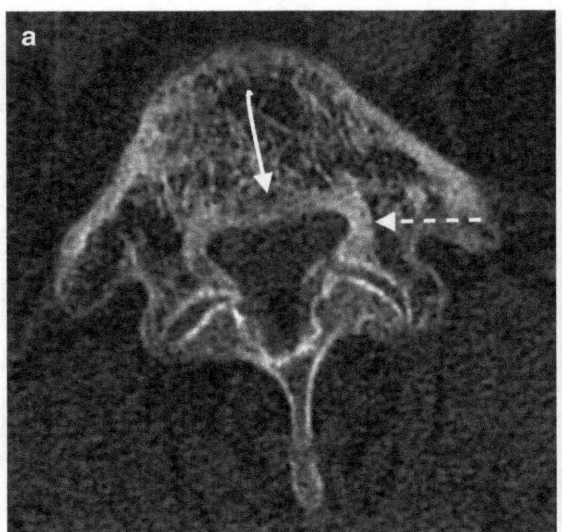

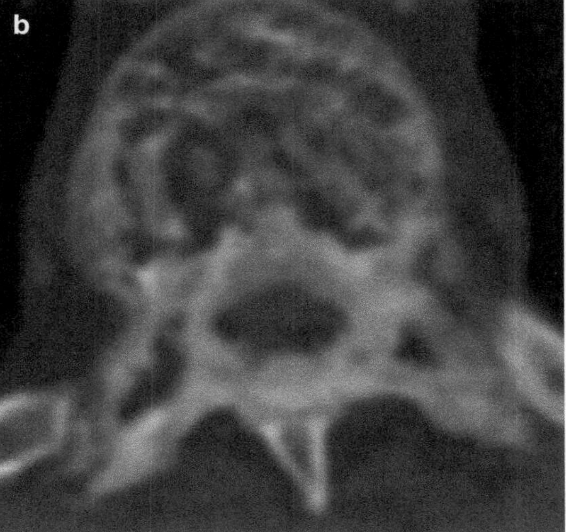

Fig. 1 (**a**) Axial CT L5: Mixed pattern in a single vertebral body where there is an area of periosteal apposition and endosteal resorption (arrow) with an area of periosteal and endosteal apposition (dotted arrow). (**b**) Axial CT T10: periosteal and endosteal apposition

is predominant (Fig. 1) (Hadjipavlou and Lander 1991; Hadjipavlou et al. 2001). Periosteal apposition usually leads to bone expansion. Changes in the endosteum will affect the marrow space. The combination of periosteal and endosteal changes will affect the cortical thickness. Periosteal and endosteal apposition will result in thickened cortex and reduced marrow size. Periosteal apposition and endosteal resorption will result in normal-thickness cortex and increased marrow size. Periosteal apposition and normal endosteum will result in thickened cortex but normal marrow size. Focal periosteal apposition will result in a focal "pumice stone"-like enlargement.

Periosteal apposition and endosteal resorption are the most frequent mechanisms of vertebral body expansion (Fig. 1). The other two mechanisms are less common in the vertebral body (Dell'Atti et al. 2007). The fourth and least common mechanism in the vertebral body is focal periosteal apposition giving rise to "pumice stone" appearance (Dell'Atti et al. 2007).

The spine is the second most common site affected by PDB (53%) after the pelvis (70%) (Fig. 2) (Langston and Ralston 2004; Dell'Atti et al. 2007). Pestka et al. reported in their sample of 101 patients of spinal PDB that the lumbar spine is the commonest site (62.3%), followed by the thoracic spine (29.6%) and least in the cervical spine (8.2%) (Pestka et al. 2012). The L4 and L5 vertebrae are the most frequently involved (Fig. 3) (Guyer and Shepherd 1980). Involvement

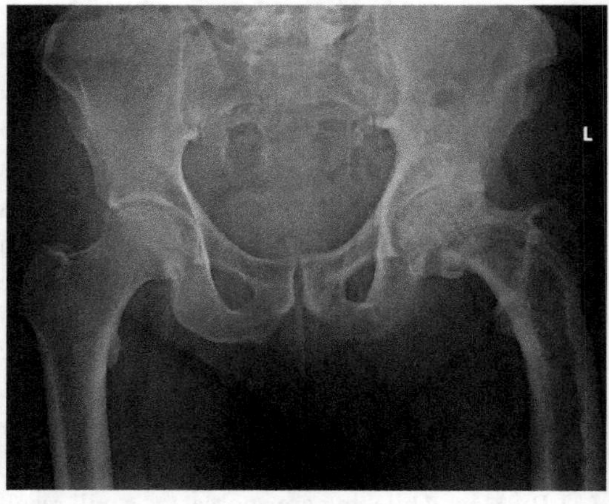

Fig. 2 Conventional radiography (CR) pelvis: note the expansion, coarsening of the trabeculae, and cortical thickening in the left hemipelvis and left proximal femur in keeping with Paget's disease. Note that the disease in long bones usually starts from an articular surface

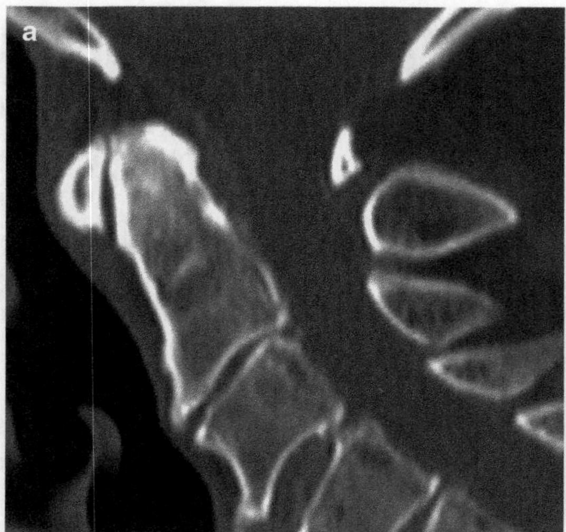

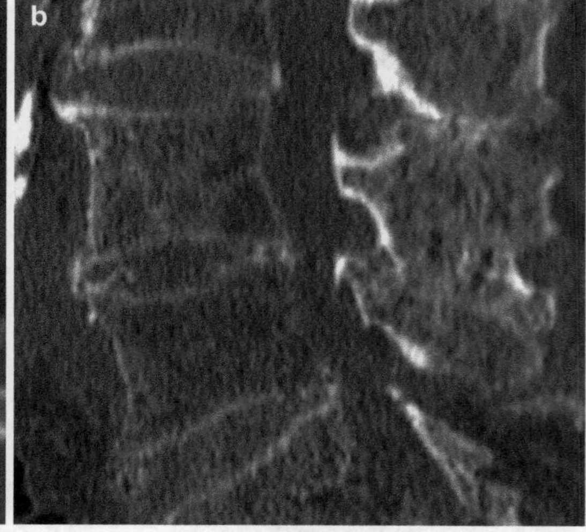

Fig. 3 (**a**) Sagittal CT C2 vertebra. Note the expansion of the peg and spinous process of C2 in comparison to the adjacent vertebrae. Also note the malalignment of the spinous process of C2. Despite the relatively normal trabeculae and cortices, the expansion together with L4 and L5 involvement is suggestive of Paget's disease. (**b**) Sagittal CT lumbar spine in same patient. Note the expansion of the spinous processes of the L4 and L5 vertebrae with trabecular and cortical thickening in keeping with Paget's disease. Note the secondary degenerative changes and fusion, which are known complications of PDB

of the atlantoaxial region is extremely rare (Brown et al. 1971; Hepple et al. 1998). The disease is polyostotic in 66% of cases, and although different stages of the disease may be found in the same bone and preexisting lesions may show progression, it is rather unusual to have involvement of a new bone after the initial diagnosis (Dell'Atti et al. 2007; Cundy and Bolland 2008; Shaker 2009; Lalam et al. 2016).

5 Clinical Features

Most patients are asymptomatic discovered incidentally when imaged for other pathologies. Back pain is the most common symptom associated with PDB of the spine. This could be due to PDB itself where the pain is dull, deep-seated, and unrelated to activity and is seen in up to 24% of cases or could be due to other complications such as osteoarthritis, fractures, spinal stenosis, neural compression, or malignant transformation (Table 1) (Dell'Atti et al. 2007). Rarely, patients may present with cardiac failure or hypercalcemia.

Table 1 Causes of neural compromise in Paget's disease of bone in the spine

- Vertebral body and/or posterior element expansion
- Facet joint arthropathy
- Degenerative disk
- Fracture retropulsion and hematomas
- Spondylolisthesis
- Neoplasia and pseudosarcoma
- Ligament ossification
- Vertebral ankylosis

6 Imaging Consideration

PDB is primarily a disease of bone involving the cortex and trabeculae rather than the marrow. Marrow involvement is only secondary. The characteristic features of bone expansion and cortical and trabecular thickening are difficult to appreciate in the spine on conventional radiography due to tissue overlap, increasing obesity in the population, and technical factors related to poor positioning and exposure. In spinal involvement in PDB, CT carries higher specificity.

The subtle cortical and trabecular changes could be quite difficult to appreciate on MRI, given the normal marrow in early stages of the disease. However, MRI is valuable in assessing for complications such as fractures and sarcomatous transformation.

Nuclear medicine may be useful in assessing the degree of metabolic activity in the affected bone.

In general, imaging modalities complement each other in spinal involvement with PDB.

7 Imaging Appearances

Practical points to consider in the imaging features of PDB in the vertebrae are the following:

- Vertebral body involvement is almost always complete, i.e., both anterior and posterior elements are affected (Fig. 4). This is, in fact, one of the most important clues and has a very high (close to 100%) negative predictive value.

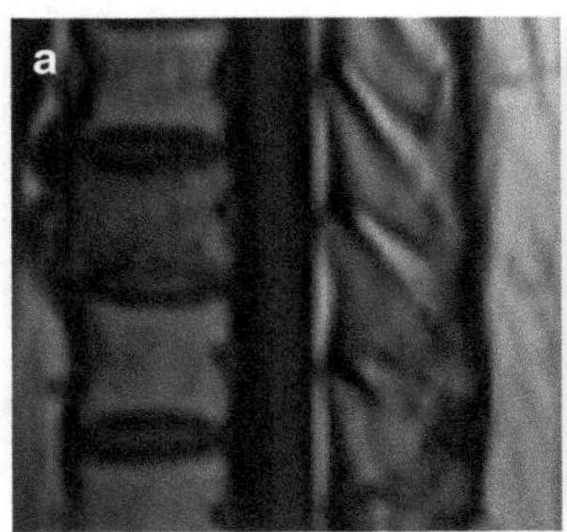

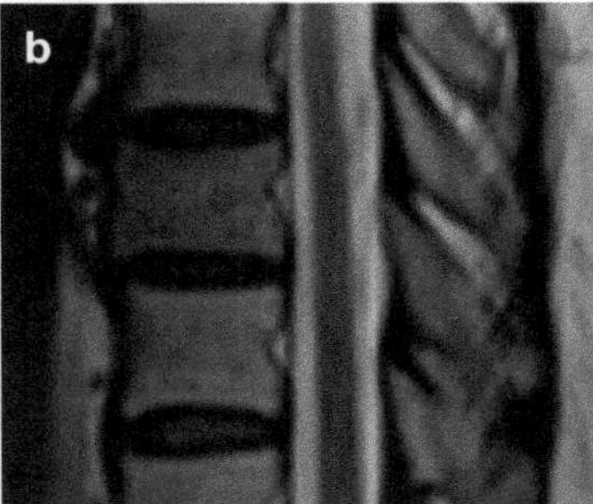

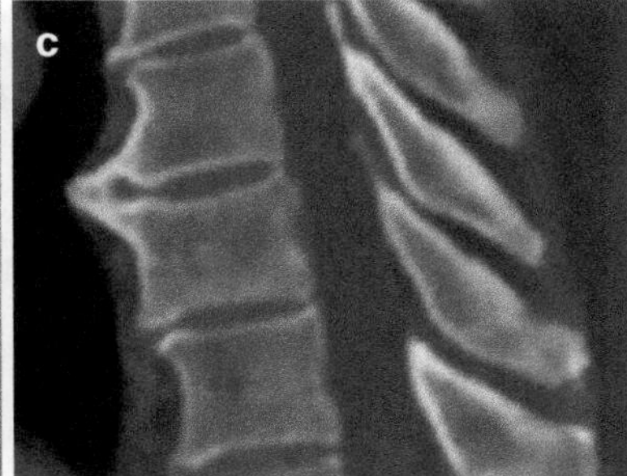

Fig. 4 (**a**) Sagittal T1-weighted image (WI), (**b**) T2-WI, and (**c**) sagittal CT images demonstrating subtle alteration in marrow signal of T9 vertebral body. Careful assessment will reveal expansion of the T9 vertebral body and, most importantly, the spinous process when compared to the adjacent vertebrae in keeping with Paget's disease. The complete vertebral body involvement (particularly the spinous process) with no soft tissue involvement is an important clue to the diagnosis

- Vertebral expansion occurs in the anteroposterior and transverse dimensions of the vertebra rather than in the craniocaudal dimension due to the fact that the vertebral end plates are trabecular condensations and do not have a periosteal-endosteal interface (Fig. 5).
- Unlike PDB in the peripheral skeleton, the initial lytic phase is very rarely seen in the vertebrae due to the high trabecular:cortex ratio in the spine (Vande Berg et al. 2001).

On radiographs and CT, the bone expansion with cortical thickening will result in a relatively sclerotic periphery and lucent center, giving the classical sing of a "picture frame" vertebra (Fig. 6). This is to be differentiated from "rugger jersey" sign seen in hyperparathyroidism where only the superior and inferior end plates of the vertebral body are sclerotic, usually involving multiple contagious vertebral bodies.

Trabecular thickening can also be seen in other conditions such as osteoporosis, hemoglo-

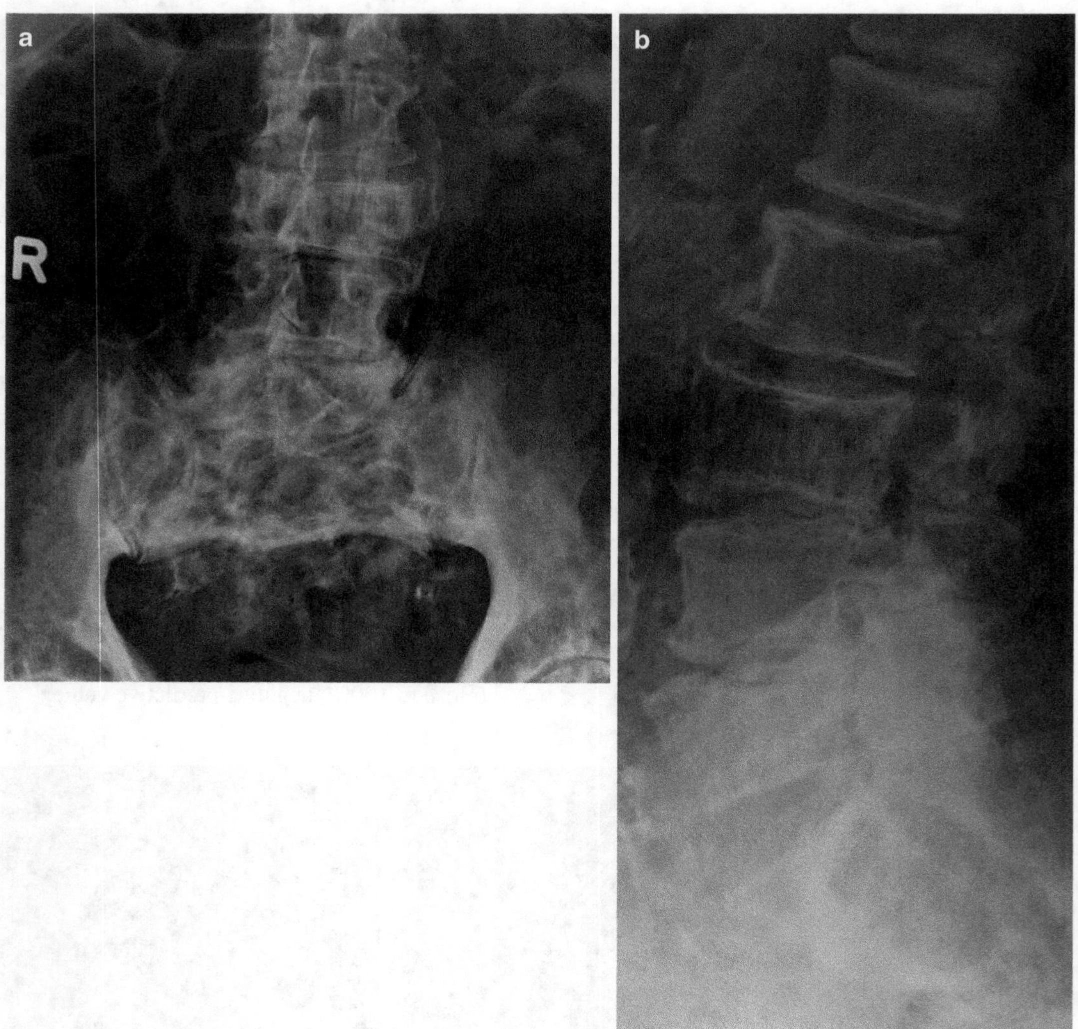

Fig. 5 (**a**) AP and (**b**) lateral CR lumbar spine. Note the expansion, coarsening of the trabeculae, and cortical thickening of the L3 and L5 vertebrae. Note that the expansion is in the anteroposterior (lateral view) and transverse (AP view) dimensions. Expansion does not occur in the craniocaudal dimension due to the lack of periosteal-endosteal interface at the vertebral end plates. Also note the extensive involvement in the pelvis

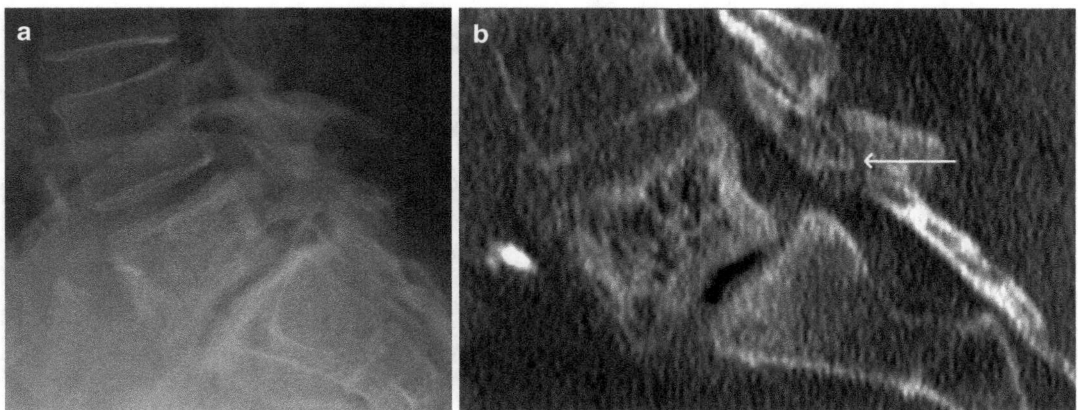

Fig. 6 (**a**) Lateral CR lumbar spine and (**b**) sagittal CT. Note the expanded L5 vertebra with trabecular thickening and cortical sclerosis giving the "picture frame" appearances. Note the anterolisthesis due to bilateral pars defects confirmed on CT (arrow)

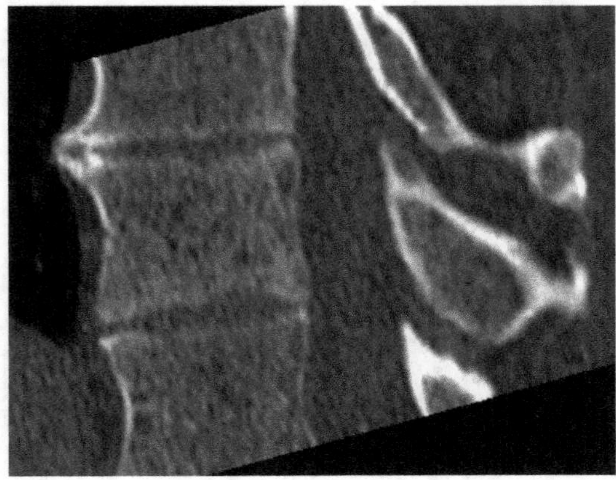

Fig. 7 Sagittal CT T10 vertebra. Note the subtle sclerotic change within the vertebral body and expansion of the spinous process when compared to the adjacent levels

binopathies, and hemangiomas, which usually results in accentuation of the vertical trabeculae (Theodorou et al. 2011). Other features of PDB like complete vertebral involvement including the posterior elements and spinous processes, expansion, and cortical thickening help in differentiation (Fig. 7).

Diffuse trabecular and cortical apposition could result in a diffusely sclerotic vertebra, "ivory vertebra." The differential diagnosis for these appearances is sclerotic metastasis, Paget's disease, and lymphoma. Involvement of the spinous processes and straitening of the anterior border of the vertebral body giving rise to a "squared vertebra" would be helpful, favoring PDB. In lymphoma, there may be anterior scalloping due to pressure erosion for the para-aortic lymphadenopathy. Biopsy may be required in some cases to achieve the final diagnosis (Fig. 8).

Pure lysis of the vertebra will result in a "ghost vertebra," which is rare in PDB but if encountered would represent a dilemma as other differential diagnosis should be considered, especially lytic metastasis (Rosen et al. 1988; Steinbach and Johnston 1993). Depicting other features of PDB on CT such as expansion and cortical and trabecular thickening with lack of destruction and extra-osseous soft tissue will aid in the diagnosis (Lalam et al. 2016). However, MRI would be extremely valuable here as demonstrating fatty marrow signal on the T1-weighted images will rule out sinister pathology since the only two lucent or osteolytic lesions on radiography that demonstrate normal marrow fat on MRI according to Sundaram et al. are intra-osseous lipomas and Paget's disease (Sundaram et al. 2001).

Osseous expansion with fatty marrow of the vertebral body posteriorly and neural arch anteriorly due to periosteal apposition and endosteal resorption will result in spinal stenosis, when the resultant cortical outline is very thin. On MRI, this may be misinterpreted as epidural fat ossification or epidural lipomatosis (Clarke and

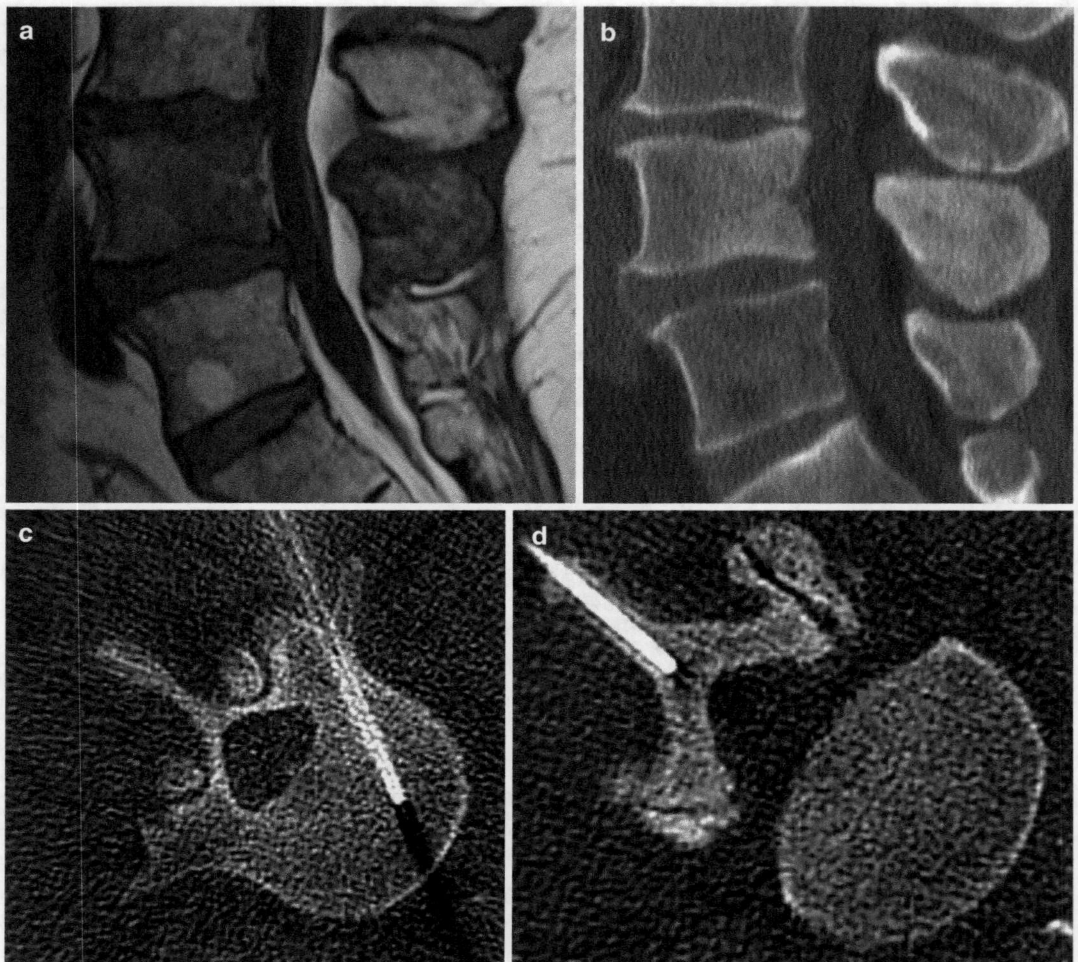

Fig. 8 (**a**) Sagittal T1-WI MRI and (**b**) sagittal CT images of the lumbar spine. MRI demonstrates subtle diffuse alteration of the marrow signal within the body and spinous process of the L4 vertebra with very subtle expansion. CT images prove the expansion and sclerosis of the spinous process of the L4 vertebra with subtle coarsening of the vertebral body trabeculae, sclerosis, and very mild expansion. Appearances are suggestive of Paget's disease. Note the complete involvement of the vertebra. (**c**, **d**) Biopsies of the L4 vertebral body and spinous process confirmed Paget's disease

Williams 1975; Koziarz and Avruch 2002). CT would be helpful in confirming the diagnosis (Fig. 9).

PDB is a disease of bone rather than marrow. Marrow changes are only secondary in the form of variable degrees of fibrosis, hypervascularity, fatty marrow replacement, and residual hematopoietic marrow. In the early stages of the disease, the marrow signal may be normal. In the lytic phase and also in the delayed phase, there is disproportionately higher marrow fat content when compared to the adjacent vertebrae. In the mixed phase, there is variable loss of the normal fatty marrow signal due to replacement by vascular tissue and increased water and cellular content. As a result, the marrow will return a heterogenous low T1 and a heterogenous high signal on the fluid-sensitive sequences. In the sclerotic phase, due to trabecular sclerosis and fibrosis, there will be low signal on all sequences.

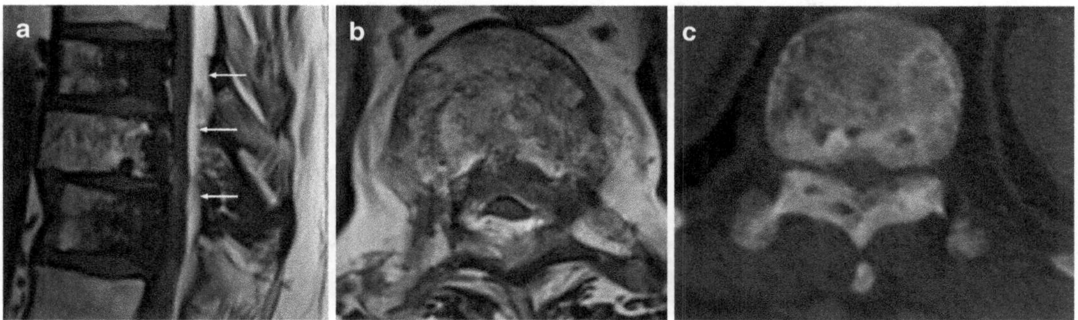

Fig. 9 (**a**) Sagittal T1-WI and (**b**) axial T2-WI MRI of the thoracic spine. Note the trabecular thickening and sclerotic changes in T9, T10, and T11 vertebrae. Note the anteroposterior expansion of T10 with involvement of the spinous processes in all three levels. Axial images demonstrate narrowing of the spinal canal and effacement of CSF due to osseous expansion of the posterior vertebral body. There is fat signal in the posterior epidural space. (**c**) CT would be helpful to assess whether this is due to marrow fat from the expanded neural arch or normal epidural fat. In this case, it was due to anterior expansion of the neural arch as demonstrated in the axial CT

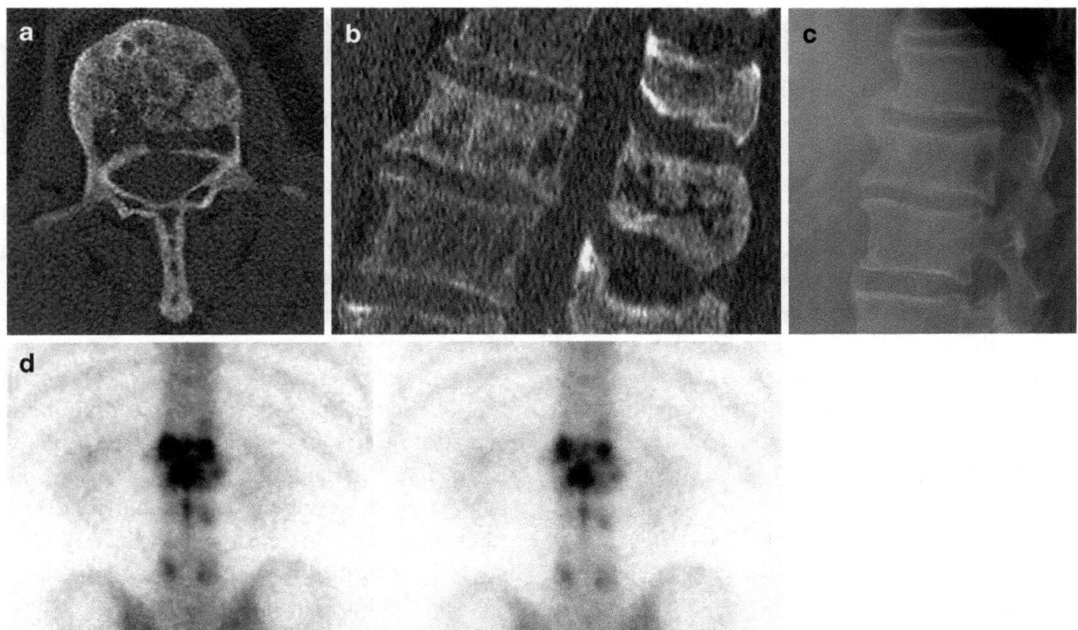

Fig. 10 (**a**) Axial and (**b**) sagittal CT, (**c**) lateral CR, and (**d**) bone scan images of L1. Note the expansion, trabecular coarsening, and thickening of the cortices of L1 vertebra. Note the expansion of the spinous process. Some intervening lucencies. Appearances are entirely in keeping with Paget's disease. Also note the anteroposterior expansion of the L1 vertebra. Bone scan demonstrates increased uptake in the Pagetic L1 vertebral body

Nuclear medicine studies will help assess the metabolic activity and extent of the disease. If a solitary lesion is detected, scintigraphy is better than whole-body MRI in detecting multifocal disease since the changes on MRI are usually very subtle and can be easily overlooked. Increased osteoblastic activity will result in increased tracer uptake on scintigraphy (Fig. 10). However, this is usually nonspecific. Depicting osseous expansion can increase confidence with the diagnosis. During the delayed dormant phase, there may not be any tracer uptake, which may be an important diagnostic marker. In the lytic phase, there may not be significant osteoblastic activity to result in increased tracer uptake (Fig. 10). PET will add the ability for better anatomic assessment in addition to metabolic status.

8 Complications

8.1 Spinal Stenosis

Spinal stenosis is seen in 33% of cases of PDB of the spine (Hadjipavlou et al. 2001). It commonly affects the lumbar spine, usually single level, less so in the thoracic spine, and rarely in the cervical spine (Saifuddin and Hassan 2003). This is not surprising given the anatomic distribution of PDB in the spine. However, it is more likely to cause neurologic dysfunction in the thoracic spine followed by the cervical spine and least so in the lumbar spine due to the relatively capacious spinal canal in the lumbar spine (Hartman and Dohn 1966; Klenerman 1966; Hadjipavlou et al. 2001). Spinal stenosis is multifactorial in PDB. It could be due to osseous expansion (complete vertebral body and neural arch, isolated vertebral body, or isolated neural arch), fact joint osteoarthritis, disk degeneration, ligamentous ossification, spondylolisthesis, fracture retropulsion, and rarely extramedullary hematopoiesis (Lalam et al. 2016). Spinal stenosis may be symptomatic in up to 33% of cases presenting with back/leg pain and/or neurological dysfunction (Hadjipavlou et al. 2001). It is important to recognize, as is the case with degenerative disk disease, that the degree of spinal stenosis does not necessarily correlate with the clinical picture. Indeed, patients with severe spinal stenosis may be asymptomatic. This is thought to be due to the chronic nature of the disease and adaptivity of the thecal sac and its neural elements (Hadjipavlou et al. 1986, 2001). Occasionally, neural dysfunction can be seen in patients with no significant spinal stenosis. This is thought to be due to "arterial steal," where the preferential blood flow to the Pagetic vertebra deprives the spinal cord from its blood supply (Herzberg and Bayliss 1980). This may respond to medical treatment with calcitonin (Douglas et al. 1980).

CT would be the best modality to assess the osseous component contributing to the central spinal canal and/or foraminal narrowing. It will also assess the degree of facet joint arthropathy. MRI is essential in assessing myelomalacia and neural compromise (Fig. 9).

8.2 Fractures

Pagetic bone is structurally weak despite the sclerotic changes due to the weakened osseous architecture from repetitive remodeling attempts. In the spine, these can be compression fractures of the vertebral body, which is the most common complication of PD in the spine, or posterior element fractures including spondylolysis (Dell'Atti et al. 2007; Lalam et al. 2016).

Compression fractures are most common in the lumbar spine, and rarely in the sacrum, coccyx, and odontoid peg (Fig. 11) (Boutin et al. 1998; Dell'Atti et al. 2007). Rarely, pathological collapse of a Pagetic vertebra could be due to long-term therapy with disodium etidronate, which inhibits mineralization (MacGowan et al. 2000).

Compression fractures present as sudden onset of back pain. Paravertebral swelling in the context of this history should raise the suspicion of a fracture. On radiographs, the fractured vertebra may appear osteolytic. This is unlikely to represent the lytic phase of PDB since this is unusually seen in the spine. It is more likely to represent fracture-induced osteolysis. CT is best in demonstrating the fracture line. It is also useful in assessing posterior bulging of vertebral body wall and whether there might be retropulsion of an osseous fragment into the spinal canal, both of which can cause neural compression. On MRI, the fracture line will demonstrate a low signal on the T1-weighted images and high signal on the fluid-sensitive sequences in the acute phase with associated marrow edema and/or paravertebral soft tissue swelling. However, in the subacute and delayed stages, the fracture line will demon-

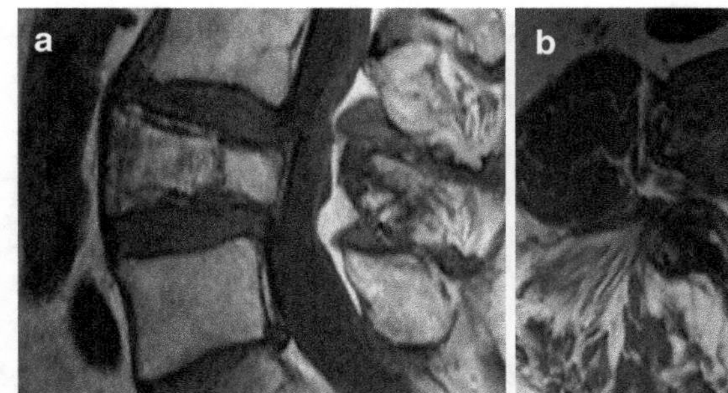

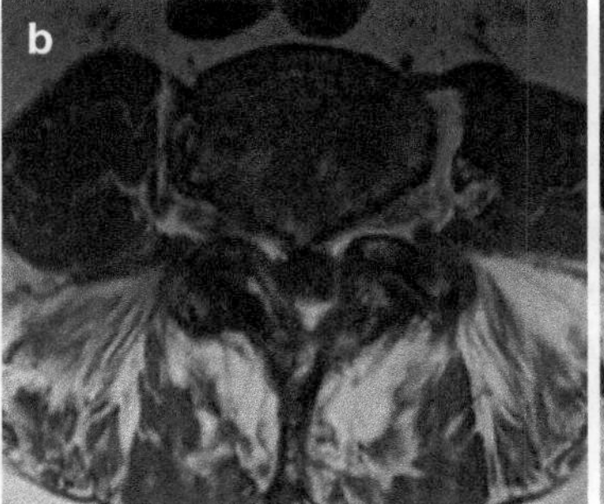

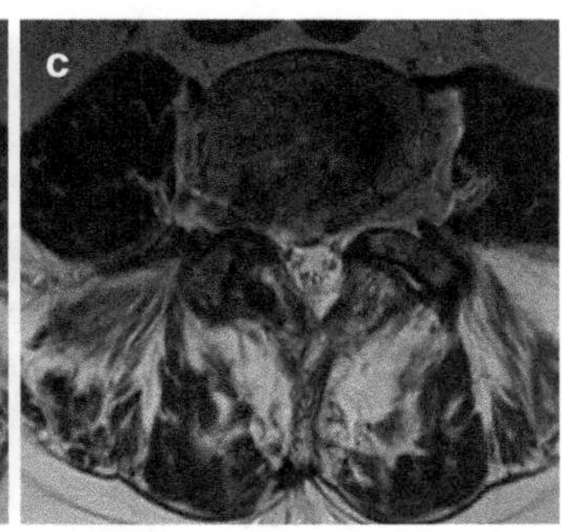

Fig. 11 (**a**) Sagittal T1 and (**b**) axial T1-WI and (**c**) T2-WI demonstrating Paget's disease in L4 vertebra with an old compression fracture. Note the expansion, coarsened trabeculae, and thickened cortices. Note the maintained normal fatty marrow signal. The axial images demonstrate narrowing of the spinal canal due to the osseous expansion and marked facet joint degeneration

strate low signal on all sequences. MRI is also useful in confirming and quantifying the degree of neural compromise. It can also be useful in differentiating between benign and malignant fractures utilizing chemical shift imaging.

8.3 Facet Joint Arthropathy

Facet joint arthropathy in PDB is secondary either to direct extension of Paget's disease into the articular cartilage or to expansion of the subchondral facet bone leading to incongruity with the opposing uninvolved facet. These changes will result in mechanical stresses and secondary degenerative changes, which may be underestimated on MRI and better depicted on CT (Zlatkin et al. 1986; Hadjipavlou et al. 2001).

Facet joint arthropathy can result in back pain characterized by pain and stiffness worst at rest and relieved by activity, which is different in nature to pain from PDB, which is usually nonmechanical dull deep-seated pain unrelated to activity (Lalam et al. 2016). Expansion of the facet joints secondary to PDB may result in lateral recess stenosis and neural compression giving rise to radicular symptoms; however, they can be asymptomatic despite the stenotic changes seen on imaging, and hence, clinical correlation is paramount (Fig. 11).

8.4 Spondylolisthesis

Spondylolisthesis in spinal PDB is either lytic or degenerative. The involved pars interarticularis is weak due to repeated remodeling and hence susceptible to insufficiency fractures. While degenerative spondylolisthesis results in spinal stenosis, spondylolytic spondylolisthesis results in widening of the spinal canal but narrowing of the neural foramina, potentially resulting in compromise of the exiting nerve roots.

Spondylolisthesis can be difficult to assess on radiographs. Anterior expansion of a Pagetic vertebral body will give a false impression of anterior slippage, while a genuinely anteriorly slipped expanded Pagetic vertebra may be overlooked due to normal alignment of the posterior vertebral body border. Pars defects may also be challenging to appreciate on radiographs. CT with sagittal reformats is the best modality in assessing for vertebral displacement and pars defects (Fig. 6).

8.5 Intervertebral Disk Involvement

Intervertebral disk degeneration in PDB may be caused by mechanical stress secondary to asymmetry at the end-plate attachment of the annulus fibrosus between a Pagetic and a normal vertebra, direct invasion of the intervertebral disk by PDB, or altered disk nutrition secondary to Pagetic involvement of the end plate (Dell'Atti et al. 2007; Beaudouin et al. 2014).

Disk involvement is more common in the lumbar spine than in the thoracic and cervical spine.

8.6 Vertebral Ankylosis

Ankylosis is the end stage of facet joint arthropathy and extension of PDB into the adjacent vertebra either by direct intervertebral disk transgression or through preexisting osteophytes. Lander et al. reported a 10.7% incidence of direct intradiscal transgression (Lander and Hadjipavlou 1991). Additionally, ossification of the spinal ligaments and paravertebral soft tissues may play a role (Dell'Atti et al. 2007).

Ankylosis has an incidence of 4.4% (Lander and Hadjipavlou 1991). It is more common in males and more common in the thoracic spine, which is involved in over 50% of cases (Marcelli et al. 1995).

8.7 Neoplasia

Pagetic bone has increased risk of sarcomatous transformation. In the spine, this is very rare (0.7%) (Hadjipavlou et al. 1986, 1988, 2001; Saifuddin and Hassan 2003). The risk increases with advancing age, longer disease duration, and more extensive involvement. The risk in elderly patients with long-standing extensive disease can increase to >10% (Lalam et al. 2016). The majority are osteosarcomatous transformation due to genetic changes on chromosome 18q (Baslé et al. 1987; Nellissery et al. 1998; Hadjipavlou et al. 2001).

However, as is the pattern with the disease prevalence, the proportion of Paget's disease patients with sarcoma has reduced. Mangham et al. showed that Pagetic sarcoma fell from 23% to 8% of primary bone sarcoma referrals in patients aged over 50 years between the decades 1986–1995 and 1996–2005. In their study of 32 patients with unequivocal Pagetic sarcoma, there was known preexisting Paget's disease in 42%. The disease was monostotic in 46% of the sample. It is therefore possible that Pagetic sarcoma could be the first presentation of PDB in a patient with monostotic disease who was previously undiagnosed of having PDB (Mangham et al. 2009).

Chondrosarcoma has been diagnosed in some cases, which may in fact represent chondroblastic osteosarcomas (Tilden and Saifuddin 2021).

Giant cell tumor (GCT) has also been reported in Paget's disease. This probably has a genetic predisposition as Rendina et al. reported a series of four cases from the same family from Southern Italy with polyostotic Paget's disease, two of which had multifocal GCT (Rendina et al. 2004). These tumors may respond to steroid therapy (Shaker 2009).

There have been two opinions regarding the affinity of Pagetic bone to develop metastases. Some authors support this claiming that the hypervascularity in PDB will increase the risk of metastatic deposits, while other authors believe that actually, Pagetic bone is less hospitable to metastatic implantation and hence has less risk of harboring metastases (Lalam et al. 2016). In either case, it is important to recognize associated metastatic deposits in Pagetic bone.

Radiologically, both on plan radiographs and on CT, the presence of a lytic lesion with aggressive features such as wide zone of transition, periosteal reaction, cortical destruction, and extra-osseous soft tissue should raise the suspicion of malignant transformation. Of course, these can be seen in other pathologies such as fractures and infection. The presence of extra-osseous soft tissue adjacent to a Pagetic bone does not necessarily imply malignancy since it may represent a hematoma next to a fracture, extra-osseous Paget's disease, pseudosarcoma, or extramedullary hematopoiesis. Presence of fat signal on T1-weighted MRI would exclude malignant transformation since malignancy and infiltrative processes would replace normal marrow fat (Figs. 12 and 13).

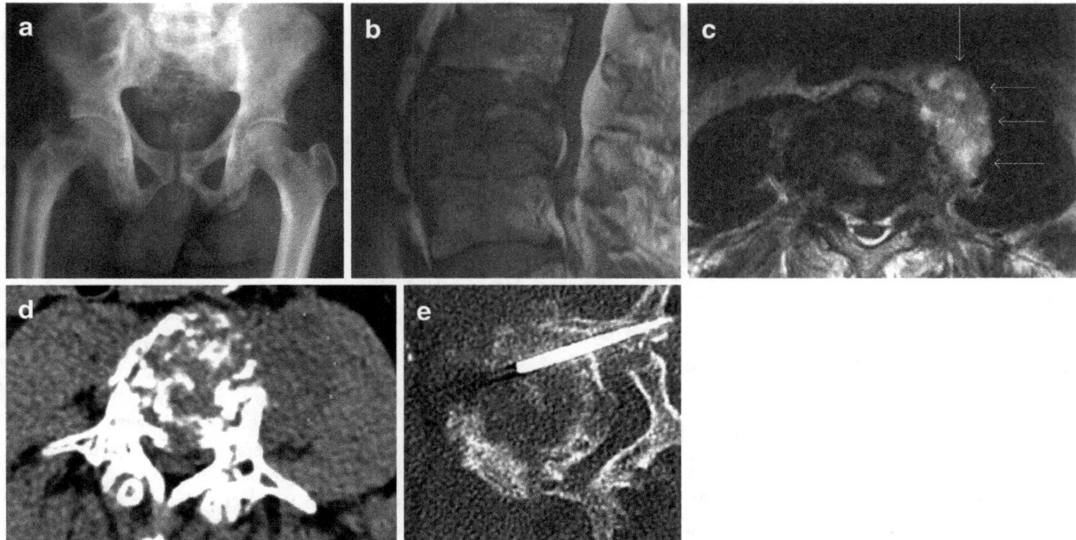

Fig. 12 (**a**) CR pelvis, (**b**) sagittal T1-WI lumbar spine, and (**c**) axial T2-WI and (**d**) axial CT through L3 vertebra. This 75-year-old male has extensive Paget's disease of the pelvis, spine, and proximal right femur. Plain radiograph of the pelvis demonstrates the typical features of bone expansion, trabecular coarsening, and cortical thickening in the pelvis, proximal right femur, and lumbosacral spine. MRI shows diffuse spinal involvement with multilevel vertebral body expansion and trabecular coarsening. Note the compression of the L3 vertebra with near-complete loss of the normal fatty marrow signal. This is concerning for edema secondary to a fracture or infiltration by tumor. Axial T2-WI through L3 demonstrates a large heterogenous extra-osseous soft tissue mass invading the left psoas muscle (arrows). Axial CT images in (**d**) soft tissue window demonstrate the cortical destruction on the left anterolateral aspect of the L3 vertebral body with an extra-osseous soft tissue component, the margin of which is highlighted by the asterisks. (**e**) CT-guided biopsy performed, which proved Pagetic sarcomatous change

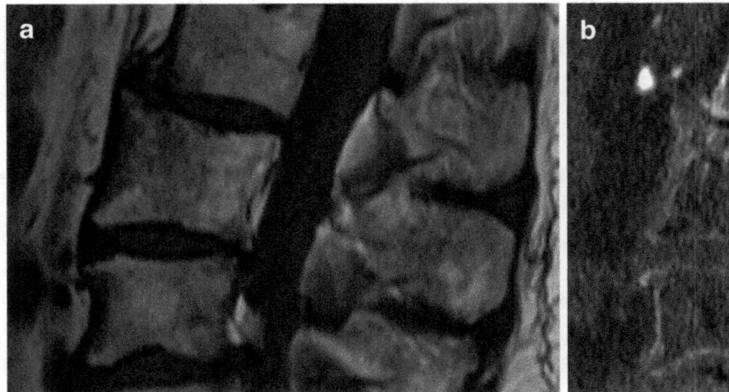

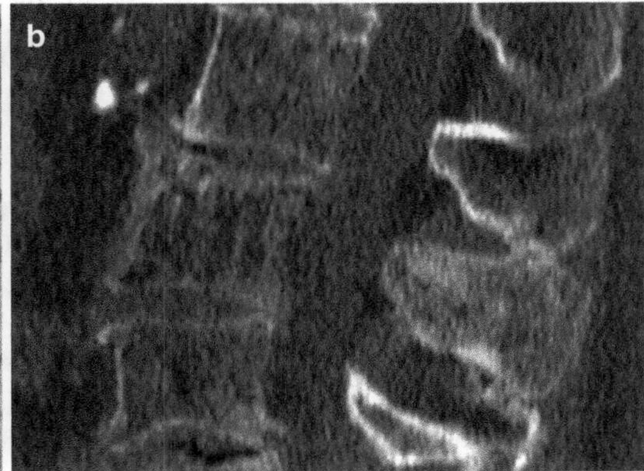

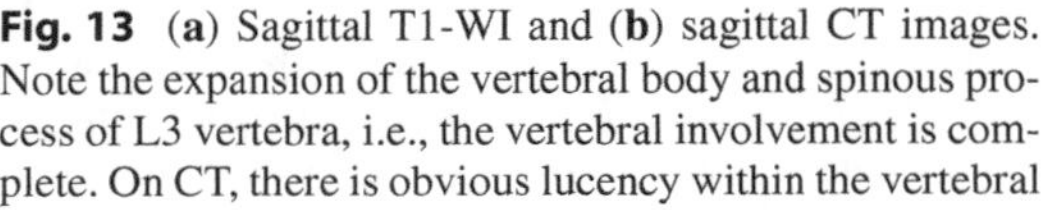

Fig. 13 (**a**) Sagittal T1-WI and (**b**) sagittal CT images. Note the expansion of the vertebral body and spinous process of L3 vertebra, i.e., the vertebral involvement is complete. On CT, there is obvious lucency within the vertebral body, which may be concerning for the interpreting radiologist or clinician. However, note the normal marrow signal within the vertebral body on the T1-WI. Appearances are of the osteolytic phase of the disease

Pseudosarcomatous lesions are unmineralized periosteal new bone formation. Despite being extremely rare, they can be confused with neoplasia like periosteal osteosarcoma. Pseudosarcoma has similar signal characteristics to normal fatty marrow (McNairn et al. 2001; Tins et al. 2001). Therefore, it can be confused with periosteal osteosarcoma. However, important distinguishing points are as follows: (1) Pagetic osteosarcoma as well as metastases are central within the affected bone and (2) periosteal osteosarcoma is not the usual type of sarcoma occurring in PDB (Lalam et al. 2016).

Extramedullary hematopoiesis is seen as paraspinal soft tissue lesions, which have similar density/signal to the normal adjacent marrow, which it usually communicates with (Relea et al. 1999).

9 Conclusion

Paget's disease of the spine is becoming less common, milder, and less extensive and affecting older population. Appearances may be very subtle on imaging particularly on radiography and MRI. Knowledge of the distribution, imaging features, and complications will aid the radiologist in achieving the correct diagnosis. CT is the best modality in assessing subtle expansion and trabecular thickening.

10 Key Points

- The prevalence, severity, and extent of PDB are reducing.
- Vertebral involvement in PDB is complete, i.e., anterior and posterior elements.
- Vertebral expansion is in the AP and transverse dimensions.
- The initial osteolytic phase of PDB is rarely seen in the vertebra. If encountered, preservation of the normal fatty marrow T1 signal on MRI is essential to differentiate it from other pathological causes of lysis.
- PDB may result in spinal stenosis, neurological compromise, fractures, degeneration, and malignant transformation.

Acknowledgments The authors would like to thank the Medical Photography Department in the Robert Jones and Agnes Hunt Orthopaedic Hospital, Oswestry, UK.

References

Al-Rashid M et al (2015) Paget disease of bone. Orthop Clin N Am 46:577. https://doi.org/10.1016/j.ocl.2015.06.008

Altman RD (2002) Epidemiology of Paget's disease of bone. Clin Rev Bone Miner Metab 1:099. https://doi.org/10.1385/bmm:1:2:099

Barker DJP et al (1980) Paget's disease of bone: the Lancashire focus. Br Med J 280:1105. https://doi.org/10.1136/bmj.280.6222.1105

Baslé MF et al (1987) On the trail of paramyxoviruses in Paget's disease of bone. Clin Orthop Relat Res 217:9–15. https://doi.org/10.1097/00003086-198704000-00003

Bastin S et al (2009) Paget's disease of bone—becoming a rarity? Rheumatology (Oxford, England). https://doi.org/10.1093/rheumatology/kep212

Beaudouin C et al (2014) Atypical vertebral Paget's disease. Skelet Radiol 43:991. https://doi.org/10.1007/s00256-013-1799-9

Boutin RD et al (1998) Complications in Paget disease at MR imaging. Radiology 209:641. https://doi.org/10.1148/radiology.209.3.9844654

Brown HP, LaRocca H, Wickstrom JK (1971) Paget's disease of the atlas and axis. J Bone Joint Surg Am 53:1441. https://doi.org/10.2106/00004623-197153070-00024

Clarke PRR, Williams HI (1975) Ossification in extradural fat in Paget's disease of the spine. Br J Surg 62:571. https://doi.org/10.1002/bjs.1800620717

Cundy T (2007) Is the prevalence of Paget's disease of bone decreasing? J Bone Miner Res 22(Suppl 2):P9. https://doi.org/10.1359/JBMR.06S202

Cundy T, Bolland M (2008) Paget disease of bone. Trends Endocrinol Metab 19:246. https://doi.org/10.1016/j.tem.2008.06.001

Dell'Atti C et al (2007) The spine in Paget's disease. Skelet Radiol 36:609. https://doi.org/10.1007/s00256-006-0270-6

Douglas DL et al (1980) Biochemical and clinical responses to dichloromethylene diphosphonate (cl2mdp) in Paget's disease of bone. Arthritis Rheum 23:1185. https://doi.org/10.1002/art.1780231017

Friedrichs WE et al (2002) Sequence analysis of measles virus nucleocapsid transcripts in patients with Paget's disease. J Bone Miner Res 17:145. https://doi.org/10.1359/jbmr.2002.17.1.145

Guyer PB, Shepherd DFC (1980) Paget's disease of the lumbar spine. Br J Radiol 53:286. https://doi.org/10.1259/0007-1285-53-628-286

Hadjipavlou A, Lander P (1991) Paget disease of the spine. J Bone Joint Surg A 73:1376. https://doi.org/10.2106/00004623-199173090-00013

Hadjipavlou A, Lander P, Srolovitz H (1986) Pagetic arthritis: pathophysiology and management. Clin Orthop Relat Res 208:15–19

Hadjipavlou A et al (1988) Pagetic spinal stenosis with extradural pagetoid ossification: a case report. Spine 13:128. https://doi.org/10.1097/00007632-198801000-00034

Hadjipavlou AG et al (2001) Paget's disease of the spine and its management. Eur Spine J 10(5):370–384. https://doi.org/10.1007/s005860100329

Hartman JT, Dohn DF (1966) Paget's disease of the spine with cord or nerve-root compression. J Bone Joint Surg Am 48:1079. https://doi.org/10.2106/00004623-196648060-00005

Hepple S, Getty JM, Douglas DL (1998) Paget's disease and odontoid peg fracture: a case report. Injury 29:323. https://doi.org/10.1016/S0020-1383(98)80216-7

Herzberg L, Bayliss E (1980) Spinal-cord syndrome due to non-compressive Paget's disease of bone: a spinal-artery steal phenomenon reversible with calcitonin. Lancet 316:13. https://doi.org/10.1016/S0140-6736(80)92891-3

Klenerman L (1966) Cauda equina and spinal cord compression in Paget's disease. J Bone Joint Surg Br 48-B: 365. https://doi.org/10.1302/0301-620x.48b2.365

Koziarz P, Avruch L (2002) Spinal epidural lipomatosis associated with Paget's disease of bone. Neuroradiology 44:858. https://doi.org/10.1007/s00234-002-0822-y

Lalam RK, Cassar-Pullicino VN, Winn N (2016) Paget disease of bone. Semin Musculoskelet Radiol 20:287. https://doi.org/10.1055/s-0036-1592368

Lander P, Hadjipavlou A (1991) Intradiscal invasion of Paget's disease of the spine. Spine 16:46

Langston AL, Ralston SH (2004) Management of Paget's disease of bone. Rheumatology 43(8):955–959. https://doi.org/10.1093/rheumatology/keh243

Layfield R (2007) The molecular pathogenesis of Paget disease of bone. Expert Rev Mol Med 9:1. https://doi.org/10.1017/S1462399407000464

Lucas GJA et al (2008) Identification of a major locus for Paget's disease on chromosome 10p13 in families of British descent. J Bone Miner Res 23:58. https://doi.org/10.1359/jbmr.071004

MacGowan JR et al (2000) Gross vertebral collapse associated with long-term disodium etidronate treatment for pelvic Paget's disease. Skelet Radiol 29:279. https://doi.org/10.1007/s002560050608

Mangham DC, Davie MW, Grimer RJ (2009) Sarcoma arising in Paget's disease of bone: declining incidence and increasing age at presentation. Bone 44:431. https://doi.org/10.1016/j.bone.2008.11.002

Marcelli C et al (1995) Pagetic vertebral ankylosis and diffuse idiopathic skeletal hyperostosis. Spine 20:454. https://doi.org/10.1097/00007632-199502001-00008

Matthews BG et al (2008) Failure to detect measles virus ribonucleic acid in bone cells from patients with Paget's disease. J Clin Endocrinol Metab 93:1398. https://doi.org/10.1210/jc.2007-1978

Mays S (2010) Archaeological skeletons support a northwest European origin for Paget's disease of bone. J Bone Miner Res 25(8):1839–1841. https://doi.org/10.1002/jbmr.64

McNairn JDK et al (2001) Benign tumefactive soft tissue extension from Paget's disease of bone simulating malignancy. Skelet Radiol 30:157. https://doi.org/10.1007/s002560000313

Mee AP et al (1998) Detection of canine distemper virus in 100% of Paget's disease samples by in situ-reverse transcriptase-polymerase chain reaction. Bone 23:171. https://doi.org/10.1016/S8756-3282(98)00079-9

Naiken VS (1971) Did Beethoven have Paget's disease of bone? Ann Intern Med 74:995. https://doi.org/10.7326/0003-4819-74-6-995

Nebot Valenzuela E, Pietschmann P (2017) Epidemiologie und Pathologie des Morbus Paget—ein Überblick. Wien Med Wochenschr 167(1–2):2–8. https://doi.org/10.1007/s10354-016-0496-4

Nellissery MJ et al (1998) Evidence for a novel osteosarcoma tumor-suppressor gene in the chromosome 18 region genetically linked with Paget disease of bone. Am J Hum Genet 63:817. https://doi.org/10.1086/302019

Paget J (1877) On a form of chronic inflammation of bones (osteitis deformans). J R Soc Med MCT-60:37. https://doi.org/10.1177/095952877706000105

Pestka JM et al (2012) Paget disease of the spine: an evaluation of 101 patients with a histomorphometric analysis of 29 cases. Eur Spine J 21(5):999–1006. https://doi.org/10.1007/s00586-011-2133-7

Relea A et al (1999) Extramedullary hematopoiesis related to Paget's disease. Eur Radiol 9:205. https://doi.org/10.1007/s003300050656

Rendina D et al (2004) Giant cell tumor and Paget's disease of bone in one family: geographic clustering. Clin Orthop Relat Res 421:218. https://doi.org/10.1097/00000118702.46373.e3

Rosen MA, Wesolowski DP, Herkowitz HN (1988) Osteolytic monostotic paget's disease of the axis: a case report. Spine 13:125. https://doi.org/10.1097/00007632-198801000-00033

Saifuddin A, Hassan A (2003) Paget's disease of the spine: unusual features and complications. Clin Radiol 58(2):102–111. https://doi.org/10.1053/crad.2002.1152

Schmorl G (1932) Über Ostitis deformans Paget. Virchows Arch Pathol Anat Physiol Klin Med 283:694. https://doi.org/10.1007/BF01887990

Shaker JL (2009) Paget's disease of bone: a review of epidemiology, pathophysiology and management. Therap Adv Musculoskelet Dis 1(2):107–125. https://doi.org/10.1177/1759720X09351779

Steinbach LS, Johnston JO (1993) Case report 777. Skelet Radiol 22. https://doi.org/10.1007/BF00206156

Sundaram M, Khanna G, El-Khoury GY (2001) T1-weighted MR imaging for distinguishing large osteolysis of Paget's disease from sarcomatous degeneration. Skelet Radiol 30:378. https://doi.org/10.1007/s002560100360

Theodorou DJ, Theodorou SJ, Kakitsubata Y (2011) Imaging of Paget disease of bone and its musculoskeletal complications: review. Am J Roentgenol 196:S64. https://doi.org/10.2214/AJR.10.7222

Tilden W, Saifuddin A (2021) An update on imaging of Paget's sarcoma. Skelet Radiol 50(7):1275–1290. https://doi.org/10.1007/s00256-020-03682-8

Tins BJ, Davies AM, Mangham DC (2001) MR imaging of pseudosarcoma in Paget's disease of bone: a report of two cases. Skelet Radiol 30:161. https://doi.org/10.1007/s002560000314

Vande Berg BC et al (2001) Magnetic resonance appearance of uncomplicated Paget's disease of bone. Semin Musculoskelet Radiol 5:69. https://doi.org/10.1055/s-2001-12919

Whitehouse RW (2002) Paget's disease of bone. Semin Musculoskelet Radiol 6:313. https://doi.org/10.1055/s-2002-36730

Zlatkin MB et al (1986) Paget disease of the spine: CT with clinical correlation. Radiology 160:155. https://doi.org/10.1148/radiology.160.1.2940618

Other Pseudotumoral Lesions of the Spine

Joan C. Vilanova, José Martel, and Cristina Vilanova

Contents

J. C. Vilanova (✉)
Department of Radiology, Clínica Girona, Institute of Diagnostic Imaging (IDI) Girona, University of Girona, Girona, Spain
e-mail: kvilanova@comg.cat

J. Martel
Department of Radiology, Hospital Universitario Fundación Alcorcón, Alcorcón (Madrid), Spain

C. Vilanova
Department of Orthopaedic Surgery, Hospital Germans Trias i Pujol, Badalona (Barcelona), Spain

Med Radiol Diagn Imaging (2023)
https://doi.org/10.1007/174_2023_436,
Published Online: 19 May 2023

Abstract

A wide variety of benign nonneoplastic bone lesions in the spine may mimic benign and malignant bone tumors. These lesions are often incidentally discovered but may also be symptomatic and diagnosed after focused imaging evaluation for pain or other symptoms. Some of these lesions (e.g., normal variants or developmental abnormalities) require no further workup once recognized. Other skeletal processes, such as stress fractures or osteomyelitis, may require semi-urgent management to prevent complication. Some osseous abnormalities may be the first indication of a more serious systemic process that warrants further evaluation and treatment. Familiarity with the spectrum of imaging features of these lesions is necessary to direct appropriate workup and management and, importantly, to avoid unnecessary tests and procedures that might result in patient morbidity. This chapter reviews the imaging characteristics and differentiating imaging features on different modalities especially including conventional radiography, computed tomography (CT), magnetic resonance imaging (MRI), and nuclear medicine of nonneoplastic lesions that could be seen in everyday practice. In most instances, the clinical history will be important in determining the true nature of the lesion.

1 Introduction

Focal lesions in spine are very common and are frequently encountered on routine imaging studies. While some lesions are true neoplasms, a number of these osseous abnormalities are not tumors. These lesions can include normal variants, congenital abnormalities, traumatic lesions, metabolic/inflammatory changes, idiopathic changes, or infection. It is important for the radiologist and clinician to be aware of this possibility and to identify the characteristic features allowing discrimination between bone tumors and bone tumor mimickers. Subjecting the patient to an inappropriate workup can lead to misdiagnosis, poor management, and anxiety for both the patient and physician. In many instances, these tumor mimickers can be left alone and no treatment is necessary; however, in other cases, they can indicate a significant disease process. However, many lesions that occur in the spine are not true tumors and may be mistaken for a neoplasm, leading to the wrong diagnosis and inappropriate treatment (Abdel Razek and Castillo 2010). A sound understanding of the appearance of bone tumor mimics and their characteristic radiologic features is essential for optimizing diagnostic accuracy. In most instances, the clinical history will be important in determining the true nature of the lesion. We will review their epidemiology, clinical presentation, anatomic distribution, differential considerations, and management. Emphasis will be placed on the imaging characteristics and differentiating imaging features, which will include findings seen on modalities to include conventional radiography, computed tomography (CT), magnetic resonance imaging (MRI), and nuclear medicine.

2 Normal Variants

2.1 Red Marrow

Erythropoietic or red marrow can be a common cause for concern on MRI. This can be particularly problematic if the area of red marrow is mass-like in appearance. Red marrow should be hyperintense to fatty marrow on fat-suppressed T2-weighted (T2W) MRI sequences and hypointense on T1-weighted (T1W) MRI sequences. The key feature is that the low signal intensity on T1W MRI sequences should be higher than that of skeletal muscle or the intervertebral disks. Chemical shift imaging with in-phase and opposed-phase T1W MRI images can be helpful in equivocal cases as red marrow should have some intermixed fatty marrow (intra-voxel fat) and, consequently, should lose signal (become darker) on out-of-phase compared to in-phase MRI (Fig. 1) (Vilanova et al. 2016). On the other hand, marrow-replacing tumors, such as many

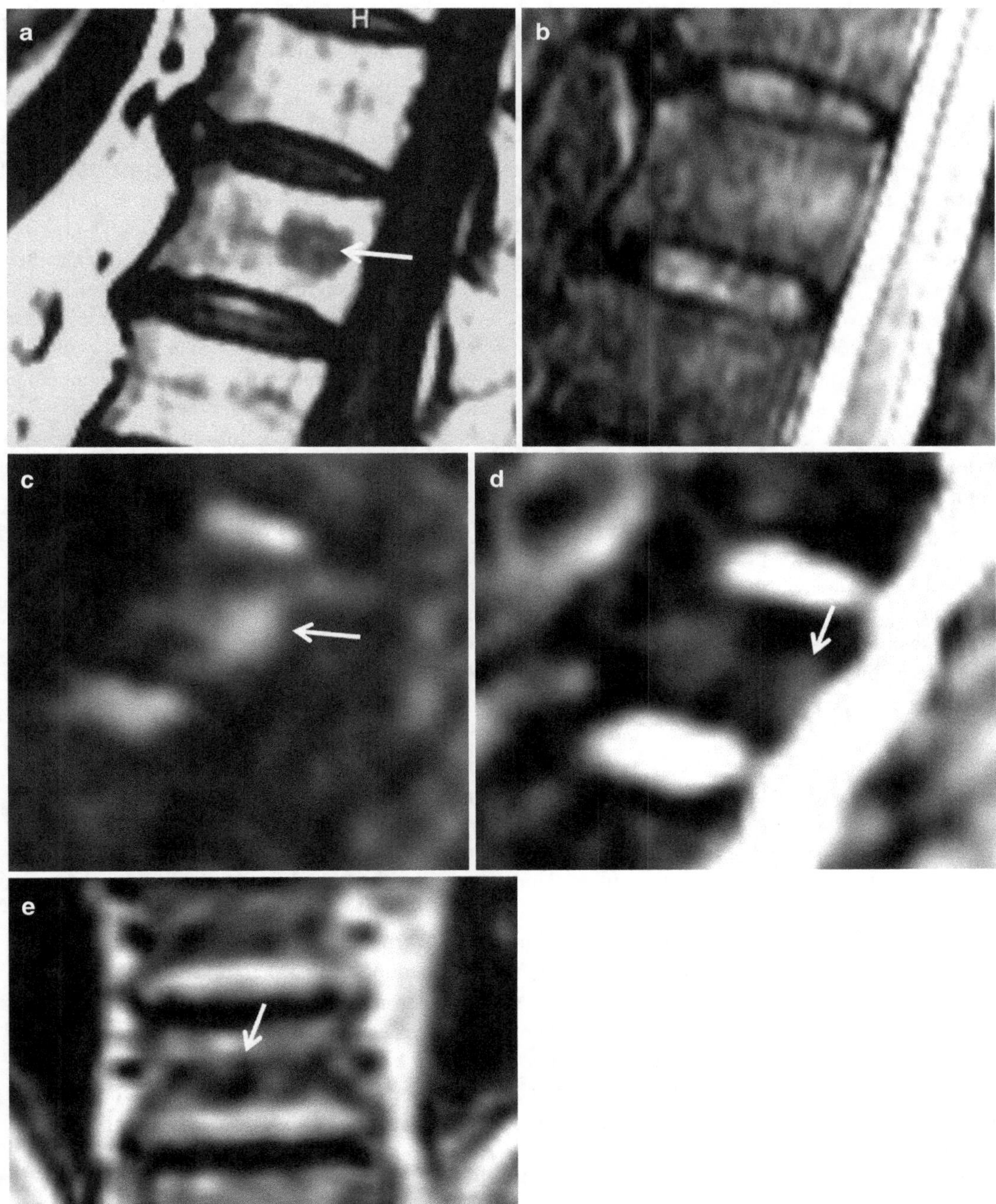

Fig. 1 Incidental focal red marrow on a 59-year-old female with breast cancer suffering from back pain. (**a**) Sagittal TSE T1W showing nodular lesion in the vertebral body with slightly higher signal than the disk and the "bull's-eye" sign, the presence of fat within a lesion (arrow). (**b**) The corresponding sagittal STIR image shows ill-defined high signal. (**c**) Sagittal DWI at b = 800 mm²/s shows the high signal of the lesion with high signal on ADC map (**d**). (**e**) The coronal opposed-phase image shows the decreased signal due to normal red bone marrow with microscopic intra-voxel fat

metastases, should replace all the fatty marrow and should not lose signal on out-of-phase T1W imaging (Broski et al. 2022). The “bull's-eye” sign is a specific feature to demonstrate the presence of fat within a lesion and exclude metastases (Fig. 1) (Schweitzer et al. 1993). The signal intensity ratio (SIR) of the marrow on the opposed-phase image to the in-phase can be calculated, creating a region of interest (ROI). It has been shown that using an SIR greater than 0.8 is suggestive of malignant process and an SIR less than 0.8 is typical of nonmalignant processes. Additionally, a signal dropout <20% on out-of-phase images is accurate to consider malignancy (Martel Villagrán et al. 2015). It is important to remember that the voxel of interest must contain both lipid and water; hence, a benign tumor such as a lipoma may show no decrease in signal intensity in opposed-phase images compared with in-phase images, even though the neoplasm is benign. Modern MR magnets can combine the in-phase and out-of-phase images with water-only (fat-suppressed image) and fat-only images, resulting in the Dixon method. The current Dixon-type sequences produce four sets of images: water only, fat only, in phase, and out of phase. The fat-only images offer the potential for fat quantification (Berglund et al. 2010). The utility of the technique is likely greater for distinguishing a true marrow replacing tumor from other processes such as edema or hematopoietic marrow than for strictly distinguishing benign and malignant bone tumor. Recognizing red marrow may pose a challenge in cases where there is marked diffuse red marrow hyperplasia, or where there is focal heterogeneity mimicking an osseous neoplasm. In both cases, T1W imaging and chemical shift sequences are useful in the differentiation.

Red marrow reconversion in adults may result from a variety of nonneoplastic conditions, including medications, smoking, anemia, and exercise. Red marrow reconversion occurs in the reverse pattern of normal regression, with increased marrow elements most often occurring first in the axial skeleton and metaphyses of long bones. Red marrow reconversion is most notable on positron emission tomography/computed tomography (PET/CT) and MR imaging. On PET/CT, this typically manifests as increased bone marrow metabolic activity.

3 Congenital/Developmental Abnormalities

Congenital vertebral deformities can be classified as defects of segmentation or defects of formation; however, a mixture of both is most common (McMaster 1984). Defects of formation include hemivertebrae, anteriorly wedged, congenital defects, and butterfly vertebrae, while defects of segmentation include unsegmented bars and block. Absence of a pedicle may be a result from neoplasm, infection, or congenital aplasia/hypoplasia. The winking owl sign occurs on AP radiographs of the spine when a pedicle is absent (Fig. 2). On a normal study, two pedicles seen end-on appear as round eyes and the spinous process represents the beak. When one pedicle is absent, one eye appears closed and the owl can be interpreted as “winking.” Differential diagnosis should also include congenital absence of pedicle, which is usually associated with hypoplastic/agenetic ipsilateral and hyperplastic contralateral pedicles, besides the neoplasm origin. “Butterfly vertebra,” also known as vertebral sagittal cleft, anterior rachischisis, and somatoschysis, is an uncommon congenital anomaly of the spine. It results from the failure of fusion of the lateral halves of the vertebral body because of persistent notochordal tissue between them forming a cleft in the center. On frontal X-ray, the two half-vertebrae resemble the wings of a butterfly while the processus spinosus represents the butterfly body. The widespread use of CT and MRI for imaging spinal disorders has led to a decrease in the use of radiography as the first imaging modality in many clinical settings, providing atypical appearances on CT or MRI (Fig. 3). The atypical appearance of the trapezoidal or anterior cuneiform morphology may be confused with osteoporotic vertebral collapse or other pathological vertebral fractures, including traumatic, infectious, or metastatic collapse (Ruiz Santiago et al. 2022).

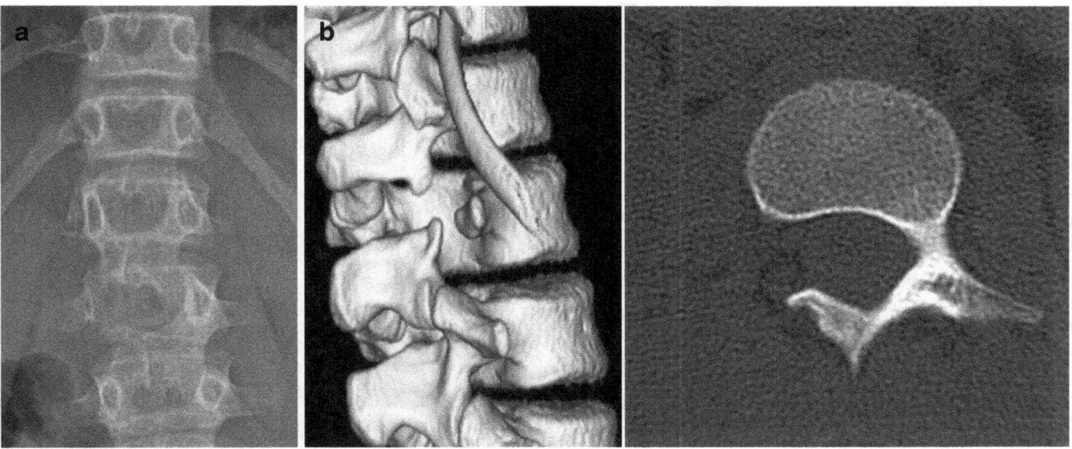

Fig. 2 Plain film of the lumbar spine. (**a**) In the AP view, we can appreciate that the right pedicle in L2 is absent. This sign is also called the winking owl sign. (**b**) Computed tomography demonstrates the congenital absence of the pedicle

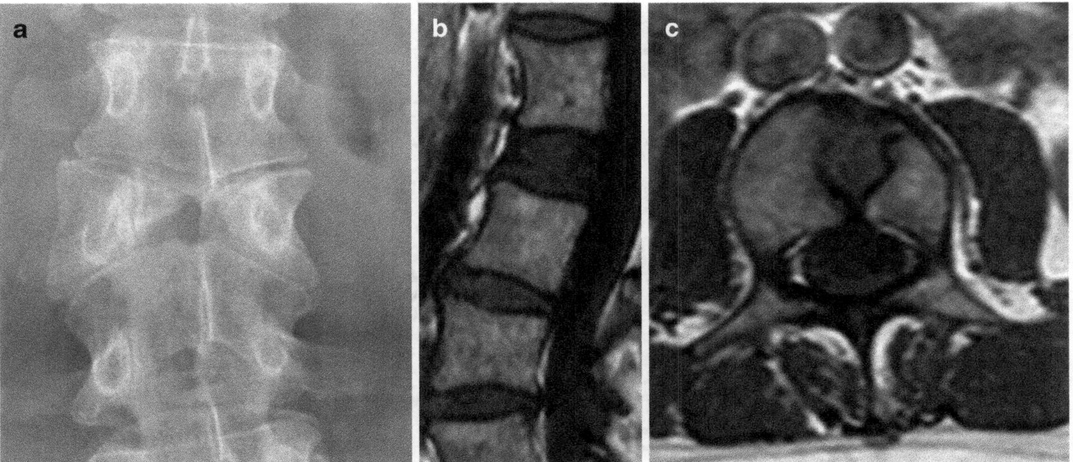

Fig. 3 Butterfly vertebra. (**a**) Plain film of the lumbar spine showing the vertebral anomaly due to failure of fusion because of persistent notochordal tissue. (**b**) Midsagittal T1W MRI of the lumbar spine showing hypointense signal on L2 vertebral body with height loss. (**c**) Corresponding axial T1-WI MRI demonstrating the hypointense midline defect

Enostosis and enostoma (bone island) (Broski et al. 2022) are considered to be developmental hamartomatous lesions. The imaging features of this benign osseous lesion to be differentiated from an osteoblastic tumor are discussed in another chapter of this book.

4 Infection/Inflammatory Disease

4.1 Spondylodiscitis

Differential diagnosis between spinal metastasis and infectious spondylodiscitis is one of the occasional challenges in daily clinical practice. The differential diagnosis of spondylodiscitis includes neoplastic processes. Radiologically, infection can occasionally mimic an osseous spinal tumor, either primary or metastatic. In general, spinal infections involve the disk whereas neoplasms involve the vertebrae and spare the disk (Hong et al. 2009). The intervertebral disk is hyperintense on T2W (Fig. 4) because of the increase in overall water content. T1W performed following intravenous infusion of gadolinium contrast may show enhancement at the end plate–disk interface fairly early in the course of the infection (Erlemann 2006). In metastatic disease, the posterior wall of the vertebral bodies, pedicles, and lamina are more commonly involved.

Awareness of the atypical imaging patterns of spinal infection is important in the appropriate clinical context. Atypical patterns of spinal infection include involvement of only one vertebral body, one vertebral body and one disk, and two vertebral bodies without the intervening disk (Skaf et al. 2010). Although it is uncommon, involvement of an isolated vertebral body without the adjacent disks or involvement of one vertebral body and one disk may be seen in MR images (Lee et al. 2015). Infection of an isolated vertebral body is thought to represent an early manifestation of a spinal infection. When two vertebral bodies are involved but not the disk, it may be difficult to differentiate infectious spondylitis from neoplastic conditions. The expression "good disk, bad news; bad disk, good news" describes the idea that a destructive bone lesion associated with a well-preserved disk space with

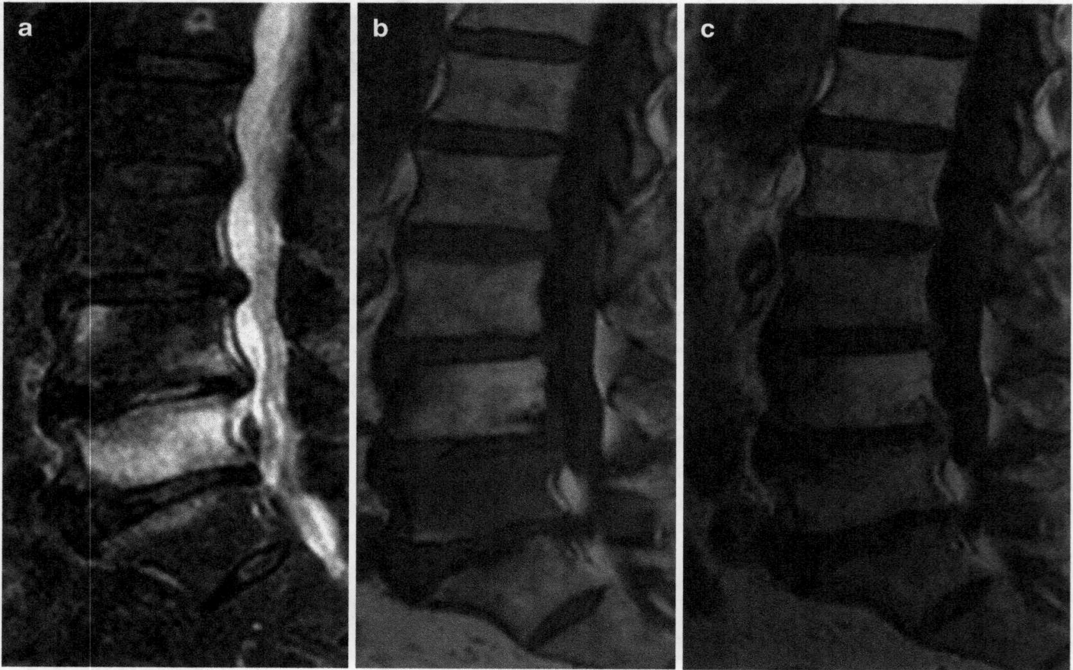

Fig. 4 Spondylodiscitis. (**a**) Sagittal STIR MRI shows diffuse hyperintense signal in L5, with high signal at the disk on L4–L5 without involvement of the posterior wall cortex. (**b**) Corresponding sagittal T1W MRI shows the hypointense diffuse signal almost completely resolved after treatment as depicted in (**c**)

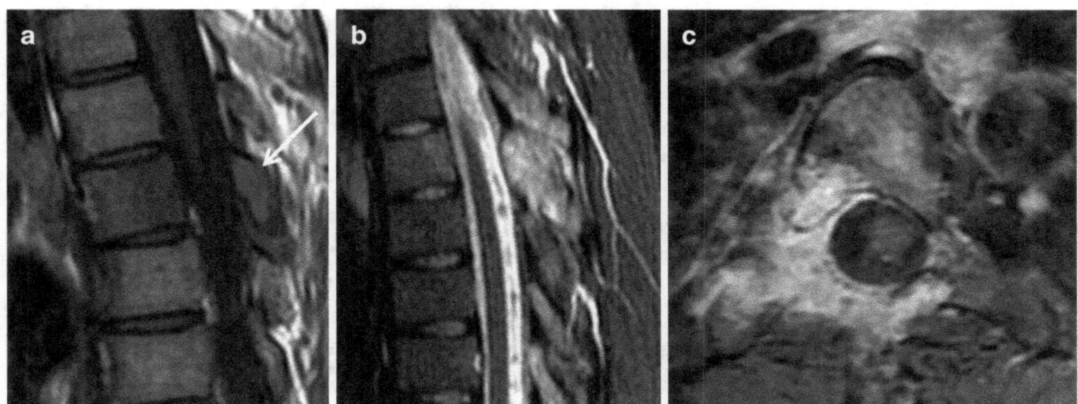

Fig. 5 Spinal tuberculosis. (**a**) Sagittal T1W MRI shows mild hypointense signal in the vertebral body extending to posterior elements with intermediate signal (arrow). (**b**) Sagittal STIR image shows the intermediate signal in the vertebral body and the lesion extending to posterior elements without involvement of the disk. (**c**) Axial T1W fat suppression with gadolinium chelate shows the lesion extending to the right pedicle and posterior elements

sharp end plates suggests neoplastic infiltration, whereas a destructive bone lesion associated with a poorly defined vertebral body end plate, with or without a loss of disk height, suggests an infection, which has a better prognosis (Hong et al. 2009).

Spinal involvement by tuberculosis is not uncommon and can differ from bacterial spinal infection in that the disk spaces are preserved until late in the disease (Fig. 5) due to the lack of proteolytic destructive enzymes by *Mycobacterium tuberculosis*. Due to the hematogenous nature of spread, multifocal lesions can occur in the spine and appendicular skeleton (De Vuyst et al. 2003; Chelli Bouaziz et al. 2021), mimicking malignancy (Mhuircheartaigh et al. 2014).

Four main radiographic patterns are observed on spinal tuberculosis: (1) a sclerotic vertebra, (2) a central round area of osteolysis with sclerosis of the remaining vertebral body, (3) a vertebral collapse, and (4) a focal destruction of the neural arch. Involvement of the neural arch in combination with the anterior vertebral elements is not infrequent. The disk space may be involved secondarily. A prevertebral abscess formation occurs frequently. Tuberculous prevertebral abscesses may extend at a great distance beneath the anterior longitudinal ligament (subligamentous tuberculosis). Spontaneous intermediate to high signal intensity on nonenhanced T1W MR images (Fig. 5) is a suggestive finding (Laredo et al. 2001). The presence of an intra-osseous and paravertebral abscess with bone fragments (sequestra) differentiates spinal tuberculosis, with normal disk height, from neoplasia. A highly characteristic feature of subacute infection to differentiate from neoplasia is the penumbra sign. The penumbra sign is a thin halo of relatively hyperintense signal in unenhanced T1 images caused by granulation tissue that rims an abscess, although this sign is described in the long bones (Davies and Grimer 2005). Skip or multifocal contiguous involvement of the spine favors neoplastic lesion.

Spinal lymphoma may manifest as paraspinal, vertebral, and epidural involvement, either in isolation or in combination simulating spinal tuberculosis with abscess. The posterior vertebral elements can be involved in spinal tuberculosis like neoplasia such as lymphoma. The appearance of vertebral lymphoma at CT and MR imaging can be nonspecific; however, lesions showing bone marrow replacement and a surrounding soft tissue mass without large areas of cortical bone destruction suggest lymphoma (Momjian and George 2014).

4.2 SAPHO Syndrome

The acronym SAPHO (synovitis, acne, pustulosis, hyperostosis, osteitis) refers to syndromes associating cutaneous and skeletal manifestations. It is a great mimicker of sclerotic bone tumors (Fig. 6). Synovitis and arthritis commonly involve the sternocostoclavicular, manubriosternal, costovertebral, and sacroiliac joints and less commonly large joints of the appendicular skeleton (Laredo et al. 2001). The spine is frequently involved in SAPHO syndrome. A large variety of radiographic appearances may be encountered in the spine in SAPHO syndrome. This syndrome is a great mimicker of vertebral tumors and infection. The radiographic appearance of spinal involvement in SAPHO syndrome includes erosion with adjacent sclerosis and hyperostosis of an anterior angle of a vertebral body similar to the Romanus lesion seen in other seronegative spondylarthritis; sclerosis of a vertebral body sometimes with involvement of the adjacent rib; exuberant osteophyte and syndesmophyte formation; and paravertebral ligamentous ossification (Laredo et al. 2007). CT scan may disclose an erosive and sclerotic arthritis of the costovertebral joint with adjacent sclerosis and hyperostosis of the vertebra, rib, and sacroiliac involvement. On MR imaging, vertebral corner erosion is a diagnostic sign that may be associated with involvement of the end plate, and the anterior cortex of the vertebral body, adjacent disk space, adjacent vertebrae, and prevertebral tissues.

4.3 Chronic Recurrent Multifocal Osteomyelitis

Chronic recurrent multifocal osteomyelitis (CRMO) is primarily a disorder of children and adolescents characterized by episodic osseous pain over several years. It is an autoinflammatory process that typically affects multiple bones with a waxing and waning course. About one-third of the patients diagnosed with CRMO have spinal involvement, which can lead to long-term morbidity. The clinical presentation and imaging features of CRMO involving the spine are nonspecific and can mimic other disease processes like infection or malignancy. Spinal CRMO involvement may be variable in appearance. The most typical manifestation is one that resembles spondylodiskitis. On radiography, these lesions exhibit vertebral plate erosion with subchondral sclerosis (Fig. 7) (Vanhoenacker et al. 1998). On MRI, CRMO typically causes irregularity of one vertebral end plate accompanied by subjacent T2-hyperintense marrow edema (Iyer et al. 2011). Spinal CRMO may also present as lytic lesions (Fig. 7) with vertebral

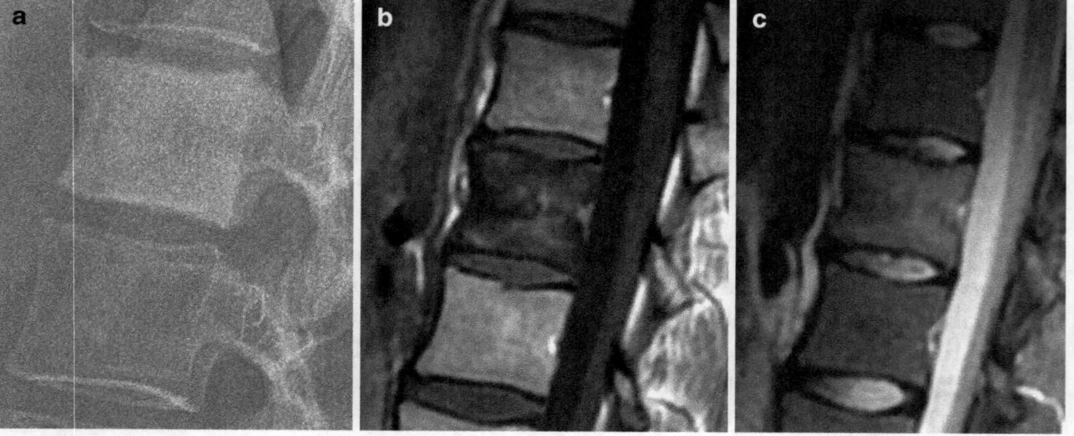

Fig. 6 SAPHO syndrome. (**a**) Plain film of the lumbar spine shows diffuse sclerotic density of the vertebral body. (**b**) Sagittal T1W shows heterogeneous hypointense signal and slightly hyperintense signal on T2W (**c**)

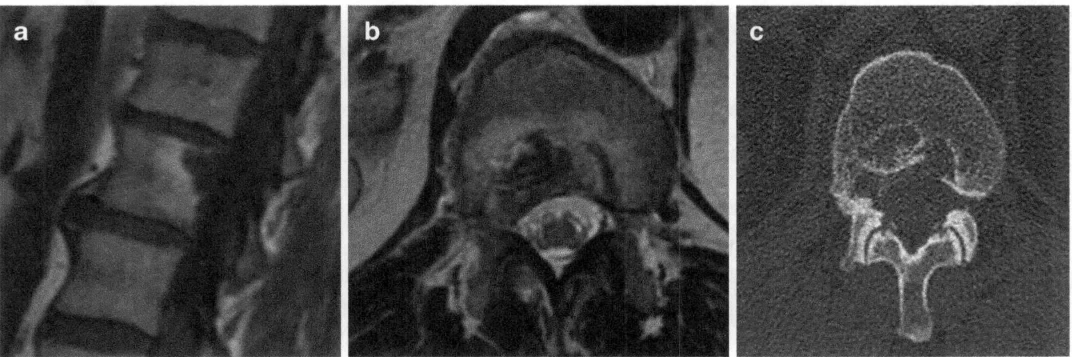

Fig. 7 Chronic recurrent multifocal osteomyelitis (CRMO). (**a**) Sagittal T1W and (**b**) axial T2W show a lesion in the vertebral body with extension to the posterior wall. (**c**) CT shows a lytic lesion with sclerotic peripheral rim anteriorly. The cortex of the posterior vertebral wall is partially absent on the left side. The perilesional high signal on T1W and T2-WI is due to fatty replacement of the bone marrow

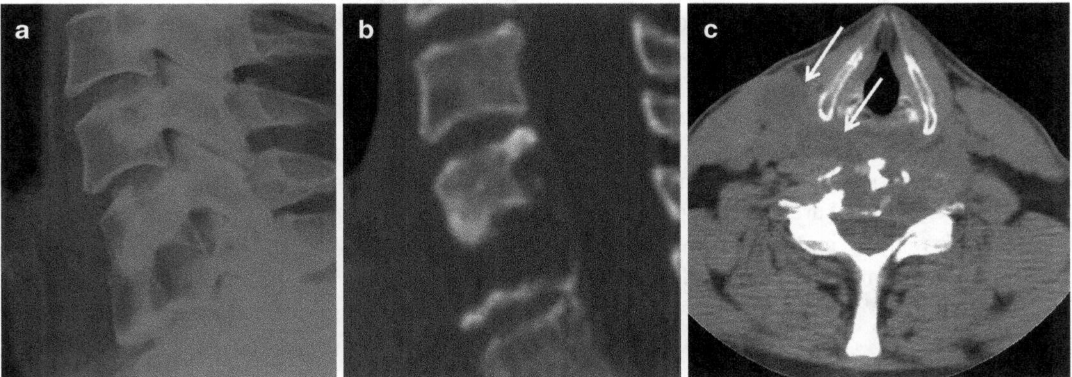

Fig. 8 Hydatid cyst. (**a**) Plain film and (**b**) sagittal CT of the neck show the lytic lesion of C5 and C6. (**c**) Axial CT shows the osteolytic vertebral lesion with adjacent soft tissue cyst extending in the prevertebral and right visceral neck space (arrows)

body collapse (Shah et al. 2022), occasionally progressing to a vertebra plana appearance. Such CRMO lesions are indistinguishable from malignancy on radiography. On MRI, the lack of additional malignant features such as soft tissue components may help in excluding tumor.

4.4 Vertebral Hydatidosis

Bone is involved in 1–2% of cases of echinococcosis (Laredo et al. 2001) and 50% of skeletal hydatid disease. Hydatidosis manifests differently in bone than in the liver or the lung because of the mechanical resistance that bone offers to the growth of hydatid cysts. Hydatid cysts proliferate by vesiculation to penetrate the bone trabeculae in the direction of least resistance and incite a slow destruction and expansion of bone. Spinal hydatid cysts are usually located in the thoracic region. A single skeletal site is usually affected, and the spine is involved in approximately 50% of the cases. The radiographic appearance may be a purely lytic lesion (Fig. 8) without reactive sclerosis or an expansile lesion with a "blownout" appearance (Abdel Razek and Castillo 2010). Hydatic cysts cause multiseptated lesions with minimal enhancement. While intra-osseous cysts show no calcification, extra-osseous cysts may calcify. Signs of nerve compression including paraplegia are frequent. The outermost adventitial layer present in visceral hydatid cysts is lacking in osseous lesions.

5 Degenerative/Metabolic Disease

5.1 Brown Tumor

Brown tumors are found in 1.5–13% of patients with renal failure and rarely involve the spine. They commonly occur in females in the third decade of life. Brown tumor is caused by increased osteoclastic activity and fibroblastic proliferation in patients with hyperparathyroidism. On radiographs, a brown tumor is seen as an area of osteolysis with jagged sharp outlines and no sclerotic rim (Abdel Razek and Castillo 2010). CT shows an osteolytic tumor of uniform tissue density replacing the cancellous bone of the vertebral body and neural arch with a spared cortex. MR imaging findings include a hypointense mass causing expansion of the involved vertebra in both T1W and T1W (Gupta et al. 2018).

5.2 Vertebral Osteonecrosis

Vertebral osteonecrosis is an uncommon disease that occurs mostly in patients with a collapsed vertebral body after major trauma or repeated microtrabecular fractures in patients with osteoporosis or long-term ingestion of glucocorticoids. Imaging shows intravertebral air alone (40%), intravertebral fluid alone (40%), or both (20%). Intravertebral vacuum cleft sign is usually seen as an irregular lesion in the central area or adjacent to an end plate of a collapsed vertebral body that exhibits low signal intensity on all sequences (Abdel Razek and Castillo 2010). Fluid appears as a well-circumscribed area of low signal intensity on T1W, with high signal intensity on T1W in the vertebral body (Fig. 9).

5.3 Degenerative Disease

A variety of degenerative diseases of the spine may present as mass lesions. Pseudotumoral lesions might show heterogenous and diverse appearances. The location of the lesion could be from the intervertebral disk (Fig. 10), facet joint, bone, or spinal ligaments (Fig. 11) (Abdel Razek

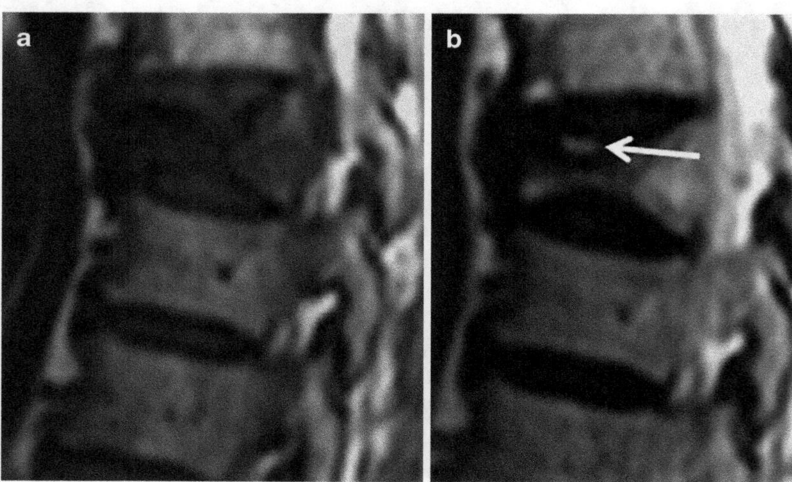

Fig. 9 A 60-year-old woman with subacute benign compression fracture of the vertebral body. (**a**) Sagittal T1-WI spin-echo MR image showing hypointense T9 vertebral body with respect to normal bone marrow. (**b**) Sagittal T2-WI fast spin-echo MR image showing T9 vertebral body fracture. The linear area of hyperintensity anterior and adjacent to the fractured superior end plate represents the fluid sign (arrow)

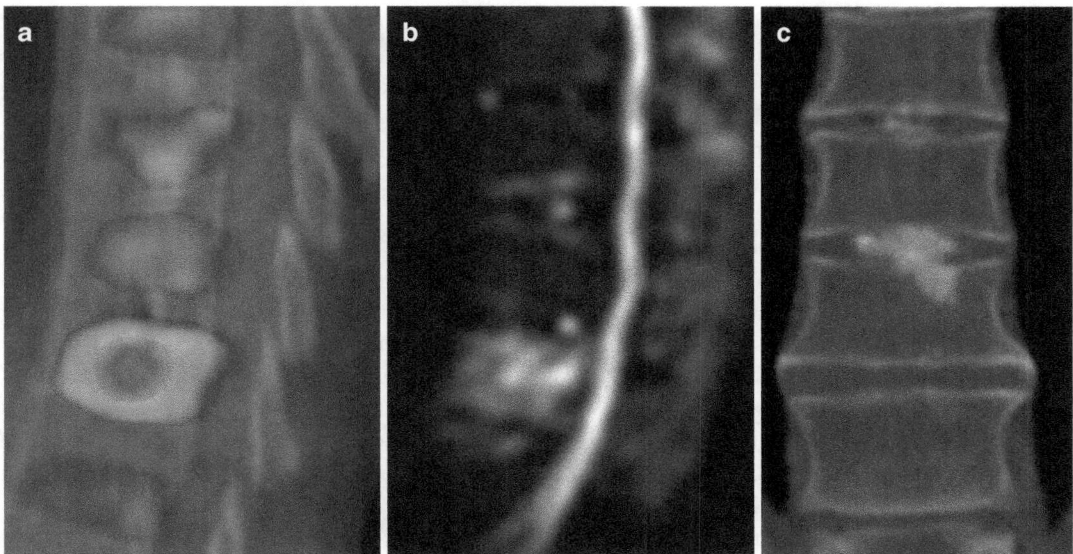

Fig. 10 Calcified disk migrating into the vertebra simulating metastasis. (**a**) PET/CT shows a lesion in T10 with a very high SUV suggesting bone metastasis in a patient with lung cancer. (**b**) Sagittal DWI shows diffuse high signal. (**c**) Coronal CT demonstrates a calcified disk migrating into the vertebral body. Biopsy to the vertebral body proved no malignancy

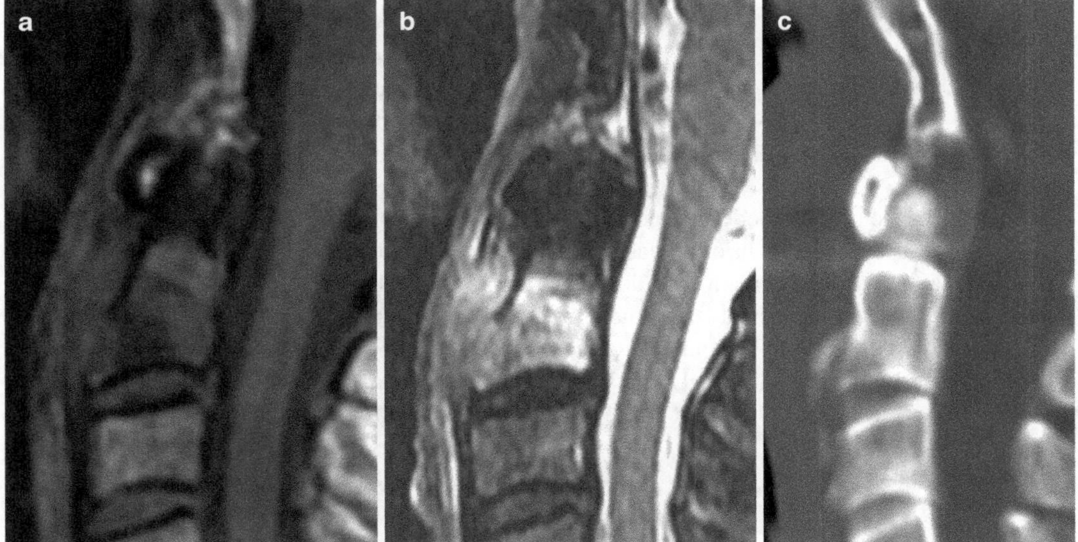

Fig. 11 Acute calcific tendinitis of the longus colli muscle simulating neoplasm. (**a**) Sagittal T1-WI shows hypointense signal in the vertebral body of C2. The lesion is hyperintense on T2-WI and STIR (**b**). Hyperintense soft tissue swelling is seen anterior to the vertebral body. (**c**) CT shows calcification in the soft tissue related to acute calcific tendinitis of the longus colli muscle

and Castillo 2010). Calcium pyrophosphate dihydrate (CPPD) deposition disease or hydroxyapatite crystal deposition disease (HADD) in the spine is a relatively uncommon entity. Atypical deposition might induce pseudotumoral appearance such as in the craniocervical junction, appearing as a radiopaque "crown" surrounding the top of the dens, described as the crowned dens syndrome (Malhotra et al. 2022). Though gouty involvement of the spine is uncommon, atypical appearance could simulate neoplasm, especially whether may harbor multiple gouty lesions (Oaks et al. 2006). A giant cystic Schmorl's node may present as a giant cystic lesion. On radiographs and CT, it appears as a benign lytic lesion with well-defined margins and surrounded by sclerotic rim. Communication with the intervertebral disk through a focal interruption of the vertebral end plate is seen. On MRI, it has a fluid signal with peripheral enhancement (Kyere et al. 2012). It is mandatory to be familiarized with atypical imaging features and correlate with the clinical history for a confident diagnosis.

5.4 Paget's Disease

Paget's disease is discussed in another chapter of this book.

The disturbance in bone modeling and remodeling because of an increase in osteoblastic and osteoclastic activity can provide a long differential diagnosis related to the osteoblastic (metastases, osteosarcoma, carcinoid, and Hodgkin's lymphoma) or lytic phase (Senthil and Balaji 2018) such as metastasis (Dell'Atti et al. 2007).

6 Trauma

6.1 Post-traumatic/Osteoporotic

Post-traumatic or osteoporotic vertebral collapse can be distinguished from malignant vertebral collapse on the basis of clinical findings and history, plain radiograph findings, and biologic tests. In some cases, however, the radiographic appearance of osteoporotic collapse may be misleading with an apparent destruction of the vertebral body (Laredo et al. 2001). The patient may also have both osteoporosis and a history of previous cancer or a biologic inflammation of variable origin. In such cases, MR imaging may be useful to differentiate osteoporotic from malignant vertebral collapse. An intravertebral vacuum phenomenon may appear on a lateral radiograph and is a strong argument for an osteoporotic origin because it almost rules out a metastatic disease as described previously. Osteoporotic collapses may be multiple, however, and are sometimes associated with other insufficiency fractures. Even in cases of a burst fracture, the vertebral cortex may be mentally reconstructed. This appearance of a burst fracture known as the puzzle sign helps to differentiate from neoplasm because there is no cortical destruction. In contrast, destruction of some parts of the vertebral body cortex is seen in malignant collapse. A benign fracture is suggested when a retropulsed bone fragment is seen, when the posterior margin of the vertebral body is angulated, when fat signal is preserved on T1W throughout the body without high signal on T2W, and when horizontal bandlike areas representing the fracture plane are seen on fluid-sensitive or Gd chelate-enhanced images. A malignant etiology of collapse is suggested when the posterior cortex is convex toward the spinal canal, when an epidural mass is seen, when the entire vertebral body or pedicles are replaced by low signal in T1-weighted images, and when high or heterogeneous signal is seen within the body in fluid-sensitive or Gd chelate-enhanced images (Table 1). Functional MRI is often used as an adjunct to morphological MRI to increase sensitivity and specificity (Vilanova et al. 2016). Diffusion MR imaging can provide additional information to differentiate acute benign collapse from malignancy, as ADC is higher in benign edema (Fig. 12), whereas malignancy shows lower ADC values (Balliu et al. 2009). Nonspecific threshold has been established, but from the previous report; ADC $< 1.0 \times 10^{-3}$ mm^2/s favors malignancy, and ADC $> 1.5 \times 10^{-3}$ mm^2/s favors benign edema. It is important to realize that functional sequences

Table 1 Magnetic resonance imaging features of benign versus malignant spine lesions

MRI feature	Benign	Malignant
Fracture line	Clearly distinct	Indistinct
Bone marrow pattern	Normal, preserved	Focal, geographic, diffuse
Morphology	Horizontal bandlike, retropulsed bone fragment, posterior cortex of vertebral body has acute angle	Rounded, diffuse, or irregular; pedicle involved, paravertebral and/or epidural mass, posterior cortex of vertebral body is smooth, convex toward canal
T2-WI	Intact posterior body wall	Disrupted posterior body wall
STIR	Lower signal intensity ratio	Higher signal intensity ratio
Dynamic intravenous contrast	No or slow enhancement	Rapid wash-in and early washout
Diffusion weighted	Higher ADC	Lower ADC
Dual-phase chemical shift (in/out of phase)	Low signal intensity ratio	High signal intensity ratio
	In phase: low SI	In phase: low SI
	Out of phase: low SI	Out of phase: high SI

SI signal intensity

are complementary; thus, it is always necessary to also obtain the morphological, T1W, and fluid-sensitive (T2W, fat suppressed, STIR, or Dixon water reconstruction) sequences. Chemical shift imaging (Dixon with in-phase and out-of-phase) may allow accurate differentiation of edema due to fracture from tumor replacement of marrow by nulling the signal from water in a local fatty environment (Vilanova et al. 2016). In difficult cases, a follow-up MR examination shows that the signal intensity of the collapse is partially or completely restored after 1–2 months in cases of osteoporotic vertebral collapse. Some cases, however, may require a percutaneous biopsy to rule out a malignant process.

6.2 Stress Lesion

Edema in the pedicle due to stress reaction may mimic osteoid osteoma on MR imaging and clinical presentation. A stress lesion appears as an infraction in the center of an area of cortical thickening, whereas osteoid osteoma appears as a round nidus (Chai et al. 2010). MRI, if obtained very early in the disease process, will initially

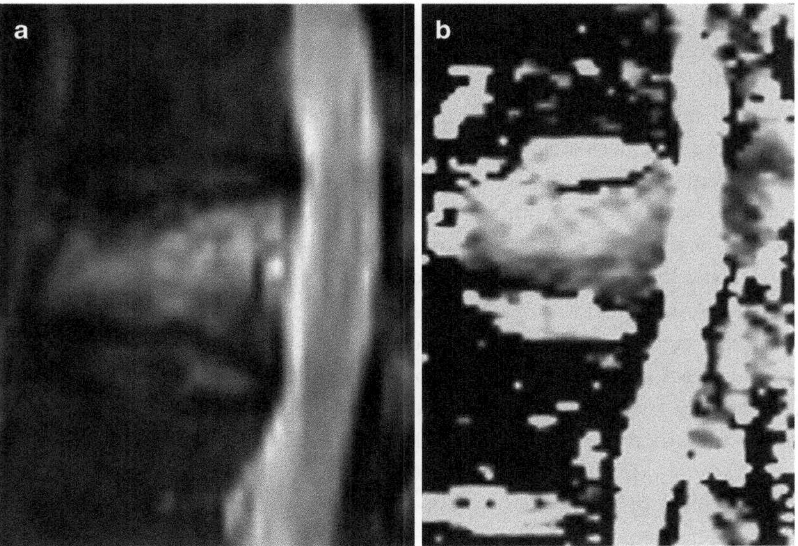

Fig. 12 A 69-year-old woman with benign acute compression fracture of the vertebral body. (**a**) Sagittal STIR image shows diffuse hyperintensity in the fractured vertebral body due to bone marrow edema. (**b**) High ADC values for the fractured vertebral body (1.809×10^{-3} mm^2/s)

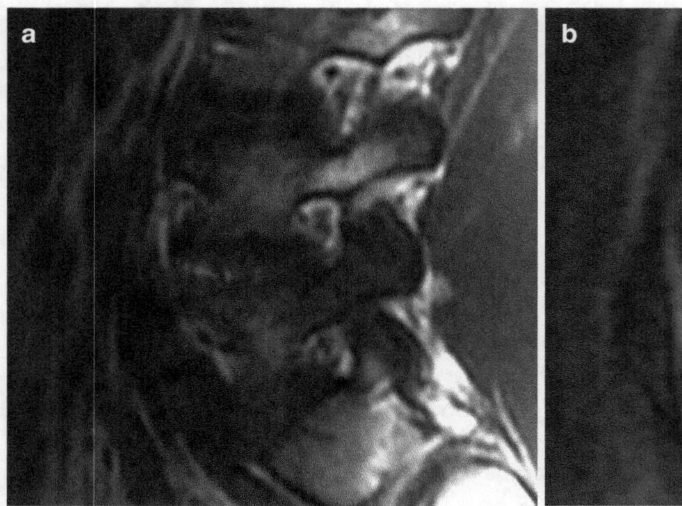
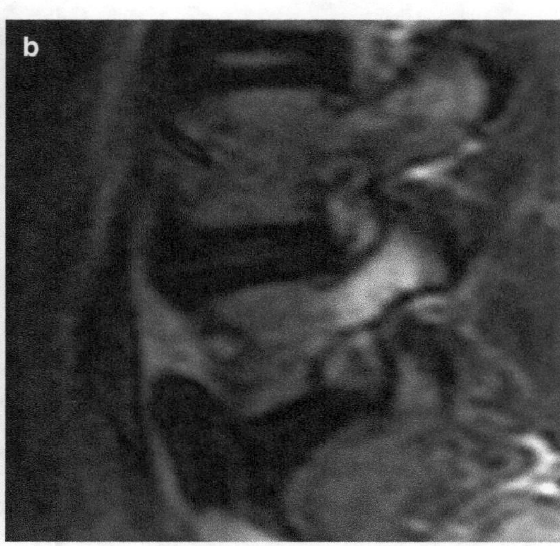
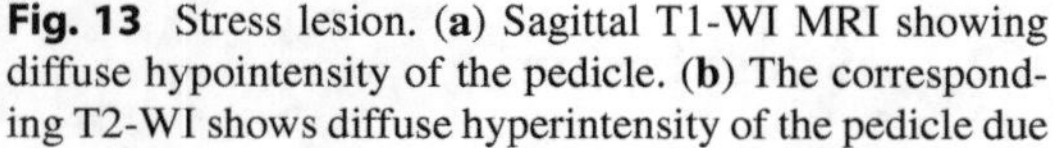

Fig. 13 Stress lesion. (**a**) Sagittal T1-WI MRI showing diffuse hypointensity of the pedicle. (**b**) The corresponding T2-WI shows diffuse hyperintensity of the pedicle due to edema stress reaction. Initial suspected diagnosis was osteoid osteoma

show only diffuse, nonspecific edema (the most common MRI finding) (Fig. 13), which may be present up to weeks before the appearance of the first radiographic findings. Initial edema appears as an ill-defined low signal region within the marrow on T1-weighted sequences and high signal on T2-weighted sequences. A fracture line is diagnostic and manifests on fluid-sensitive sequences as a linear area of hypointense signal with surrounding ill-defined high T2 signal. MRI generally offers more information compared with skeletal scintigraphy, to include demonstration of a fracture line, periosteal reaction, and bone marrow edema. Care should be taken not to mistake early bone marrow edema, adjacent soft tissue edema, and periosteal reaction as evidence of a neoplastic process. Lack of an associated soft tissue mass, a clinical history suggestive of a stress fracture, and appropriate clinical follow-up lead to a correct diagnosis, avoiding biopsy (which has a risk of false-positive histopathologic diagnosis of sarcoma) (Gould et al. 2007). CT adds value to exclude the nidus, and bone scintigraphy may help to differentiate a stress fracture from osteoid osteoma. On scintigraphy, a stress fracture demonstrates linear, intense uptake of the tracer, whereas osteoid osteoma displays the "double-density" sign, in which intense central uptake is seen at the site of the nidus and moderate uptake is seen in the surrounding area. A stress-induced unilateral arch hypertrophy with contralateral deficiency should not be confused with some tumoral lesion (Maldague and Malghem 1976).

7 Idiopathic

7.1 Sarcoidosis

Sarcoidosis is an inflammatory disorder characterized by the development of noncaseating granulomas that can affect multiple-organ systems, most commonly the lungs and skin, but may also manifest in bone. Osseous involvement by sarcoidosis occurs in approximately 5% of patients (range between 1% and 13%). Osseous involvement by sarcoidosis has been well described in the hands and feet, where there can be bilateral but asymmetric osteolytic destruction with a latticework or honeycomb pattern in the small bones (Broski et al. 2022). In cases with classic hilar sarcoidosis involvement, a presumptive diagnosis of osseous sarcoidosis can be made on the basis of the clinical and imaging features. However, when osseous involvement is the presenting finding or is an incidental finding, the diagnosis can be considerably more problematic. With the increased usage of MRI as imaging modality, osseous sarcoidosis is detected more commonly. It has been shown that in cases of multifocal bone lesions on MRI and an established diagnosis of sarcoidosis (Sarvesvaran and Chandramohan 2021), a diagnosis of bone sarcoidosis can be made presumptively; however, differentiation from metastasis cannot be achieved by morphologic criteria (Moore et al. 2012). Discussion between the radiologist and clinician on a per-case basis is recommended to determine the advisability of follow-up imaging or biopsy in such cases.

7.2 Osteopoikilosis

Osteopoikilia, also referred to as osteopoikilosis, is an asymptomatic osteosclerosing dysplasia, of nonspecific etiology first described by Albers-Schönberg. The most common locations of occurrence seen are the carpal and metacarpal phalanges, phalanges of the foot, metatarsals, tarsus, pelvis, femur, sacrum, humerus, and tibia. The involvement of the ribs, clavicles, spine, and skull is uncommon. The diagnosis is radiological because the image is very indicative, characterized by foci of sclerosis, rarely over 10 mm, without affecting cortical bone (Fig. 14) (Yang et al. 2022). Patients are usually asymptomatic and most often found incidentally on radiographic imaging. Bone scan shows no pathological data, which is very useful in making the differential diagnosis with other osteocondensing lesions. Histologically, there is an increase in the number and thickness of the trabeculae of the spongious bone. The differential diagnosis includes osteoblastic bone metastases, mastocytosis (Leone et al. 2021), tuberous sclerosis, osteopathia striata, melorheostosis, osteopetrosis, sclerosteosis, Erdheim–Chester disease, or fluorosis (Vanhoenacker et al. 2000).

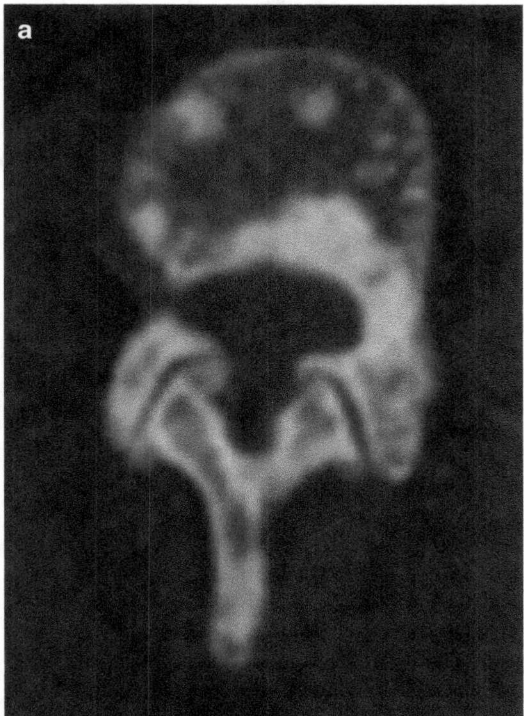

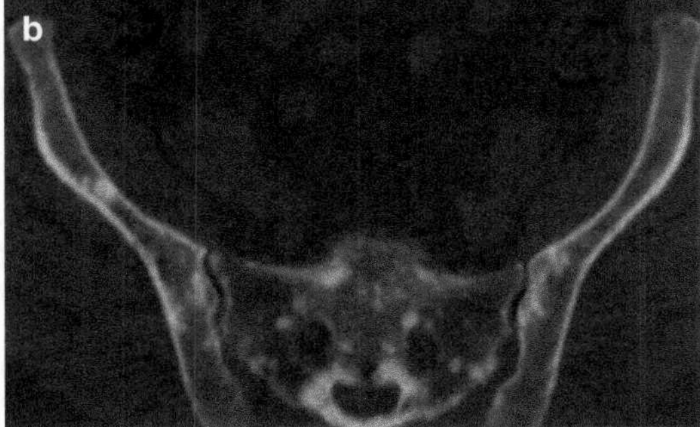

Fig. 14 Osteopoikilosis. Multiple rounded sclerotic lesions from the spine (**a**) and the pelvis (**b**)

7.3 Osteomesopyknosis

Osteomesopyknosis is a rare autosomal dominant condition that manifests with sclerotic bone lesions confined to the axial skeleton and proximal long bones (Fig. 15). Few cases have been published in the medical literature. The typical radiologic findings seen in a large number of patients are thickened end plates of the vertebral bodies

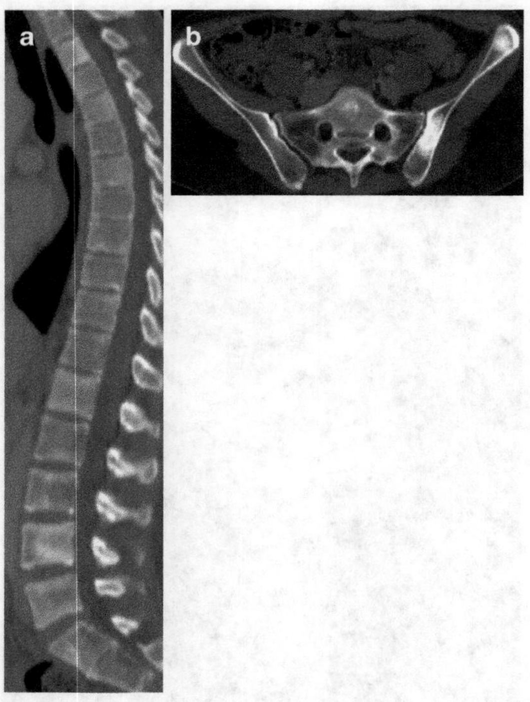

Fig. 15 Osteomesopyknosis. Multiple sclerotic lesions in the axial skeleton. (**a**) Sagittal reconstruction of the spine and axial image of the pelvis (**b**) show patchy sclerotic lesions with well-defined margins that are located in the bone marrow

(Heursen et al. 2016). Dense end plates can be confounded with the so-called rugger jersey spine seen in patients with hyperparathyroidism. Some authors mistakenly consider osteomesopyknosis as a mild form of osteopetrosis (Albers-Schönberg disease), because it can show similar hyperdense end plates or a "bone-in-a-bone" appearance (increased central density within a vertebral body). In some cases of osteomesopyknosis, the most salient radiologic findings are patchy sclerotic lesions located in the vertebral bodies and posterior elements of the spine rather than dense end plate radiologic presentation that can misleadingly raise the suspicion of blastic metastasis. Osteomesopyknosis is a benign axial hyperostosis with a good prognosis that appears not to progress significantly over time. Clinical presentation could be diffuse back pain, although patients may be asymptomatic. Blood analysis is usually normal. Scintigraphy may show an increased uptake of radiotracer. Most of the patients have additional lesions in the iliac bones, femoral head, scapula, or humerus. The diagnostic key to differentiate osteomesopyknosis from other sclerosing bone disorders such as osteopoikilosis or osteopetrosis is that the head and distal extremities are not involved and that there are no associated abnormalities (Yao and Camacho 2014). It is important to know this benign entity in order to avoid anxiety and overdiagnosis.

7.4 Gorham-Stout Disease

Gorham-Stout disease (GSD) is a rare disease characterized by progressive osteolysis and angiomatosis, known as vanishing bone disease or phantom bone disease. It is an idiopathic musculoskeletal disorder characterized by spontaneous and progressive osteolysis replaced by lymphatic vessels, angiomatous proliferation, and soft tissue swelling without new bone formation (Liu et al. 2016). The exact etiology and pathophysiology remain poorly understood. Major features of GSD are nonspecific symptoms, including bone pain, muscular weakness, and skeletal deformity. The radiologic appearance of bone lesions reveals intramedullary and subcortical radiolucency as osteolysis (Fig. 16). Different locations within the skeleton have been reported: mandible, tibia, ribs, pelvis, femur, clavicle, and spine. Laboratory findings are usually normal and only helpful in the differential diagnosis. Prognosis and complications of GSD vary depending on the extent and sites of bone destruction. Osteolysis might be polyostotic or monostotic. Generally, GSD is a self-limited disease but potentially may be fatal. Bisphosphonates and radiotherapy can contribute to the clinical stabilization in bone lesion of GSD. Case complicated by chylothorax possibly indicates poor prognosis.

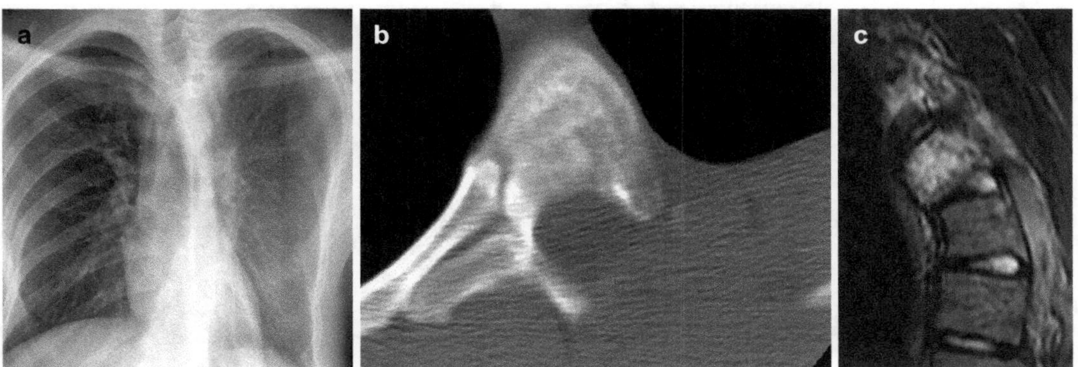

Fig. 16 Gorham-Stout syndrome. (**a**) Plain film shows osteolysis of the left ribs extending to vertebral bodies, as seen on CT (**b**). (**c**) Sagittal STIR image shows heterogeneous vertebral edema with multinodular appearance, as a proliferative angiomatous pattern, simulating infiltrative lesions

8 Posttreatment Changes

8.1 Post-radiotherapy Osteonecrosis

Initially, radiotherapy causes vascular congestion, edema, and decreased cellularity in the bone marrow. This will cause decreased signal on T1W sequences and increased signal on T2W sequences (Fig. 17). With time, the bone marrow will be replaced with fat and occasionally with fibrosis, with high signal on T1W and intermediate signal on T2W sequences (Mhuircheartaigh et al. 2014). There can be a clear demarcation along the borders of the radiation field. Irradiated bone can be at increased risk for insufficiency factures, osteonecrosis, bone erosion (Fig. 17), and radiation-induced sarcomas.

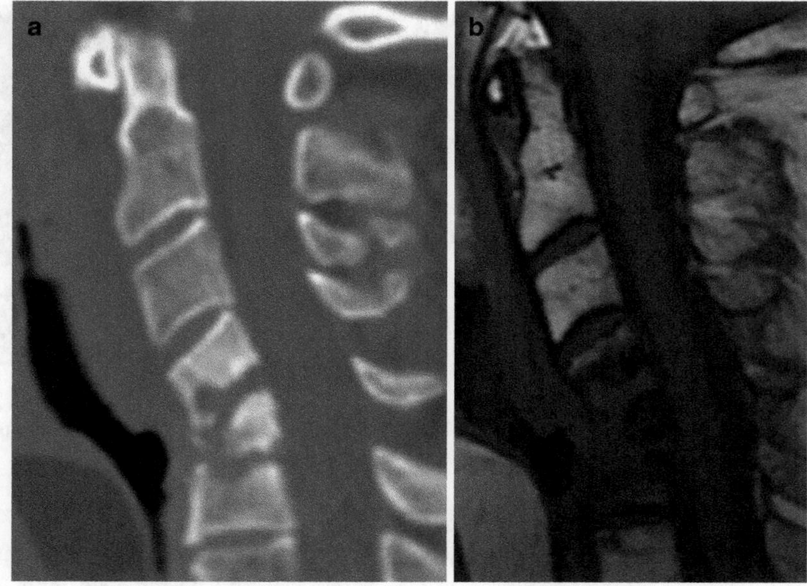

Fig. 17 Post-radiotherapy changes in C4–C5–C6. (**a**) Sagittal view at CT shows erosion of the vertebral bodies with wedging of C5. (**b**) Sagittal MRI shows hypointensity of the vertebral bodies with bone erosion and reduced height

9 Miscellaneous

Occasionally, soft tissue lesions located paravertebral and extending to and eroding the bone could raise possible differential diagnosis for a primary or secondary bone tumor originated from the spine. Pigmented villonodular synovitis—currently designated as diffuse-type tenosynovial giant cell tumor (TSGCT)—is a benign proliferative joint disease that rarely involves the spine (Oh et al. 2014). TSGCT of the spine may originate from the posterior facet joint, causing bone erosion. In this scenario, a differential diagnosis with a primary bone should be considered (Fig. 18).

Extramedullary hematopoiesis can result in paravertebral masses caused by compensatory expansion of bone marrow in patients with severe anemia caused by inadequate production or excessive destruction of blood cells. Radiographically, lobulated paravertebral masses, usually multiple and bilateral in the lower thoracic vertebra, are typically seen (Haidar et al. 2010). They appear well marginated. The bones may be normal or may show an altered lacelike trabecular pattern caused by marrow expansion (Fig. 19). The masses are usually of homogeneous soft tissue attenuation on CT (Fig. 19), although, occasionally, when the anemia resolves, a fatty component may be visible. Usually, the masses are bilateral and reasonably symmetrical (Georgiades et al. 2002).

Hemophilic pseudotumor involving the spine is extremely uncommon and presents a challenging problem. Hemophilic pseudotumor can extend to the vertebra showing bone destruction mimicking bone tumor (Nachimuthu et al. 2014).

Cystic lesions have been described in another chapter of this book. It is uncommon to find a simple cyst in a vertebra, but its specific features should not be confused with a bone tumor (Fig. 20).

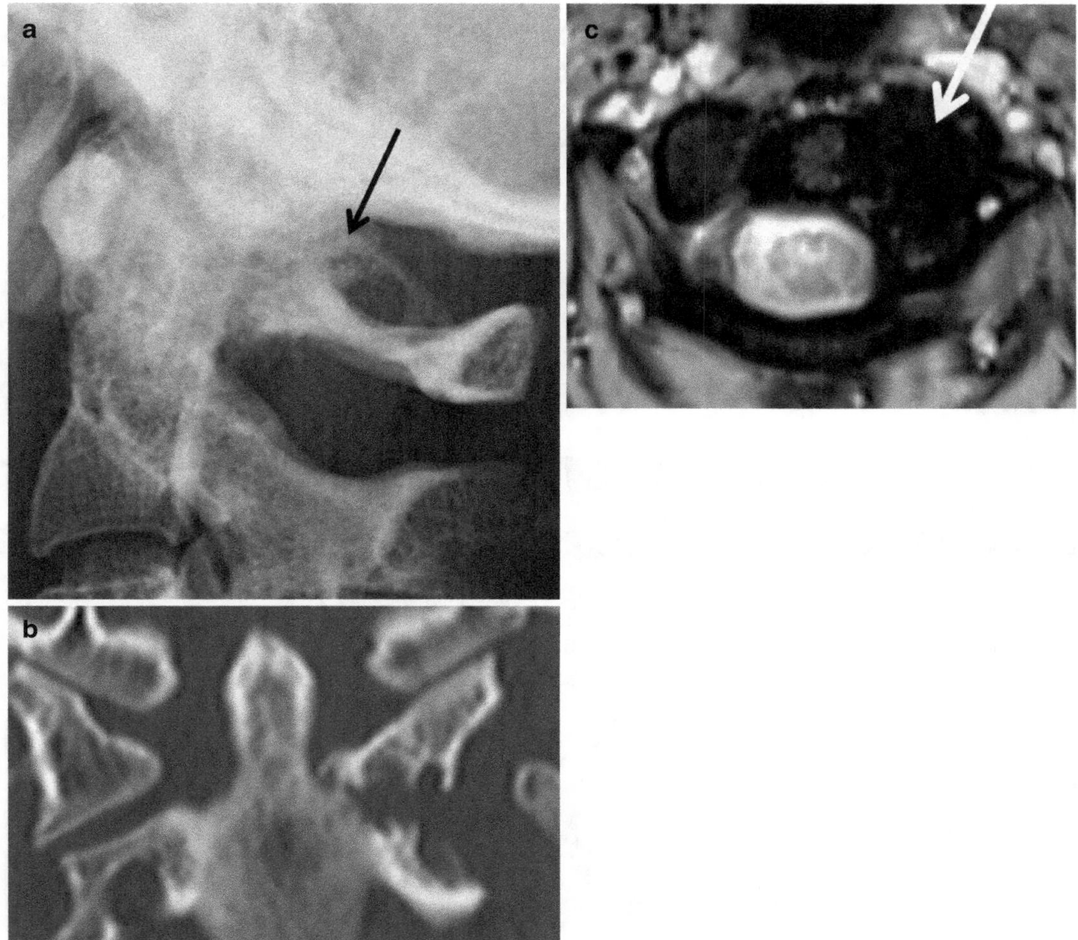

Fig. 18 Pigmented villonodular synovitis/diffuse-type TSGCT. (**a**) The lesion is difficult to depict on conventional radiography, with subtle poorly defined margins of C1 and intralesional lytic area (arrow). (**b**) CT image shows the lytic lesion in the left lateral mass of C1, extending toward the joint with the body of C2. It shows a distinct transition zone with thin, sclerotic margins (characteristic of slow-growing benign lesions). (**c**) Axial Gradient-echo T2WI shows signal decay (T2*-effect) of hemosiderinladen from thickened synovium (arrow)

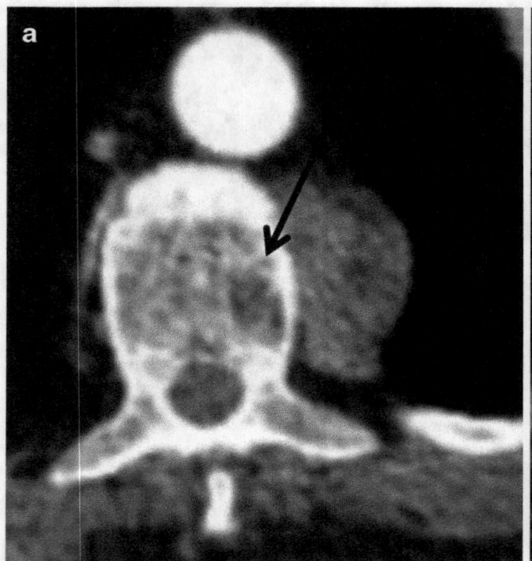

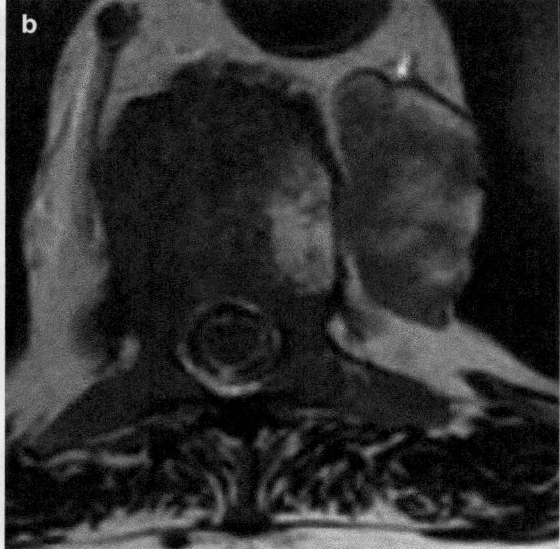

Fig. 19 Extramedullary hematopoiesis. (**a**) CT image shows a soft tissue mass around a thoracic vertebral body with lytic lesion in the vertebral body (arrow). (**b**) Corresponding axial T2-WI shows the soft tissue mass extending to the bone marrow of the vertebral body

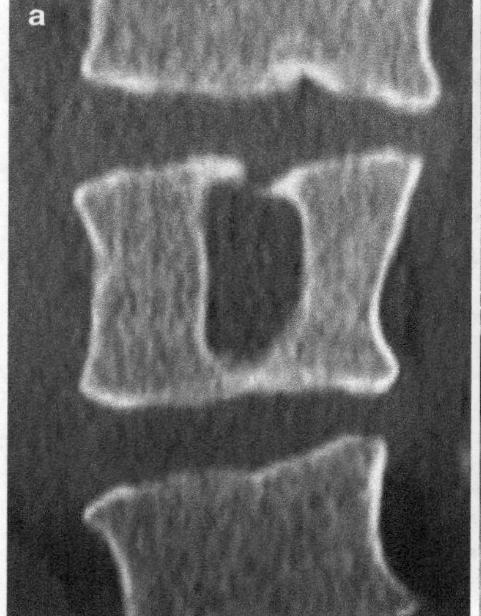

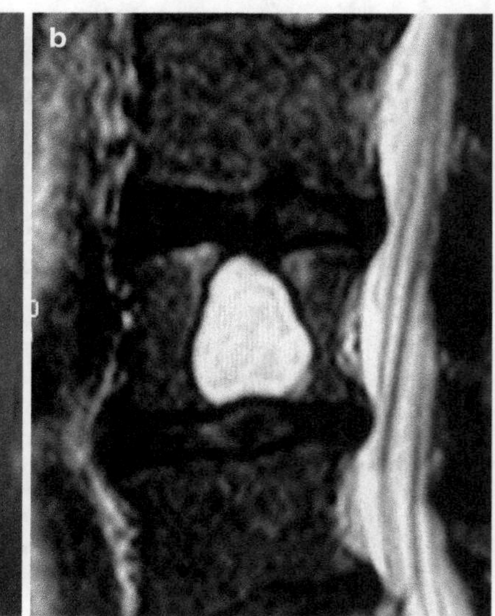

Fig. 20 Simple vertebral cyst. (**a**) Sagittal CT image showing well-delineated vertebral lesion. (**b**) Corresponding sagittal T2-WI showing the hyperintense signal of the lesion with well-defined margins

10 Key Points

- A variety of benign, nonneoplastic bone lesions may mimic benign and malignant bone tumors. Usually, a combination of lesion location, patient demographics, and imaging features allows distinction from neoplastic bone disease.
- Most nonneoplastic lesions exhibit characteristic imaging features that can allow for confident distinction from neoplastic bone disease.
- In some cases, distinguishing benign nonneoplastic lesions from bone tumors may be difficult on radiographs, but usually cross-sectional imaging with CT, MR imaging, or nuclear medicine imaging allows for accurate diagnosis.

References

Abdel Razek AAK, Castillo M (2010) Imaging appearance of primary bony tumors and pseudo-tumors of the spine. J Neuroradiol 37:37–50. https://doi.org/10.1016/j.neurad.2009.08.006

Balliu E, Vilanova JC, Peláez I et al (2009) Diagnostic value of apparent diffusion coefficients to differentiate benign from malignant vertebral bone marrow lesions. Eur J Radiol 69:560–566. https://doi.org/10.1016/j.ejrad.2007.11.037

Berglund J, Johansson L, Ahlström H, Kullberg J (2010) Three-point Dixon method enables whole-body water and fat imaging of obese subjects. Magn Reson Med 63:1659–1668. https://doi.org/10.1002/mrm.22385

Broski SM, Littrell LA, Howe BM, Wenger DE (2022) Bone tumors. Radiol Clin North Am 60:239–252. https://doi.org/10.1016/j.rcl.2021.11.004

Chai JW, Hong SH, Choi J-Y et al (2010) Radiologic diagnosis of osteoid osteoma: from simple to challenging findings. Radiographics 30:737–749. https://doi.org/10.1148/rg.303095120

Chelli Bouaziz M et al (2021) Imaging of spinal tuberculosis. In: Ladeb MF, Peh WC (eds) Imaging of spinal infection, Medical radiology. Springer, Cham

Davies AM, Grimer R (2005) The penumbra sign in subacute osteomyelitis. Eur Radiol 15:1268–1270

De Vuyst D, Vanhoenacker F, Gielen J et al (2003) Imaging features of musculoskeletal tuberculosis. Eur Radiol 13:1809–1819. https://doi.org/10.1007/s00330-002-1609-6

Dell'Atti C, Cassar-Pullicino VN, Lalam RK et al (2007) The spine in Paget's disease. Skeletal Radiol 36:609–626. https://doi.org/10.1007/s00256-006-0270-6

Erlemann R (2006) Imaging and differential diagnosis of primary bone tumors and tumor-like lesions of the spine. Eur J Radiol 58:48–67. https://doi.org/10.1016/j.ejrad.2005.12.006

Georgiades CS, Neyman EG, Francis IR et al (2002) Typical and atypical presentations of extramedullary hemopoiesis. AJR Am J Roentgenol 179:1239–1243. https://doi.org/10.2214/ajr.179.5.1791239

Gould CF, Ly JQ, Lattin GE et al (2007) Bone tumor mimics: avoiding misdiagnosis. Curr Probl Diagn Radiol 36:124–141. https://doi.org/10.1067/j.cpradiol.2007.01.001

Gupta M, Singhal L, Kumar A (2018) Hyperparathyroidism mimicking metastatic bone disease: a case report and review of literature. J Adolesc Young Adult Oncol 7:400–403. https://doi.org/10.1089/jayao.2017.0114

Haidar R, Mhaidli H, Taher AT (2010) Paraspinal extramedullary hematopoiesis in patients with thalassemia intermedia. Eur Spine J 19:871–878. https://doi.org/10.1007/s00586-010-1357-2

Heursen E-M, González Partida MC, Paz Expósito J, Navarro Díaz F (2016) Osteomesopyknosis—a benign axial hyperostosis that can mimic metastatic disease. Skeletal Radiol 45:141–146. https://doi.org/10.1007/s00256-015-2216-3

Hong SH, Choi J-Y, Lee JW et al (2009) MR imaging assessment of the spine: infection or an imitation? Radiographics 29:599–612. https://doi.org/10.1148/rg.292085137

Iyer RS, Thapa MM, Chew FS (2011) Chronic recurrent multifocal osteomyelitis: review. AJR Am J Roentgenol 196:S87–S91. https://doi.org/10.2214/AJR.09.7212

Kyere KA, Than KD, Wang AC et al (2012) Schmorl's nodes. Eur Spine J 21:2115–2121. https://doi.org/10.1007/s00586-012-2325-9

Laredo J-D, Quessar AEI, Bossard P, Vuillemin-Bodaghi V (2001) Vertebral tumors and pseudotumors. Radiol Clin North Am 39:137–163. https://doi.org/10.1016/S0033-8389(05)70267-0

Laredo J-D, Vuillemin-Bodaghi V, Boutry N et al (2007) SAPHO syndrome: MR appearance of vertebral involvement. Radiology 242:825–831. https://doi.org/10.1148/radiol.2423051222

Lee C-M, Lee S, Bae J (2015) Contiguous spinal metastasis mimicking infectious spondylodiscitis. J Korean Soc Radiol 73:408. https://doi.org/10.3348/jksr.2015.73.6.408

Leone A, Macagnino S, D'Ambra G et al (2021) Systemic mastocytosis: radiological point of view. Mediterr J Hematol Infect Dis 13:e2021056. https://doi.org/10.4084/MJHID.2021.056

Liu Y, Zhong D-R, Zhou P-R et al (2016) Gorham-Stout disease: radiological, histological, and clinical features of 12 cases and review of literature. Clin Rheumatol 35:813–823. https://doi.org/10.1007/s10067-014-2780-2

Maldague BE, Malghem JJ (1976) Unilateral arch hypertrophy with spinous process tilt: a sign of arch deficiency. Radiology 121:567–574. https://doi.org/10.1148/121.3.567

Malhotra AK, Malhotra AR, Landry AP et al (2022) Calcium pyrophosphate dihydrate crystal deposition disease and retro-odontoid pseudotumor rupture managed via posterior occipital cervical instrumented fusion: illustrative case. J Neurosurg Case Lessons 3:CASE21662. https://doi.org/10.3171/CASE21662

Martel Villagrán J, Bueno Horcajadas Á, Pérez Fernández E, Martín Martín S (2015) Accuracy of magnetic resonance imaging in differentiating between benign and malignant vertebral lesions: role of diffusion-weighted imaging, in-phase/opposed-phase imaging and apparent diffusion coefficient. Radiologia 57:142–149. https://doi.org/10.1016/j.rxeng.2013.11.002

McMaster MJ (1984) Occult intraspinal anomalies and congenital scoliosis. J Bone Joint Surg Am 66:588–601

Mhuircheartaigh JN, Lin Y-C, Wu JS (2014) Bone tumor mimickers: a pictorial essay. Indian J Radiol Imaging 24:225–236. https://doi.org/10.4103/0971-3026.137026

Momjian R, George M (2014) Atypical imaging features of tuberculous spondylitis: case report with literature review. Radiol Case 8:1–14. https://doi.org/10.3941/jrcr.v8i11.2309

Moore SL, Kransdorf MJ, Schweitzer ME et al (2012) Can sarcoidosis and metastatic bone lesions be reliably differentiated on routine MRI? AJR Am J Roentgenol 198:1387–1393. https://doi.org/10.2214/AJR.11.7498

Nachimuthu G, Arockiaraj J, Krishnan V, Sundararaj GD (2014) Hemophilic pseudotumor of the first lumbar vertebra. Indian J Orthop 48:617–620. https://doi.org/10.4103/0019-5413.144238

Oaks J, Quarfordt SD, Metcalfe JK (2006) MR features of vertebral tophaceous gout. AJR Am J Roentgenol 187:W658–W659. https://doi.org/10.2214/AJR.06.0661

Oh SW, Lee MH, Eoh W (2014) Pigmented villonodular synovitis on lumbar spine: a case report and literature review. J Korean Neurosurg Soc 56:272. https://doi.org/10.3340/jkns.2014.56.3.272

Ruiz Santiago F, Láinez Ramos-Bossini AJ, Wáng YXJ et al (2022) The value of magnetic resonance imaging and computed tomography in the study of spinal disorders. Quant Imaging Med Surg 12:3947–3986. https://doi.org/10.21037/qims-2022-04

Sarvesvaran M, Chandramohan M (2021) Skeletal sarcoidosis; an uncommon mimic of metastatic disease. BMJ Case Rep 14:e238493. https://doi.org/10.1136/bcr-2020-238493

Schweitzer ME, Levine C, Mitchell DG et al (1993) Bull's-eyes and halos: useful MR discriminators of osseous metastases. Radiology 188:249–252. https://doi.org/10.1148/radiology.188.1.8511306

Senthil V, Balaji S (2018) Monostotic Paget disease of the lumbar vertebrae: a pathological mimicker. Neurospine 15:182–186. https://doi.org/10.14245/ns.1834922.461

Shah A, Rosenkranz M, Thapa M (2022) Review of spinal involvement in chronic recurrent multifocal osteomyelitis (CRMO): what radiologists need to know about CRMO and its imitators. Clin Imaging 81:122–135. https://doi.org/10.1016/j.clinimag.2021.09.012

Skaf GS, Domloj NT, Fehlings MG et al (2010) Pyogenic spondylodiscitis: an overview. J Infect Public Health 3:5–16. https://doi.org/10.1016/j.jiph.2010.01.001

Vanhoenacker FM, Baekelandt J, Vanwambeke K et al (1998) Chronic recurrent multifocal osteomyelitis. J Belge Radiol 81:84–86

Vanhoenacker FM, De Beuckeleer LH, Van Hul W et al (2000) Sclerosing bone dysplasias: genetic and radioclinical features. Eur Radiol 10:1423–1433. https://doi.org/10.1007/s003300000495

Vilanova JC, Baleato-Gonzalez S, Romero MJ et al (2016) Assessment of musculoskeletal malignancies with functional MR imaging. Magn Reson Imaging Clin N Am 24:239–259. https://doi.org/10.1016/j.mric.2015.08.006

Yang Y-F, Kang Y-J, Zheng B-W (2022) Spinal vertebral osteopoikilosis: a case report. Asian J Surg 45:2293–2295. https://doi.org/10.1016/j.asjsur.2022.05.016

Yao ALM, Camacho PM (2014) Osteomesopyknosis: a case report and review of sclerosing bone disorders. Endocr Pract 20:e106–e111. https://doi.org/10.4158/EP13352.CR

Part IV

Treatment of Tumors and Tumor-Like Conditions of the Osseous Spine

Primary Bone Tumors of the Spine: Surgical Management

Mouadh Nefiss, Anis Teborbi, Ramzi Bouzidi, and Khelil Ezzaouia

Contents

M. Nefiss (✉) · A. Teborbi · R. Bouzidi · K. Ezzaouia
Orthopedic Surgery Department, Mongi Slim University Hospital, La Marsa, Tunisia

Faculty of Medicine of Tunis, Tunis-El Manar University, Tunis, Tunisia

Abstract

Surgical management of primary bone tumors of the spine, whether malignant or benign, requires a good preoperative analysis with staging according to recently updated systems. The surgical planning must take into account the risk-benefit ratio for the patient and skill level of the surgical team. En bloc vertebrectomy seems to be correlated with the best prognosis whether for malignant or benign tumors; however, invasion of the spinal canal or large vessels makes this surgery too aggressive and illusory. Advances in chemotherapy modalities and new radiotherapy techniques are particularly important in case of incomplete resection in reducing the risk of recurrence. Osteosynthesis and reconstruction of the frontal and sagittal balance of the spine after tumor resection have benefited from the evolution of instrumentation in spinal surgery.

1 Introduction

Primary bone tumors of the spine (PBTSs) are rare tumors that include both benign and malignant lesions, accounting for 5% of all primary bone tumors (Kerr and Dial 2019). Localization in the thoracic and lumbosacral spine is more frequent than in the cervical segment (Choi and Crockard 2010). Osteosarcoma, chondrosar-

Med Radiol Diagn Imaging (2023)
https://doi.org/10.1007/174_2023_455,
Published Online: 24 September 2023

coma, Ewing's sarcoma, chordoma, and plasmacytoma are the most represented malignant PBTSs (Patnaik and Jyotsnarani 2016). Hematological malignancies with multiple localizations such as multiple myeloma and lymphoproliferative tumors are excluded from this chapter. Surgical management of PBTS is associated with a high morbidity rate, up to 35% in some series in the literature.

The management of PBTS has undergone a significant evolution over the last 20 years in terms of diagnosis, therapy, and prognosis. Coordination of an interprofessional team and close collaboration with the patient and his family are mandatory to ensure the best results.

Although en bloc resection with wide healthy margins remains the best technique to cure malignant tumors, it is challenging in spinal localization due to proximity of dura, nerve root, and major vascular structures. Tremendous progress has been made either for reconstruction techniques or for stabilization procedures at all levels of the spine, including vertebroplasty and kyphoplasty, which have further allowed palliation of pain and symptom relief (Sundaresan and Rosen 2009).

This increasingly enthusiastic surgical approach has also benefited from the evolution of radiotherapy techniques, which has made it possible to better control the tumoral disease and improve the quality of life and survival. Advanced radiation techniques (intensity-modulated radiation therapy, stereotactic radiation therapy, or proton beam radiation therapy) have also allowed better sterilization of the tumor remnant often present after PBTS resection with a lower rate of complications and side effects.

This chapter reviews current management modalities of primary bone tumors of the spine and presents cases treated in our department as examples.

2 Surgical Considerations in Primary Bone Tumors of the Spine

Due to the rarity of these tumors, there is a lack of guidelines in the literature. The aims of surgical management are:

- Complete resection of the tumor with safe margins if feasible particularly in malignant PBTS
- Minimum morbidity with respect to neurological structures
- Stabilization of the vertebral column with a good sagittal and frontal alignment

To achieve these objectives, the correct analysis of the tumor, its limits, as well as the correct staging are fundamental steps.

Imaging analysis is mainly based on conventional radiography (CR) and MRI. Nowadays, the CT/PET scan association has shown advantages as well regarding sensitivity and specificity in the analysis of malignant bone tumors, including malignant bone tumors of the spine (Steffner and Jang 2018).

The most used staging systems and scores nowadays in the classification of PBTS and in the planning of surgery are the following (see also chapter "Local and Distant Staging"):

- **The Enneking staging system of bone sarcomas**: It remains the most used by orthopedic and spine surgeons since its first publication in 1980 and its validation by the Musculoskeletal Tumor Society (MSTS) (Enneking and Spanier 1980; Steffner and Jang 2018).
- **The American Joint Committee on Cancer (AJCC) staging system**: It includes much more precision than the Enneking classifica-

tion, and it aligns with the classifications of other tumors, which makes it more universal although it is not popular in the orthopedic community (American Joint Committee on Cancer 2017).

- **The Weinstein-Biagini-Boriani classification**: It is also widely used in the surgical planning of spinal bone tumors in general but specifically in PBTS where a curative treatment is aimed (Boriani and Weinstein 1997).

Although biopsy is not required in vertebral metastases from a known primary tumor, it is mandatory in PBTS. Ideally, this biopsy will be done percutaneously (CT-guided biopsy) with tattooing of the trajectory. If this is technically not feasible or in case of failure, a surgical biopsy will be performed. It should preferably be performed in the same reference center that will perform the definitive surgery to include it in the resection specimen.

In addition to oncological objectives, achieving stabilization of the spine after tumor resection is very important, and for this, the spine surgeon can use **the Spine Instability Neoplastic Score (SINS)** (Fisher and DiPaola 2010), which evaluates the instability that the spinal tumor can cause and thus helps to plan the best instrumentation and grafting techniques to ensure good stabilization of the spine. Surgical stabilization is strongly recommended from a score greater than or equal to 7 (see also chapter "Local and Distant Staging").

Posterior stabilization is traditionally done with pedicle screws or articular screws for the cervical spine with a transverse device. Anterior bone loss can be filled by a simple bone graft taken from the iliac crest or the fibula; otherwise, a Pyramesh cage or an expandable cage can be used.

3 Surgical Management of Malignant Primary Bone Tumors of the Spine

En bloc resection with safe margins is the ultimate goal of any curative surgical treatment of malignant PBTS. This objective is sometimes difficult to achieve in the axial skeleton due to specific anatomical constraints.

The decision to sacrifice a nerve root or other paraspinal soft tissue depends in the majority of cases on intraoperative findings. In case of a major functional risk (paraplegia, tetraplegia) or a vascular risk that could compromise the patient's vital prognosis (in tumors in contact with major vessels), marginal resection is always preferred.

Overall, the decision of the type of surgery to perform (en bloc resection, piecemeal resection, or curettage) and the choice of the approach (anterior, posterior or combined) depends on the morphological analysis of the tumor on the imaging and its staging according to systems described previously in this chapter. This decision is often on a case-by-case basis as we will detail in our illustrative cases.

All these elements form the basis of the preoperative planning together with a meticulous and careful execution of the surgical procedure that yields the best possible results and prognosis.

3.1 Surgical Management of Chordoma

Chordomas (see chapter "Notochordal Tumors") are neoplasms that arise from notochordal remnants. They were the most common mPBTS in the study of the National Cancer Database of the United States, representing 37% of the cohort.

They are most commonly low-grade, slow-growing neoplasms, with metastatic disease only reported in 3% of patients (Kerr and Dial 2019). However, they are locally aggressive. About 50% of chordomas are sacral, 35% occur in the skull base, and 15% occur in the vertebral bodies of the mobile spine, most commonly the second cervical vertebra followed by the lumbar and thoracic spine (Tenny et al. 2023).

Clinical signs depend on the specific location of the chordoma; thus, the localization at the level of skull base and clivus can manifest itself by headaches or cranial nerve dysfunctions. In the mobile spine, symptoms are nonspecific such as localized pain and radiculopathy. Sacral chordomas, however, can give sometimes confusing symptoms such as constipation or dysfunction of the bladder.

Surgical management is challenging either for en bloc resection or for reconstruction. In fact, complete resection with clean margins is difficult to obtain due to proximity of vascular, neurological, and digestive structures. A double approach is often necessary to control the neurovascular elements, to avoid bleeding, and to respect the safety margins.

Five-year survival of chordomas is approximately 50% overall but improved with complete resection with negative margins to a 65% 5-year survival rate. Surgical resection with positive margins is approximately 50% 5-year survival, and if the chordoma is inoperable, 5-year survival rate is approximately 40%. Thus and despite their well-known radioresistance, most physicians recommend radiotherapy for chordomas due to the high risk of recurrence. Highly conformal radiotherapy including proton beam radiation or radiosurgery is a promising technique and increasingly used today (Tenny et al. 2023).

If complete resection is not feasible, intratumoral resection and local debulking can relieve symptoms and provide a smaller target volume for radiation therapy. Surgical abstention remains a wise choice in many cases.

Case Presentation

Chordoma in a 42-year-old patient who suffered from a painful mass in the sacrum. Diagnosis was suspected on imaging (Fig. 1a) and confirmed by biopsy. The tumor involved the fourth and fifth sacral vertebrae (Fig. 1a).

According to the WBB system, there was an involvement of anterior elements (4–9 sections) and posterior elements (1–3, 10–12 sections). There was also invasion of different layers (A–D) since it is a circumferential lesion.

The SINS score was calculated at 6, reflecting a stable lesion with no instrumentation or graft requirement.

Complete tumor resection was obtained by a double approach allowing trans-S3 sacrectomy while sacrificing bilateral S3–S5 sacral roots. The resection margins were free of tumor on histological examination. There was no local recurrence at the last follow-up (Fig. 1b). Surgery-associated morbidity included persistent unresolved bladder and sphincter disorders.

Six years after surgery, the patient consulted for a painful back mass. Imaging (Fig. 2a,b) and biopsy confirmed a distant recurrence of chordoma in the thoracic spine. According to the WBB system, there was an involvement of anterior elements (4–5 sections) and posterior elements (1–3 sections). There was also invasion of layers A–D.

The SINS score was calculated at 9, reflecting a potentially unstable lesion requiring instrumentation and graft. En bloc resection of T5 vertebra (Fig. 2c) with instrumented graft through a double approach was performed (Fig. 2d, e).

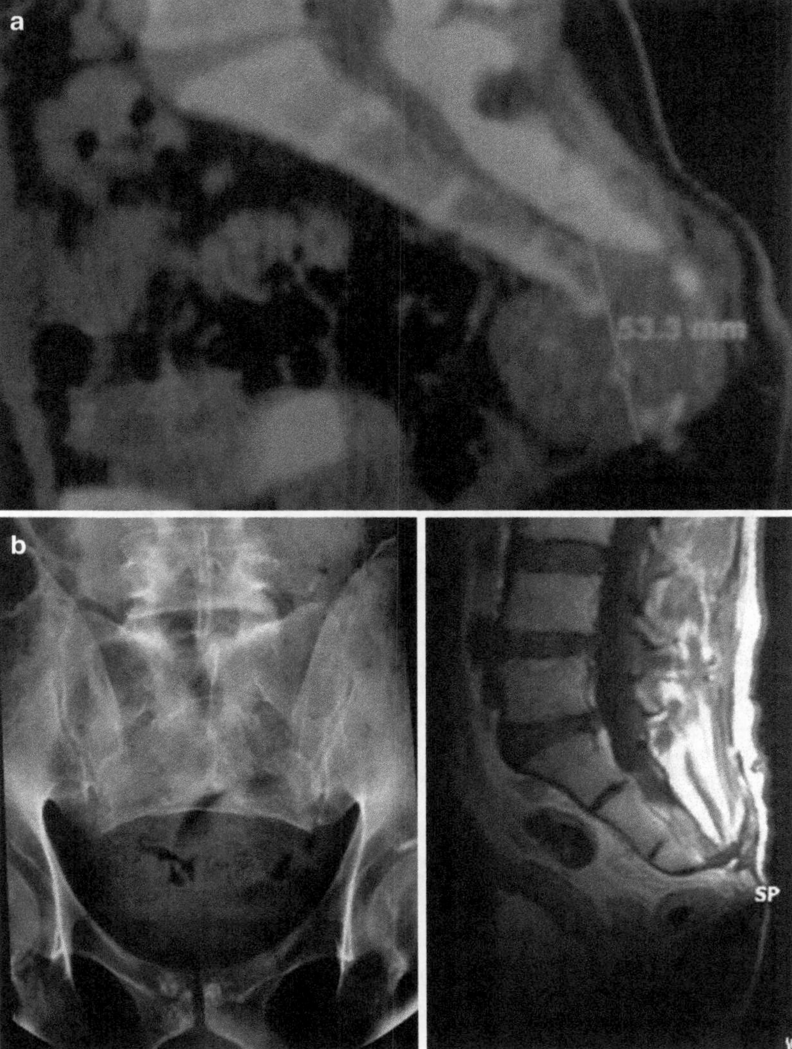

Fig. 1 Chordoma in a 42-year-old man. (**a**) CT scan sagittal image: hypodense mass of the fourth and fifth sacral vertebrae. (**b**) CR frontal view and MRI sagittal T1-weighted image (WI). Seven years after sacrectomy. No local recurrence was found

3.2 Surgical Management of Ewing's Sarcoma

Ewing's sarcomas (see chapter "Ewing's Sarcoma/PNET") are small, round-cell neoplasms that commonly present during the first and second decades of life. There are no known predisposing factors; however, there is a slightly higher incidence in males and exceedingly higher rate in Caucasian descent compared to African descent. The most common locations are the metaphyses of the long bones and the flat bones of the shoulder and pelvis.

Primary Ewing's sarcoma (EWS) of the spine is rare and highly proliferative and has a confusing variety of imaging manifestations in adult patients. According to the National Cancer Database of the United States, Ewing's sarcoma accounts for 27% of all PBTSs among which 97% were reported as high grade, and the rate of metastatic disease was 18% (Kerr and Dial 2019).

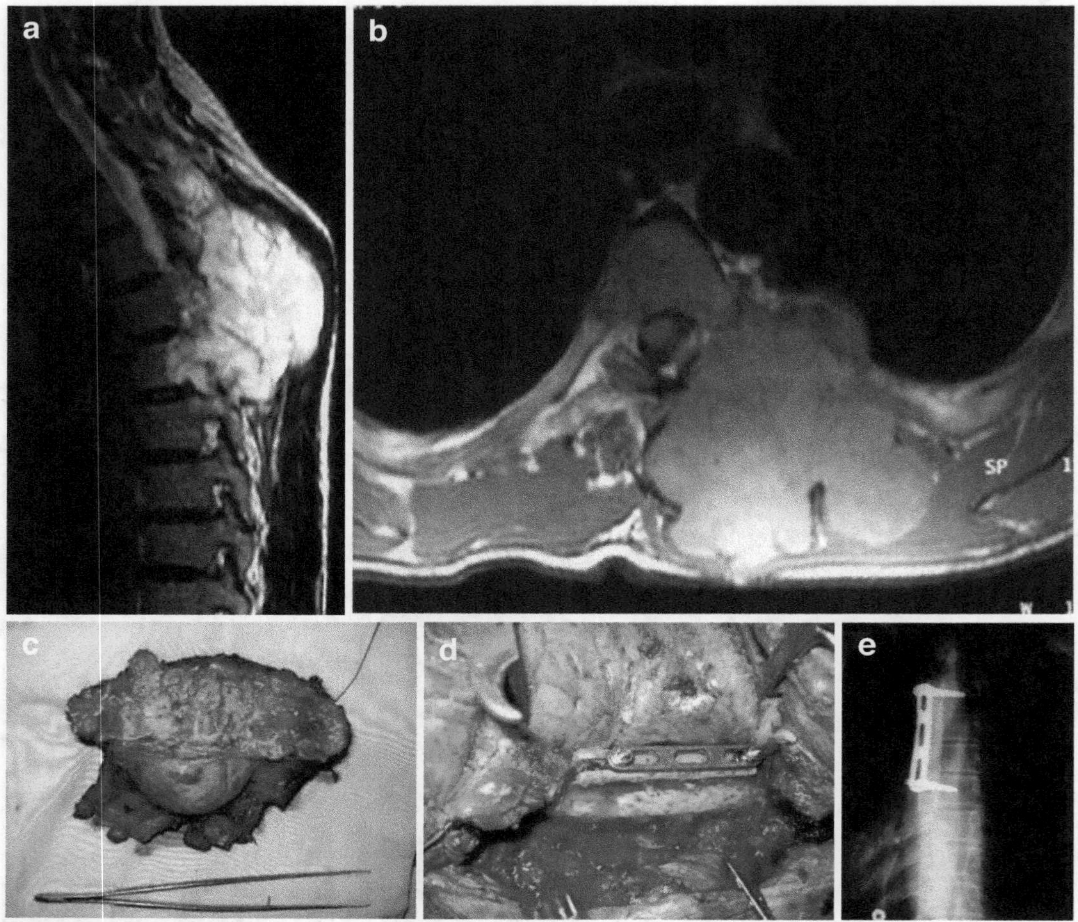

Fig. 2 Thoracic recurrence of the chordoma 6 years after surgery. (**a**) MRI sagittal T2-WI of the thoracic mass. (**b**) MRI axial enhanced T1-WI axial view: left dorsal paravertebral mass next to T5 measuring 10 cm in size extending to the spinal canal. (**c**) Resected mass of the recurrent chordoma through a double approach and after embolization of the seventh intercostal artery. (**d**) Grafting and fixation. (**e**) Postoperative CR

Nonspecific symptoms with insidious onset and a clinical-biological presentation mimicking osteomyelitis may cause delay of the accurate diagnosis. Indeed, EWS can present with fever, an increased white blood cell count, elevated erythrocyte sedimentation rate, an elevated C-reactive protein level, and even presence of pus on the biopsy puncture, hence the rule to submit the biopsy samples for histological study even when infection is strongly suspected.

Given the rarity of the spinal localization, treatment is based on that of the appendicular skeleton EWS including neoadjuvant chemotherapy, surgical resection, radiation therapy, and adjuvant chemotherapy.

The aim of surgery is a complete tumor removal and spinal column stability restoration. Although this goal is often achieved in the appendicular skeleton, it is rarely obtained in the spinal located tumors due to anatomical complexity and the often locally advanced tumor at diagnosis. Thus, spinal EWS has a worse prognosis compared to other locations.

Case Presentation

EWS of 12th thoracic vertebra in a 30-year-old man diagnosed after 7 months of nonspecific pain of the thoracolumbar junction with right intercostal neuralgia.

Imaging showed a mass affecting the right hemivertebral body and posterior arch of T12 with paravertebral soft tissue extension and spinal cord compression (Fig. 3).

CT-guided biopsy confirmed the diagnosis of EWS.

Staging of this tumor showed that there was an involvement of anterior elements (6–9 sections) and posterior elements (10–12 sections) according to the WBB system. There was also invasion of layers A–D (Fig. 4). The SINS score was calculated at 9.

Management consisted of neoadjuvant chemotherapy, double-approach vertebrectomy with posterior stabilization and anterior bone grafting, radiation, and adjuvant chemotherapy. At the last follow-up (4 years), there was no local recurrence. However, the patient died from pulmonary metastasis (Fig. 5).

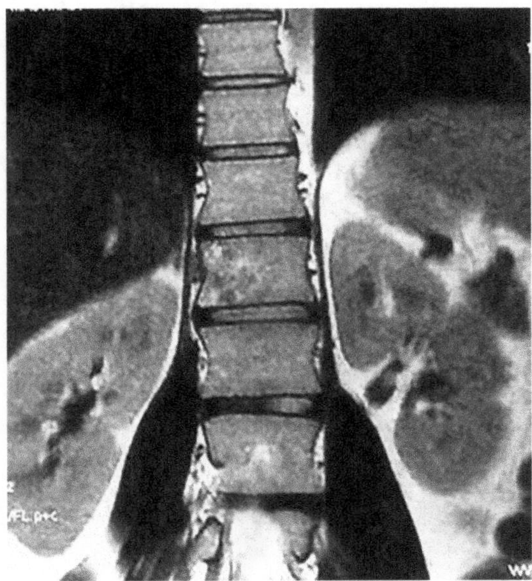

Fig. 3 EWS of T12: MRI T1-WI: A vascularized mass affecting the right hemivertebral body and posterior arch of T12 with right paravertebral soft tissue extension and spinal cord compression

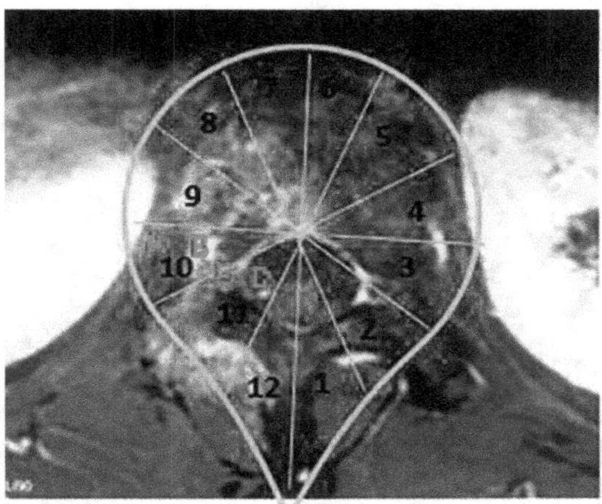

Fig. 4 Staging of the EWS according to WBB system on an axial enhanced T1-WI post-neoadjuvant chemotherapy

3.3 Surgical Management of Plasmacytoma

Solitary bone plasmacytoma (SBP) is a rare hematologic malignant disease, which is defined by the presence of a single osteolytic lesion due to monoclonal plasma cell infiltration, with or without soft-tissue extension (Tan and Gu 2021) (see also chapter "Plasmacytoma").

More precisely, the International Myeloma Working Group (IMWG) has defined four basic criteria for the diagnosis of solitary plasmacytoma: (1) biopsy-proven solitary lesion of bone or soft tissue with evidence of clonal plasma cells, (2) normal bone marrow with no evidence of clonal plasma cells, (3) normal skeletal survey and MRI (or CT) of spine and pelvis (except for the primary solitary lesion), and (4) absence of end-organ damage such as hypercalcemia, renal insufficiency, anemia, or bone lesions (CRAB) that can be attributed to a lymphoplasma cell proliferative disorder. The use of much more sophisticated techniques has allowed the IMWG in recent years to revise the diagnostic criteria for solitary plasmacytoma in general and SBP in particular. Thus, the use of flow cytometry may be helpful in the distinction of the true SBP (negative flow cytometry) with a very low rate of evolution to MM from those with high risk of

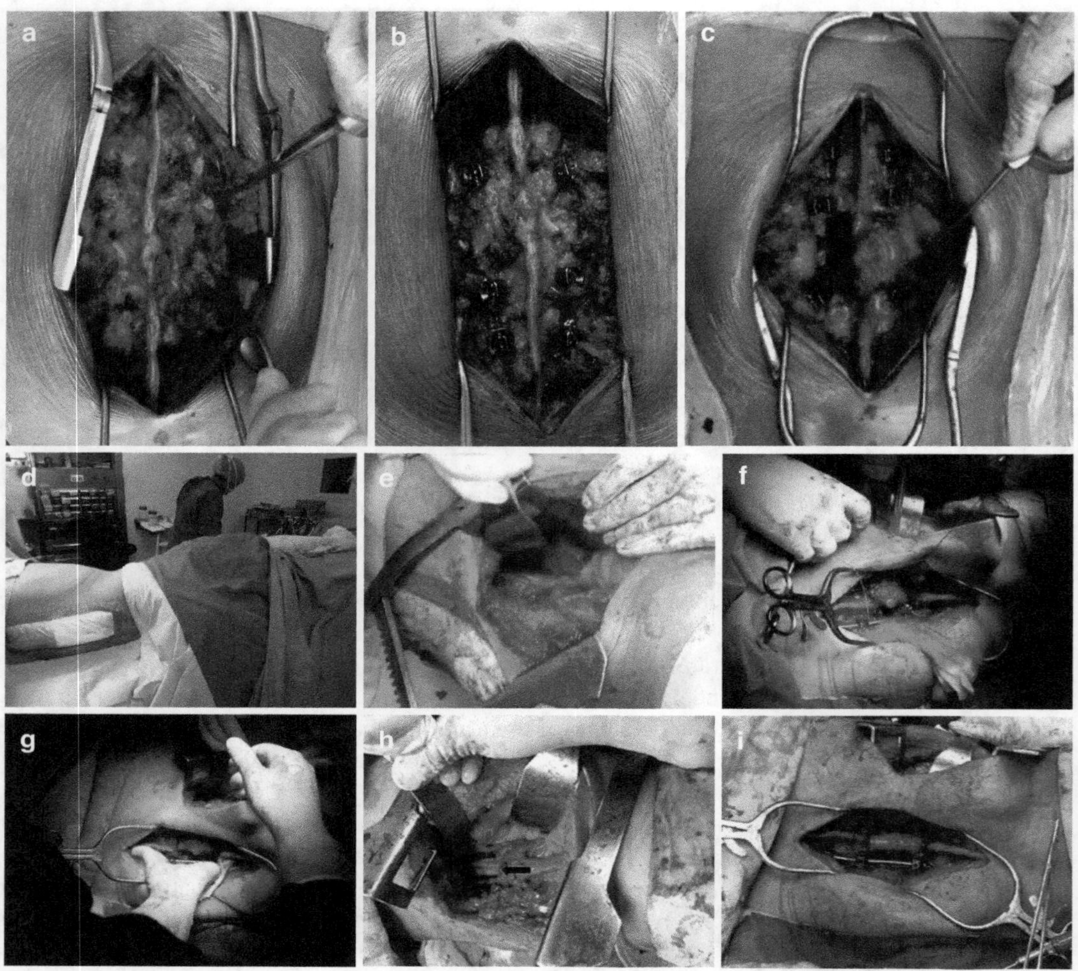

Fig. 5 Surgical management of primary Ewing's sarcoma of T12. (**a**) Step 1: posterior approach respecting a safety margin within paravertebral soft tissues on the right side and including the biopsy path. (**b**) Step 2: pedicle screw insertion 2 levels above and 2 levels below the EWS. (**c**) Step 3: release of the spinal cord. Soft tissue margins on the right side were respected. (**d**) Step 3: positioning for the anterolateral approach. Identification of the level under fluoroscopy. Installation of the lower limb to harvest the fibular graft. (**e**) Anterolateral approach (thoraco-phreno-lobotomy) to separate the anterior part of the tumor and control the segmental arteries. (**f**) Cutting of the upper and inferior level (inferior end plate of T11 and superior end plate of L1) using a Gigli saw. (**g**) Extraction of the vertebra released from all its attachments was possible through a simple rotation of the specimen. (**h**) Anterior graft using a nonvascularized fibula (black arrow). (**i**) Final appearance after tumor extraction and vertebral column stabilization. (**j**) Clinical appearance of the extracted vertebrae. (**k**) Radiographs of the extracted vertebrae. (**l**) Postoperative AP and lateral radiographs of the thoracolumbar spine

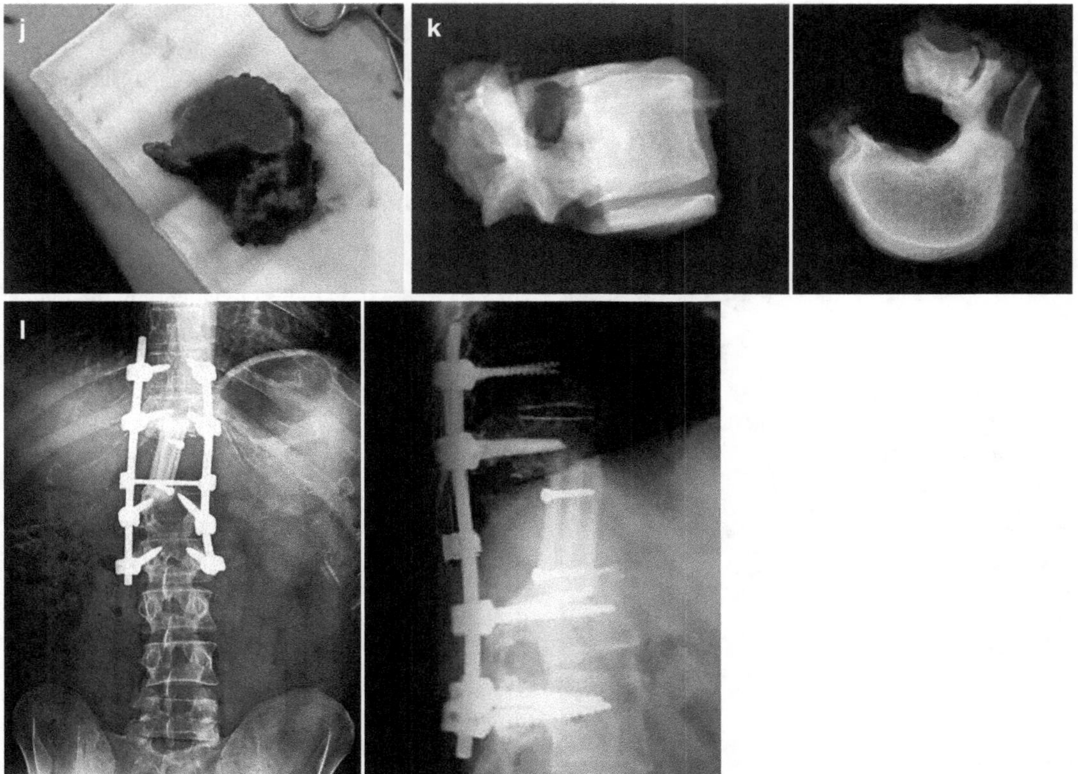

Fig. 5 (continued)

progression to myeloma (positive flow cytometry) where close attention should be given during routine follow-up (Caers and Paiva 2018; Rajkumar and Dimopoulos 2014).

This lesion occurs in middle-aged or elderly patients, and males are more frequently affected; it can remain single as it can progress to multiple myeloma (MM). Approximately 50% of patients with SBP develop MM within 10 years after the initial diagnosis (Kilciksiz and Karakoyun-Celik 2012).

The axial skeleton and the skull are preferable locations, and the thoracic spine is the most frequently involved segment. Involvement of the upper cervical spine is rare and a more challenging condition because it may cause atlantoaxial dislocation and cranio-vertebral junction (CVJ) instability (Tan and Gu 2021).

Clinical signs are often nonspecific and vary according to the localization, which delays the diagnosis.

Diagnosis can be difficult even after biological explorations and biopsy. Indeed, laboratory examinations (white blood cell count, erythrocyte sedimentation rate, and C-reactive protein) are nonspecific, and histological examination can miss the diagnosis in 18% of cases. Likewise, CT scan-guided percutaneous biopsy has a sensitivity of 52% for the diagnosis of spinal infections according to the meta-analysis of Pupaibool and Vasoo (2015).

SBP is highly sensitive to radiotherapy according to initial clinical trials; however, the evidence of effectiveness was based on retrospective studies. Current recommendations value radiotherapy as the first-line treatment in plasmacytoma with a minimum dose of 4000 cGy without exceeding 5000 cGy due to the risk of toxicity.

The use of chemotherapy remains controversial in the literature, especially in the borderline cases between solitary plasmacytoma and multiple myeloma.

Literature remains controversial whether surgery is needed or not in solitary spinal plasmacytoma; however, in cases where there is spinal instability or neural compression secondary to tumor proliferation, surgery is frequently indicated and thus consists of either decompression alone or decompression with fixation and fusion. In case of craniovertebral localization, the majority advises fixation and fusion to avoid instability.

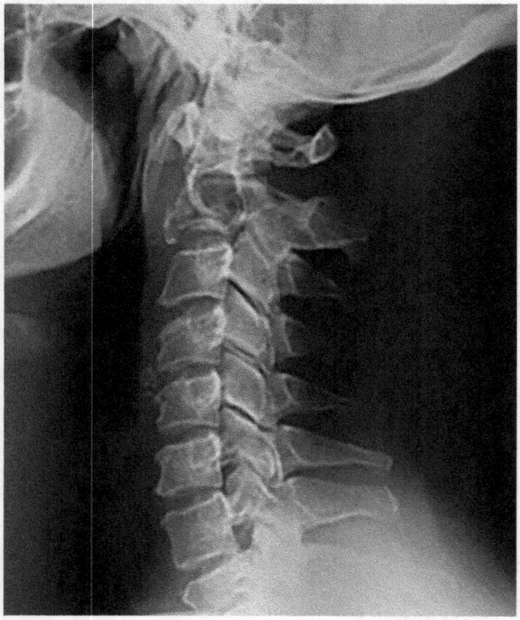

Fig. 6 CR at initial presentation. Lateral view showed the extension of the bone lysis to the vertebral body and odontoid process with a preserved sagittal alignement

Case Presentation

A 59-year-old man was referred to our institution for neck pain and numbness of both hands not resolving under symptomatic treatment.

CR showed a lytic lesion of the odontoid process and the vertebral body of C2 (Fig. 6), and CT scan revealed extension to the posterior arch. MRI identified extension in the spinal canal and prevertebral soft tissues (Fig. 7). Laboratory examinations were negative, and histological examination of the CT scan-guided biopsy was inconclusive.

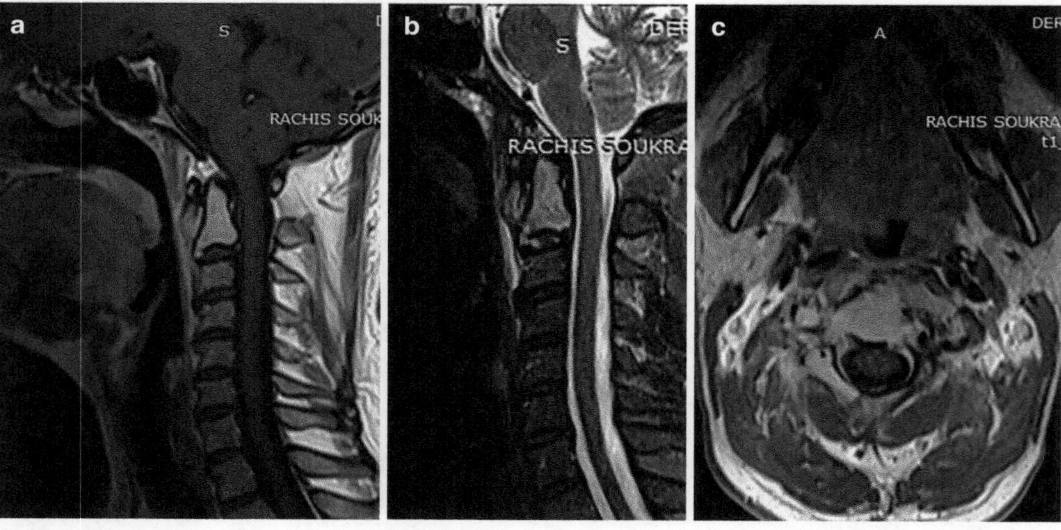

Fig. 7 MRI. (**a**) High signal on sagittal T1-WI. (**b**) High signal on sagittal T2-WI. (**c**) Local extension is better assessed on axial images, showing extension to the right posterior lamina

Surgical management consisted of surgical biopsy with curettage of the tumor invading the posterior arch. At the same time, occipito-C4 fixation was performed, and fusion with an autologous bone graft taken from the posterior iliac crest was done and fixed with a screw to avoid instability of the craniovertebral junction (Fig. 8) (as the lesion was considered instable with a SINS score of 11). The diagnosis of solitary bone plasmacytoma of C2 was confirmed on histological examination. The diagnosis of multiple myeloma was ruled out following biological and radiological assessment.

The patient was subsequently followed up by oncologists and had 45 G radiotherapy as well as chemotherapy. At 3 years of follow-up, he is doing well without neurologic deficit or progression to multiple myeloma. However, limitation of the cervical spine range of motion persisted as well as limited mouth opening. Imaging showed slight calcification of the tumor with a good fusion of the posterior bone graft (Fig. 9).

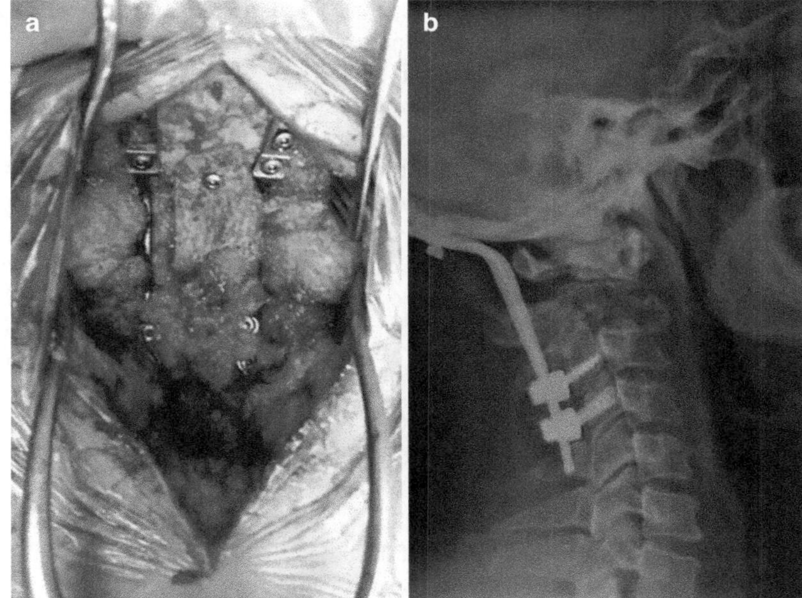

Fig. 8 Surgical management. (**a**) Perioperative image of occipito-cervical fixation and fusion. (**b**) Postoperative CR

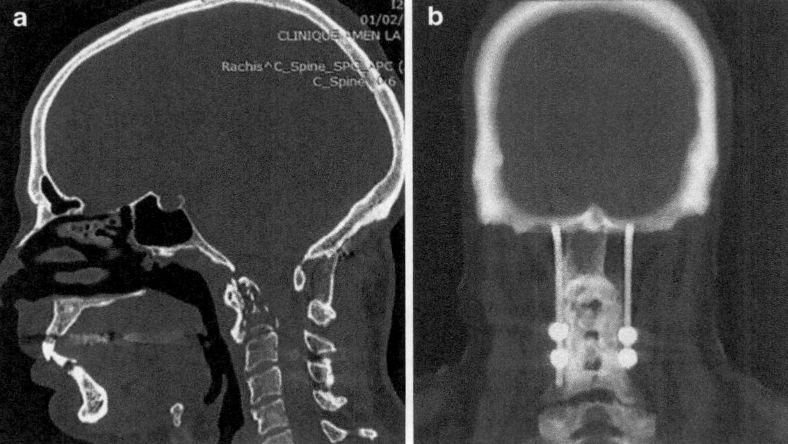

Fig. 9 Imaging at 4-year follow-up. (**a**) Sagittal CT scan image showed partial calcification of the tumor with a good sagittal alignment and no further extension to adjacent levels. (**b**) Coronal CT scan image showing the good quality of fusion

3.4 Surgical Management of Chondrosarcoma

Chondrosarcomas (see also chapter "Cartilaginous Tumors") are neoplasms producing cartilaginous matrix without osteoid. According to the National Cancer Database of the United States, chondrosarcomas accounted for 22% of the PBTS. The majority of chondrosarcomas were reported as low or intermediate grade, and only 4% of patients were reported to have metastatic disease (Kerr and Dial 2019).

Unlike other malignant tumors of the spine which tend to have an anterior localization at the vertebral body, this tumor can originate in the vertebral body, the posterior arch, or both. The radiological appearance varies according to the histological grade of the tumor. The second difference of chondrosarcomas with other malignant tumors is that it does not respond to chemotherapy and radiotherapy. Thus, adequate surgical treatment is often the only alternative to avoid the risk of recurrence, and the outcome is based on the margins achieved (Katonis and Alpantaki 2011).

The spine surgeon must carefully analyze the limits of the tumor to achieve surgery objective. Classification according to the Enneking system and the Weinstein-Boriani-Biagini (WBB) system is of indisputable contribution in this stage. It is also necessary to respect the rules of the biopsy and to discuss its pathway with the radiologist in order to include it in the definitive surgery.

En bloc resection with safe margins can offer the patient a good result with a low risk of recurrence estimated at 3–8% compared to intralesional resection where the risk of recurrence can reach 100%. In case of incomplete resection, proton beam radiation or focused photon radiotherapy can be prescribed in order to control the risk of recurrence even without proven effectiveness (Pennington and Ehresman 2021).

Reconstruction and stabilization after tumor resection correspond to the same principles described above.

3.5 Surgical Management of Osteosarcoma

Osteosarcomas (see chapter "Osteosarcoma") are neoplasms producing osteoid. In the spine, it represented the least common malignant PBTS according to the study of the National Cancer Database of the United States accounting for 13%. In the same study, the majority of osteosarcomas in the mobile spine were high grade at diagnosis (79%), and metastatic disease was reported in 15% of patients (Kerr and Dial 2019).

This tumor has a poor prognosis because of its significant local aggressiveness, the high risk of recurrence, and the strong metastatic potential. Thus, the management must be multidisciplinary including oncologists, spine surgeons, radiotherapists, radiologists, and pathologists.

Feng and Yang (2013), in their cohort study of 16 cases of primary osteosarcoma of the spine, found a similar distribution between the different regions of the mobile spine (six cases in the cervical, six in the thoracic, and four in the lumbar spine). Local recurrence rate was estimated at 37.5% and metastasis at 56.3% despite wide surgical resection, neoadjuvant and postoperative chemotherapy, as well as radiotherapy. They concluded that the association between patient outcome and various treatments for osteosarcoma of the spine is not known.

Prognosis is poor with fatal outcome in most of the cases in spite of aggressive surgery; however, en bloc resection with wide margins can increase the overall survival with an average of 6.8 years compared to 3.7 years for those with intralesional resection (Dekutoski and Clarke 2016).

While the role of neoadjuvant and postoperative chemotherapy was underscored in different studies dealing with osteosarcoma of the appendicular skeleton, this could not be confirmed for spinal localization in view of its rarity. However, the same therapeutic protocols have been extrapolated for spinal localization and are widely used. On the other hand, the role of radiotherapy remains unclear despite the optimistic expectations from new radiotherapy techniques that are more precise and less damaging to the surrounding tissues regarding the reduction of local recurrence. This remains to be confirmed in further studies.

4 Surgical Management of Benign Primary Bone Tumor of the Spine

The majority of benign PBTSs are discovered incidentally; however, some localizations may be symptomatic presenting with back pain, radicular pain, rarely spinal deformation, or a neurological deficit.

Malignancy must be ruled out before retaining the diagnosis of a benign tumor. Imaging and biopsy when necessary are of an important contribution in the differentiation between the two types.

Giant cell tumor (GCT), osteochondroma, osteoid osteoma, osteoblastoma, aneurysmal bone cyst (ABC), neurofibroma, eosinophilic granuloma, and hemangioma are the most described benign PBTSs. In this chapter, we will detail the first five tumors that require surgical treatment more than the others.

4.1 Surgical Management of Giant Cell Tumor

GCT of the spine (see chapter "Giant Cell Tumor") is a rare entity accounting for 1–1.5% of all GCT of bone (Redhu and Poonia 2012). It is considered as the most aggressive benign PBTS with a high risk of recurrence and an unpredictable outcome. The risk of developing neurological signs is very high because of its potential to invade the spinal canal and compress the spinal cord.

En bloc resection of the vertebra would be the perfect solution; however, this is often difficult since diagnosis is mostly made at locally advanced stage. Thus, intralesional resection or curettage is often the reasonable technique with the best risk-benefit ratio. The choice of approach (anterior, posterior, or double approach) essentially depends on the location of the tumor and its relationship with the vessels and nerves. The recurrence risk is the major drawback of this technique, and additional postoperative radiotherapy and use of cement or a metal cage instead of bone grafts can reduce this risk (Bhojraj and Nene 2007).

Denosumab is currently widely used whether for GCT of the long bones or the spine without proven effectiveness (Luengo-Alonso and Mellado-Romero 2019; Li and Gao 2020).

Lung metastasis of spinal GCT seems to be more frequent than that of long bones (Donthineni and Boriani 2009). Special attention must be given to these patients during postoperative follow-up in order to detect these metastases and treat them in time.

Case Presentation

A 38-year-old woman, with no past medical history presented with thoracolumbar spinal pain evolving for 8 months with recent onset of neurological deficit class C according to the Frankel-ASIA score.

CR showed a lytic lesion of T12 with moderate kyphosis. MRI showed a mass invading the vertebral body of T12 as well as its pedicles (predominantly the left side) with spinal cord compression (Fig. 10).

According to the WBB system, there was an involvement of the anterior (5–8 sections) and posterior elements (2–4, 9–10 sections). There was also invasion of extra-osseous space (paravertebral, layer A), intra-osseous deep space (layer C), and epidural space (layer D) (Fig. 11).

The SINS score was calculated at 15, so it is an unstable lesion that requires instrumentation with a graft. At first, an emergency spinal decompression surgery with biopsy was needed. Histopathology confirmed the diagnosis of giant cell tumor. A second surgery with the aim of fur-

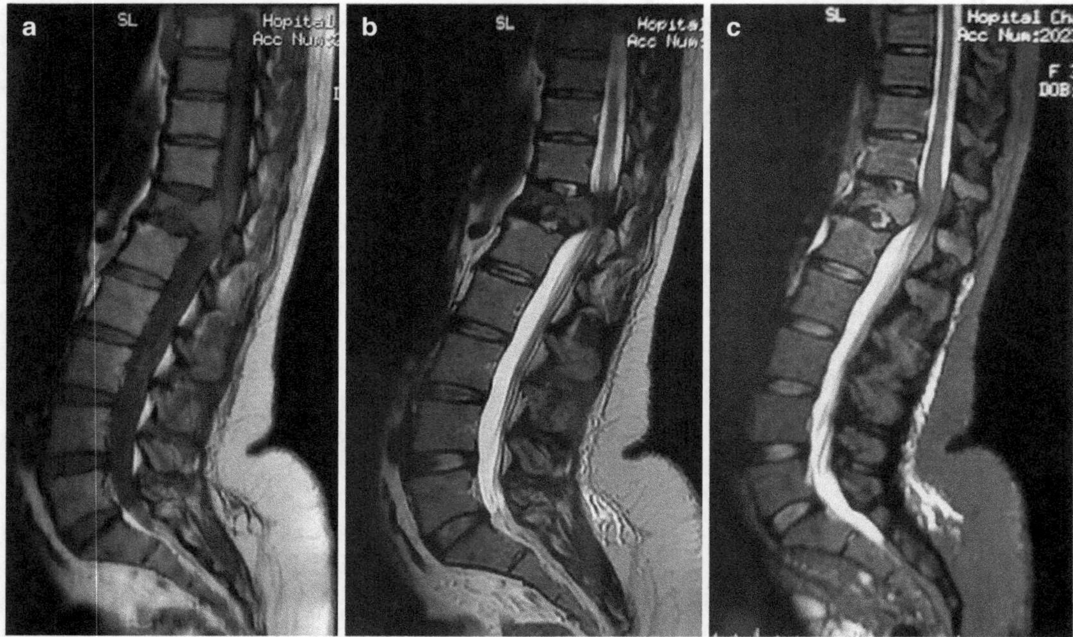

Fig. 10 Sagittal T1-WI (**a**), T2-WI (**b**), and fat-sat T2-WI (**c**) showing vertebral collapse of intermediate signal on all sequences and spinal cord compression

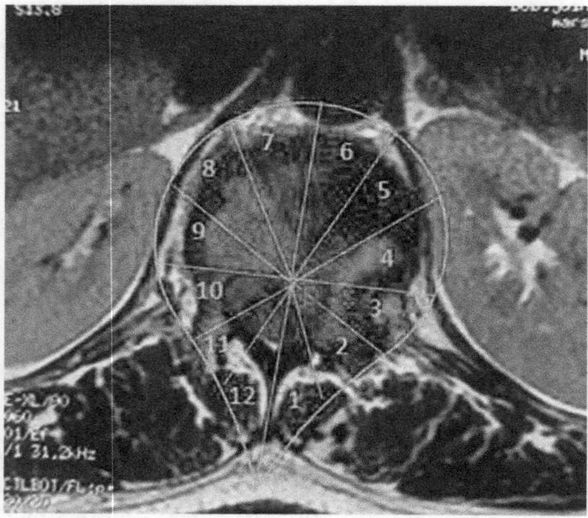

Fig. 11 Planning of compartment to resect according to the WBB system

ther excision of the posterior arch and fixation with pedicle screws was performed (Fig. 12).

The last step was an anterolateral thoracotomy with resection of T12 vertebral body and filling of the empty space with a resected rib graft although a fibula graft was considered previously (Figs. 13 and 14).

Surgery achieved the goals of spinal decompression and stabilization (Fig. 15).

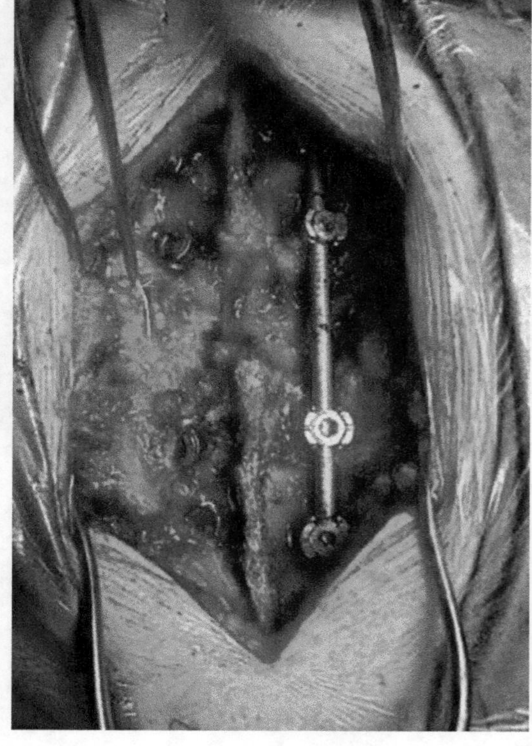

Fig. 12 Posterior arch resection, spine decompression, and fixation with two pedicular screws above and two below T12

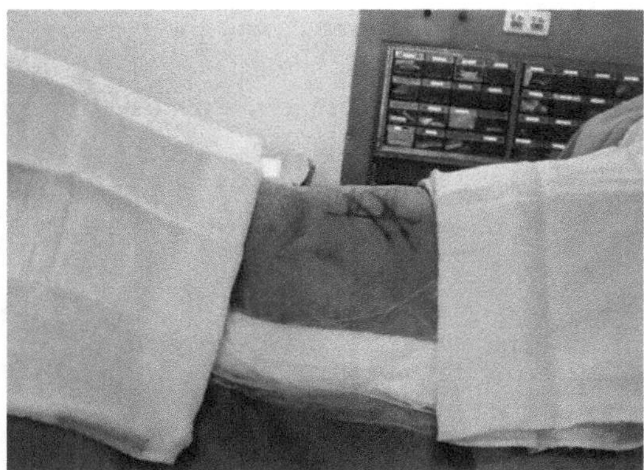

Fig. 13 Patient positioning and fluoroscopic identification of the affected vertebra and the rib to be resected

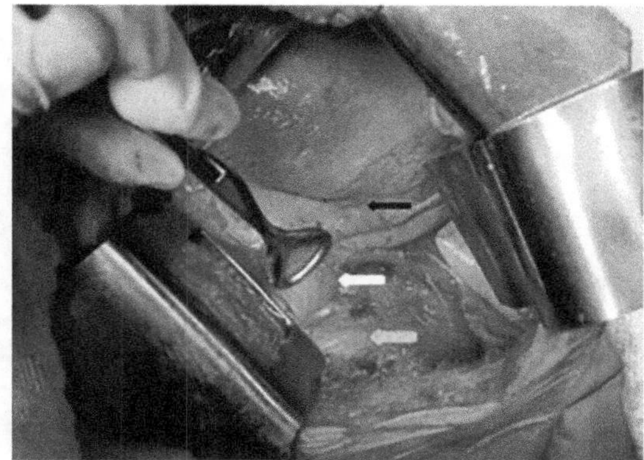

Fig. 14 Exposure of T12 vertebral body (yellow arrows) through the tenth rib and after overelevating of the pleura (white arrow). The diaphragm was respected (black arrow)

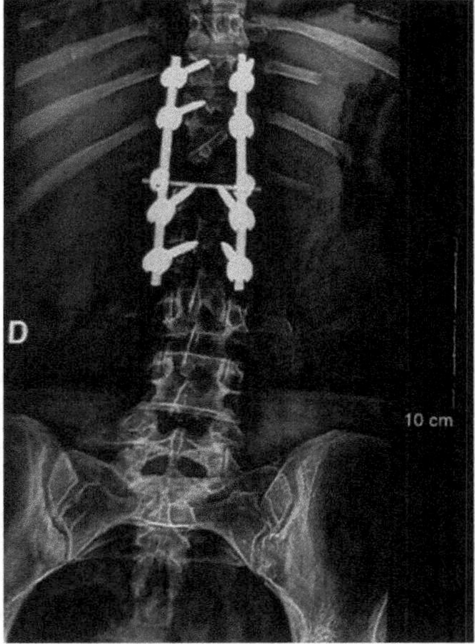

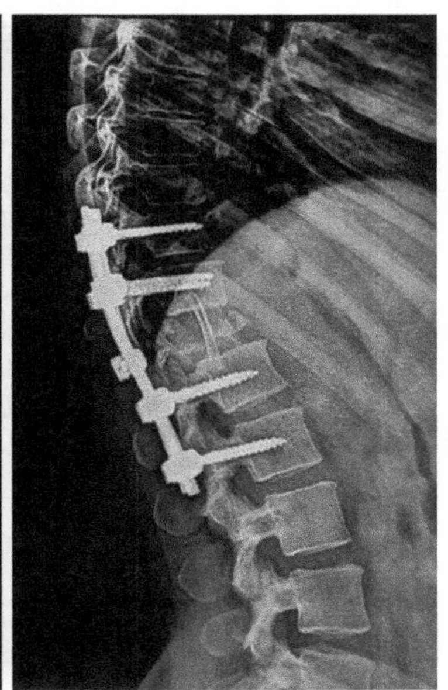

Fig. 15 Postoperative AP and lateral radiographs with posterior fixation and anterior graft

The patient recovered a normal Frankel E neurological status and was referred for denosumab and radiotherapy as adjuvant treatment to minimize the risk of recurrence.

4.2 Osteoid Osteoma and Osteoblastoma

Osteoid osteoma (OO) and osteoblastoma (see chapter "Osteoid Osteoma and Osteoblastoma") are histologically and clinically similar tumors, although osteoblastoma is larger and more aggressive (Kan and Schmidt 2008). A painful scoliosis in an adolescent is the most common clinical presentation. The localization in the posterior vertebral elements is characteristic. Thus, posterior approach is often sufficient for resection.

While intralesional excision of the nidus was the most practiced procedure for a long time, en bloc resection of OO has a low recurrence rate. CT-guided radiofrequency ablation of OO is a mini-invasive option that can be performed while paying attention to the risk of thermal damage to adjacent neurovascular structures (Mallepally and Mahajan 2020).

Sometimes, resection includes removal of a facet joint or a pedicle leading to instability of the level affected requiring fixation and fusion.

Osteoblastoma due to its larger size and recurrence risk may require more complex surgical management similar to that of malignant tumors.

4.3 Aneurysmal Bone Cyst

Aneurysmal bone cyst (ABC) (see chapter "Aneurysmal Bone Cyst and Other Cystic Lesions") is a benign hemorrhagic bone tumor that invades the bone giving the appearance of lytic cavities separated by septa. The appearance on imaging is variable depending on its stage of maturation at the time of diagnosis, and the most characteristic form is the soap bubble appearance (Riahi and Mechri 2018).

It represents 15% of all primary spinal tumor, and 30% of ABCs are localized in the spine occurring more often in children and young adults (Codd and Riesenburger 2006).

Compared to the ABC of the long bones, the spinal localization presents several particularities. In fact, contact with the vertebral canal and the greater risk of recurrence make curettage or simple osteosynthesis inappropriate for the spine. Thus, the most complete resection possible is the ideal choice to hope for a good prognosis and avoid the risk of recurrence.

4.4 Chondroblastoma

Spinal chondroblastoma (see chapter "Cartilaginous Tumors") is a rare condition accounting for about 1.4% of all chondroblastoma cases. It is the rarest among the bPBTS, and its first differential diagnosis remains the giant cell tumor. The World Health Organization (WHO) defined it as a locally aggressive tumor with low risk of metastasis (<2%) and high risk of recurrence (38%) (Jia and Liu 2018; Zheng and Huang 2023).

As with other benign bone tumors of the spine, spinal chondroblastoma, despite being considered a benign bone tumor, is locally aggressive with high risk of recurrence and a worse prognosis compared to chondroblastomas of the long bones. Thus, the current surgical trend is to resect them as completely as possible with an R0 margin if possible; otherwise, a resection is done removing most of the tumor while considering the risk-benefit ratio regarding the vascular and nervous elements. Adjuvant radiotherapy with its new techniques would have a (still to be confirmed) advantage in controlling the risk of local recurrence.

4.5 Benign Notochordal Cell Tumor

This entity has been recently described. It originates from the same precursors as chordoma (notochordal remnant). The difference with chordoma and remnants of notochord has been proven by multiple histological studies as well as the risk of malignant transformation of these benign tumors (Yamaguchi and Suzuki 2004; Yamaguchi and Iwata 2008) (see chapter "Notochordal Tumors").

In view of this confusion with chordomas on imaging and almost similar histological appearance, this tumor was often treated by complete surgical excision (en bloc vertebrectomy), which is not proven mandatory nowadays. Thus, the current management is, once the histological diagnosis is confirmed, to monitor the clinical and imaging evolution in order to detect malignant degeneration requiring surgical resection, in case of persistent pain, instability, or spinal compression. A less aggressive surgery surgical can always be proposed (Ma and Xia 2014).

5 Conclusion

PBTS, whether malignant or benign, requires a good preoperative analysis with staging according to recently updated systems. The management must be discussed with the patient and within a multidisciplinary staff.

En bloc vertebrectomy seems to be correlated to the best prognosis; however, the invasion of the spinal canal or large vessels makes this type of surgery difficult to perform. Incomplete resection with new radiotherapy techniques can reduce the risk of recurrence with promising results.

6 Key Points

- Primary bone tumors of the spine are a rare condition needing a high level of suspicion.
- Biopsy should be performed to confirm the benign or malignant nature of the tumor except when the imaging appearance is specific like in osteoid osteoma.
- Staging systems that are currently most used for PBTS are the Enneking system, the American Joint Committee on Cancer (AJCC) system, and the Weinstein-Biagini-Boriani classification. The Spine Instability Neoplastic Score (SINS) is used to evaluate the risk of instability after tumor resection.
- For malignant tumors, en bloc resection with wide healthy margins offers the best prognosis; however, this achievement remains challenging due to proximity of dura, nerve root, and major vascular structures. Advanced radiation techniques allowed better sterilization of the tumor remnant with a lower rate of recurrence and side effects.
- Spinal benign bone tumors are more demanding in terms of surgery compared to other locations for the same reasons mentioned above, and the most complete resection possible is the only guarantee to avoid the risk of recurrence and subsequent surgical revisions' morbidity.

References

Bhojraj SY, Nene A (2007) Giant cell tumor of the spine: a review of 9 surgical interventions in 6 cases. Indian J Orthop 41(2):146–150. https://doi.org/10.4103/0019-5413.32047

Boriani S, Weinstein JN (1997) Primary bone tumors of the spine: terminology and surgical staging. Spine 22(9):1036–1044. https://doi.org/10.1097/00007632-199705010-00020

Caers J, Paiva B (2018) Diagnosis, treatment, and response assessment in solitary plasmacytoma: updated recommendations from a European Expert Panel. J Hematol Oncol 11(1):10. https://doi.org/10.1186/s13045-017-0549-1

Choi D, Crockard A (2010) Review of metastatic spine tumour classification and indications for surgery: the consensus statement of the Global Spine Tumour Study Group. Eur Spine J 19(2):215–222. https://doi.org/10.1007/s00586-009-1252-x

Codd PJ, Riesenburger RI (2006) Vertebra plana due to an aneurysmal bone cyst of the lumbar spine. Case report and review of the literature. J Neurosurg 105(6 Suppl):490–495. https://doi.org/10.3171/ped.2006.105.6.490

Dekutoski MB, Clarke MJ (2016) AOSpine knowledge forum tumor. Osteosarcoma of the spine: prognostic variables for local recurrence and overall survival, a multicenter ambispective study. J Neurosurg Spine 25(1):59–68. https://doi.org/10.3171/2015.11.SPINE15870

Donthineni R, Boriani L (2009) Metastatic behaviour of giant cell tumour of the spine. Int Orthop 33:497–501. https://doi.org/10.1007/s00264-008-0560-9

Enneking WF, Spanier SS (1980) A system for the surgical staging of musculoskeletal sarcoma. Clin Orthop Relat Res 2003:4–18. https://doi.org/10.1097/01.blo.0000093891.12372.0f

Feng D, Yang X (2013) Osteosarcoma of the spine: surgical treatment and outcomes. World J Surg Oncol 11(1):89. https://doi.org/10.1186/1477-7819-11-89

Fisher CG, DiPaola CP (2010) A novel classification system for spinal instability in neoplastic disease: an evidence-based approach and expert consensus from the Spine Oncology Study Group. Spine (Phila Pa 1976) 35(22):E1221–E1229. https://doi.org/10.1097/BRS.0b013e3181e16ae2

Jia Q, Liu C (2018) Clinical features, treatments and long-term follow-up outcomes of spinal chondroblastoma: report of 13 clinical cases in a single center. J Neuro-Oncol 140(1):99–106. https://doi.org/10.1007/s11060-018-2935-0

Kan P, Schmidt MH (2008) Osteoid osteoma and osteoblastoma of the spine. Neurosurg Clin N Am 19(1):65–70. https://doi.org/10.1016/j.nec.2007.09.003

Katonis P, Alpantaki K (2011) Spinal chondrosarcoma: a review. Sarcoma 2011:378957. https://doi.org/10.1155/2011/378957

Kerr DL, Dial BL (2019) Epidemiologic and survival trends in adult primary bone tumors of the spine. Spine J 19(12):1941–1949. https://doi.org/10.1016/j.spinee.2019.07.003

Kilciksiz S, Karakoyun-Celik O (2012) A review for solitary plasmacytoma of bone and extramedullary plasmacytoma. Sci World J 2012:895765. https://doi.org/10.1100/2012/895765

Li H, Gao J (2020) Denosumab in giant cell tumor of bone: current status and pitfalls. Front Oncol 10:580605. https://doi.org/10.3389/fonc.2020.580605

Luengo-Alonso G, Mellado-Romero M (2019) Denosumab treatment for giant-cell tumor of bone: a systematic review of the literature. Arch Orthop

Trauma Surg 139(10):1339–1349. https://doi.org/10.1007/s00402-019-03167-x

Ma X, Xia C (2014) Benign notochordal cell tumor: a retrospective study of 11 cases with 13 vertebra bodies. Int J Clin Exp Pathol 7(7):3548–3554

Mallepally AR, Mahajan R (2020) Spinal osteoid osteoma: surgical resection and review of literature. Surg Neurol Int 11:308. https://doi.org/10.25259/SNI_510_2020

Patnaik S, Jyotsnarani Y (2016) Imaging features of primary tumors of the spine: a pictorial essay. Indian J Radiol Imaging 26:279–289. https://doi.org/10.4103/0971-3026.184413

Pennington Z, Ehresman J (2021) Chondrosarcoma of the spine: a narrative review. Spine J 21(12):2078–2096. https://doi.org/10.1016/j.spinee.2021.04.021

Pupaibool J, Vasoo S (2015) The utility of image-guided percutaneous needle aspiration biopsy for the diagnosis of spontaneous vertebral osteomyelitis: a systematic review and meta-analysis. Spine J 15:122–131. https://doi.org/10.1016/j.spinee.2014.07.003

Rajkumar SV, Dimopoulos MA (2014) International myeloma working group updated criteria for the diagnosis of multiple myeloma. Lancet Oncol 15(12):e538–e548. https://doi.org/10.1016/S1470-2045(14)70442-5

Redhu R, Poonia R (2012) Giant cell tumor of dorsal vertebral body. J Craniovertebr Junction Spine 3(2):67–69. https://doi.org/10.4103/0974-8237.116542

Riahi H, Mechri M (2018) Imaging of benign tumors of the osseous spine. J Belg Soc Radiol 102(1):13. https://doi.org/10.5334/jbsr.1380

Steffner RJ, Jang ES (2018) Staging of bone and soft-tissue sarcomas. J Am Acad Orthop Surg 26:e269–e278. https://doi.org/10.5435/JAAOS-D-17-00055

Sundaresan N, Rosen G (2009) Primary malignant tumors of the spine. Orthop Clin North Am 40:21–36, v. https://doi.org/10.1016/j.ocl.2008.10.004

Tan H, Gu J (2021) Solitary bone plasmacytoma of spine with involvement of adjacent disc space: a case report. Medicine (Baltimore) 100(37):e27288

Tenny S, Varacallo M (2023). Chordoma. In StatPearls. StatPearls Publishing

Yamaguchi T, Iwata J (2008) Distinguishing benign notochordal cell tumors from vertebral chordoma. Skelet Radiol 37(4):291–299. https://doi.org/10.1007/s00256-007-0435-y

Yamaguchi T, Suzuki S (2004) Benign notochordal cell tumors: a comparative histological study of benign notochordal cell tumors, classic chordomas, and notochordal vestiges of fetal intervertebral discs. Am J Surg Pathol 28(6):756–761. https://doi.org/10.1097/01.pas.0000126058.18669.5d

Zheng BW, Huang W (2023) Clinicopathological and prognostic characteristics in spinal chondroblastomas: a pooled analysis of individual patient data from a single institute and 27 studies. Global Spine J 13(3):713–723. https://doi.org/10.1177/21925682211005732

Interventional Radiology in Primary Spinal Tumors

Manraj Kanwal Singh Heran
and Michal Krolikowski

Contents

Abstract

Primary tumors of the spinal axis are rare, with the majority being benign in nature. Most are asymptomatic and are often found incidentally on imaging. For these, conservative management may be all that is required, with or without the potential need for clinical and/or imaging follow-up. However, some may warrant active management, such as if the spinal tumor is malignant, or if there is concern of local complications, such as neural compromise, or in the setting of pain or other symptoms, regardless of histology. Although surgery remains an important treatment option, especially in the management of primary spinal malignancy, advances in interventional radiology techniques have expanded the role for minimally invasive image-guided approaches, whether it be to assist surgery or as independent curative or symptom-based management strategies. Indeed, these advances now allow for more primary spinal tumors to be treated, with many benign tumors no longer requiring surgical intervention. The role of interventional radiology in the diagnosis and management of primary spinal tumors will be discussed, including percutaneous and endovascular techniques, with case examples highlighting some of these options.

M. K. S. Heran (✉)
Division of Neuroradiology, Department of Radiology, Vancouver General Hospital, University of British Columbia, Vancouver, BC, Canada
e-mail: manraj.heran@vch.ca

M. Krolikowski
Richmond Hospital, University of British Columbia, Vancouver, BC, Canada
e-mail: Michal.krolikowski@vch.ca

Med Radiol Diagn Imaging (2023)
https://doi.org/10.1007/174_2023_449,
Published Online: 24 September 2023

1 Introduction

Primary tumors of the spinal axis are rare. The majority are benign in nature, with malignant spinal tumors comprising only a small percentage of primary spinal lesions (Ariyaratne et al. 2023; Chalamgari et al. 2023). Most primary spinal tumors are asymptomatic and are often found incidentally on imaging. Conservative management may be all that is required for benign spinal tumors, with or without the potential need for clinical and/or imaging follow-up. However, it is critical to avoid misdiagnosis, as malignant spinal tumors and infectious lesions may require dramatically different approaches in their management. Although clinical history and imaging may allow for accurate diagnosis to be made, in some instances, biopsy may be required for pathologic diagnosis (Fig. 1). This requires discussion with the spinal surgeon before the biopsy, to understand the indications for biopsy and to ensure the appropriate path for obtaining tissue so as not to violate critical tissue planes. The biopsy will help distinguish malignant from benign lesions and infection from neoplasm or determine the histologic/pathologic features of the malignancy. There may be need for larger sample acquisition, especially if personalized oncogenomics is being considered to tailor adjuvant therapies (see also chapter "Image-Guided Biopsy").

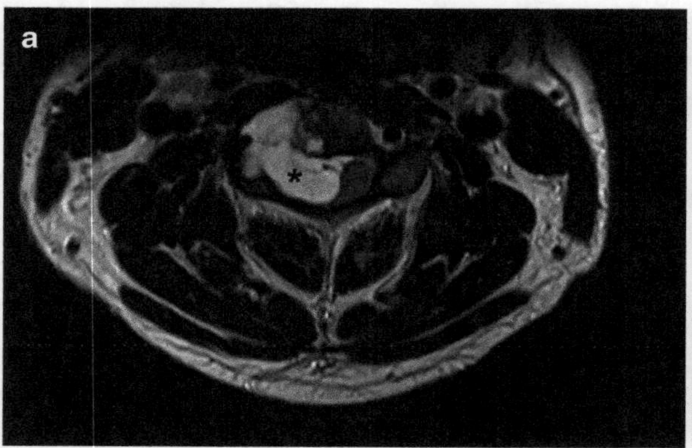

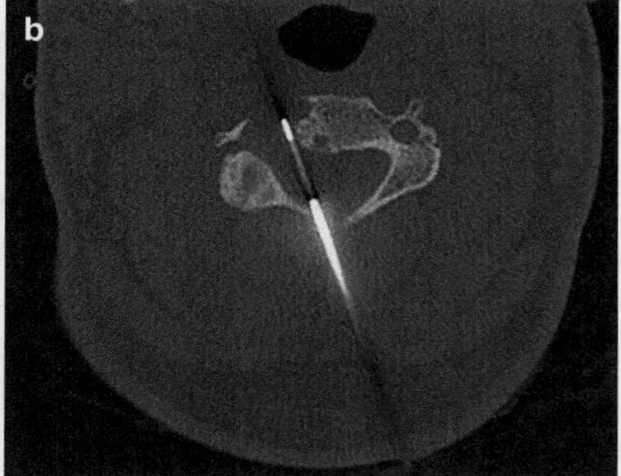

Fig. 1 (**a**) Axial T2 FSE MRI scan of the cervical spine demonstrating a hyperintense mass originating from the vertebral body and extending into the spinal canal (asterisk) with resultant marked mass effect upon the spinal cord. (**b**) Axial CT bone window, with anesthesia-sedation-assisted coaxial 18-gauge biopsy performed of the mass using a posterior interlaminar approach. Diagnosis was chordoma

2 General Considerations

Most primary benign spinal tumors are osteogenic, vascular, or chondrogenic. Imaging features usually (but not always) are helpful in characterizing these lesions. Hemangiomas and osteomas represent the most common benign spinal tumors with an estimated incidence between 11% and 14% of all primary tumors of the spine. Other benign bone tumors, such as osteoid osteoma, aneurysmal bone cyst, and giant cell tumor, can also be seen in the spinal axis. A more complete list can be found in Table 1.

Although, as mentioned, many of these are incidentally found and are asymptomatic, some may warrant active management, especially if there is concern for local complications, such as neural compromise, or in the setting of pain or other symptoms.

Primary malignant spinal tumors are relatively rare in the spine, with the majority being osteosarcoma, Ewing's sarcoma, and chondrosarcoma. Another important one involving the spinal axis is chordoma. Although surgery remains the mainstay for management of primary malignant spinal tumors, advances in interventional radiology techniques have expanded the role for minimally invasive image-guided approaches, whether they be as assists to surgery or as independent curative or symptom-based management strategies (Table 2) (Sgalambro et al. 2022). Challenges in IR are the complex anatomy of the spine, especially in the cervical region and sacrum, and risk of damage to adjacent structures, including nerve roots and spinal cord. Close communication with the spinal surgeon is critical in determining the best treatment.

The usual factors appropriate to any patient procedure must be considered. These include coagulation parameters, preferred imaging modality, and whether there is a need for sedation or anesthetic support of the patient while performing the procedure. Where possible, it is preferred to minimize the need for general anesthesia; however, this may be required, especially for those who cannot remain still through their pro-

Table 1 Classification of primary benign spinal tumors

Osteogenic
Osteoma (enostosis)
Osteoid osteoma
Osteoblastoma
Chondrogenic
Osteochondroma
Chondroblastoma
Vascular
Hemangioma
Aggressive hemangioma
Osteoclastic giant cell-rich
Aneurysmal bone cyst
Benign giant cell tumor
Notochordal
Notochordal rest
Other mesenchymal tumors of bone
Simple bone cyst
Fibrous dysplasia
Hematopoietic
Eosinophilic granuloma

Table 2 IR techniques in management of primary spinal tumors

Diagnostic
Biopsy
Therapeutic
Nonvascular
Injections/blocks
Ablation
Energy-based (i.e., thermal)
Radiofrequency
Cryoablation
Microwave
High-intensity focused ultrasound (HIFU)
Laser
Chemical-based (i.e., sclerotherapy)
Alcohol
Doxycycline
Bleomycin
Sodium tetradecyl sulfate
Other (e.g., calcitonin and methylprednisolone for ABC)
Stabilization
Cementoplasty
Percutaneous device fixation
Vascular
Embolization
Particulate
Liquid
n-Butyl cyanoacrylate
Ethylene vinyl alcohol copolymer
Chemotherapeutic
Sclerotherapy
Alcohol

cedures, for procedures that are expected to be more complex or longer in duration, or when significant pain may be encountered during the procedure itself.

3 Nonvascular Procedures

The main indications for performing these procedures are management of pain, or to provide locoregional control/cure. These procedures can be done without the need for additional treatment or surgery; however, they can be combined with more complex management strategies.

3.1 Simple Spinal Procedures

Image-guided spinal pain procedures are commonly performed for a variety of indications. The most common of these are nerve blocks, epidural injections, and procedures done for facet-mediated pain (Fig. 2). Although the vast majority of spinal pain procedures are done for non-tumoral indications, it is important to consider them whenever encountering someone with pain associated with their spinal axis primary tumor. Depending on the location of the pain generator, there may be a role for more than one type of injection, with the local anesthetic component of the injection serving as an important diagnostic tool, helping determine the appropriateness and efficacy of the procedure. The imaging modalities most commonly used are fluoroscopy, CT, and sometimes ultrasound. The choice of which imaging modality a proceduralist uses is often determined by factors such as access to imaging tools, comfort and experience with the modalities, and suitability for visualization of the target area. The usual considerations with respect to performing these procedures apply, as do choice and dosing of corticosteroids.

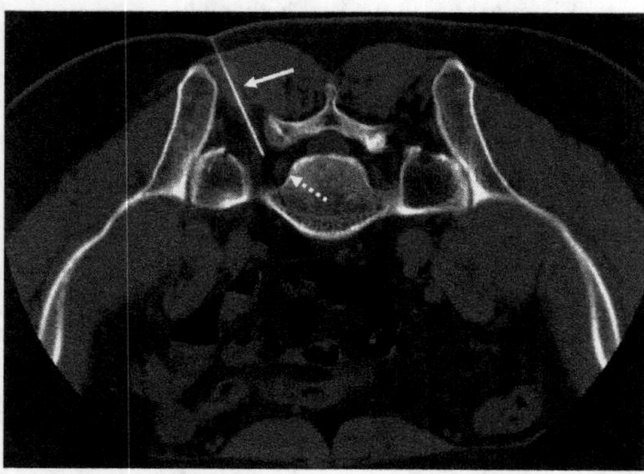

Fig. 2 CT-guided nerve root block of the left S1 nerve (dotted arrow) using a 22-gauge spinal needle (solid arrow), performed in the setting of mass effect on the S1 nerve root at the L5 level due to a benign primary spinal tumor at the L5 level (not shown)

3.2 Complex Spinal Procedures

3.2.1 Ablation

In many instances, management of pain associated with primary spinal tumors requires more than simple blocks or injections. This may be due to local inflammation (as in the case of osteoid osteoma or osteoblastoma) or because of local mass effect or invasion of adjacent structures (including traversing or exiting nerve roots). In these situations, local ablative options may be suitable to treat the offending problem. As outlined, there are several methods for performing ablation, with the most common being radiofrequency ablation (RFA) and cryoablation (Tsoumakidou et al. 2016; Tomasian et al. 2017; Cazzato et al. 2020; Lindquester et al. 2020; Izzo et al. 2021). Microwave ablation may be an option, in selected cases. These are all examples of "needle-based" procedures, requiring placement of needles or probes into the tumor or target area for subsequent delivery of energy for local tissue destruction. In some instances, the needle systems used to access the lesion may actually even allow for removal of the entire primary spinal tumor (e.g., trephine ablation of osteoid osteoma). Needleless techniques are also emerging, such as magnetic resonance imaging-guided high intensity focused ultrasound (HIFU). This allows for passage of an ultrasound beam through tissue, focusing on the target for ablation, conceptually like focusing sunlight with a magnifying glass. The benefit of this is being able to ablate tissue without needing direct access, either percutaneously or via an open approach; however, institutions with the required equipment are very limited.

An important consideration in performing these procedures in the spinal axis is the potential for thermal injury to critical structures, including the spinal cord and nerve roots. Many factors play into this, including the degree and duration of thermal effect, presence or absence of intact osseous cortex, and distance of the critical structures from the margins of the ablation zone. The sensitivity of the tissue at risk may vary depending on the tissue type, as well as the clinical significance of the damage (e.g., esophageal perforation or permanent neural injury). As transient motor and sensory dysfunction can occur at temperatures between 0 and 5 °C; thermal monitoring and thermal protection have become important tools when performing ablation procedures (Tomasian et al. 2017). Thermal insulation can be achieved by using air or fluid. As saline for hydrodissection in the setting of RFA procedures can result in ablation zone expansion, nonionic fluids such as dextrose 5% in water are recommended. Thermal monitoring should be considered whenever ablation temperatures may exceed 45 °C or be less than 10 °C. This is done through the placement of thermocouples close to the critical structures at risk during the procedure. Neurophysiologic monitoring may also be useful in selected settings. If there is risk of thermal skin injury, maneuvers such as active warming of the skin surface through application of warm saline during cryoablation can help reduce this risk.

3.2.2 Radiofrequency Ablation

RFA is widely used for treatment of tumors throughout the body, including the spine. With respect to primary spinal tumors, it can be used with curative intent, or for local tissue ablation, with the aim being to reduce or eliminate pain. As a heat-based technique, the procedure is painful, with patients often supported with monitored anesthetic care, and possible need for intubation and general anesthesia. Ablation size is determined through the choice of appropriate probes, with ablation times typically being short (typically less than 10 min), with tissue temperatures in the ablation zone usually between 70° and 95°. RFA has been a popular choice in the management of benign primary spinal tumors, such as osteoid osteoma and osteoblastoma (Fig. 3). This is primarily due to the precise ablation zone achieved, especially if there is a shell of cortical bone surrounding the lesion, which acts as a boundary for limiting heat propagation. However, it can be used for other spinal tumors, both for cure and for palliation. RFA can also be used for deliberate ablation of neural structures in the setting of neuritic pain associated with spinal tumors, especially in advanced malignancy (Fig. 4).

3.2.3 Cryoablation

Cryoablation has become an increasingly popular ablation method. It relies on freezing the water within the tissues local to the probe placed to temperatures between 0 and −40 °C. It is crucial to understand the sizes of the isotherms achieved in the ice ball (i.e., <−40°, −40° to −20°, −20° to 0°), as each can have local tissue effects. Temperatures of <−40 °C are typically necessary to achieve complete cellular death (Tomasian

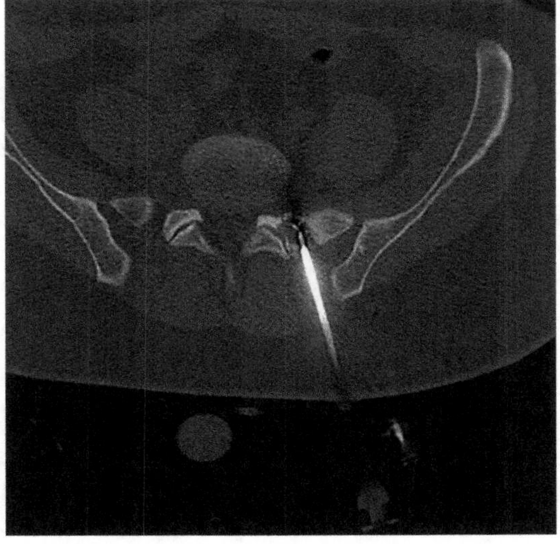

Fig. 3 Axial CT scan demonstrating an osteoid osteoma situated in the left sacral ala at the S1 segment level. An umbrella RFA probe has been placed through a coaxial needle for heat-based thermal ablation of the lesion

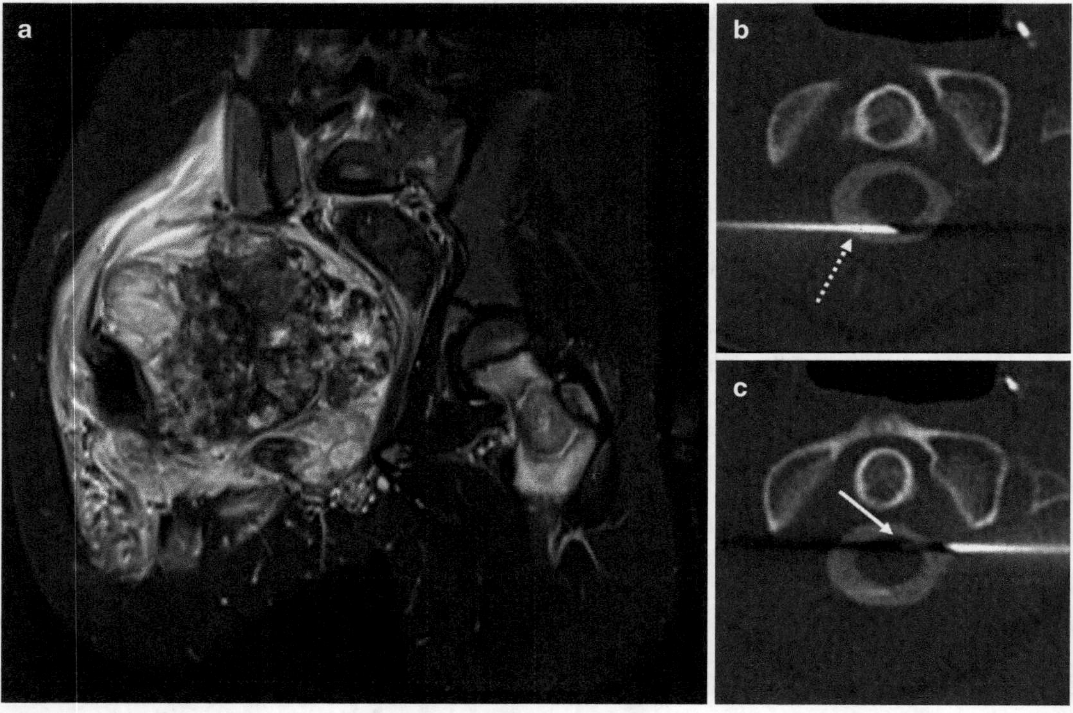

Fig. 4 (**a**) Coronal T2 fat-saturation MRI of the pelvis in a 10-year-old male. This shows an advanced and inoperable osteogenic sarcoma, with marked local mass effect, and multiple metastases (not shown). The patient had right-sided pain refractory to all oral and intravenous medications. (**b**) Axial imaging from a cordotomy procedure shows a right-sided 22-gauge spinal needle access into the subarachnoid space posterior to the spinal cord at the C1/2 level (dotted arrow) for purposes of performing a cervical myelogram. (**c**) With visualization of the spinal cord achieved, a radiofrequency probe has been placed through a coaxial needle into the left spinothalamic tract (solid arrow), with subsequent cordotomy performed

et al. 2017). Cryoablation generally allows for larger ablation zones, which is one of its main advantages. This can be done through selecting specific probes, which allow for creation of larger ice balls, or through the placement of multiple probes, which will allow for coalescence of the adjacent ice balls and the ability to "sculpt" the cryoablation zone (Fig. 5) (Tsoumakidou et al. 2015; Li et al. 2020). Another advantage of cryoablation is the relative lack of discomfort associated with the actual thermal ablation procedure, as well as post-procedurally. The ice ball can be visualized on conventional or cone-beam CT, and even with ultrasound (in the setting of more superficial lesions). Cryoablation is especially useful when the primary spinal tumor does not have critical structures immediately adjacent to the ablation zone; however, instilled air can be useful as a thermal protector in appropriate locations, if there is concern of thermal injury (Fig. 6). Flowing blood or fluid (such as cerebrospinal fluid within the thecal sac) can also alter the ice ball size and appearance and serve as thermal protectors.

3.2.4 Sclerotherapy

Sclerotherapy is commonly performed for vascular lesions situated in various soft tissue compartments throughout the body. This can be for vascular neoplasms, as well as vascular malformations. Selected primary spinal tumors, such as aneurysmal bone cysts or vertebral hemangio-

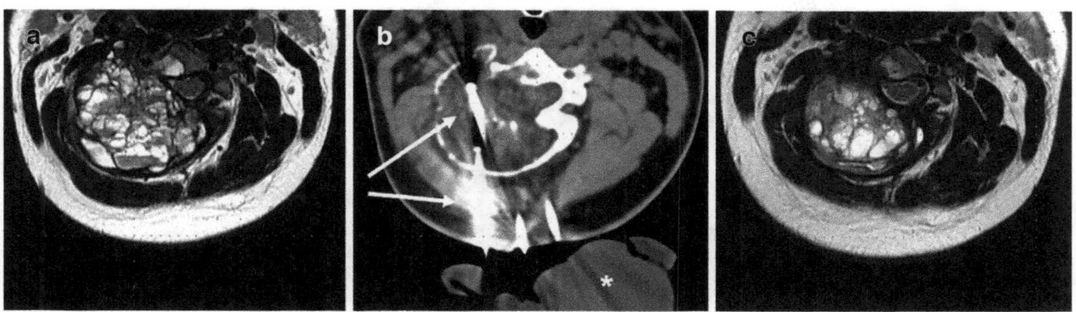

Fig. 5 (**a**) Axial T2 MRI of the cervical spine in a 22-year-old male presenting with upper neck pain, demonstrating a multicystic tumor involving the C2 vertebra with innumerable serum-hematocrit levels, with a large exophytic component extending into the right posterior paraspinal musculature. Imaging features are compatible with an aneurysmal bone cyst. There is narrowing of the adjacent spinal canal. (**b**) Axial CT through the lesion at the time of cryoablation of the ABC, performed under general anesthesia, demonstrates multiple cryoablation probes placed in the lesion (white arrows), with a halo of low attenuation seen around the periphery of the lesion, representing the sculpted ice ball. Thermal protection of the skin using warmed saline placed into sterile gloves (asterisk) is also seen. (**c**) Follow-up T2 axial MRI performed 3 months post-procedure shows considerable shrinkage of the ABC, with coalescence of many of its cystic components, and elimination of the previously noted deformation of the spinal canal adjacent to the spinal cord. The patient had complete relief of his pre-procedure pain, with no palpable mass

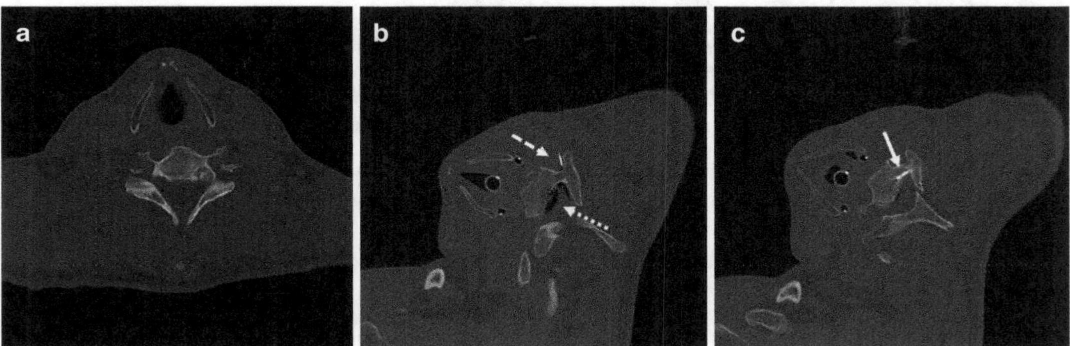

Fig. 6 (**a**) Axial CT scan of a 37-year-old male presenting with left-sided neck pain radiating into his shoulder and left arm demonstrates an osteoid osteoma involving the posterior left lateral aspect of the C6 vertebra. (**b**) At the time of cryoablation performed with endotracheal intubation and general anesthesia, a 22-gauge Tuohy needle was first placed adjacent to the exiting left C6 nerve root (long dashed arrow), with air injected for purposes of providing thermal protection (short, dashed arrow). (**c**) Ice Seed probe (solid white arrow, Boston Scientific Inc.) placed into the osteoid osteoma for cryoablation. Patient awoke neurologically intact, with complete relief of pre-procedural symptoms 1 week following the procedure

mas, can be treated in a similar fashion. However, there are important differences to consider, including access techniques and approaches, as well as awareness of location-specific critical structures, and how to minimize the risk of non-target tissue damage. Transarterial administration of sclerosant agents can be done (Fig. 7), as well as percutaneous delivery of these medications (Fig. 8). Combined strategies may also be appropriate (Srinivasan et al. 2021; Tonosu et al. 2023). It is essential that the interventionalist be knowledgeable in the spinal vascular anatomy, espe-

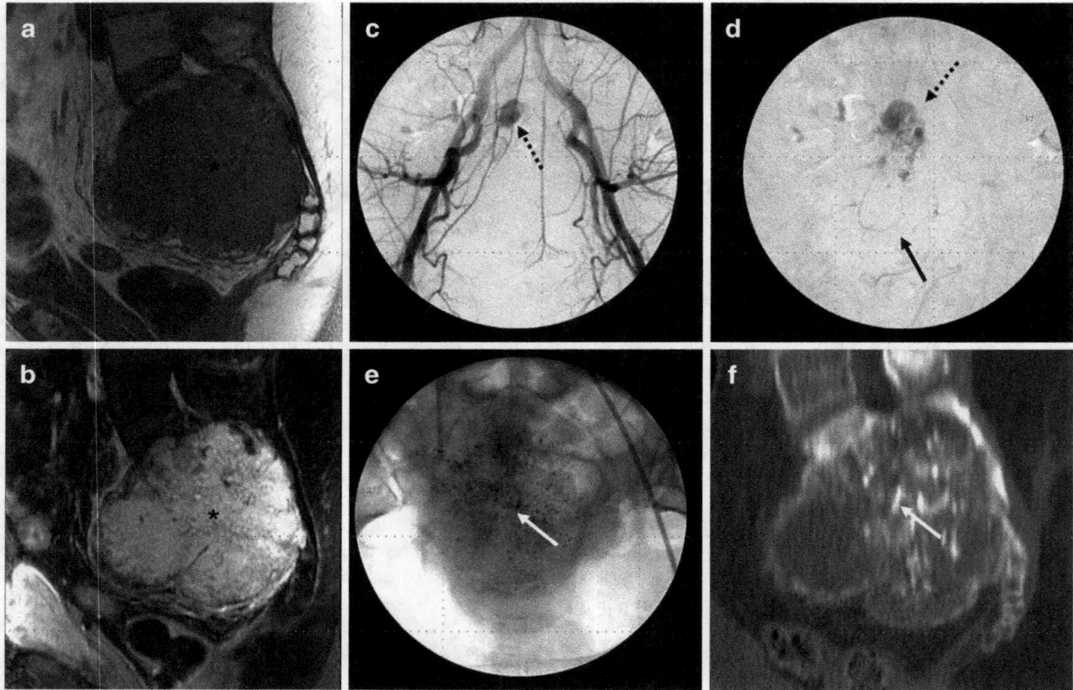

Fig. 7 Pre-procedural sagittal T1 axial (**a**) and T2 fat-saturation MRI (**b**) demonstrates a giant aggressive hemangioma involving the upper and mid-sacrum (asterisk) in a middle-aged woman presenting with profound coccydynia and pelvic congestion symptoms. (**c, d**) Transarterial alcohol sclerotherapy of the tumor performed under general anesthetic, with initial digital subtraction angiography of the pelvis demonstrating the vascular supply arising from the right lateral sacral artery (dashed black arrow), with placement of a microcatheter in this artery (solid black arrow), and super-selective angiography done to confirm its supply of the lesion (dashed black arrow). (**e**) Unsubtracted fluoroscopic image at the end of the procedure, demonstrating the oil-based contrast agent used to opacify the medical grade alcohol during the embolization/sclerotherapy procedure (solid white arrow). (**f**) Post-procedure sagittal CT reformat, again demonstrating the oil-based contrast (solid white arrow). After several sessions, the patient's symptoms significantly improved

cially with respect to the circulation to the spinal cord, as inadvertent sclerosant passage into radiculomedullary arteries can result in devastating neurologic complications. Medical grade alcohol is a very powerful sclerosing agent, with doxycycline being a suitable medication for treatment of selected aneurysmal bone cysts (Lyons et al. 2019). Bleomycin, an antimitotic agent, is not a true sclerosant. However, its mechanism of action can result in fibrosis and subsequent treatment/healing of lesions in which it is administered. Its use in the management of low- and high-flow malformations in non-osseous locations is increasing, with emerging experience in its use for treatment of similar lesions involving the skeletal structures, including the spine.

3.2.5 Stabilization Procedures

3.2.5.1 Cementoplasty

Cementoplasty has an established role in the management of painful spinal fractures not responding to conservative therapy, or for those demonstrating progressive instability and/or collapse. The procedure consists of image-guided delivery of polymethyl methacrylate (PMMA) into the vertebra, with resultant filling and fixation of fracture lines (Fig. 9). This provides stabilization, with reduced mechanical pain. The procedure itself is usually quite straightforward and can be done on an outpatient basis, with sedation support provided by the anesthesia service. Risk of cement leak has been dramatically

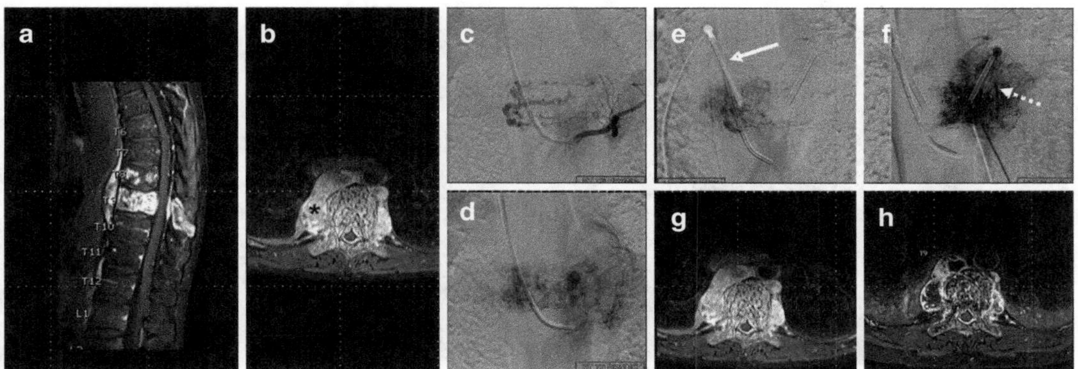

Fig. 8 (**a**, **b**) Pre-procedural T1 axial FS contrast-enhanced MR demonstrates avid enhancement associated with a T9 aggressive hemangioma involving the entire vertebra, with a large extra-osseous component (asterisk), and circumferential intra-canal extradural disease. (**c**, **d**) With the patient positioned prone and with monitoring, angiography performed of the T9 segmental arterial circulation via a left radial arterial approach. (**e**, **f**) Bilateral transpedicular access was obtained to the T9 vertebra, with contrast injection confirming satisfactory position (**dashed arrow**), followed by administration of medical grade alcohol through the cannulae (solid arrow) for purposes of intralesional sclerotherapy. (**g**, **h**) Post-procedural follow-up T1 FS axial contrast-enhanced MR shows marked reduction in enhancement and size of the aggressive hemangioma, in keeping with interval sclerosis. Note the improved caliber of the thecal sac

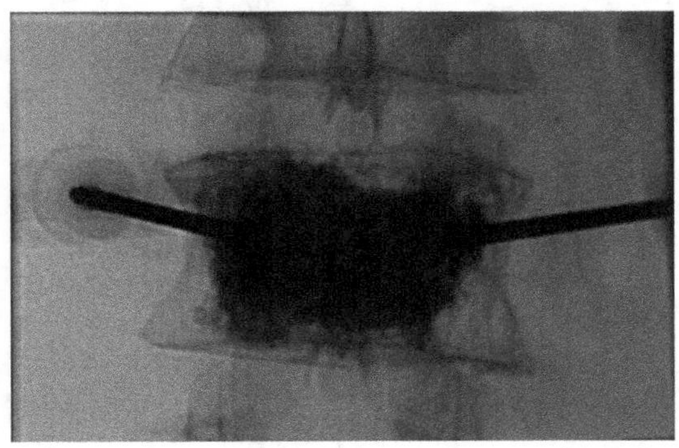

Fig. 9 Posterior-anterior fluoroscopic image during lumbar vertebroplasty, demonstrating bi-pedicular access and instillation of PMMA

reduced since the introduction of high-viscosity cements, with the procedure usually able to be performed quickly. It is most often done using fluoroscopic guidance; however, selected primary spinal tumors may be better treated using CT. Although it is primarily used for treating mechanical pain associated with the diseased vertebra, other treatment methods can be combined with cementoplasty to provide even greater pain control or to provide locoregional tissue destruction (Premat et al. 2017). This may be especially useful when dealing with primary malignant spinal tumors that have an instability component to them due to fracture.

4 Vascular Procedures

4.1 Embolization

Transarterial embolization is a very important IR tool in the management of primary spinal tumors (Facchini et al. 2021). This is most often done via a transfemoral arterial approach; however, there is growing experience in performing some of these procedures from a trans-radial arterial approach (Eesa et al. 2022). The overwhelming majority of patients with primary spinal tumors in which this is performed have it done as a pre-operative strategy to reduce vascularity of the lesion (Yang et al. 2010; Ozkan and Gupta 2011; Nair et al. 2013; Ashour and Aziz-Sultan 2014; Griessenauer et al. 2016; Eichberg et al. 2018; Omid-Fard et al. 2019; Zhang et al. 2019). The goal of embolization is complete devascularization of the tumor. This allows for reduced intra-operative blood loss and improvements in lesion

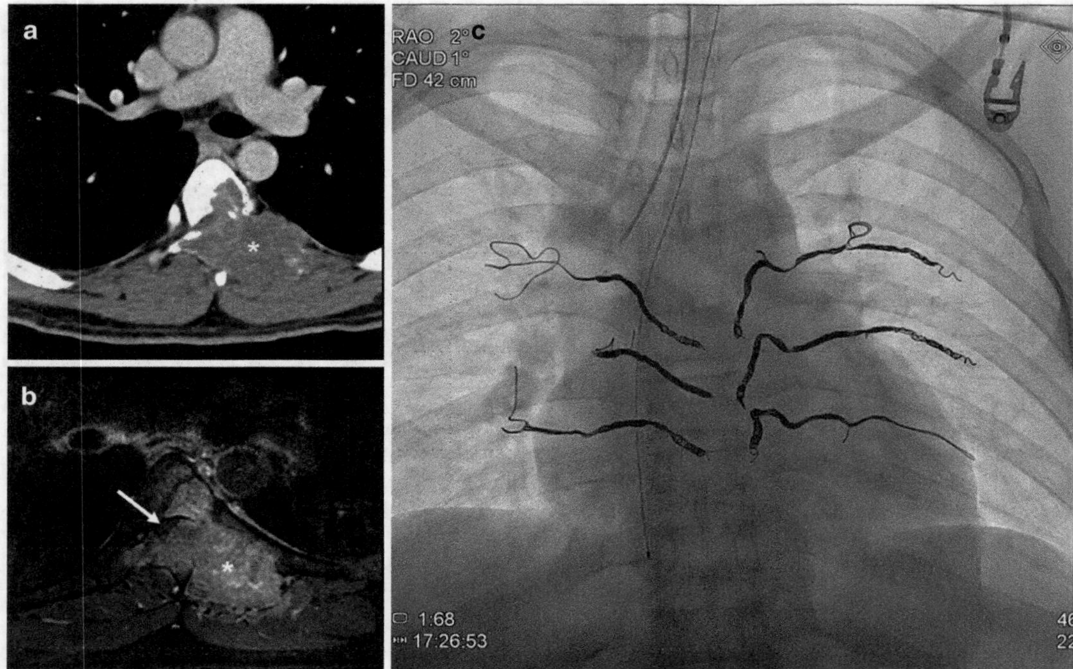

Fig. 10 (**a**) CT and (**b**) MRI axial imaging demonstrating a biopsy-proven osteogenic sarcoma at T7 (asterisk), with marked spinal cord compression (white arrow) in a 28-year-old male presenting with rapidly progressive lower limb paralysis. (**c**) Post-embolization AP fluoroscopic image shows bilateral segmental artery embolization of the hypovascular tumor, in preparation for en bloc resection

resection/removal while often shortening total operative time. Transarterial embolization can also be performed if en bloc resection is to be performed by providing endovascular occlusion of segmental arteries and surrounding vasculature, which will be encountered upon tumor removal. Preoperative embolization of hypervascular primary spinal tumors is classically done within 72 h of the planned surgery, with a variety of embolic agents available to the interventionalists. One of the most common are particulate agents, such as polyvinyl alcohol, or trisacryl gelatin, which are administered into the target circulation through catheters or microcatheters, thereby obstructing blood flow, typically at the precapillary level. The addition of permanent embolic agents such as metallic coils or occluder devices may enhance the durability of the embolization while aiding in resectability if segmental artery ligation/sectioning is required. Other temporary embolic agents, such as Gelfoam, may also be appropriate in selected settings, as can liquid embolization materials, such as *n*-butyl cyanoacrylate (*n*BCA) or ethylene vinyl alcohol copolymer (EVOH) (Ghobrial et al. 2013; Grandhi et al. 2015). Preoperative embolization of hypovascular primary spinal tumors does not necessarily need to be done within the same time window as that for their hypervascular counterparts as the goal is typically to aid the surgeon in en bloc removal, rather than assisting in resection where an intralesional approach may be necessary (Figs. 10 and 11) (Ogungbemi et al. 2015).

Prior to performing transarterial embolization, it is critical to discuss the goals and objectives of surgery with the surgeon, as well as what is going to be most beneficial to them from the IR procedure. It is essential that the interventionalist be

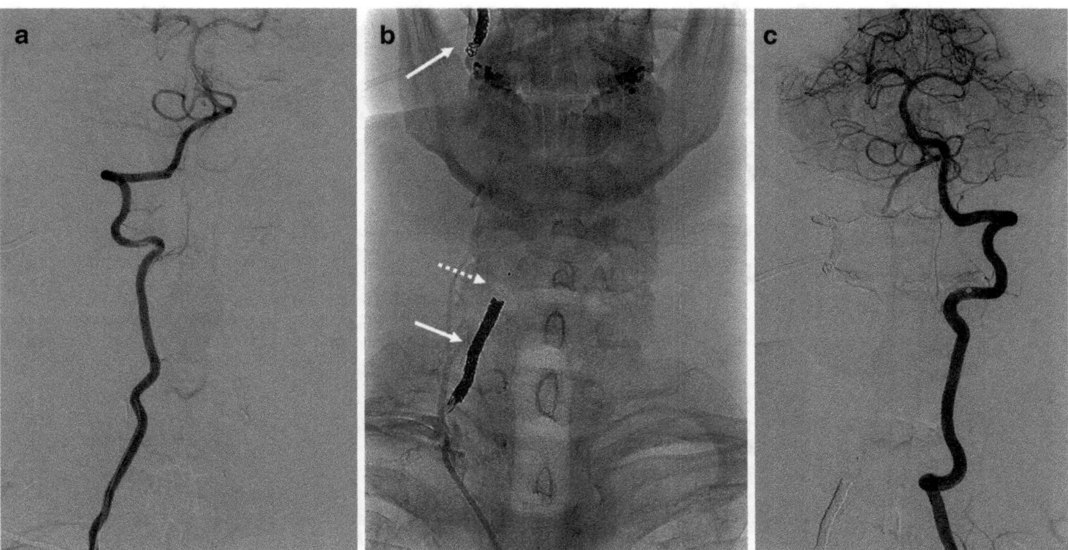

Fig. 11 (**a**) Digital subtraction angiogram of right vertebral artery prior to vessel sacrifice in preparation for en bloc removal of cervical chordoma shown in Fig. 1, demonstrating no vascularity to the tumor. (**b**) Fluoroscopic image post-right vertebral artery occlusion, with coil embolization performed cranial and caudal to the tumor level (solid arrows), with an occluder device assisting in the lower embolization (dotted arrow). Note the lack of embolic material through the window of access for the en bloc resection, deliberately done at the request of the oncology spine surgeon. (**c**) Digital subtraction angiogram performed of the left vertebral artery demonstrates maintained perfusion of the posterior circulation intracranially, including retrograde filling into the right posterior inferior cerebellar artery

knowledgeable in the spinal vascular anatomy, especially with respect to the circulation to the spinal cord. Understanding the appearance and location of important radiculomedullary arteries, such as the artery of Adamkiewicz, can help minimize the risk of spinal cord ischemia as a complication of the embolization procedure.

Transarterial embolization can also be performed as a primary strategy for the management of specific primary spinal tumors (Boriani et al. 2014; He et al. 2017; Ehlers et al. 2020). This may ameliorate symptoms or provide locoregional tumor control through devascularization and subsequent tissue infarction. In addition, transarterial embolization can be combined with other IR techniques to increase the efficacy of therapy, whether it be to devascularize the tumor prior to surgery or to provide symptom control or lesion treatment/volume reduction. A unique strategy of percutaneous intralesional embolization can also be done via access derived from cementoplasty techniques allowing for administration of embolic agents such as EVOH or *n*BCA to enhance devascularization (Fig. 12) (Yao and Malek 2013). This may be especially helpful when intralesional resection of hypervascular primary spinal lesions is contemplated.

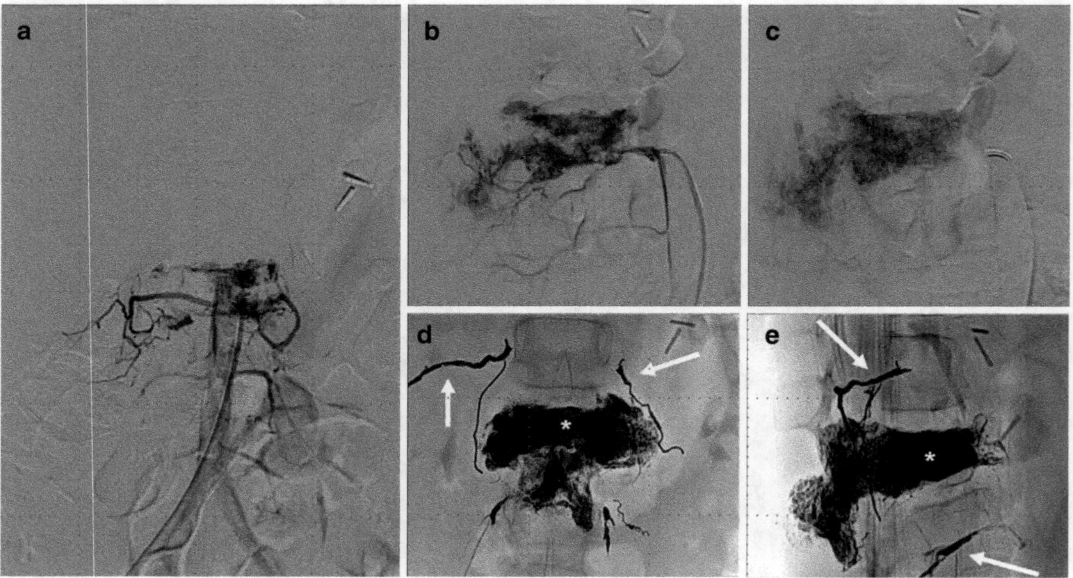

Fig. 12 Twelve-year-old female presenting with progressively worsening back pain, with biopsy-proven aggressive hemangioma at L2. Digital subtraction angiography at the time of preoperative embolization demonstrates considerable vascular blush, as seen on (**a**) AP view, and lateral (**b**) early and (**c**) late projections. Transarterial and percutaneous intralesional embolization performed, with (**d, e**) frontal and lateral images immediately following the embolization showing embolic coils placed in the segmental arteries above and below the tumor level, as well as EVOH completely filling the L2 vertebra (asterisk), as performed through multiple percutaneous needle placements (not shown)

5 Conclusion

Advances in interventional radiology techniques have expanded the role for minimally invasive image-guided procedures for primary spinal tumors, whether it be to assist surgery or as independent curative or symptom-based management strategies. Percutaneous and transarterial approaches provide opportunities for improved diagnosis, greater efficacy of preoperative devascularization, and pain control. These advances now allow for more primary spinal tumors to be treated, with many benign tumors no longer requiring surgical intervention. Enhancement of currently available ablative techniques, greater availability of niche treatment tools such as HIFU, and development of new devices and medical therapies able to be delivered through IR techniques will continue to advance the care of benign and malignant primary spinal tumors (Costăchescu et al. 2022). Through collaboration with spine surgeons and other specialties, and using a multidisciplinary approach, the future of IR in this field of spinal care is exciting, with IR remaining integral in these patients' care.

6 Key Points

- Interventional radiology techniques can be used to treat benign and malignant primary spinal tumors.
- Strategies for treatment can be for curative or palliative intent.
- Multidisciplinary approach is often very important to determine goals of procedure.
- Combining treatment strategies can be helpful in achieving the desired outcome.
- Developing technologies will expand the role of IR in the treatment of primary spinal tumors.

References

Ariyaratne S, Jenko N, Iyengar KP, James S, Mehta J, Botchu R (2023) Primary benign neoplasms of the spine. Diagnostics (Basel) 13(12):2006

Ashour R, Aziz-Sultan A (2014) Preoperative tumor embolization. Neurosurg Clin N Am 25(3):607–617

Boriani S, Lo SF, Puvanesarajah V, Fisher CG, Varga PP, Rhines LD, Germscheid NM, Luzzati A, Chou D, Reynolds JJ, Williams RP, Zadnik P, Groves M, Sciubba DM, Bettegowda C, Gokaslan ZL (2014) Aneurysmal bone cysts of the spine: treatment options and considerations. J Neurooncol 120(1):171–178

Cazzato RL, Auloge P, De Marini P, Boatta E, Koch G, Dalili D, Rao PP, Garnon J, Gangi A (2020) Spinal tumor ablation: indications, techniques, and clinical management. Tech Vasc Interv Radiol 23(2):100677

Chalamgari A, Valle D, Palau Villarreal X, Foreman M, Liu A, Patel A, Dave A, Lucke-Wold B (2023) Vertebral primary bone lesions: review of management options. Curr Oncol 30(3):3064–3078

Costăchescu B, Niculescu AG, Iliescu BF, Dabija MG, Grumezescu AM, Rotariu D (2022) Current and emerging approaches for spine tumor treatment. Int J Mol Sci 23(24):15680

Eesa M, Mitha AP, Lewkonia P (2022) Distal transradial access for targeted spinal angiography and embolization. Interv Neuroradiol. https://doi.org/10.1177/15910199221097489

Ehlers LD, McMordie J, Lookian P, Surdell D, Puccioni M (2020) Cervical spine aneurysmal bone cyst in a pediatric patient: embolization considerations and potential pitfalls. World Neurosurg 139:163–168

Eichberg DG, Starke RM, Levi AD (2018) Combined surgical and endovascular approach for treatment of aggressive vertebral haemangiomas. Br J Neurosurg 32(4):381–388

Facchini G, Parmeggiani A, Peta G, Martella C, Gasbarrini A, Evangelisti G, Miceli M, Rossi G (2021) The role of percutaneous transarterial embolization in the management of spinal bone tumors: a literature review. Eur Spine J 30(10):2839–2851

Ghobrial GM, Chalouhi N, Harrop J, Dalyai RT, Tjoumakaris S, Gonzalez LF, Hasan D, Rosenwasser RH, Jabbour P (2013) Preoperative spinal tumor embolization: an institutional experience with onyx. Clin Neurol Neurosurg 115(12):2457–2463

Grandhi R, Hunnicutt CT, Harrison G, Zwagerman NT, Snyderman CH, Gardner PA, Hartman DJ, Horowitz M (2015) Comparing angiographic devascularization with histologic penetration after preoperative tumor embolization with onyx: what indicates an effective procedure? J Neurol Surg A Cent Eur Neurosurg 76(4):309–317

Griessenauer CJ, Salem M, Hendrix P, Foreman PM, Ogilvy CS, Thomas AJ (2016) Preoperative embolization of spinal tumors: a systematic review and meta-analysis. World Neurosurg 87:362–371

He SH, Xu W, Sun ZW, Liu WB, Liu YJ, Wei HF, Xiao JR (2017) Selective arterial embolization for the treatment of sacral and pelvic Giant cell tumor: a systematic review. Orthop Surg 9(2):139–144

Izzo A, Zugaro L, Fascetti E, Bruno F, Zoccali C, Arrigoni F (2021) Management of osteoblastoma and giant osteoid osteoma with percutaneous thermoablation techniques. J Clin Med 10(24):5717

Li L, Jiang XF, Sun LJ, Fu YF, Zhang W (2020) Computed tomography-guided argon-helium cryoablation for sacrum chordoma. Medicine (Baltimore) 99(42):e22604

Lindquester WS, Crowley J, Hawkins CM (2020) Percutaneous thermal ablation for treatment of osteoid osteoma: a systematic review and analysis. Skelet Radiol 49(9):1403–1411

Lyons KW, Borsinger TM, Pearson AM (2019) Percutaneous doxycycline foam injections: novel treatment method for vertebral aneurysmal bone cysts. World Neurosurg 125:3–5

Nair S, Gobin YP, Leng LZ, Marcus JD, Bilsky M, Laufer I, Patsalides A (2013) Preoperative embolization of hypervascular thoracic, lumbar, and sacral spinal column tumors: technique and outcomes from a single center. Interv Neuroradiol 19(3):377–385

Ogungbemi A, Elwell V, Choi D, Robertson F (2015) Permanent endovascular balloon occlusion of the vertebral artery as an adjunct to the surgical resection of selected cervical spine tumors: a single center experience. Interv Neuroradiol 21(4):532–537

Omid-Fard N, Fisher CG, Heran MK (2019) The evolution of pre-operative spine tumour embolization. Br J Radiol 92(1100):20180899

Ozkan E, Gupta S (2011) Embolization of spinal tumors: vascular anatomy, indications, and technique. Tech Vasc Interv Radiol 14(3):129–140

Premat K, Clarençon F, Cormier É, Mahtout J, Bonaccorsi R, Degos V, Chiras J (2017) Long-term outcome of percutaneous alcohol embolization combined with percutaneous vertebroplasty in aggressive vertebral hemangiomas with epidural extension. Eur Radiol 27(7):2860–2867

Sgalambro F, Zugaro L, Bruno F, Palumbo P, Salducca N, Zoccali C, Barile A, Masciocchi C, Arrigoni F (2022) Interventional radiology in the management of metastases and bone tumors. J Clin Med 11(12):3265

Srinivasan G, Moses V, Padmanabhan A, Ahmed M, Keshava SN, Krishnan V, Joseph BV, Raju KP, Rajshekhar V (2021) Utility of spinal angiography and arterial embolization in patients undergoing CT guided alcohol injection of aggressive vertebral hemangiomas. Neuroradiology 63(11):1935–1945

Tomasian A, Wallace AN, Jennings JW (2017) Benign spine lesions: advances in techniques for minimally invasive percutaneous treatment. AJNR Am J Neuroradiol 38(5):852–861

Tonosu J, Yamaguchi Y, Higashikawa A, Watanabe K (2023) Ethanol sclerosis therapy for aggressive vertebral hemangioma of the spine: a narrative review. J Clin Med 12(12):3926

Tsoumakidou G, Too CW, Garnon J, Steib JP, Gangi A (2015) Treatment of a spinal aneurysmal bone cyst using combined image-guided cryoablation and cementoplasty. Skelet Radiol 44(2):285–289

Tsoumakidou G, Koch G, Caudrelier J, Garnon J, Cazzato RL, Edalat F, Gangi A (2016) Image-guided spinal ablation: a review. Cardiovasc Intervent Radiol 39(9):1229–1238

Yang HL, Chen KW, Wang GL, Lu J, Ji YM, Liu JY, Wu GZ, Gu Y, Sun ZY (2010) Pre-operative transarterial embolization for treatment of primary sacral tumors. J Clin Neurosci 17(10):1280–1285

Yao KC, Malek AM (2013) Transpedicular N-butyl cyanoacrylate-mediated percutaneous embolization of symptomatic vertebral hemangiomas. J Neurosurg Spine 18(5):450–455

Zhang J, Kumar NS, Tan BWL, Shen L, Anil G (2019) Pre-operative embolisation of spinal tumours: neither neglect the neighbour nor blindly follow the gold standard. Neurosurg Rev 42(4):951–959

Part V

Posttreatment Evaluation

Assessment of Postoperative Posttreatment Changes: General Considerations

Olympia Papakonstantinou, Filip Vanhoenacker, and Iris-Melanie Nöebauer-Huhmann

Contents

O. Papakonstantinou (✉)
2nd Department of Radiology, National and Kapodistrian University of Athens, Chaidari, Greece

F. Vanhoenacker
Department of Radiology, AZ Sint-Maarten Mechelen, Mechelen, Belgium

University Hospital Antwerp, Antwerp, Belgium

University Antwerp, Ghent, Belgium
e-mail: filip.vanhoenacker@telenet.be

I.-M. Nöebauer-Huhmann
Division of Neuroradiology and Musculoskeletal Radiology, Department of Biomedical Imaging and Image-Guided Therapy, Medical University of Vienna, Vienna, Austria
e-mail: iris.noebauer@meduniwien.ac.at

Abstract

This chapter deals with the general principles of posttreatment imaging of tumors of the osseous spine. Prerequisites for post-therapeutic imaging include clinical presentation and familiarity with the tumor histology, surgical technique, previous radio- or chemotherapy, and access to the preoperative imaging. The recommended time interval for local and distant posttreatment imaging depends on the tumor histology.

MRI is the preferred technique for local surveillance and should include conventional MRI, diffusion-weighted imaging, and dynamic contrast-enhanced imaging. In the presence of metal implants, the imaging parameters should be adjusted.

1 Introduction

Aggressive spinal tumors comprise a heterogeneous spectrum of bone tumors with variable recurrence rates associated with the type, the histologic grade, the size of the tumor and the presence of metastases (Ariyaratne et al. 2018; Cho and Chang 2013). Recent advances in the diagnosis and treatment of malignant bone tumors of the spine have led to prolonged survival and quality of life of patients (Lange et al. 2022; Munoz-Bendix et al. 2015). Effective follow-up is based

https://doi.org/10.1007/174_2024_480,
Published Online: 28 March 2024

upon imaging that should enable evaluation of posttreatment response as well as early detection of tumor recurrence and discrimination between tumor recurrence and anticipated therapy-associated changes or complications (Fayad et al. 2012; Garner et al. 2011; Garner and Kransdorf 2016).

According to the ESSR recommendations, the diagnostic workup and treatment of bone tumors are optionally performed in a dedicated sarcoma center and attended by multidisciplinary team including orthopedic surgeons with expertise in musculoskeletal oncology, musculoskeletal radiologists and pathologists, radiotherapists, and oncologists (Lalam et al. 2017). For spinal tumors, a neurosurgeon and vascular surgeon should be incorporated in the interdisciplinary team.

The current standard framework for treatment of aggressive spinal tumors is an evolving field and includes "en bloc resection" of the tumor comprising total surgical removal with negative resection margins that is with a shell of healthy tissue contiguous to the tumor (Yamazaki et al. 2009; Charest-Morin et al. 2019). Prerequisites for "en bloc resection" comprise a good general condition of the patient and the absence of metastases or other systemic diseases, since this procedure represents an extensive surgery carrying significant morbidity (Janu et al. 2023). Placement of instrumentation supplemented by bone grafts, like peroneal struts in sacrectomy, ensues (Charest-Morin et al. 2019). To cover the empty space after resection of a bulky bone tumor, reconstructive surgery is performed using vascularized myocutaneous flaps. These can be rotational flaps from the adjacent paraspinous muscles (Franck et al. 2018) to form a deep layer, whereas a more superficial layer is usually mobilized from the musculus (m.) latissimus dorsi for the thoracic, m. trapezius for the cervical, and thoracolumbar fascia for the lumbar spine. Gluteal muscles are mobilized after medium defects in the sacral region, whereas rectus abdominis flaps or free flaps are harvested for larger defects (Deskoulidi et al. 2023). Myocutaneous flaps fill the dead space, protect instrumentation, provide vascularized tissue that promotes healing, and decrease tension and CSF leaks, thus preventing wound dehiscence and infection (Franck et al. 2018). Surgical procedures are elaborated in the chapter "Surgical Treatment of Primary Tumors of the Spine" in this book.

Administration of chemo- and/or radiotherapy before (neoadjuvant) or after (adjuvant) surgery significantly decreases local recurrence rates of excised malignant vertebral tumors. The therapeutic strategy depends on the type, size, and histologic grade of the tumor; the proximity to vital structures; the age of the patient; and the presence of metastases. Response to chemo- or radiotherapy varies in different tumor types. Chemotherapy is usually administered in osteosarcoma and Ewing's sarcoma (Katonis et al. 2013; Zhang et al. 2018). Chordomas and chondrosarcomas are radio- and chemoresistant tumors; however, preoperative (neoadjuvant) radiotherapy with high radiation dose up to 70 Gy can be employed to shrink the tumor before or for local control in inoperable cases (Lange et al. 2022; Shao et al. 2023).

Lymphoma of the osseous spine is usually secondary, whereas primary lymphoma of the vertebrae is rare. Chemotherapy with the CHOP scheme is traditionally used (cyclophosphamide, doxorubicin, vincristine, prednisolone) with the addition of monoclonal antibody rituximab (R-CHOP) (Barz et al. 2021). Plasmacytoma is radiosensitive; therefore, radiotherapy of the tumor with a 2 mm tumor margin remains the treatment of choice. Intensity-modulated radiation therapy (IMRT) can be used in case of close proximity of critical structures, whereas chemotherapy has been additionally administered in large tumors >5 cm. Spinal surgery is performed in spinal lymphoma and plasmacytoma in case of spinal instability or compression of neurological structures (Janu et al. 2023).

Treatment of spinal GCTs includes "en bloc resection" of the tumor and neoadjuvant treatment with denosumab. Administration of denosumab as a standalone definite treatment remains controversial (Legget et al. 2022).

Imaging after neoadjuvant treatment and during surveillance and regular follow-up is critical for prompt detection of local recurrence and response to treatment while affecting the time of surgery and decisions concerning probable alteration of therapeutic regimens and schemes (Garner and Kransdorf 2016; Pennington et al. 2019). The radiologist should be aware of the most appropriate imaging technique to reveal relapsed neoplastic tissue as well as the anticipated postoperative or after-treatment findings and complications that might be confused with neoplasms (Bloem et al. 2020; Inarejos Clemente et al. 2022; Liu et al. 2023).

2 Prerequisites Preceding Postoperative Post-therapeutic Imaging

Before imaging, it is necessary for the radiologist to be aware of the type of surgical procedure, resection margins, administration of and time elapsed from previous radiation therapy or chemotherapy, and current clinical presentation (Garner et al. 2009). Since local recurrences most often present similar morphologic features with the primary tumor, preoperative imaging should be available to assess the exact site, size, and tissue characteristics of the primary tumor (Garner et al. 2011). Inspection of the area that is going to be imaged is recommended, for obvious superficial changes, palpable mass, or signs of inflammation or fibrosis, whereas a marker can be placed over ulcerations (Noebauer-Huhmann et al. 2020).

3 Time Intervals for Imaging Evaluation of Therapy Response and for Surveillance Follow-Up

Imaging is recommended to be performed for all tumor types after neoadjuvant chemo- or radiotherapy before surgery and after surgery. Time intervals for imaging follow-up depend on the histological type and grade of the spine tumor. Figure 1 shows a flowchart for imaging surveillance including baseline, preoperative, and postoperative/post-therapeutic imaging. Postoperative/post-therapeutic imaging should be performed approximately 3 months postoperatively or after the end of treatment to avoid misinterpretation of early post-therapeutic changes as recurrent tumor. Table 1 shows the recommended time intervals for imaging surveillance for the most common primary spinal tumors, whereas Table 2 summarizes recommendations for time intervals for imaging of chest for investigation of metastases according to

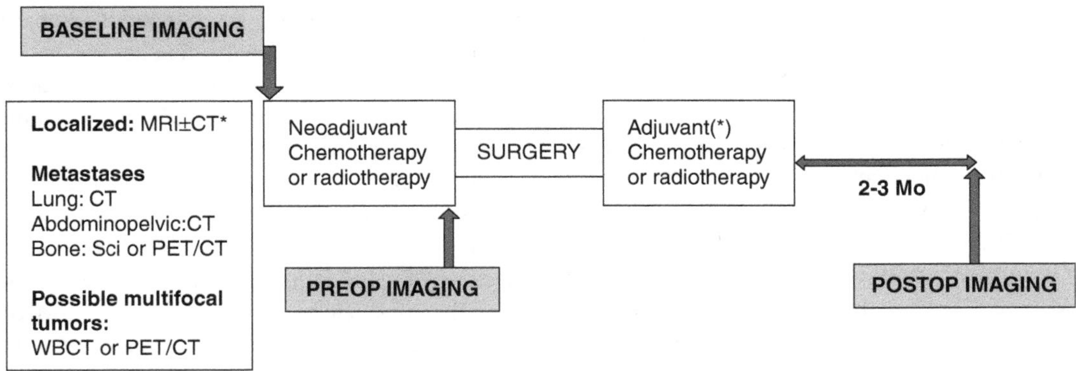

Fig. 1 Flowchart of imaging in relation to treatment of spinal tumors. (Asterisk) If adjuvant treatment is not administered, postoperative imaging can be performed 2–3 months after surgery

Table 1 Time interval[a] for locoregional surveillance by imaging[b] of common primary spinal bone tumors

	First 5 years	5 years[c]
Chordoma	6 months	6–15 years: 12 months
Chondrosarcoma		
Low grade	2 years: 6 months 3–5 years: 12 months	12 months
High grade	At clinical indication	
Ewing's sarcoma	2 years: 3 months 3–5 years: 6 months	12 months
Osteosarcoma	First 2 years: 3 months Third year: 4 months 4–5 year: 6 months	12 months

[a] Time intervals for imaging can be modified according to clinical presentation
[b] Imaging modalities: Radiography, MRI ± CT
[c] Minimum time for surveillance: 10 years

Table 2 Time interval for surveillance of lung metastases of common primary spinal bone tumors

	Chest
Chordoma	≤5 years: 6 months >5 years: 12 months
Chondrosarcoma	
Low grade	1–2 years: 6 months >2 years: 12 months
High grade	1–5 years: 3–6 months >5 years: 12 months
Ewing's sarcoma	1–2 years: 2–3 months
Osteosarcoma	2–5 years: 3–12 months >5 years: 12 months

the National Comprehensive Cancer Network (NCCN) guidelines v.1.2024, the European Society for Medical Oncology (ESMO) (Janu et al. 2023), and the Chordoma Global Consensus Group (Stacchiotti et al. 2017). Radiographs and MRI ± CT are indicated for imaging the local site. CT is recommended for follow-up imaging of chest and abdomen, whereas scintigraphy or positron emission tomography/CT (PET/CT) should be considered for bone metastases (Liu et al. 2023).

As a general rule, for high-grade bone sarcomas, imaging of the primary site together with chest CT scan should be performed approximately every 3 months for the first 2 years, every 6 months for years 3–5, every 6–12 months for years 5–10, and thereafter every 6 months to 1–2 years. For low-grade bone tumors, the frequency of imaging is lower, approximately 6 months for 2 years and then annually (Janu et al. 2023). Modifications of time intervals from guidelines can be performed according to clinical indications, such as occurrence of neurological symptoms.

4 Imaging Techniques

Conventional radiography (CR) or even better postoperative *CT* with sagittal and coronal reformats can provide an overall inspection of the osseous changes and defects, the position of the grafts, and the relation between them and adjacent soft tissues. CT is preferable in spine and pelvis avoiding overprojection of anatomic structures. Moreover, the presence and type of calcifications either within the tumor matrix or as dystrophic ones can be delineated with more specificity as well as the development of sclerosis in certain tumors as a marker of good response after treatment (Oguro et al. 2018; Lalam et al. 2017).

MR imaging, comprising both morphological and functional MR imaging, is the most used imaging modality for the assessment of response to treatment and post-therapeutic changes and of possible complications and for early detection of local recurrence due to superior contrast capabilities for characterization of different tissues. Furthermore, MRI can reveal the relation between the vertebral tumor and critical neural structures of the spine. If MR imaging is inconclusive because of metal-induced artifacts or due to contraindications, such as presence of non-MRI-conditional devices for cardiac conductivity or ear implants, *PET/CT* can be performed in PET-avid tumors. *PET/MRI* is a powerful sensitive tool for detection of local recurrence and metastases at the same time in PET-avid lesions, but the availability of this technique remains limited worldwide. In certain tumors such as lymphoma, with a strong probability of recurrence at other parts of the body, PET/CT is recommended for evaluation of treatment (Messina et al. 2015). In such cases, PET/CT is usually performed before treatment for tumor staging, and the posttreatment study is compared with it (see chapter "PET/CT" in this book).

4.1 MR Imaging

4.1.1 Conventional (Morphological) MR Imaging

Before starting imaging, markers should be placed at the borders of the postoperative scars. The field of view must be large enough to visualize the surgical bed and adjacent tissues, in three orthogonal planes. A fluid-sensitive sequence and a T1-weighted (T1-W) sequence should be applied in long and short axes (Noebauer-Huhmann et al. 2020). T2-weighted images (T2-WI) without fat suppression are often helpful for visualization of intralesional matrix detail such as fibrosis, substance deposits, or calcifications and for hypercellular tumors like Ewing's sarcoma (Papakonstantinou et al. 2019). Contrast-enhanced T1-WI, with or without fat suppression, is strongly recommended to be included in the imaging protocol with the same sequence being obtained before the administration of the paramagnetic contrast. Subtraction images show enhancing lesions more conspicuously and are mostly helpful to differentiate subacute hemorrhage from enhancing lesions (Fayad et al. 2012).

Dixon technique is increasingly used as it can be implemented with any type of sequence (SE, TSE, or GRE), T1, PD, or T2 weighting, and provides a set of four in- and opposed-phase images, and water-only and fat-only images in a single acquisition, while achieving homogenous fat suppression (Del Grande et al. 2014a, b). Magnetic resonance myelography (MRM) has also been advocated as a complementary technique for the evaluation of cord and nerve root compression, often showing more conspicuously to the surgeon the level and degree of thecal, cord, and nerve compression by the extrinsic osseous tumor. It is based on heavily T2-WI with fat suppression sequence depicting hyperintense CSF against hypointense nerve roots and cord; though this appearance resembles CT myelography, it is noninvasive (Patel et al. 2015). Additional T2 GRE* sequences can be applied to confirm the presence of blood products but should be avoided in the presence of metallic implants. Metallic implants also distort chemically selective fat-suppressed images; therefore, subtraction T1-WI without fat suppression is preferable after gadolinium contrast administration. Adaptation of imaging parameters is necessary to eliminate metal artifact as much as possible such as increase of matrix size, avoid GRE T2* sequences, apply FSE, and increase receiver bandwidth (Bancroft 2011). Nowadays, imaging protocols for eliminating metal-induced artifacts are usually provided by the manufacturers, whereas medium magnetic field strength (1.5 T) is preferable to high field (3 T). If the images are still inconclusive due to strong metal artifacts despite adjustments, then an alternative method such as PET/CT should be recommended (Pennington et al. 2019).

4.1.2 Functional MR Imaging

Functional MR techniques including diffusion-weighted imaging (DWI) and dynamic contrast-enhanced MR imaging (DCE MRI) constitute an integral part of the MR imaging protocol in oncologic imaging, as they offer the additional benefit of assessment of metabolic activity and neovascularity of tumors providing both qualitative and quantitative data during follow-up (Verstraete 2009; Del Grande et al. 2014a, b; Vilanova et al. 2016).

Diffusion imaging reflects tissue cellularity and membrane integrity. High *b*-values are most suitable for detection of pathology of fatty marrow; employment of *b*-values of 0, 50, and 800 s/mm^2 is most suitable for DWI of bone tumors (Subhawong et al. 2014; Yao and Troupis 2016; Chaturvedi 2021a, b). However, ADC calculation is affected by hardware, vendor-specific software, and employed MR sequences. It has been advocated that DW metrics to be performed on the same MR imager in order to afford comparison of values during and after treatment (Lecouvet et al. 2022). Histograms based on ADC calculations, with estimation of skewness and kurtosis of data, have been proposed as a more objective and user-friendly technique; flat, wide, and asymmetric distribution reflects significant heterogeneity and tumor necrosis, whereas sharp and high histograms indicate viable neoplastic tissue (Liu et al. 2023). However, conventional DWI that is based on EPI sequences is susceptible to distortion effects and local inhomogeneities produced from different interfaces between fat, bone, and water that coexist in bone tumors. Shortened echo-train length, modified radiofrequency pulses, and correction algorithms along with parallel imaging have been used to eliminate these effects. *b*-Values should be high enough to provide contrast and less shine-through effect (Kim et al. 2023; Liu et al. 2023). Moreover, local inhomogeneities are accentuated by metallic implants; application of specific sequences such as 2D-MSI PROPELLER (2D periodically rotated overlapping parallel lines with enhanced reconstruction) DWI may eliminate artifacts (Gao et al. 2023).

The capabilities *of dynamic contrast-enhanced MRI* (*DCE-MRI*) in the identification of viable tumor and discrimination from post-therapeutic/postoperative changes have been extensively referred to during the last two decades. The most widely used parameters in the follow-up of MSK tumors include the type of the tissue-time intensity curve (TIC), the time to peak (TTP), the maximum signal intensity, and the maximum slope (Verstraete et al. 1996; Inarejos Clemente et al. 2022). The type of TIC is indicative of the nature of the lesions (Fig. 2): Type 1 (no enhancement) represents necrosis or cystic change, type II corresponds to mildly enhancing benign lesions, types III and IV represent rapidly enhancing lesions which most often (but not always) are malignant, whereas type V is usually correlated with fibrosis and granulation tissue (Van Rijswijk et al. 2004; Verstraete 2009).

Time-resolved 3D MR or 2D imaging sequences are used although the former may be more representative of tumor necrosis. Total scan time is usually less than 6 min. Commonly used temporal resolution is 4–8 s although there is a large variability of temporal resolution in various reports (Liu et al. 2023). Parameters that are less commonly used in clinical practice include the area under the curve, the extravascular extracellular space (EES) volume, the plasma volume fraction (Vp), and the volume transfer constant from plasma to the extracellular space (Ktrans) (Tofts et al. 1999). However, the more sophisticated DCE MRI parameters are affected by various factors and have not been standardized in different MR equipment, while different post-processing models have been used. Therefore, these parameters should preferably be estimated on the same MR system during the follow-up of an individual patient.

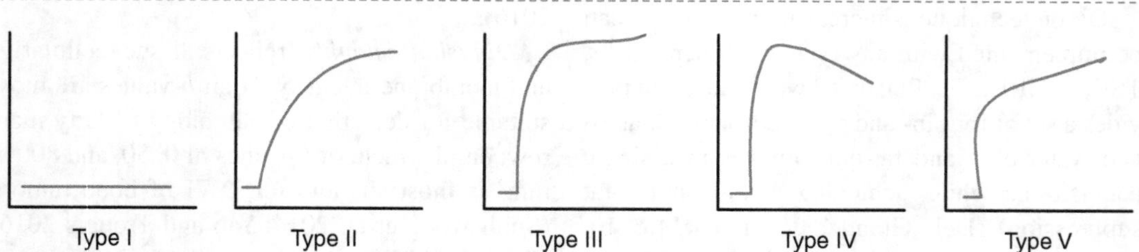

Fig. 2 Dynamic contrast-enhanced MRI (DCE MRI): Time-intensity curves (TIC). Type I: absence of enhancement, consistent with necrosis or cystic changes or necrosis; type II: slow wash-in and progressive enhancement consistent with benign edema; types III and IV: rapid wash-in followed by plateau (type III) or rapid washout (type IV) in keeping with viable tumor tissue; type V: rapid wash-in followed by late increasing enhancement mostly indicative with granulation tissue or fibrosis

5 Key Points

- The radiologist should be aware of the histology of the primary tumor, surgical technique, and previous radio- or chemotherapy and should have access to the preoperative imaging before interpreting the posttreatment imaging.
- The recommended time interval for local and distant posttreatment imaging depends on the tumor histology.
- MRI is most commonly used for imaging of response to treatment and surveillance; if inconclusive or due to contraindications, PET/CT can be performed in PET-avid tumors.
- Conventional MRI is performed by a combination of T1-WI and T2-WI without and with fat suppression and subtraction images before and after administration of gadolinium contrast.
- Functional imaging techniques including DCE MRI and DWI should be part of the postoperative imaging protocol.
- Adaptation of imaging parameters is necessary to eliminate metal artifacts.
- Ideally, postoperative imaging should be performed with the same MR equipment as the preoperative imaging.

References

Ariyaratne S, Jenko N, Iyengar KP et al (2018) Primary osseous malignancies of the spine. Diagnostics 13(10):1801

Bancroft LW (2011) Postoperative tumor imaging. Semin Musculoskelet Radiol 15(4):425–438

Barz M, Aftahy K, Janssen I et al (2021) Spinal manifestation of primary malignant (PLB) and secondary bone lymphoma (SLB). Curr Oncol 28(5):3891–3899

Bloem JL, Vriens D, Krol ADG et al (2020) Therapy-related imaging findings in patients with sarcoma. Semin Musculoskelet Radiol 24:676–691

Charest-Morin R, Fischer CG, Sahgal A et al (2019) Primary Bone tumor of the spine—an evolving field: what a general spine surgeon should know. Global Spine J 9(IS):108S–116S

Chaturvedi A (2021a) Pediatric skeletal diffusion-weighted magnetic resonance imaging: Part 1—Technical considerations and optimization strategies. Pediatr Radiol 51:1562–1574

Chaturvedi A (2021b) Pediatric skeletal diffusion-weighted magnetic resonance imaging: Part 2: Current and emerging applications. Pediatr Radiol 51:1575–1588

Cho W, Chang UK (2013) Survival and recurrence rate after treatment for primary spinal sarcomas. J Korean Neurosurg 53:228–234

Del Grande F, Santini F, Herzka DA et al (2014a) Fat-suppression techniques for 3-T MR imaging of the musculoskeletal system. Radiographics 34(1):217–233

Del Grande P, Subhawaong T, Weber C et al (2014b) Detection of soft tissue sarcoma recurrence: added value of functional MR imaging techniques at 3.0T. Radiology 271:499–511

Deskoulidi P, Stavrianos SD, Mastorakos D et al (2023) Anatomical considerations and plastic surgery reconstruction options of sacral chordoma resection. Cureus 15(4):e37965

Fayad LM, Jacobs MA, Carrino JA, Bluemke DA (2012) Musculoskeletal tumors: how to use anatomic, functional and metabolic MR techniques. Radiology 265:340–356

Franck P, Bernstein JL, Cohen LE et al (2018) Local muscle flaps minimize post-operative wound morbidity in patients with neoplastic disease of the spine. Clin Neurol Neurosurg 171:100–105

Gao MA, Tan ET, Neri JP et al (2023) Diffusion-weighted MRI of total hip arthroplasty for classification of synovial reactions: a pilot study. Magn Reson Imaging 96:108–115

Garner HW, Kransdorf MJ (2016) Musculoskeletal sarcoma: update on imaging of the post-treatment patient. Can Assoc Radiol J 67:12–120

Garner HW, Kransdorf MJ, Bancroft LW et al (2009) Benign and malignant soft-tissue tumors: posttreatment MR imaging. Radiographics 29:119–134

Garner HW, Kransdorf MJ, Peterson JJ (2011) Posttherapy imaging of musculoskeletal neoplasms. Posttherapy imaging of musculoskeletal neoplasms. Radiol Clin North Am 49(6):1307–1323

Inarejos Clemente EJ, Navarro OM, Navallas M et al (2022) Multiparametric MRI evaluation of bone sarcomas in children. Insights Imaging 13:33

Janu A, Patra A, Kumar M et al (2023) Imaging recommendations for diagnosis, staging and management of bone tumors. Indian J Med Paediatr Oncol 44:257–260

Katonis P, Datsis G, Karantanas A et al (2013) Spinal osteosarcoma. Clin Med Insights Oncol 7:199–208

Kim Y, Lee SK, Kim JY, Kim JH (2023) Pitfalls of diffusion-weighted imaging: clinical utility of T2-shine-through and T2-black-out for musculoskeletal diseases. Diagnostics 13(9):1647

Lalam R, Bloem JL, Noebauer-Huhmann IM et al (2017) ESSR consensus document for detection, characterization, and referral pathway for tumors and tumor-like lesions of bone. Semin Musculoskelet Radiol 21:630–647

Lange N, Jorger AK, Ryang YM et al (2022) Primary bone tumors of the spine—proposal for treatment based on a single center experience. Diagnostics 12(9):2264

Lecouvet FE, Vekemans MC, Van Den Berghe T et al (2022) Imaging of treatment response and minimal residual disease in multiple myeloma: state of the art WB-MRI and PET/CT. Skeletal Radiol 51(1):59–80

Legget AR, Berg AR, Hullinger H, Benevenia JB (2022) Diagnosis and treatment of lumbar giant cell tumor of the spine: update on current management strategies. Diagnostics 12(4):857

Liu X, Duan Z, Fang S, Wang S (2023) Imaging assessment of the efficacy of chemotherapy in primary malignant bone tumors: recent advances in qualitative and quantitative magnetic resonance imaging and radiomics. J Magn Reson Imaging 59:7–31

Messina C, Christie D, Zucca E et al (2015) Primary and secondary bone lymphomas. Cancer Treat Rev 41:235–246

Munoz-Bendix C, Slotty PJ, Ahmadi SA et al (2015) Primary bone tumors of the spine revisited: a 10-year single-center experience of the management and outcome in a neurosurgical department. J Craniovert Junction Spine 16(1):91–104

Noebauer-Huhmann IM, Chaudhary SR, Papakonstantinou O et al (2020) Soft tissue sarcoma follow-up imaging: strategies to distinguish post-treatment changes from recurrence. Semin Musculoskelet Radiol 24:627–644

Oguro S, Okuda S, Sugiura H et al (2018) Giant cell tumor of the bone: change in image features after denosumab administration. Magn Reson Med Sci 17:325–333

Papakonstantinou O, Isaac A, Dalili D, Noebauer-Huhmann IM (2019) T2 hypointense tumors and tumor like lesions. Semin Musculoskelet Radiol 23:58–75

Patel A, James SL, Davies AM, Botchu R (2015) Spinal imaging update: an introduction to techniques for advanced MRI. Bone Joint J 97-B(12):1683–1692

Pennington Z, Ahmed AK, Cottrill E et al (2019) Systematic review on the utility of magnetic resonance imaging for operative management and follow-up for primary sarcoma—lessons from extremity sarcomas. Ann Transl Med 7(10):225

Shao Y, Wang Z, Shi X, Wang Y (2023) Development and validation of nomograms predicting overall and cancer-specific survival for non-metastatic primary malignant bone tumor of spine patients. Sci Rep 13:3503

Stacchiotti S, Gronchi A, Fossati P et al (2017) Best practices for the management of local-regional recurrent chordoma: a position paper by the Chordoma Global Consensus Group. Ann Oncol 28:1230–1242

Subhawong TK, Jacobs MA, Fayad LM (2014) Diffusion-weighted imaging for characterizing musculoskeletal lesions. Radiographics 34(5):1163–1177

Tofts PS, Brix G, Buckley DL et al (1999) Estimating kinetic parameters from dynamic contrast-enhanced T(1)-weighted MRI of a diffusable tracer: standardized quantities and symbols. J Magn Reson Imaging 10:223–232

Van Rijswijk CS, Geirnaerdt MJ, Hogendoorn PC (2004) Soft tissue tumors: value of static and dynamic gadopentetate dimeglumine-enhanced MR imaging in prediction of malignancy. Radiology 233:493–502

Verstraete K (2009) Assessment of response to chemotherapy and radiotherapy. In: Davies AM, Sundaram M, James SLJ (eds) Imaging of bone tumors and tumor-like lesions. Techniques and applications. Springer, Berlin

Verstraete KL, Van der Woude HJ, Hogendoorn PC et al (1996) Dynamic contrast-enhanced MR imaging of musculoskeletal tumors: basic principles and clinical applications. J Magn Reson Imaging 6:311–321

Vilanova JC, Baleato-Gonzalez S, Romero M et al (2016) Assessment of musculoskeletal malignancies with functional MR imaging. Magn Reson Imaging Clin N Am 24:239–259

Yamazaki T, McLoughlin GS, Patel S et al (2009) Feasibility and safety of en bloc resection for primary spine tumors: a systematic review by the Spine Oncology Group. Spine (Phila Pa 1976) 34(22 Suppl):S31

Yao K, Troupis JM (2016) Diffusion-weighted imaging and the skeletal system: a literature review. Clin Radiol 71(11):1071–1082

Zhang J, Huang Y, Lu J et al (2018) Impact of first-line treatment on outcomes of Ewing sarcoma of the spine. Am J Cancer 8:1262–1272

Assessment of Locally Recurrent Disease, Response to Chemo- and Radiotherapy, and Special Considerations

Olympia Papakonstantinou, Snehansh Roy Chaudhary, Smilla Pusitz, and Iris-Melanie Nöebauer-Huhmann

Contents

O. Papakonstantinou (✉)
2nd Department of Radiology, Attikon Hospital, National and Kapodistrian University of Athens, Chaidari, Greece

S. R. Chaudhary
Nuffield Orthopaedic Centre, Oxford University Hospitals NHS Foundation Trust, Oxford, UK

S. Pusitz
Department of Biomedical Imaging and Image-Guided Therapy, Vienna General Hospital, Medical University of Vienna, Vienna, Austria

I.-M. Nöebauer-Huhmann
Division of Neuroradiology and Musculoskeletal Radiology, Department of Biomedical Imaging and Image-Guided Therapy, Medical University of Vienna, Vienna, Austria
e-mail: iris.noebauer@meduniwien.ac.at

Med Radiol Diagn Imaging (2024)

https://doi.org/10.1007/174_2024_478,

Published Online: 29 March 2024

Abstract

This chapter gives a short overview of the expected imaging appearance of postoperative findings, postoperative recurrence, and potential postoperative complications that may occur after treatment of tumors of the osseous spine. Furthermore, assessment of response to chemo- and radiotherapy is discussed. Magnetic resonance imaging (MRI), including morphological sequences, dynamic contrast-enhanced imaging, and diffusion-weighted imaging, is the preferred technique to differentiate expected postoperative changes such as edema and fibrosis from local recurrence. Complementary computed tomography (CT) may add information by demonstrating osteolysis, detection of chondroid calcifications in recurrent cartilage tumors of chordoma, and calcified osteoid matrix in recurrent osteosarcoma. Positron emission tomography (PET)/CT and WBMRI have a complementary role in the posttreatment evaluation of lymphoma. PET/CT also has a role in the evaluation of posttreatment response of plasmacytoma.

Complications such as damage to neural structures, flap reconstruction failure, CSF leak with formation of pseudomeningocele, vascular injury, wound-related complications such as tissue necrosis, wound dehiscence, hematomas, seromas, infections, and development of extensive fibrosis are also best evaluated on MRI. CT is, however, the mainstay for hardware and bone graft failure.

Mimickers of poor response to chemotherapy include early granulation tissue, bone marrow changes due to chemotherapy or irradiation, radiation necrosis, and insufficiency fractures.

1 Expected Postoperative Findings

Relapsed tumor must be differentiated from expected postoperative changes such as edema, fibrosis, and granulation tissue that develop in the surgical bed and may coincide with the relapsed tumor. Both relapsed neoplasms and early postoperative changes can share similar radiologic features in terms of low signal intensity on T1-weighted images (WI), high signal intensity on water-sensitive sequences, and enhancement after static intravenous administration of contrast medium (Verstraete 2009; Fayad et al. 2012), whereas late fibrosis shows decreased signal on both T1-WI and water-sensitive sequences and mild late enhancement (Fig. 1). Occasionally, granulation tissue or fibrosis may have a mass-like appearance (Griffiths et al. 1997), whereas plaque-like lesions cannot confidently exclude local recurrence (Noebauer-Huhmann et al. 2020). T1-WI is the most useful to show the anatomy of the surgical bed.

Myocutaneous flaps (MCFs) are initially of increased signal intensity on fluid-sensitive sequences for approximately 2 years and maintain the muscle texture, while most of them present with diffuse enhancement that subsides after 18 months. The flaps progressively undergo fatty replacement and atrophy due to denervation and disuse (Fox et al. 2006; Garner et al. 2011).

Instrumentation, vascularized bone autografts, or allografts are used to provide structural support in spine (Fig. 2) after resection of involved spinal segments by the tumor (Bancroft 2011) (see chapter "Surgical Treatment of Primary Tumors of the Spine" in this book). Host cells invade the autografts or allografts inciting vascularization of the grafts, which gradually leads to osseous remodeling comprising resorption and bone formation. Vascularized autografts usually appear like normal bone on CT and MR imaging; however, heterogenous low signal intensity on T1-WI and hyperintensity on fluid-sensitive sequences are not uncommon due to development of necrotic areas and granulation tissue. Ossification at the osteotomy site extending to soft tissues may resemble recurrent osteosarcoma (Bloem et al. 2020; Gupta et al. 2018). Allografts exhibit low signal intensity on all sequences and no enhancement in the immediate postoperative period. Persistence of low signal implies lack of graft incorporation (Beaman et al. 2006). With progressive incorporation, the graft displays red

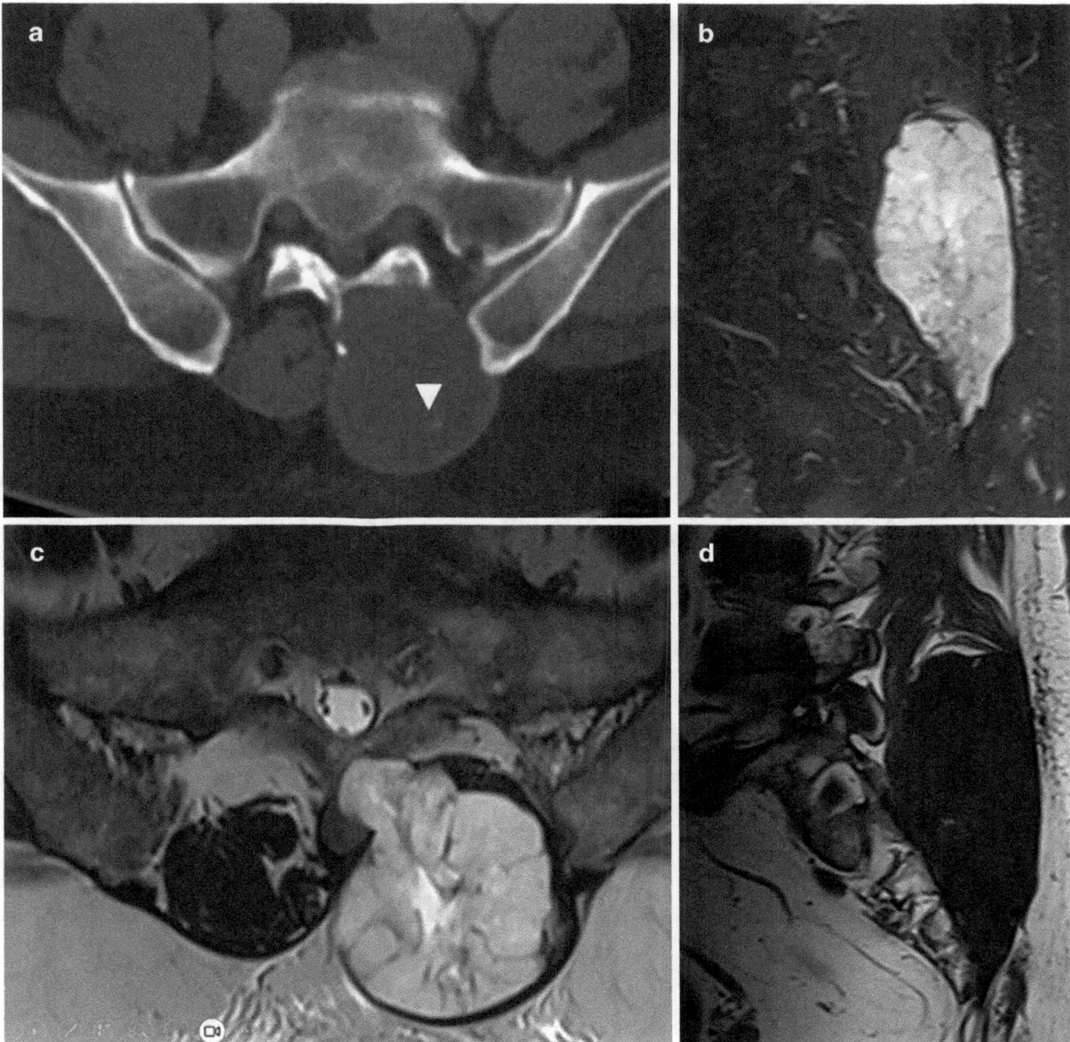

Fig. 1 Sixty-one-year-old male patient with biopsy-confirmed chondrosarcoma. Preoperative CT (**a**, axial reformation) shows a geographic osteolytic lesion with minor intralesional mineralization (arrowhead) in the dorsal elements of the sacrum. MRI shows a multiseptated markedly hyperintense tumor, which involves L5 and spans to S5 (**b**, sagittal TIRM image), which is markedly hyperintense on T2-WI (**c**), and unspecifically hypointense, almost without contrast enhancement, on T1-WI (**d**). The tumor was resected in sano. Two years post-surgery, routine follow-up imaging revealed a lobulated hyperintense lesion (arrow) at the border of the resection (**e**, coronal TIRM), which also shows almost fluidlike signal, with marked hyperintensity on nonfat-saturated T2-WI (**f**). This light-bulb appearance resembles the original tumor being typical for the chondroid matrix and corresponds to a high ADC (**g**). The lesion is unspecifically hypointense on T1-WI without visible contrast enhancement (**h**, arrow) even in the water images of the Dixon sequence (**h**). This is confirmed on the dynamic contrast enhancement sequence (**i**), where the wash-in curve of the lesion (blue) is even lower than that of the unaffected muscle (pink); arterial enhancement is shown in orange. Repeat surgery was performed. One year later, routine follow-up (**j**: coronal TIRM; **k**: axial T2-WI; **l**: axial water images of the Dixon sequence) shows a small postoperative retention (arrows), while the signal intensity may be similar; both the shape of the retention and the surrounding rim of postoperative scarring (thin arrows) are helpful in the differentiation from recurrence, which is not present. Scar tissue is hypointense in all images and presents mild late enhancement (thin arrows)

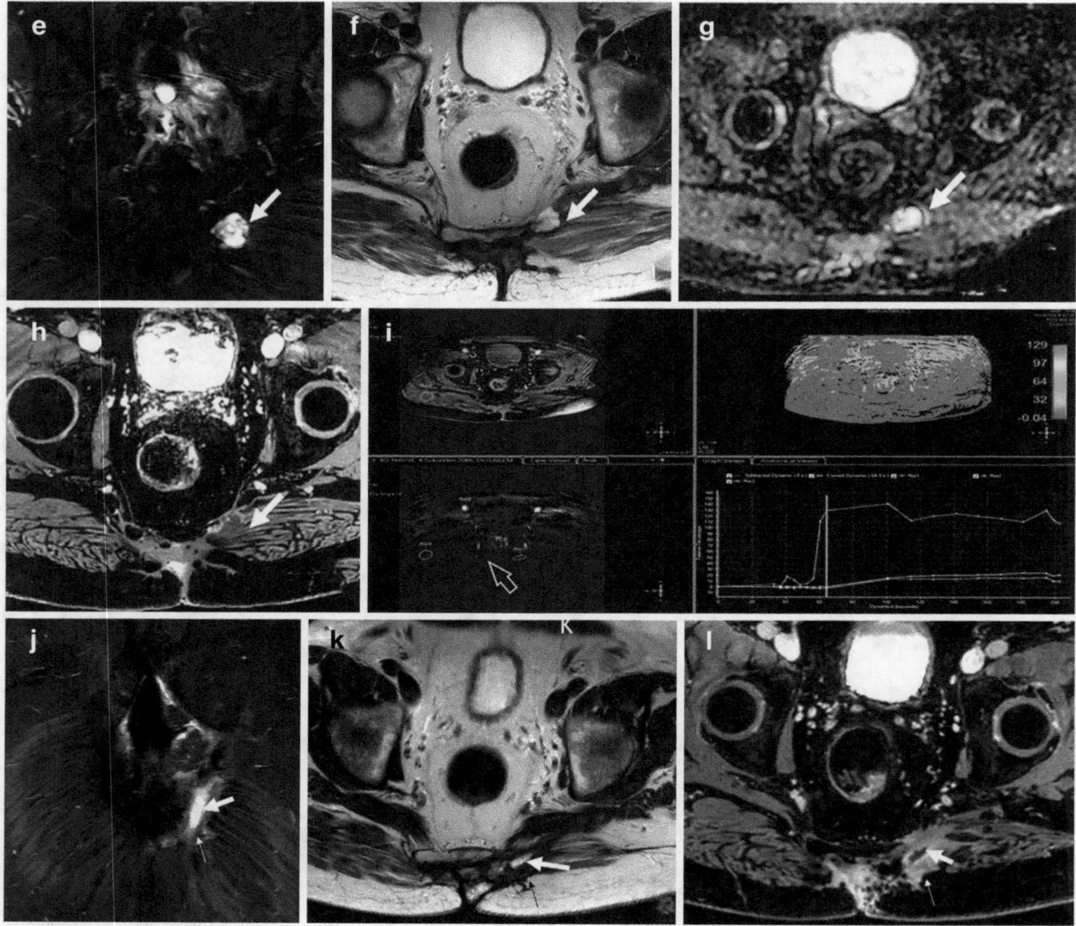

Fig. 1 (continued)

marrow signal intensity. In the intermediate post-operative period between 3 months and 2 years, a thin hypervascular tissue is seen in the margins of the allograft that resolves after more than 2 years after the graft has been incorporated. Small focal areas hypointense on T1-WI and hyperintense on water-sensitive sequences may be seen corresponding to necrosis or fibrous changes (Kattapuram et al. 1999).

2 Imaging of Local Recurrence

Recurrent musculoskeletal tumors—if large—can be easily seen even on non-contrast morphologic images and most often share similar features with the initial tumor (Figs. 1 and 3). Thus, pre-operative MR imaging scans should be available for comparison (Garner and Kransdorf 2016). A relapsed conventional chordoma, that is the commonest primary malignant tumor of the sacrum, typically presents with lobulated high T2 signal with hypointense fibrous septa (Figs. 2, 3, and 4). Both the original and the relapsed tumor may be indolent and present as a bulky mass extending across the sacroiliac joint to the iliac bones, to the posterolateral pelvic muscles, and to the sciatic foramen invading the sciatic nerve and (Lee et al. 2022) anteriorly adjacent to mesorectum (see also chapter "Notochordal Tumors" in this book). Relapsed chordomas usually demonstrate mild heterogenous honeycomb pattern of enhance-

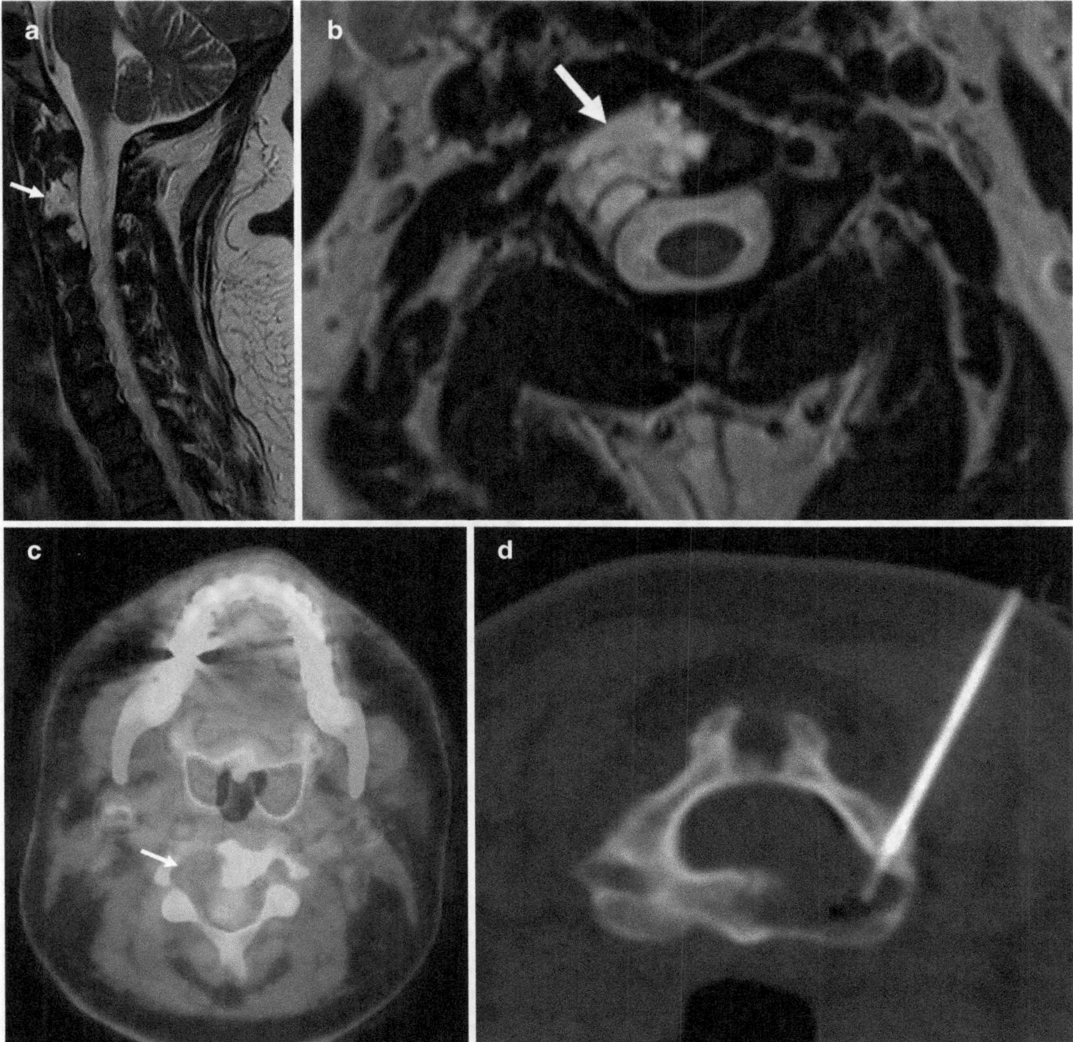

Fig. 2 A 28-year-old female patient, presenting with 1-year history of right-sided neck pain. Sagittal (**a**) and axial (**b**) T2-WI reveal a hyperintense lobulated mass in the C2–C3 vertebral bodies and right arch (arrows). The lesion demonstrated background FDG-PET avidity on PET/CT (**c**). On CT, the lesion was destructive (**d**), whereas CT-guided biopsy did not reveal any abnormal cells. The patient was addressed to a tertiary center 6 months later. Repeated MRI did not reveal any morphological changes of the lesion (**e**, STIR sagittal image, arrow), whereas an ADC map (**f**) demonstrated restricted diffusion (arrow). Open biopsy and posterior cervical stabilization surgery were subsequently planned. Lateral and AP view radiographs of the cervical spine (**g**, **h**) demonstrating posterior cervical fixation. Subsequently, the right-sided metalwork was removed (**i**) to facilitate preoperative proton beam therapy (PBT). However, repeat MRI (not shown) after PBT revealed no significant interval change. Surgical removal of the tumor was performed subsequently. Postoperative CT of the cervical spine, sagittal reconstructions showing en bloc resection, i.e., C2–C3 corpectomy with resection of right-sided posterior elements, which has been replaced with bone graft (**g**, arrows) from iliac crest and fixed with anterior C1–C4 plate and screws (**g**, arrowhead). Additionally, left occipitocervical fusion from C0–C5 for stabilization was performed (**k**, arrow). Postoperative MRI, 1 month after surgery, shows cord edema (new finding) on a sagittal T2-WI (**l**), whereas an axial T2-WI with fat suppression (**m**) shows a large fluid collection projecting into adjacent soft tissues (arrow)

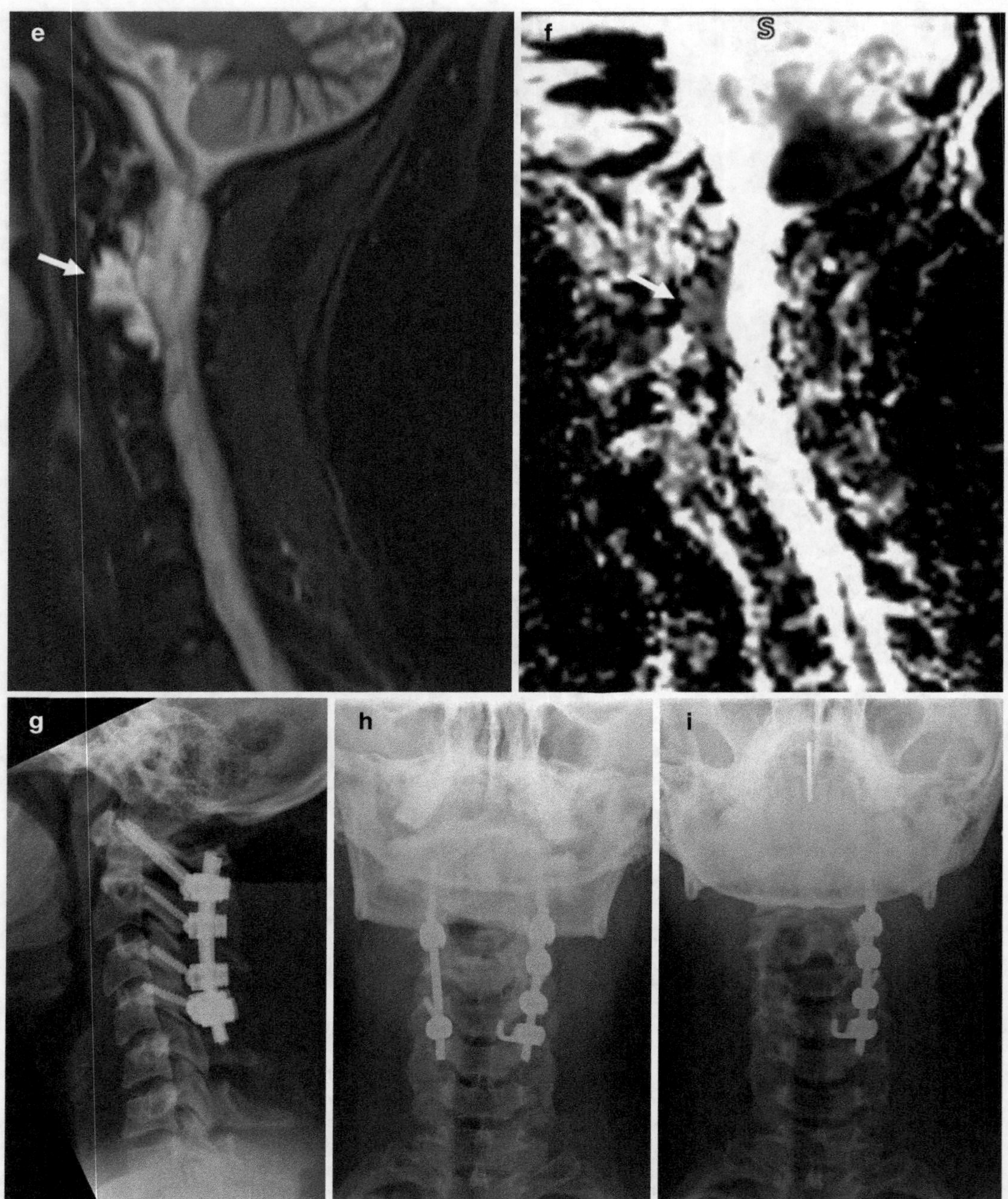

Fig. 2 (continued)

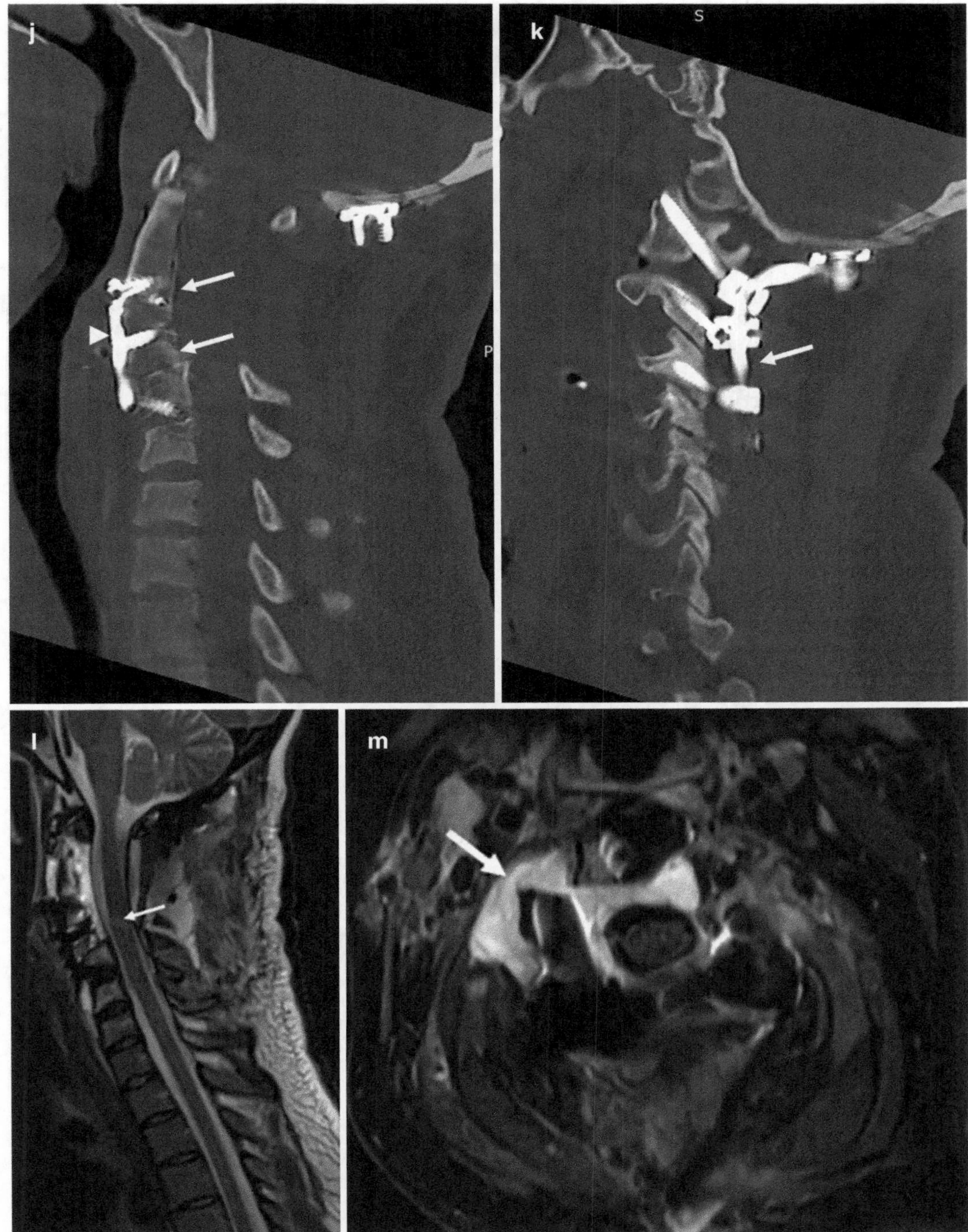

Fig. 2 (continued)

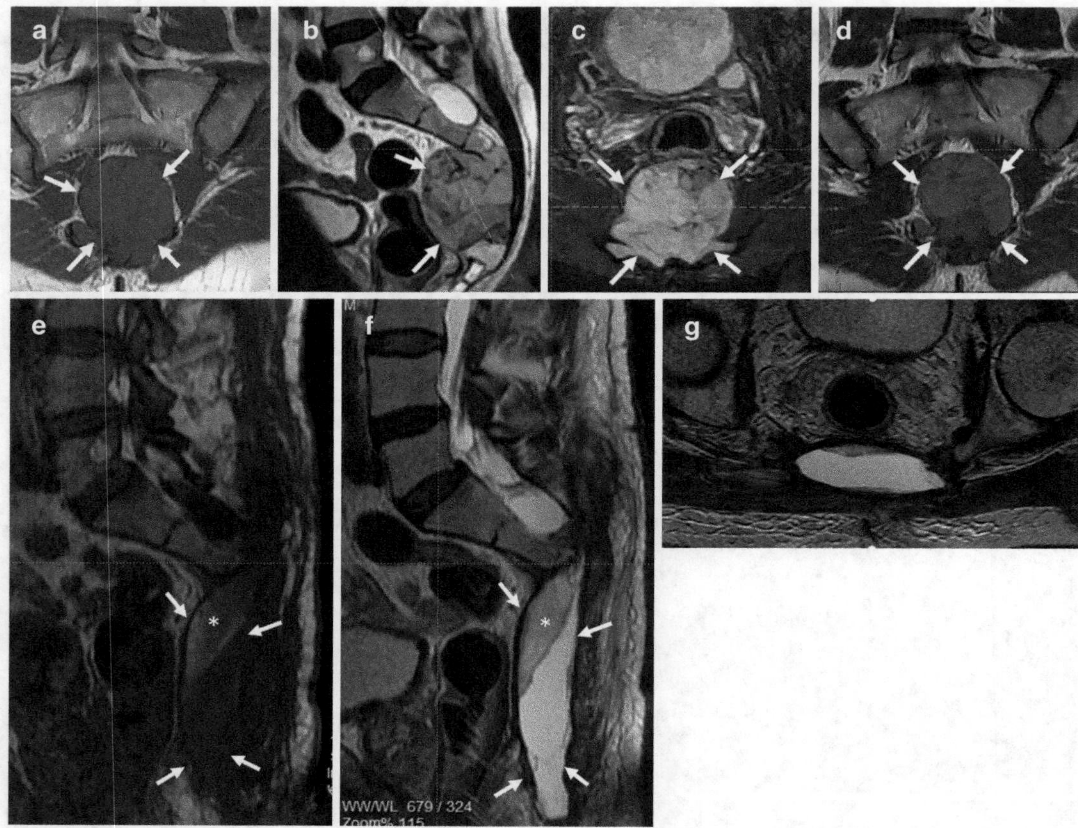

Fig. 3 Preoperative imaging in a 58-year-old male with sacral chordoma. The tumor (arrows) is isointense to muscles (**a**, coronal oblique T1-WI) and mildly hyperintense (**b**, sagittal T2-WI; **c**, oblique axial STIR image) with typical mild enhancement (**d**, coronal oblique CE T1-WI). Two months after surgery, a fluid collection is seen (**e–g**) in surgical bed (arrows) with a thrombus attached on the anterior wall (asterisk). The thrombus shows a hyperintense periphery (**e**, sagittal T1-WI) and is mildly hypointense on sagittal T2-WI (**f**). No lesion suggestive of residual tumor was shown. Fourteen months after surgery, MRI (**h**, oblique axial T2-WI with FS; **i**: axial CE T1-WI with FS; **j**: ADC map; **k**: axial DWI, b = 1000) shows a T2-hyperintense nodule (**h**) adjacent to the anterior wall of the fluid collection (white arrow—compare with image (**g**) at the same level) that shows nonsignificant contrast enhancement (**i**) and restricted diffusion (**j**). The nodule was suspicious but not definite for local recurrence because of its very bright signal on DWI b = 1000 (**k**). After 12 months, the patient underwent repeat MR imaging on a sarcoma center. Images at the same level (**l**: oblique axial T2-WI with FS; **m**: axial CE T1-WI with FS; **n**: ADC map; **o**: axial DWI, b = 1000) exhibit increased size of the anterior nodule, which shows faint peripheral enhancement (**m**), restricted diffusion (**n**), and inhomogeneity on DWI, b = 1000 (**o**). In addition, a new second nodule is seen, adjacent to the posterior wall of the fluid collection (curved arrow) with similar features to the anterior one. The fluid collection decreased in size, and the thrombus (thin black arrows) has been shrunk and is seen hypointense in all sequences (thin arrow). The final diagnosis was recurrent chordoma confirmed on histology

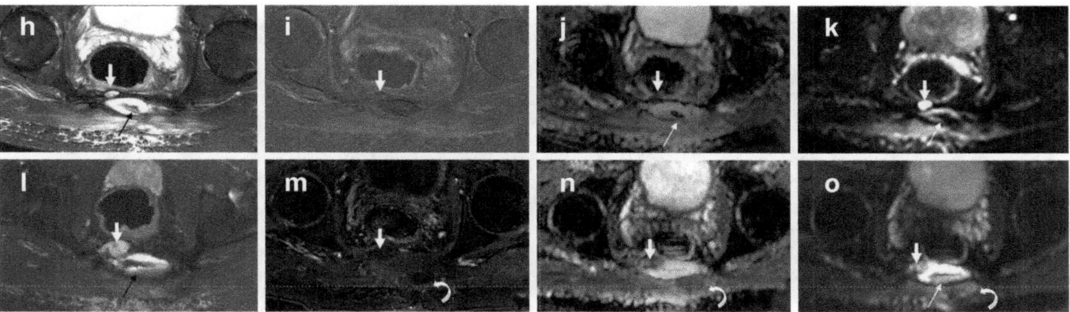

Fig. 3 (continued)

ment, like the primary tumors, while more intense enhancement may represent more aggressive tumor areas (Lin et al. 2018). As encasement of neural and arterial structures is frequent, additional CT or MR angiography can be of help to evaluate the patency of vessels.

Chondrosarcomas usually involve the thoracic spine and less frequently the sacral alae. Non-mineralized chondrosarcomas are usually more aggressive and are more prone to local recurrence (Rodallec et al. 2008). It should be noted that water-rich tumors such as cartilaginous or myxoid-type tumors, or tumors with more sparse cellularity, like chondrosarcomas and chordomas, usually present with less restricted diffusion and mild enhancement (Fig. 1) (Baur et al. 2001); however, poorly differentiated chordomas show decreased ADC values (Sasaki et al. 2018) (Fig. 3). Morphologic and functional data should be interpreted in conjunction for evaluation of tumor recurrence. Complementary CT can be performed, if necessary, to verify novel osteolysis and cortical disruption indicative of recurrence as well as the presence and type of mineralization (see also chapter "Cartilaginous Tumors" in this book).

Ewing's sarcoma typically presents with a soft tissue mass larger than the osseous counterpart (Albano et al. 2019) often presenting the typical wraparound sign (Fig. 5). Imaging following neoadjuvant therapy aims primarily to evaluate the decrease of soft tissue component and the residual viable tumor tissue prior to or after surgery. Viable tumor shows early uptake of contrast (time-intensity curve: type III or IV—see chapter "General Considerations of Posttreatment Evaluation" in this book). Diffusion-weighted imaging (DWI) can further indicate the malignant nature of locally recurrent Ewing's sarcoma presenting with restricted diffusion shown as hyperintensity on high *b*-value images and low ADC values (Inarejos Clemente et al. 2022; Vilanova et al. 2016).

Spinal osteosarcomas have a high rate of recurrence after excision presenting as a sclerotic mass with cloud-like osteoid matrix mineralization around the prosthesis. CT can confidently visualize this mineralization (Gupta et al. 2018). Functional imaging including DCE-MRI can reveal small areas of local recurrence that may not be visible on morphologic imaging (Dyke et al. 2003).

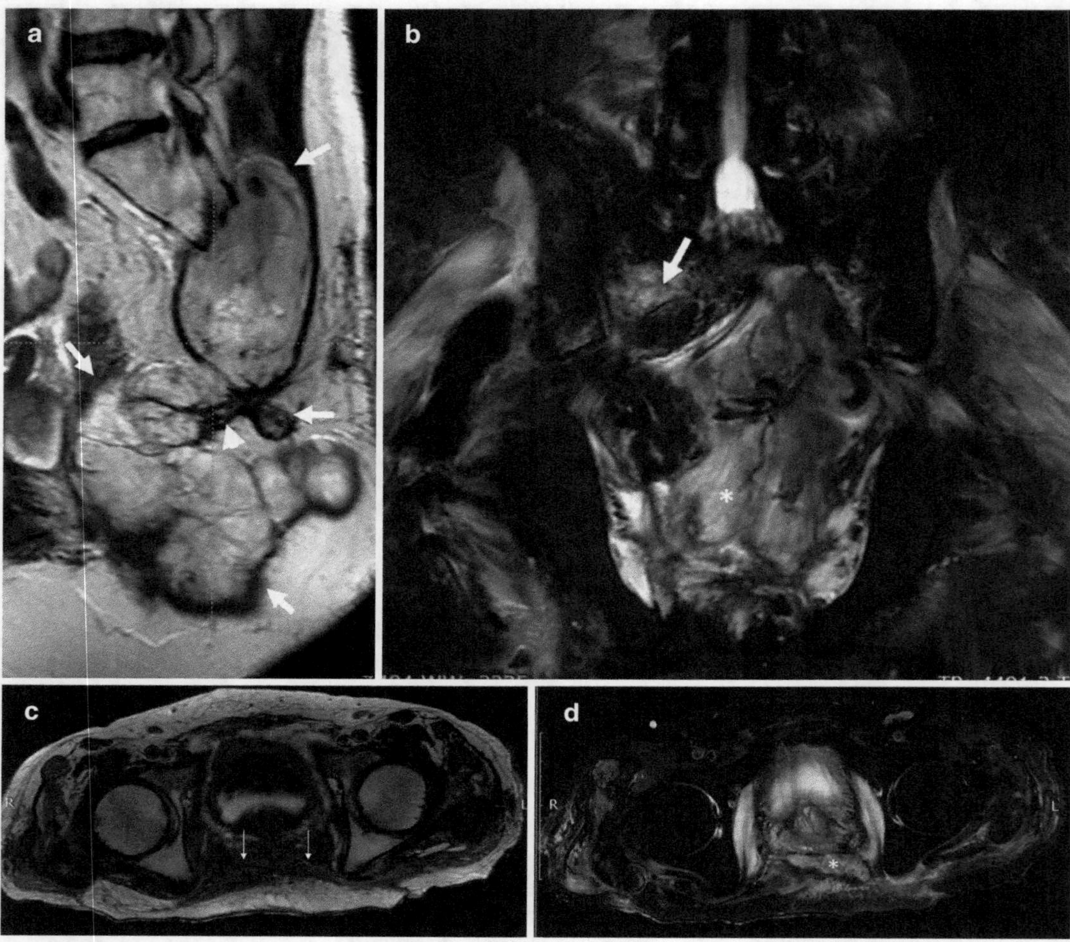

Fig. 4 A 62-year-old man with relapsed chordoma, 7 years after resection of the original tumor. Previous imaging studies were not available. MRI illustrates a bulky relapsed tumor which occupied the surgical bed and adjacent soft tissues (**a**, sagittal T2-WI), being typically lobulated and hyperintense (arrows). Hypointense bands between tumor lobules represent scar tissue (arrowhead). Neoadjuvant radiotherapy was administered, and repeat surgery was performed with resection of the relapsed tumor and reconstruction surgery with free myocutaneous flap. MR imaging performed 12 months after surgery and 9 months after radiotherapy shows diffuse postradiation edema of gluteal and pelvic muscles, which maintain their feathery pattern (**b**, coronal T2-WI with FS; **d**, axial T2-WI Dixon, water only). The myocutaneous flap (asterisk) exhibits also diffuse edema, whereas some tiny linear T1 hyperintensities (**c**, axial non-contrast-enhanced T1-WI) represent mild fatty replacement (thin arrows). At the right sacral ala (**b**, arrow), there is a barely seen hypointense line surrounded by bone marrow edema (arrow), representing a stress fracture. No new recurrence was seen

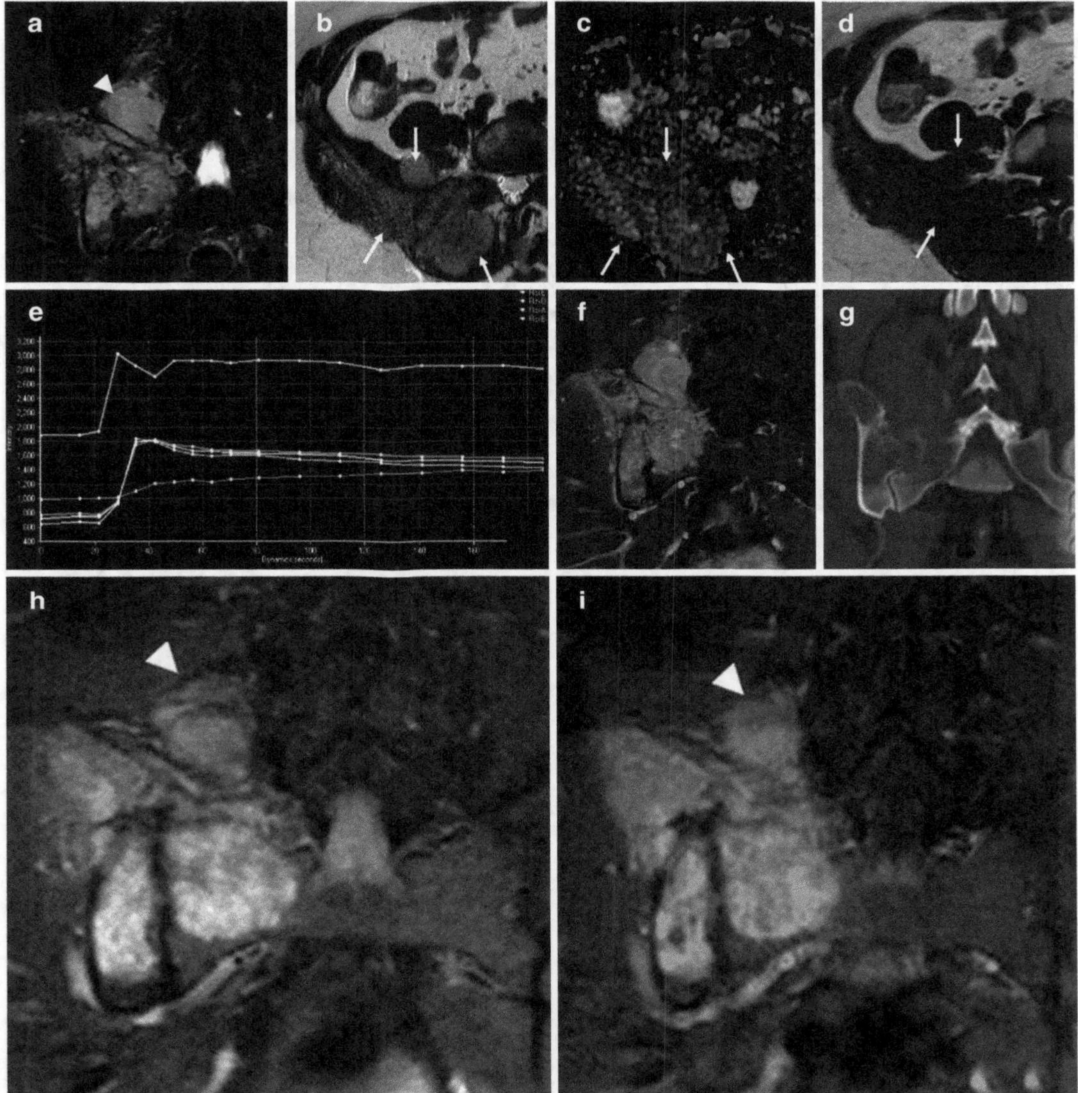

Fig. 5 Forty-one-year-old female patient with Ewing's sarcoma. Coronal STIR image (**a**) shows infiltration of the iliosacral right pelvis, with partly preserved cortical architecture of the sacroiliac joint, due to the highly aggressive tumor growth. Note the large extra-osseous component (arrowhead) while the cortex appears partly preserved (typical "wrapped-around sign"). The tumor exhibits intermediate T2 signal intensity (**b**, axial T2-WI, arrows), due to its high cellular content, which also leads to diffusion restriction on the ADC map (**c**). An axial T1-WI (**d**) shows unspecific low signal. The time-intensity curve (TIC) during gadolinium contrast administration (**e**) reveals an early wash-in (white, blue, and pink curves of different tumor areas), which starts simultaneously with arterial enhancement (green curve), compared to very little enhancement of an unaffected muscle (red curve). The static CE T1-WI with FS shows enhancement of the tumor (**f**). The aggressive bone destruction with partially preserved cortex is demonstrated by CT (**g**—coronal reconstruction). The patient received chemotherapy. *Three months later*, MR imaging denotes decrease of the extra-osseous tumor volume (**h**, coronal STIR image; **i**, coronal CE T1 with FS). TIC during gadolinium contrast administration (**j**) reveals later and slower wash-in (white, blue, and pink curves of different tumor areas, white curve, artery, and blue curve, muscle). Due to the sacral extent, rebiopsy was performed, which showed treatment response; it was decided to perform definitive radiochemotherapy. *Six months after initial imaging*, decrease of the extra-osseous tumor volume is even more pronounced (arrowhead) (**k**, coronal STIR image; **l**, axial T2-WI; **m**, coronal CE T1-WI with FS). An axial CT image (**n**) shows cortical remineralization

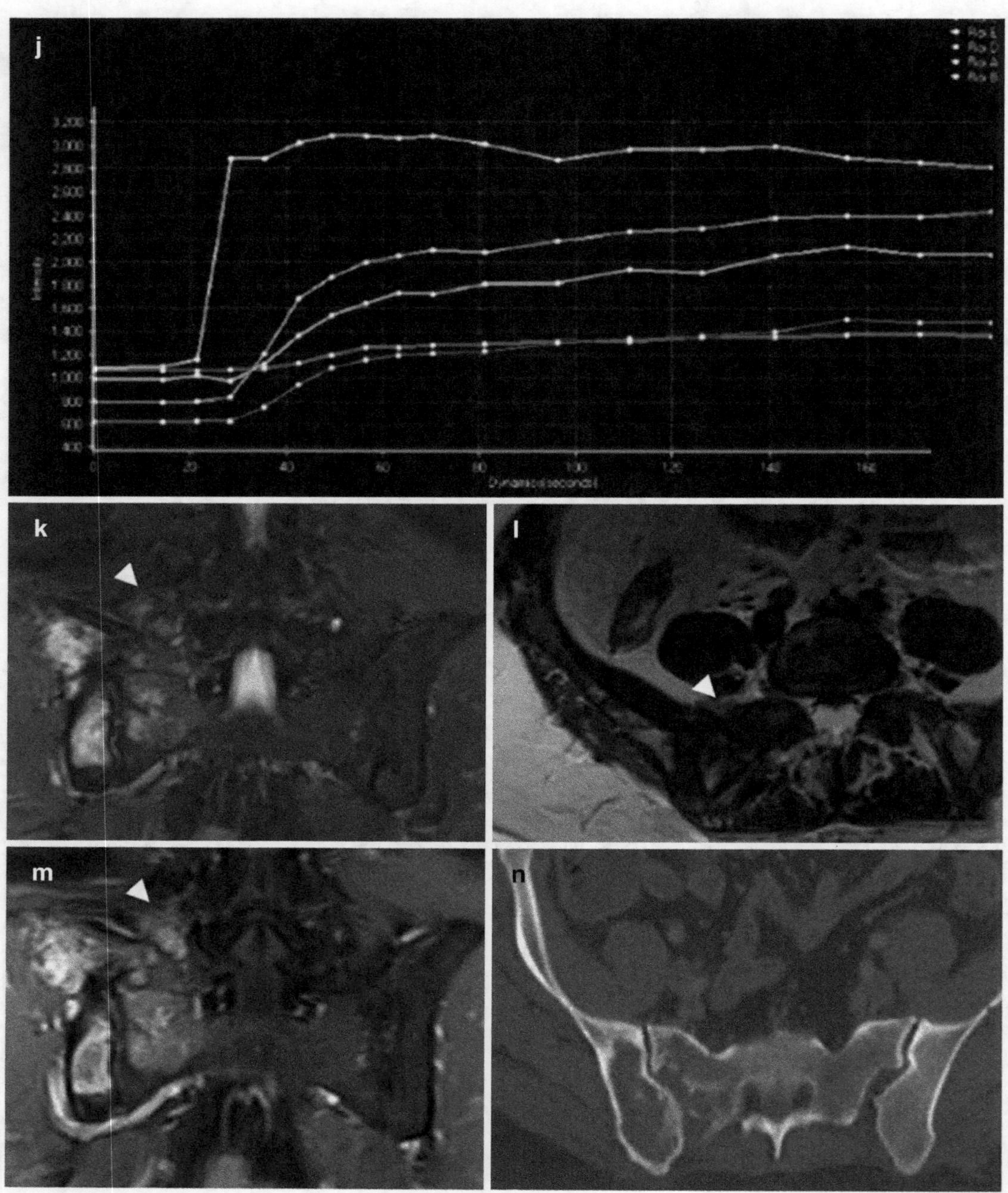

Fig. 5 (continued)

3 Postoperative Complications

En bloc resection with wide margins of primary vertebral tumors is a major operation with high rates of complications, up to 58%, even in most experienced centers (Yamazaki et al. 2009). The most frequent complications include damage to neural structures, failure of hardware, bone graft or myocutaneous flaps (approximately 12% each), cerebrospinal fluid (CSF) leak (approximately 10%), vascular injury and hemorrhage, as well as wound-related complications that comprise tissue necrosis, wound dehiscence, hematomas, seromas, infections, and development of extensive fibrosis (Shapeero et al. 2008; Li et al. 2023). Instrumentation, prior (neoadjuvant) radiation, and diabetes constitute risk factors for the development of complications (Schilling et al. 2020).

Infections not infrequently complicate spinal surgery during the early or late postoperative period. Superficial soft tissue infections present with typical clinical symptoms of redness, pain, swelling, and often a draining sinus tract and usually appear earlier than deeper infections (Noebauer-Huhmann et al. 2020). MRI can depict the extent of infection in the involved tissues, either bone marrow or soft tissues. Infected tissue is hyperintense on water-sensitive sequences and enhances after administration of gadolinium contrast. Indistinctness of bone cortex and low signal intensity of bone marrow on T1-WI are additional typical findings of bone infection, whereas destruction of bone is seen in late stages of infection. In the presence of infection of the surgical bed, areas of devitalized tissue show absence of enhancement with an abrupt enhancing geographic border (Ledermann et al. 2002). Deep infections may extend to intervertebral disks or sacroiliac joints causing spondylodiscitis or sacroiliitis, respectively. Abscesses and sinus tracts are common (Young et al. 2007).

A cutaneous fistula draining CSF is due to a tear of the arachnoid and dura during surgery and is frequently accompanied by a collection of CSF, known as pseudomeningocele, which typically projects into the surrounding soft tissues (Fig. 2). Most of these dural tears heal spontaneously, but some of them persist and result in the development of pseudomeningocele by means of valve-ball mechanism. Previous irradiation, large size of the defect, and weak adjacent musculature favor the development of pseudomeningoceles. Less frequently pseudomeningoceles leak into the epidural space spanning several levels and causing spinal stenosis with spinal cord and nerve root compression. Intradural fibrous tissue due to postoperative scars may lead to arachnoiditis shown as traction and clumping of nerve roots (Young et al. 2007; Jain et al. 2014). Other fluid collections presenting as cystic space-occupying lesions include seromas, hematomas, and abscesses, which are common complications after spine surgery. The fluid contents of pseudomeningocele, seromas, and abscesses are typically hypointense on T1-WI and hyperintense on water-sensitive images (Fig. 2m), whereas the signal intensity of hematomas depends on the evolutionary stage of blood degradation products (Fig. 3e–g) (Garner and Kransdorf 2016; Garner et al. 2011). Hematomas, abscesses, and sinus tracts display peripheral enhancement after contrast administration that is more intense in abscesses, while pseudomeningoceles and CSF fistulas show only faint linear peripheral enhancement. CSF fistulas contain beta-2 transferrin (Hawk and Kim 2000), whereas sinus tracts discharge purulent fluid (Herrera et al. 2013; Radcliff et al. 2016). ADC values of pseudomeningoceles and seromas show the unrestricted diffusion of water, whereas DWI with ADC can be misleading in case of abscess or hematomas/thrombus in the hyperacute (oxyhemoglobin, <24 h) or late subacute (extracellular methemoglobin) stage showing increased signal on high *b*-value DWI and low ADC values, like hypercellular tumors (Chaturvedi 2021; Kim et al. 2023). Occasionally, locoregional recurrence may coexist with hematomas or abscesses and cannot be discriminated based on morphologic features, especially in case of the nodular wall thickening of an expanding hematoma (Noebauer-Huhmann et al. 2020). Functional imaging can be helpful (Fig. 3), although in this scenario, biopsy or resection of the whole lesion should be performed.

Fibrosis or more superficial scar tissue may be bulky, especially after resection of large spinal tumors like chordomas, and most often is band-like although nodular type may occur without maintenance of viable tumor (Garner et al. 2011). Chronic fibrosis typically shows late enhancement on DCE-MRI (Papakonstantinou et al. 2019).

Hardware failure and inadequate incorporation of the bone grafts may lead to spinal instability and pseudarthrosis. MRI denotes bone marrow edema at the site of mechanical instability, whereas a linear hyperintensity on water-sensitive images is shown in case of pseudarthrosis (Bloem et al. 2020). MDCT with multiplanar reformations and capabilities of suppression hard beam artifacts can delineate the integrity of instrumentation and grafts (Fig. 2). Malpositioning of hardware can lead to compression of neural structures and myelopathy (Fig. 2) or vascular structures (Young et al. 2007). Complications of reconstructive surgery include venous congestion followed by necrosis of the flap (Franck et al. 2018).

4 Assessment of Response to Chemotherapy

4.1 Histologic Criteria

Assessment of tumor necrosis on histology is the most accurate predictor of tumor responsiveness to chemotherapy. According to the widely used Huvos classification, tumor necrosis is rated as grade 1 for less than 50% of the total tumor volume, grade II for 50–89%, grade II for 90–99%, and grade IV for 100% tumor necrosis. Positive response to chemotherapy is considered when more than 90% of the tumor cells present necrosis on histology (grades Huvos II and IV) (Huvos et al. 1977). In alignment with Huvos classification, the WHO classification suggests a more simplified assessment of necrosis of ≥90% for good response and <90% for poor response, based on the histologic evaluation of necrosis in the total volume of the surgically resected tumor (Wardelmann et al. 2016). Preoperative estimation of necrosis after neoadjuvant treatment with imaging is of paramount importance for the evaluation of the efficacy of treatment and therapeutic decisions regarding possible change of regimens and schemes as well as time and planning of surgery (Garner and Kransdorf 2016).

4.2 Imaging

Imaging criteria being used for tumor response to treatment include RECIST criteria, which are traditionally used in oncologic imaging for response assessment of solid tumors and rely on reduction of the size of solid tumors and target sites, such as lymph nodes (Eisenhauer et al. 2009). Choi criteria are based on the size of the soft tissue component along with the density of the bone tumor on CT images since increased density/sclerosis of bone tumors associates with better response (Choi et al. 2007; Alothman et al. 2020). Subsequent mRECIST modified criteria incorporated functional information based on early arterial enhancement on MR or CT to identify the "viable tumor" (Fournier et al. 2014), whereas PERCIST take into consideration the FDG uptake on PET/CT (Wahl et al. 2009; Bauckneht et al. 2019). We should note that there is a paucity of series including exclusively posttreatment imaging of spinal bone tumors after neoadjuvant or adjuvant chemotherapy; most information provided herein are extrapolated from appendicular tumor counterparts.

Reduction of the size of the extra-osseous component, sharp demarcation, and sclerosis are indicators of favorable response of bone tumors after chemotherapy (Henderson et al. 2020). MRI can delineate tumor margins and size of extra-osseous component due to superior soft tissue and bone marrow contrast resolution, whereas sclerosis is best seen on conventional radiography (CR) or CT (Figs. 5 and 6). RECIST criteria have limited value for bone tumor response, since they apply only for the soft tissue component, whereas the response of bone component depends upon the tumor type; furthermore, there is inconsistency even for the same type of bone tumor between various studies (Holscher et al. 1992; Laux et al. 2015). For example, in Ewing's sarcoma, good response is usually indicated by significant reduction in size of the soft tissue component (Fig. 5) and development of necrosis,

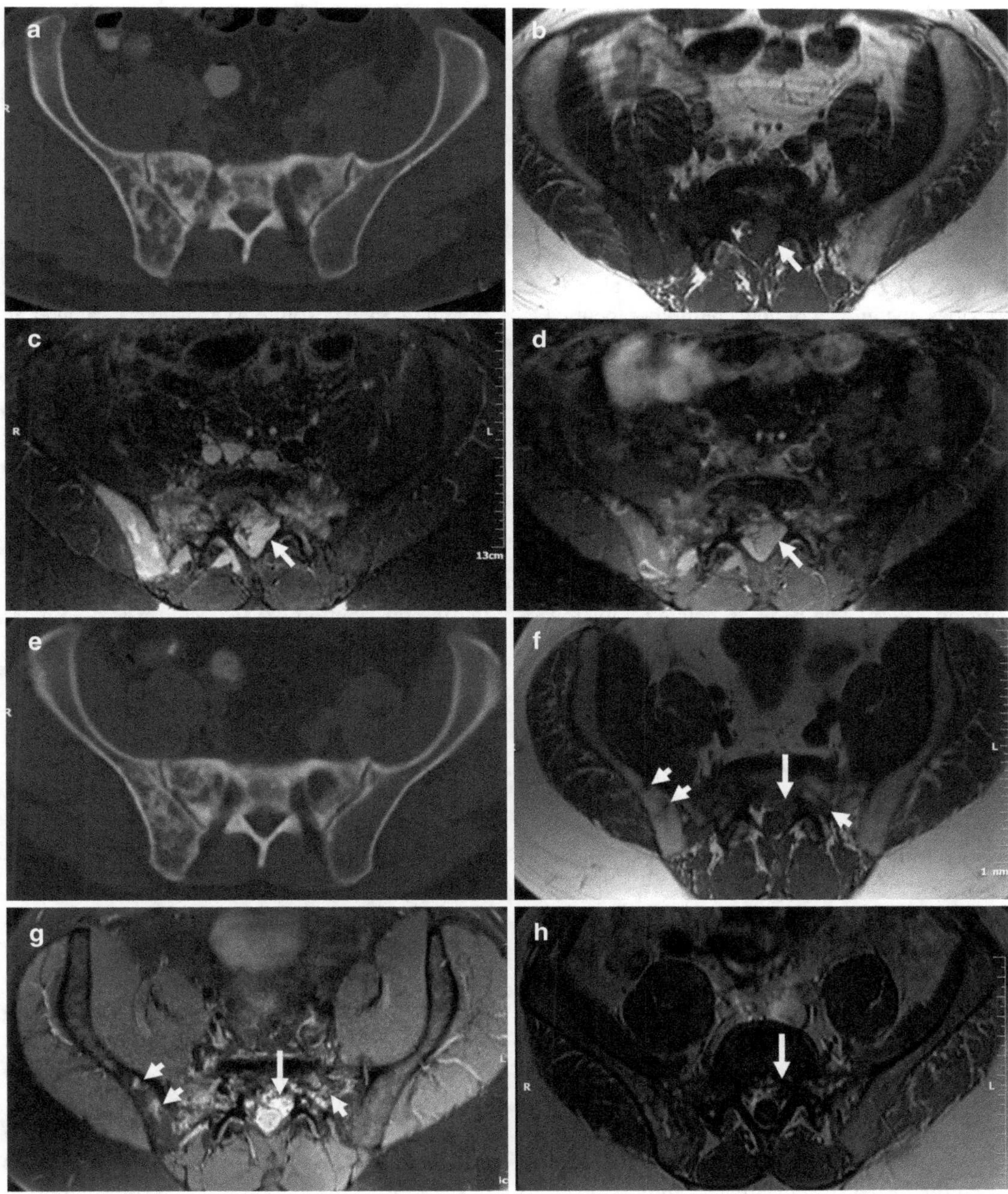

Fig. 6 CT image in a 40-year-old male with non-Hodgkin's lymphoma (**a**) illustrates a mixed lytic-sclerotic pattern, occupying the sacrum and adjacent right iliac bone. On MR imaging, the tumor extends into and obliterates the spinal canal (arrow) and spans partly the right sacroiliac joint. Involved osseous areas and soft tissue epidural mass are T1 hypointense (**b**, axial T1-WI) and T2 hyperintense (**c**, axial PD-WI with FS), presenting gadolinium enhancement (**d**, axial CE T1-WI with FS). The patient received chemotherapy (R-CHOP). *Six months later*, CT shows decrease of the osteolytic areas which are mostly sclerotic after treatment (**e**). MR imaging reveals remission of the abnormal signal in the right ileum and left sacral wing and replacement with fatty marrow, i.e., hyperintense on T1-WI (**f**) and hypointense on PD-WI with FS (**g**) with scattered foci of abnormal signal (small arrows), which represent either residual disease or granulomatous/fibrotic tissue. The soft tissue epidural component has considerably decreased occupying only the left lateral recess (arrows), exhibiting marked hyperintensity on PD-WI with FS (**g**) but absence of contrast enhancement on a CE T1-WI (**h**) implying cystic change of the epidural tumor tissue

whereas poor response is suggested by reduction of tumor volume <25% with residual soft tissue component (Aghighi et al. 2016). On the other hand, the osteoid matrix prevents shrinkage of the intra-osseous osteosarcomas (Henry et al. 2006); vice versa, the increase of the size of a bone tumor can be due to poor response to treatment but is not specific since intratumoral hemorrhage may also cause tumor expansion (Fayad et al. 2012; Inarejos Clemente et al. 2022). Besides, the impact of new chemotherapeutic targeting drugs or immunotherapy on the size of spinal bone tumors is not adequately explored (Hu et al. 2022). Choi criteria have been mainly applied to the response of giant cell tumors (GCTs) to denosumab and are based on the size of the soft tissue component along with the density of the bone tumor on CT images (Alothman et al. 2020).

On morphologic imaging, high signal intensity on T2-WI has been associated with mucomyxoid degeneration, tumor necrosis, granulation, or fibrotic tissue (Erlemann et al. 1990; Roberge et al. 2010). However, Holscher et al. argued that high T2 signal does not exclude viability of the tumor (Holscher et al. 1992). Viable tumor areas typically show paramagnetic contrast enhancement; however, granulation or early fibrotic tissue can share similar signal intensity and enhancement on static contrast-enhanced MRI (Verstraete 2009). Therefore, viable tumor cannot be always discriminated based solely on morphologic criteria; additional functional data are required.

Functional MR techniques including DWI and DCE-MRI, reflecting tumor cellularity and type of blood perfusion, are noninvasive alternatives to histological evaluation of tumor recurrence. Destruction of cellular membranes and reduction of cellular density in treated tumors lead to increased water diffusion within the tissue, indicated by increased ADC values. DWI can provide more objective quantitative metrics based on ADC calculation in addition to qualitative information on DWI using various *b*-values (Subhawong et al. 2014; Bhojwani et al. 2015). A large number of studies have documented that increased ADC values either in selected ROIs or as mean ADC of the whole tumor are superior to morphologic features such as tumor size and signal intensity, for the evaluation of responsiveness to chemotherapy (Wang et al. 2013; Asmar et al. 2020; Saleh et al. 2020; Sasaki et al. 2018). Ratios of ADC post- and pre-chemotherapy (ADC post-chem–ADC pre-chem)/ADC pre-chem have been suggested as a more accurate index for the prediction of the outcome of the treatment than absolute ADC values (Kayal et al. 2023; Kubo et al. 2017). Based on previous studies, the mean ADC of a tumor shows the overall efficacy of chemotherapy, whereas minimum ADC reflects areas of viable tumor that should be followed longitudinally (Uhl et al. 2006; Oka et al. 2010). In good responders after chemotherapy for osteosarcoma, ADC has been found to increase both within the tumor and in the peritumoral area (Hao et al. 2021). Histograms presenting the distribution of ADC can provide a more objective and user-friendly assessment: a flat and wide histogram implies tumor inhomogeneity and necrosis, whereas a sharp and high histogram reflects nonresponse (Liu et al. 2024). Advanced DWI techniques such as intravoxel incoherent motion (IVIM) and diffusion kurtosis (DKI) have been reported to correlate with early responsiveness to chemotherapy in patients with osteosarcoma (Kubo et al. 2016).

However, we should bear in mind the pitfalls of DWI: that in the pediatric skeleton, DWI can be misleading since pediatric bone marrow is more cellular, leading to higher ADC normal values (Chan et al. 2016; Chaturvedi 2021). Calcifications or hemosiderin due to hemorrhage is not uncommon in osseous tumors of the spine and is characterized by low T2 signal and also low SI on DWI and low ADC values due to T2 blackout effect (Dietrich et al. 2009); therefore, interpretation of DWI and ADC maps should be performed in conjunction with conventional morphologic MR images.

Dynamic contrast-enhanced MRI (DCE MRI) has been extensively employed in the posttreatment imaging of bone tumors, particularly osteosarcoma and Ewing's sarcoma (Zeng et al. 2022) (see chapter "General Considerations of Posttreatment Evaluation" in this book). A meta-analysis on DCE MRI documented that a decrease of 60% of the slope of TIC predicted responsiveness of osteosarcomas and Ewing's sarcomas with 73% sensitivity and 83% specificity (Kubo et al. 2016). Other studies documented that viable malignant tissue presents rapid enhancement ≤3 s after the bolus injection, higher slope than necrotic areas (16.1%/min versus 1.5%/min), and decreased time to peak (TTP) (mean 55 s versus 131 s) although overlapping existed (Dyke et al. 2003; Uhl et al. 2006). Possible differences in pharmacokinetic behavior between appendicular bone tumors and their spinal counterparts have not been explored. Employment of 3D isotropic sequences can allow visualization of the whole tumor area allowing improved accuracy over 2D sequences in the estimation of the necrotic regions (Son et al. 2022). A potential false-positive finding for tumor recurrence on DCE MRI is the pattern of enhancement of early reactive granulation tissue that may mimic viable tumor, if the DCE MRI is performed within 4 weeks or less following the end of chemotherapy (Fayad et al. 2012; Verstraete 2009). Therefore, time elapsed between last chemotherapy and posttreatment imaging should be performed 3 months after the end of the neoadjuvant chemotherapy when the revascularization of the granulation tissue has subsided, preferably in the same MR imager employing the same pre- and posttreatment MR acquisition and injection protocol (Liu et al. 2024).

Advanced quantitative perfusion parameters, including extravascular extracellular space (EES), volume transfer constant (Ktrans), and plasma volume fraction (Vp), have been found to correlate with histologic necrosis (Baidya Kayal et al. 2019). However, these parameters are complex with equivocal reproducibility to be used in everyday clinical practice. Alternatively, DCE MRI's more simple imaging protocols including dual-phase postcontrast acquisitions of a late arterial and delayed phase have been recently employed (Son et al. 2022).

5 Assessment of Response to Radiotherapy

5.1 Types of Radiotherapy Used in Spinal Bone Tumors

Radiotherapy is not used as the treatment of choice in most spinal bone tumors. Conventional radiotherapy with volumes of radiation with photon beams ~50 Gy is employed for plasmacytoma; if the tumor invades or is adjacent to critical structures, then focused radiotherapy with intensity-modulated radiation therapy (IMRT) or the more advanced particle beam therapy is applied. Focused radiotherapy with IMRT or particle beam radiotherapy employs larger volumes of precise radiation either with photon beams (IMRT) or with charged particles (particle beam therapy) while minimizing radiation of adjacent normal tissues. Particle beam therapy includes proton beam therapy (PBT), carbon-ion beam therapy (CIBT), and the more advanced boron neutron capture therapy (BNCT) that employ beams of protons or other charged particles (Matsumoto et al. 2021; Klish et al. 2004). Particle beam therapy is preferred in radioresistant tumors and tumors resistant to chemotherapy such as chordoma and chondrosarcoma, which need large volumes of radiation (>70 Gy) before surgery to avoid damage of critical neural structures (Frisch and Timmermann 2007). In spinal osteosarcoma and Ewing's sarcoma, radiotherapy is administered in bulky tumors in order to achieve shrinkage before surgical resection. Low-dose radiation therapy has also been utilized in LCH and in large spinal GCT as focused adjuvant treatment after surgery (Ariyarante et al. 2023).

5.2 Imaging

In general, signs indicative of poor response include more extensive bone marrow involvement or a new soft tissue mass or both, persistence of peritumoral edema, persistence of low

ADC values, and fast and early enhancement. Like chemotherapy, radiation may induce neovascularization initially leading to early and increased contrast enhancement of the radiated tissue similar to viable tumor. In good responders, neovascularization and early enhancement subside after 2–3 months (Verstraete 2009). Reduction of tumor size in Ewing's sarcoma and osteosarcoma is an indicator of good response, but there is paucity of data for the less frequent osseous tumors of the spine.

On the other hand, the size and signal intensity of chordomas after neoadjuvant radiation do not relate with response to treatment. Responsiveness of chordomas has been associated with increased diffusivity (increased ADC values) and decreased DCE MRI parameters such as plasma volume (Vp) and vascular permeability (Ktrans) after neoadjuvant radiation of bulky tumors (Yeom et al. 2013; Santos et al. 2017). Sasaki et al. found that decreased ADC values of chordomas, with a cutoff $<1.494 \times 10^{-3} \times \mathrm{mm}^2/\mathrm{s}$, correlate with poor response and prognosis (Sasaki et al. 2018). However, further studies with larger number of patients should be conducted.

6 Expected Changes and Complications Posttreatment That May Mimic Poor Response

6.1 Post-chemotherapy and Supportive Medication

6.1.1 Bone Marrow Changes

Chemotherapy initially provokes marrow congestion and cellular death leading to increase of extracellular space and thus decreased signal intensity of bone marrow on T1-WI and increased SI on water-sensitive sequences. Gradually, the diffuse inflammatory response subsides leading to predominance of fat within the bone marrow that is seen as increase of marrow signal intensity on T1-WI and decrease SI on the water-sensitive sequences. After the end of interruption of chemotherapy, bone marrow cellularity is restored, approximately in 4 weeks (Ollivier et al. 2006). Granulocyte-colony-stimulating factor (G-CSF), that is usually administered as adjuvant medication to stimulate the suppressed bone marrow after chemotherapy, further enhances bone marrow reconversion (Hartman et al. 2004; Gu et al. 2019). Occasionally, reconversion may be patchy or nodular mimicking metastases. PET/CT and DWI may be confusing showing increased uptake or decreased ADC values, respectively, reflecting increased bone marrow cellularity that may be due to either bone marrow reconversion or neoplastic tissue (Bloem et al. 2020). DCE MRI is more specific to differentiate reconverted marrow that does not display rapid and intense enhancement compared to neoplastic tissue.

Gelatinous transformation of bone marrow (alternative term serous atrophy of bone marrow) is an infrequent chronic complication after chemotherapy or radiotherapy or combination of both (Hwang et al. 2009). It denotes hypoplasia of fat cells, focal loss of hematopoietic cells, and deposition of extracellular gelatinous substances, such as mucopolysaccharides (Lee et al. 2018), and is illustrated as hyperintensity of bone marrow on water-sensitive and T2-WI and hypointensity on T1-WI MR images, like neoplastic tissue (Boutin et al. 2015), but it lacks contrast enhancement and diffusion restriction. In good responders, cystic change of the soft tissue or epidural part of the osseous tumor shares similar features (Fig. 6g, h). T2-WI without fat saturation may be more specific than water-sensitive sequences as non-necrotic bone neoplasms rarely show such a high signal as in gelatinous transformation.

Multiple small bone infarcts associated with chemotherapy and adjuvant corticosteroid therapy are not uncommon in the appendicular skeleton (Ollivier et al. 1991) and may also occur in the spine. Chemotherapy, especially methotrexate either high dose or long-term lower dose, may induce osteoporosis, whereas multifocal osteomyelitis can be seen in granulocytic patients having received intensive chemotherapy (Ollivier et al. 2006). Rebound hyperplasia of thymus and spleen is not infrequent after the end of chemotherapy (Bloem et al. 2020).

6.2 Post-radiotherapy Changes

Changes induced by radiotherapy in bone and soft tissues adjacent to the tumor depend on characteristics of radiation such as the type of radiation, i.e., proton beam or photon, total dose, number of fractions, dose per fraction, and interval between them as well as time elapsed from radiation (Capps et al. 1997). Therefore, it is important to be aware of the time and type of administered radiotherapy.

6.2.1 Bone Marrow Changes

Similar to chemotherapy, irradiation has early effects on bone marrow inciting initially edema and inflammatory reaction of bone marrow within the first 1–6 weeks followed by gradual substitution with fat (Ollivier et al. 2006); in approximately 6 weeks after the end of treatment, these changes exhibit similar MR features to post-chemotherapy changes (Bloem et al. 2020). Late fibrotic areas are not uncommon within the irradiated bone marrow presenting as low signal on all sequences (Noebauer-Huhmann et al. 2020).

Gelatinous transformation of bone marrow can occur approximately 9 months after the end of radiotherapy and, usually, disappears after 2 years, but data are mainly based on extremity bone marrow after irradiation of soft tissue sarcoma (Hwang et al. 2009).

6.2.2 Late Bone Changes: Radiation Osteitis, Avascular Necrosis, Osteoporotic Fractures

Expected late bone changes have been referred to as radiation osteitis and include osteopenia, occurring approximately 1 year after irradiation, coarsening of trabeculae and bone cortex, sclerosis, and heterogenous bone density resembling Paget-like changes (Brown et al. 1983; Bluemke et al. 1994). Postradiation avascular necrosis (AVN) after a latent period of 1–5 years has been reported in sacrum and spine after radiation of abdominal malignancies (Capps et al. 1997; Jin et al. 2020), but data on postradiation AVN in patients with vertebral tumors are sparse. Insufficiency fractures of the sacrum are common in patients with chordoma who have received radiation treatment, especially proton beam therapy (Bostel et al. 2018). They are usually bilateral and multiple (seen as hypointense lines on all sequences surrounded by bone marrow edema) (Fig. 4b). Fractures in osteoporotic bone are self-limiting and have a better prognosis than fractures due to osteonecrosis as the latter often evolve to nonunion and pseudoarthrosis (Meixel et al. 2018).

6.2.3 Soft Tissue Changes

Diffuse edema of soft tissues appears early within the first week of the radiation portal. The septa within the subcutaneous fat and the intermuscular septa are thickened, hypointense on T1-WI and hyperintense on fluid-sensitive sequences, whereas edematous muscles typically retain their feathery pattern (Fig. 4c, d). It is noteworthy that postirradiation muscle edema is more intense after 12–18 months and may persist for years, whereas postirradiation edema of the subcutaneous tissue and thickening of intermuscular septa may increase over time (Richardson et al. 1996). Granulation tissue and fibrosis in soft tissue may develop after surgery and become worse if radiotherapy has been additionally administered (Noebauer-Huhmann et al. 2020). Early granulation tissue may depict more intense and early enhancement mimicking viable tumoral tissue. After 4 weeks, vascularity of the postradiation changes subsides, and enhancement turns to be late and usually mild (Verstraete 2009); therefore, imaging should be performed at least after 4 weeks after the end of radiotherapy.

Neoadjuvant radiation predisposes to wound healing complications such as seromas, dehiscence, and infections, while soft issue edema and fibrosis are more frequent with adjuvant radiation (O'Sallivan et al. 2002).

6.2.4 Complications of Radiation Therapy in Developing Skeleton

Complications of radiation therapy on the developing skeleton occur late but are not infrequent and include delayed ossification and alignment deformities such as kyphosis, scoliosis, and lordosis, whereas late development of osteochondromas, soft tissue myxomas, and schwannomas includes other well-recognized complications (Hoeben et al. 2019). Fortunately, primary vertebral tumors are rare in pediatric population.

6.2.5 Complications in the Spinal Cord

Postradiation myelopathy (radiation myelitis) consists of demyelination and necrosis of spinal cord, due to damage of the endothelial cells of feeding blood vessels. This complication is not frequent nowadays thanks to the application of new targeted radiotherapy methods that eliminate damage to the adjacent critical neural structures (Schultheiss 2008). Inflammatory pseudotumor in epidural space of the spine, that compresses the spinal cord, has been reported (Hoeben et al. 2019), whereas spinal cord hypoplasia has been referred to in children and adolescents (Chokshi et al. 2018).

6.2.6 Postradiation Sarcomas

Postradiation sarcoma is a rare late complication of radiotherapy within the radiation field, after a latency period of 4–40 years. Predisposing factors include high radiation dose, younger age, and administration of combined chemo- and radiotherapy. Since radiation therapy in osseous bone tumors of the spine is rare, there is sparsity of data concerning postradiation sarcomas (Sheppard and Libshitz 2001; Patel 2000).

7 Special Considerations to Lymphoma, Plasmacytoma, GCT

7.1 Lymphoma

The spine is a rare site of primary osseous lymphoma, but secondary lymphoma is common (Barz et al. 2021), necessitating whole-body imaging, either PET/CT or whole-body MRI (WBMRI) (Lim and Ong 2013). PET/CT has been established as the method of choice for staging of lymphomas and early response to treatment (see chapters "PET/CT" and "Lymphoma" in this book). A hypermetabolic activity of >2.5 SUV is an established threshold indicative of viable tumor (Fig. 6) (Seam et al. 2007; Johnson et al. 2015). Whole-body MR imaging, including T1, water-sensitive, and diffusion images, is also well suited for this purpose. DWI can assess response to treatment earlier than conventional MR imaging and similar to PET/CT (Albano et al. 2021). PET/CT is superior to MRI in detecting viable disease in extraskeletal sites where WBMRI has poor sensitivity in body parts such as the lung parenchyma (Mayerhoefer et al. 2020; Yamamoto et al. 2009). However, PET/CT can be false positive especially in the evaluation of progressive disease because benign conditions, such as inflammation or infection, can be PET-avid and mimic lymphoma (Barrington and O'Doherty 2003). Benefits of MRI are the lack of radiation mostly helpful in pediatric population, more availability, and less total time of the examination compared to PET/CT (Rahmouni et al. 2003).

Findings indicative of good response include decrease of osteolytic and increase of sclerotic areas on CT and reduction of the soft tissue component. Bone marrow of responders exhibits decreased signal intensity on water-sensitive images and hyperintensity on T1-WI due to substitution of tumor cells by fatty marrow (Fig. 7) as well as increase of diffusivity of affected tissues reflected by increased ADC values (Albano et al. 2021). Posttreatment complications such as infections can also be easily depicted on MRI.

7.2 Plasmacytoma/Multiple Myeloma

Although low-dose CT has largely substituted radiographic screening, the capability of CT to discriminate between response to treatment and stable or progressive disease remains limited (Hillengass et al. 2017). Measurement of Hounsfield units as an indicator of viable disease is further confounded by alterations induced by adjuvant therapies, such as bisphosphonates (Schulze et al. 2014). Implementation of dual-energy CT with the additional benefit of bone marrow imaging on non-calcium images may

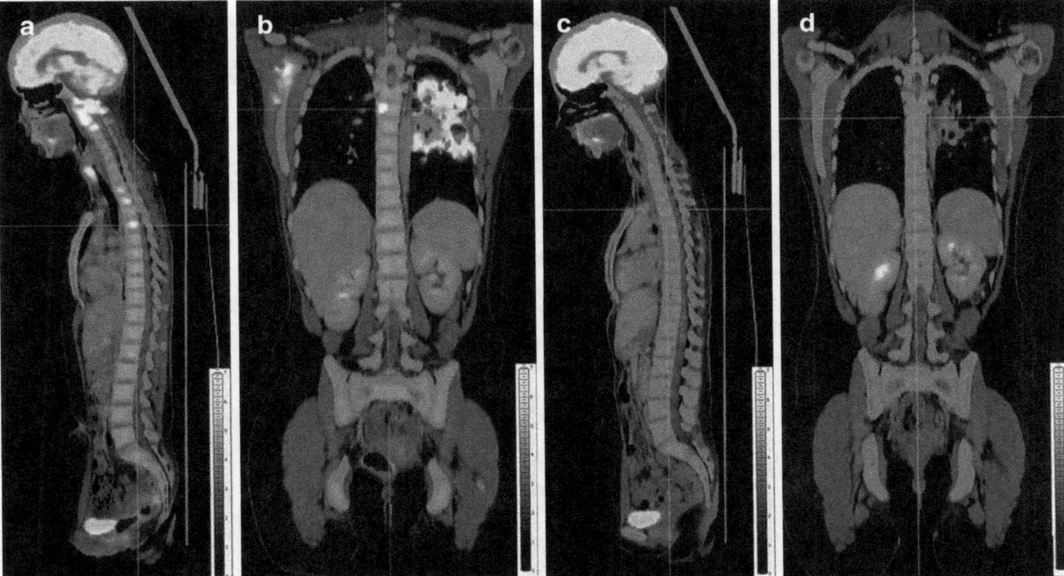

Fig. 7 A 24-year-old female with diffuse B-cell lymphoma. PET/CT shows FDG hotspots in C1–C3, Th3, Th4, and Th6 vertebrae (**a**) without morphologic correlation. The scapula and periscapular muscles are clearly FDG-avid with SUV max: 22.2 (**b**). There are also multiple FDG-avid lymphoma manifestations in both lungs. *Two months later and after three cycles of chemotherapy*, PET/CT shows regression of scapular infiltration and surrounding FDG-avid tissue (**c**); further remission of focal FDG positivity in Th3, Th4, and Th6 vertebrae; and minimal residual activity of the lymphoma manifestations in lungs (**d**)

improve CT performance (Reinert et al. 2020) (see also chapter "Plasmacytoma" in this book).

WBMRI or MRI of the axial skeleton using T1 and water-sensitive morphological sequences along with DWI can also provide quantitative evaluation of the response to treatment (Lecouvet et al. 2022; Koutoulidis et al. 2017). Dixon technique can be particularly useful in the evaluation of remission or progress of disease. On the other hand, despite initial encouraging results, DCE MRI is not recommended in myeloma investigation due to lack of standardization and clinical validation (Lecouvet et al. 2022).

Although WBMRI has been advocated as a more sensitive modality for initial diagnosis, FDG-PET/CT is considered the imaging modality of choice for evaluation of posttreatment response according to recent consensus statement (NICE 2016; Chen et al. 2019). If PET/MRI is available, it can be beneficial for the follow-up evaluation of diffuse marrow infiltration since lifetime radiation exposure is not as high as by PET/CT, whereas combined data from PET and MRI can be obtained (Fig. 8) (Mule et al. 2020).

Again, for evaluation of response, pre- and posttreatment examinations obtained with the same protocol should be compared regarding morphologic and functional features (Lecouvet et al. 2022). Regarding solitary lesions, reduction of size and appearance of a "fatty halo" around the lesion, progressive restoration of the normal bone marrow signal and ADC values, and elimination of the soft tissue component are indicators of good response. On the other hand, malignant compression fractures, increase of the extra-osseous component, and appearance of new lesions or diffuse marrow infiltration indicate poor response (Baur-Melnyk and Reiser 2009). False-positive interpretation may result from fibrotic/granulomatous tissue or cystic necrosis of a lesion that appears hyperintense on T2-WI and on high *b*-value DWI due to shine-through effect; in this case, high ADC values indicate a benign etiology (see chapter "Plasmacytoma" in

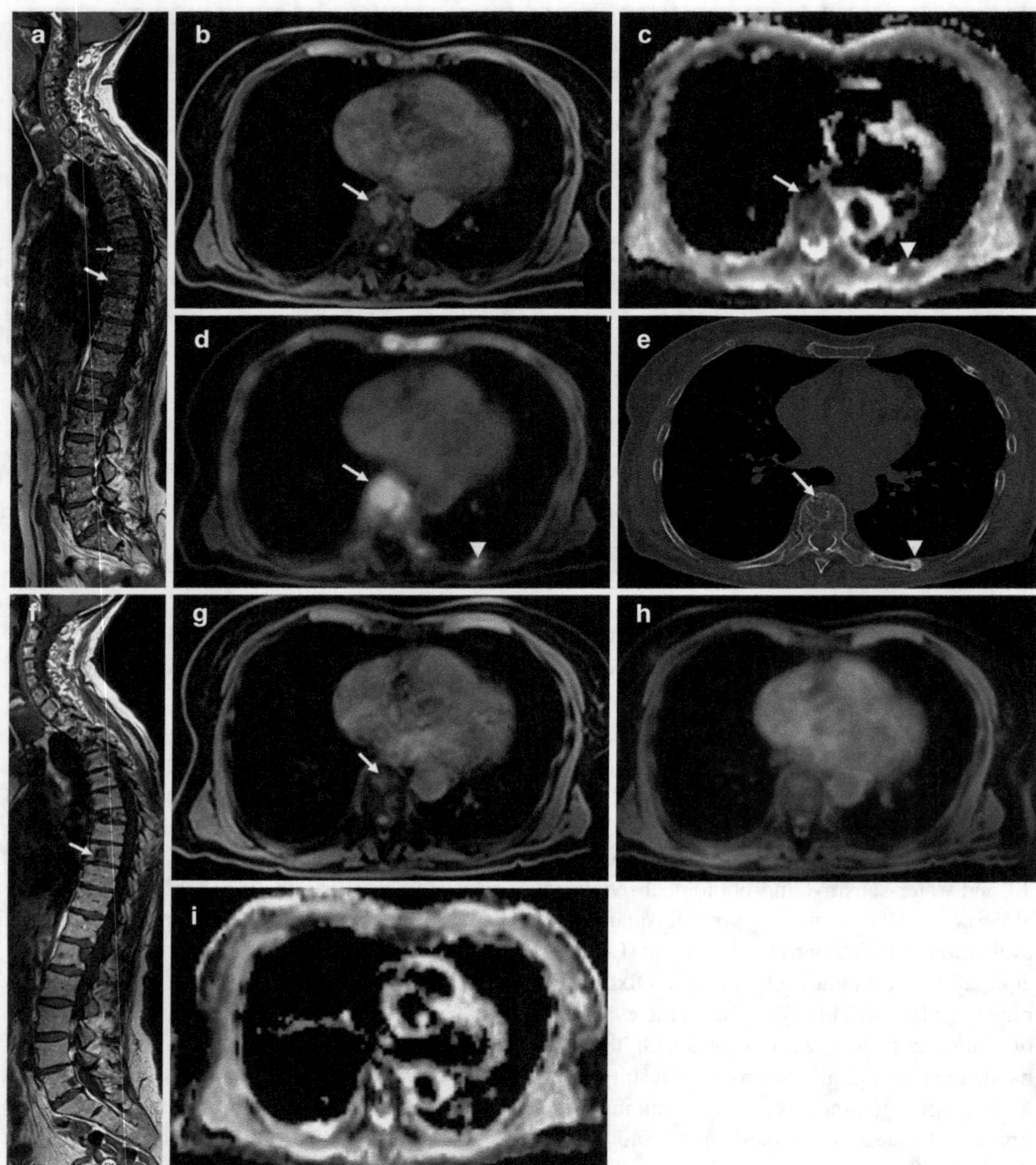

Fig. 8 A 69-year-old female patient with relapse of multiple myeloma. FDG-PET/MRI demonstrates disseminated involvement of the spine on sagittal T1-WI (**a**), with fractures of the third (not shown) and seventh thoracic vertebrae (small arrow), and several larger lesions, such as the one at Th9 (arrow). Axial T1-WI Dixon (**b**, water only) shows the large lesion in Th9, with diffusion restriction on the ADC map (**c**) and intense PET avidity in the fused co-registered reconstruction (**d**) (arrows). CT (**e**), performed for another reason, showed multiple osteolytic lesions; the lesion in Th9 shows a partial sclerotic rim (arrow), likely due to previous therapy, and a rib lesion with pathologic fracture and callus formation (arrowhead). The rib fracture also shows diffusion restriction and PET avidity (arrowheads, **c**, **d**). Repeat FDG-PET/MRI was performed 9 months after the initiation of a therapy with bortezomib-cyclophosphamide-dexamethasone. Sagittal T1-WI (**f**) demonstrates more homogeneous, mainly fat-isointense appearance of the spinal bone marrow. Also, substantial decrease of the larger lesions, including the one in Th9 (arrow) (**g**, axial T1-WI Dixon water only). Also, there is no longer diffusion restriction in the ADC map (**h**), whereas the lesion and the rib fracture have become PET negative (**i**) with complete metabolic response of the patient in PET. Later, the patient received stem cell transplantation

this book). Estimation of the change in fat fraction based on Dixon fat and water images has been found to correlate inversely with early response to treatment. The fat fraction is defined as SI (fat image) = SI (fat image)/[SI (fat image) + SI (water image)] (Koutoulidis et al. 2022; Latifoltojar et al. 2017).

7.3 Giant Cell Tumor (GCT)

Choi criteria have been widely applied in GCTs where morphologic alterations concerning reduction in size and osteosclerosis correlate with response to denosumab administration. Denosumab is a human monoclonal antibody against RANKL that inhibits osteoclastic activity and provokes bone mineralization (see chapter "Giant Cell Tumor" in this book). CT can directly show the degree and distribution of increased mineralization of the tumor as early as 2 weeks after the administration of denosumab (Oguro et al. 2018; Lejoly et al. 2024). On MR imaging, morphologic criteria indicative of good response include shrinkage of the cystic part of the tumor and reduced signal intensity on T1- and T2-WI due to new bone formation (Parmeggiani et al. 2021) (Fig. 9). Campanacci et al. proposed a CT-based classification considering size and peripheral and internal ossification as indicators of GCT response. According to this system, progressive disease presents >25% increase of the

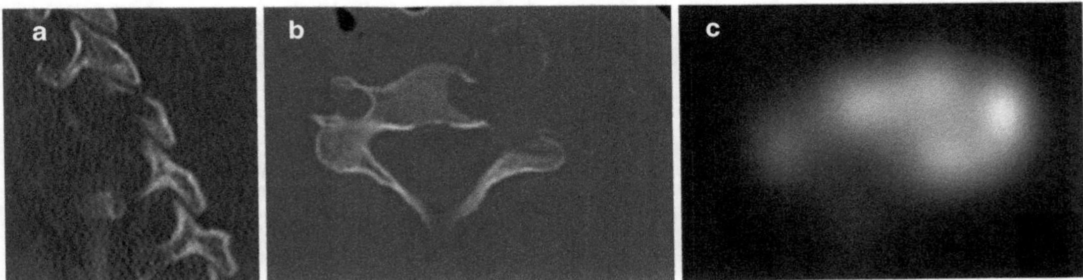

Fig. 9 A 16-year-old male with biopsy-confirmed giant cell tumor (GCT) with secondary aneurysmal bone cyst. Initial CT (**a**, sagittal, and **b**, axial CT reformations) shows geographical expansile osteolysis of C5 without sclerotic rim, with thin neocortex, corresponding with grade II aggressiveness according to the modified Lodwick-Madewell classification, which is typical for GCT. The lesion is scintigraphically positive (**c**). MRI shows involvement of the left part of the body, left pedicle, and transverse process of C5 (**d**, coronal TIRM; **e**, axial T2-WI); the lesion extends to C4 and C6 (**d**, coronal T2-WI), obliterates the left C5–C6 neuroforamen (**e**, **f** arrows), and surrounds the still perfused left vertebral artery circumferentially (**f**, axial CE T1-WI with FS, small black arrow). Intralesional fluid-fluid levels (**e**, small white arrow) are seen, corresponding to the presence of secondary ABC; after contrast agent administration (**f**), solid areas are revealed as well as peripheral enhancement around the cystic components, and considerable perilesional edema-like changes in the bone and soft tissues. GCT with secondary aneurysmal bone cyst was diagnosed based on imaging findings and biopsy. The patient came to the tumor center where imaging was repeated, 3 months after the first MRI. The tumor had led to a pathological height loss of C5 (**g**, coronal TIRM) and had grown, now extending to the right side of the vertebral body and the lamina of C5 (**h**, axial T2-WI). Systemic therapy with denosumab was started. *Six weeks later*, CT (**i**, axial reformation) reveals some sclerosis, mainly rim-like, and some regression of the cystic areas (**j**, axial T2-WI). *Nine months later*, CT shows progressive sclerosis also within the lesion (**k**). The corresponding MRI shows minor progression in height loss (arrow) and (**l**, coronal TIRM), complete regression of the cystic areas (**m**, axial T2-WI), and conversion zones with more homogeneous contrast enhancement (**n**, axial CE T1-WI with FS, arrow). The patient was then referred to a center in his home country and *presented again 18 months after therapy initiation*; the lesion was stable (not shown), and the patient was almost symptom free, so that the board decided not to perform surgery. Denosumab was paused; follow-up imaging was performed and revealed no growth (not shown). *Three and a half years later*, C5 shows remodeling and is fused with C4 (**o**, axial, and **p**, sagittal CT reformatted images); the residual lesion is smaller (arrows) and more hypointense on MRI (**q**, axial T2-WI) and only shows minor contrast enhancement (**r**, coronal CE T1-WI with FS arrow)

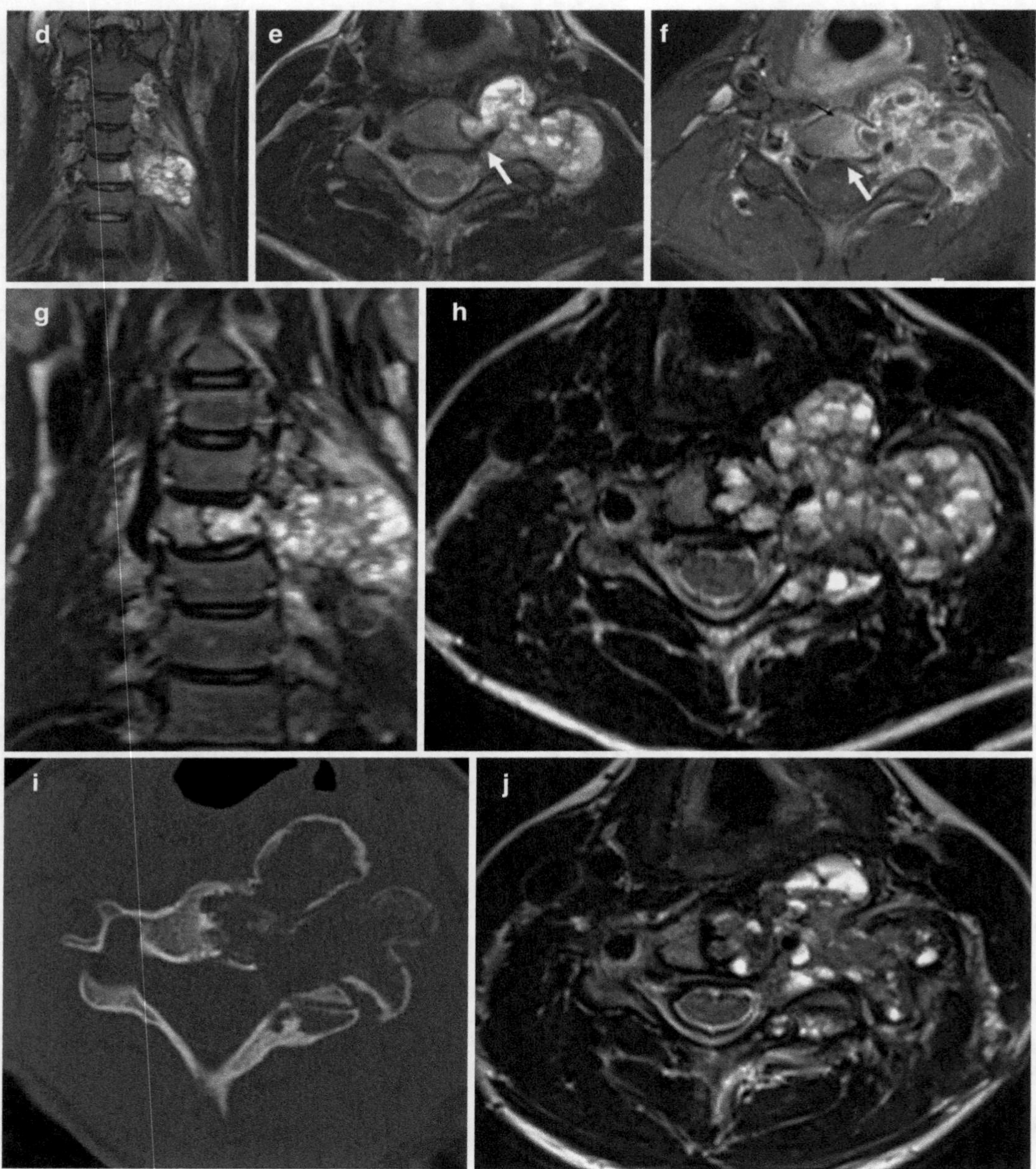

Fig. 9 (continued)

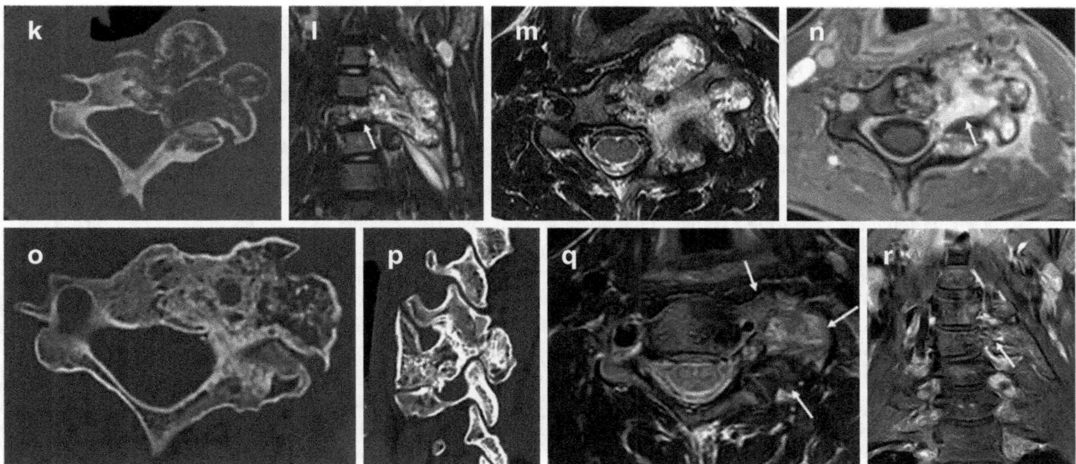

Fig. 9 (continued)

tumor size, whereas stable tumor shows <25% increase in size, and partial response is determined based on the presence and degree of ossification with or without reduction in size (Campanacci et al. 2019). GCT is a hypermetabolic tumor showing increased FDG uptake (Engellau et al. 2018). According to Engelau et al., favorable response is indicated by significantly reduced activity. The same authors found that PET modified criteria and inverse Choi density/size (ICDS) criteria are accurate methods for assessment of early response, whereas reduction of tumor size alone, evaluated by RECIST criteria, was a poor indicator of the outcome.

8 Key Points

- MRI is the preferred technique to differentiate expected postoperative changes such as edema and fibrosis from local recurrence and other postoperative complications.
- In addition to conventional sequences, dynamic contrast-enhanced imaging and diffusion-weighted imaging are mandatory for detection of recurrence.
- Water-rich tumors such as cartilaginous or myxoid tumorlike chordoma or chondrosarcoma or tumors with more sparse cellularity usually present with increased ADC values due to less restricted diffusion compared to other malignant tumors.
- CT is useful for detection of chondroid calcifications in recurrent cartilage tumors of chordoma and calcified osteoid matrix in recurrent osteosarcoma and for evaluation of hardware and bone graft failure.
- Mimickers of poor response to chemotherapy include early granulation tissue, bone marrow changes due to chemotherapy or irradiation, and insufficiency fractures.
- PET/CT and WBMRI have a complementary role in the posttreatment evaluation of lymphoma.
- FDG-PET/CT is the imaging modality of choice for evaluation of posttreatment response of plasmacytoma.
- PET modified criteria and ICDS are accurate methods for assessment of early response of denosumab therapy in GCT.

References

Aghighi M, Boe J, Rosenberg J et al (2016) Three-dimensional radiologic assessment of chemotherapy response in Ewing sarcoma can be used to predict clinical outcome. Radiology 280:905–915

Albano D, Messina C, Gitto S et al (2019) Differential diagnosis of spine tumors—my favorite mistake. Semin Musculoskelet Radiol 23:26–35

Albano D, Micci G, Patti C et al (2021) Whole-body magnetic resonance imaging: current role in patients with lymphoma. Diagnostics 11:1007

Alothman M, Althobaity W, Asiri Y et al (2020) Giant cell tumor of bone following denosumab treatment: assessment of tumor response using various imaging modalities. Insights Imaging 11(1):41

Ariyarante S, Jenko N, Iyengar KP et al (2023) Primary osseous malignancies of the spine. Diagnostics 13(12):2006

Asmar K, Saade C, Salman R et al (2020) The value of diffusion weighted imaging and apparent diffusion coefficient in primary osteogenic and Ewing sarcomas for the monitoring of response to treatment: initial experience. Eur J Radiol 124:108855

Baidya Kayal E, Kandasamy D, Khare K et al (2019) Intravoxel incoherent motion (IVIM) for response assessment in patients with osteosarcoma undergoing neoadjuvant chemotherapy. Eur J Radiol 119:108635

Bancroft LW (2011) Postoperative tumor imaging. Semin Musculoskelet Radiol 2011(15):425–438

Barrington SF, O'Doherty MJ (2003) Limitations of Pet for imaging lymphoma. Eur J Nucl Med Mol Imaging Suppl 1:S117–127

Barz M, Aftahy K, Janssen I et al (2021) Spinal manifestation of primary malignant (PLB) and secondary bone lymphoma (SLB). Curr Oncol 28(5):3891–3899

Bauckneht M, Capitanio S, Donegani MI et al (2019) Role of baseline and post-therapy 18F-FDG PET in the prognostic stratification of metastatic castration-resistant prostate cancer (mCRPC) patients treated with radium-223. Cancers 12:31

Baur A, Huber A, Arbogast S et al (2001) Diffusion-weighted imaging of tumor recurrencies and posttherapeutical soft-tissue changes in humans. Eur Radiol 11:828–833

Baur-Melnyk A, Reiser MF (2009) Multiple myeloma. Semin Musculoskelet Radiol 13:111–119

Beaman FD, Bancroft LW, Peterson JJ et al (2006) Imaging characteristics of bone graft materials. Radiographics 26(2):373–388

Bhojwani N, Szpakowski P, Partovi S et al (2015) Diffusion-weighted imaging in musculoskeletal radiology—clinical applications and future directions. Quant Imaging Med Surg 5:740–753

Bloem JL, Vriens D, Krol ADG et al (2020) Therapy-related imaging findings in patients with sarcoma. Semin Musculoskelet Radiol 24:676–691

Bluemke DA, Fishman EK, Scott WW Jr (1994) Skeletal complications of radiation therapy. Radiographics 14:111–121

Bostel T, Nicolay NH, Welzel T et al (2018) Sacral insufficiency fractures after high-dose carbon-ion based radiotherapy of sacral chordomas. Radiat Oncol 13:154

Boutin RD, White LM, Laor T et al (2015) MRI findings of serous atrophy of bone marrow and associated complications. Eur Radiol 25:2771–2778

Brown KT, Rosental DI, Rosenberg A (1983) Case report 247. Post-radiation osteitis of the sacrum. Skeletal Radiol 10:269–272

Campanacci L, Sambri A, Medellin MR et al (2019) A new computerized tomography classification to evaluate response to denosumab in giant cell tumors in the extremities (2019) Acta Orthop Traumatol Turc 53:376–380

Capps GW, Fulcher AS, Szucs RA, Turner MA (1997) Imaging features of radiation-induced changes in the abdomen. Radiographics 17:1455–1473

Chan BY, Gill KG, Rebsamen SL, Nguyen JC (2016) MR imaging of pediatric bone marrow. Radiographics 36:1911–1930

Chaturvedi A (2021) Pediatric skeletal diffusion-weighted magnetic resonance imaging: Part 2: Current and emerging applications. Pediatr Radiol 51:1575–1588

Chen J, Li C, Tian Y et al (2019) Comparison of whole-body DWI and (18)F-FDG PET/CT for detecting intramedullary and extramedullary lesions in multiple myeloma. AJR Am J Roentgenol 213:514–523

Choi H, Charnsangavej C, Faria SC et al (2007) Correlation of computed tomography and positron emission tomography in patients with metastatic gastrointestinal stromal tumor treated at a single institution with imatinib mesylate: proposal of new computed tomography response criteria. J Clin Oncol 25:1753–1759

Chokshi FH, Low M, Gibbs WN (2018) Conventional and advanced imaging of spine oncologic disease, nonoperative post-treatment effects and unique spinal conditions. Neurosurgery 82:1–23

Dietrich O, Biffar A, Reiser MF, Baur-Melnyk A (2009) Diffusion-weighted imaging of bone marrow. Semin Musculoskelet Radiol 13:134–144

Dyke JP, Panicek DM, Healey JH et al (2003) Osteogenic and Ewing sarcomas: estimation of necrotic fraction during induction chemotherapy with dynamic contrast enhanced MR imaging. Radiology 228:271–278

Eisenhauer EA, Therasseb P, Bogaerts J et al (2009) New response evaluation criteria in solid tumours: revised RECIST guideline (version 1.1). Eur J Cancer 45:228–247

Engellau J, Seeger L, Grimer R et al (2018) Assessment of denosumab treatment effects and imaging response in patients with giant cell tumor of bone. World J Surg Oncol 16:191

Erlemann R, Sciuk J, Bosse A et al (1990) Response of osteosarcoma and Ewing sarcoma to preoperative chemotherapy: assessment with dynamic and static MR imaging and skeletal scintigraphy. Radiology 75:791–796

Fayad LM, Jacobs MA, Carrino JA, Bluemke DA (2012) Musculoskeletal tumors: how to use anatomic, functional and metabolic MR techniques. Radiology 265:340–356

Fournier L, Ammari S, Thiam R, Cuénod CA (2014) Imaging criteria for assessing tumour response: RECIST, mRECIST, Cheson. Diagn Interv Imaging 95:689–703

Fox MG, Bancroft LW, Peterson JJ (2006) MRI appearance of myocutaneous flaps commonly used in orthopedic reconstructive surgery. Am J Roentgenol 187:800–806

Franck P, Bernstein JL, Cohen LE et al (2018) Local muscle flaps minimize post-operative wound morbidity in patients with neoplastic disease of the spine. Clin Neurol Neurosurg 171:100–105

Frisch S, Timmermann B (2007) The evolving role of proton beam therapy for sarcomas. Clin Oncol 29:500–506

Garner HW, Kransdorf MJ (2016) Musculoskeletal sarcoma: update on imaging of the post-treatment patient. Can Assoc Radiol J 67:12–120

Garner HW, Kransdorf MJ, Peterson JJ (2011) Posttherapy imaging of musculoskeletal neoplasms. Posttherapy imaging of musculoskeletal neoplasms. Radiol Clin North Am 49(6):1307–1323

Griffiths HJ, Thompson RC, Nitke SJ et al (1997) Use of MRI in evaluating postoperative changes in patients with bone and soft tissue tumors. Orthopedics 20:215–220

Gu L, Madewell JE, Aslam R, Mujtba B (2019) The effects of granulocyte growth stimulating factor on MR images of bone marrow. Skeletal Radiol 48:209–218

Gupta S, Stinson ZS, Marco RA, Dormans JP (2018) Single stage en bloc resection of a recurrent metastatic osteosarcoma of the pediatric lumbar spine through multiple exposures—a novel approach. SICOT-J 4:32

Hao Y, An R, Xue Y (2021) Prognostic value of tumoral and peritumoral magnetic resonance parameters in osteosarcoma patients for monitoring chemotherapy response. Eur Radiol 31:3518–3529

Hartman RP, Sundaram M, Okuno SH, Sim FH (2004) Effect of granulocyte-stimulating factors on marrow of adult patients with musculoskeletal malignancies. AJR Am J Roentgenol 183:645–653

Hawk MW, Kim KD (2000) Review of spinal pseudomeningoceles and cerebrospinal fluid fistulas. Neurosurg Focus 9(1):e5

Henderson ER, Xu X, Pogue BW et al (2020) Osteosarcoma mineralization changes on radiographs have moderate correlation to chemotherapy response using bone subtraction methodology. Ann Jt 5:38

Henry TD, McCarville ME, Hoffer FA (2006) Diagnostic imaging of pediatric bone and soft tissue sarcomas. In: Pappo A (ed) Pediatric bone and soft tissue sarcomas. Springer, Berlin, pp 35–69

Herrera IH, Dela Presa RM, Gutierrez RG et al (2013) Evaluation of the post operative lumbar spine. Radiologia 55(1):12–23

Hillengass J, Moulopoulos LA, Delorme S et al (2017) Whole-body computed tomography versus conventional skeletal survey in patients with multiple myeloma: a study of the International Myeloma Working Group. Blood Cancer J 7:e599

Hoeben BA, Carrie C, Timmermann B et al (2019) Management of vertebral radiotherapy dose in paediatric patients with cancer: consensus recommendations from the SIOPE Radiotherapy Working Group. Lancet Oncol 20:e155–e166

Holscher HC, Bloem JL, Vanel D et al (1992) Osteosarcoma: chemotherapy-induced changes at MR imaging. Radiology 182:839–844

Hu Z, Wen S, Huo Z et al (2022) Current status and prospects of targeted therapy for osteosarcoma. Cells 11:3507

Huvos AG, Rosen G, Marcove RC (1977) Primary osteogenic sarcoma: pathologic aspects in 20 patients after treatment with chemotherapy en bloc resection and prosthetic bone replacement. Arch Pathol Lab Med 101:14–18

Hwang S, Lefkowitz R, Landa J et al (2009) Local changes in bone marrow at MRI after treatment of extremity soft tissue sarcoma. Skeletal Radiol 38:11–19

Inarejos Clemente EJ, Navarro OM, Navallas M et al (2022) Multiparametric MRI evaluation of bone sarcomas in children. Insights Imaging 13:33

Jain NK, Dao K, Ortiz AO (2014) Radiologic evaluation and management of postoperative paraspinal fluid collections. Neuroimaging Clin N Am 24(2):375–389

Jin C, Xie M, Liang W, Qian Y (2020) Lumbar vertebral osteoradionecrosis: a rare case report with 10-year follow-up and brief literature review. BMC Musculoskelet Disord 21:7

Johnson SA, Kumar A, Matasar MJ et al (2015) Imaging for staging and response assessment in lymphoma. Radiology 276:323–338

Kattapuram SV, Rosol MS, Rosenthal DI et al (1999) Magnetic resonance imaging features of allografts. Skeletal Radiol 28:383–389

Kayal EB, Alampally JT, Sharma R et al (2023) Chemotherapy response evaluation using diffusion weighted MRI in Ewing sarcoma: a single center experience. Acta Radiol 64:1508–1517

Kim Y, Lee SK, Kim JY, Kim JH (2023) Pitfalls of diffusion-weighted imaging: clinical utility of T2-shine-through and T2-black-out for musculoskeletal diseases. Diagnostics 13(9):1647

Klish MD, Watson GA, Shrieve DC et al (2004) Radiation and intensity-modulated radiotherapy for metastatic spine tumors. Neurosurg Clin N Am 15(4):481–490

Koutoulidis V, Fontara S, Terpos E et al (2017) Quantitative diffusion-weighted imaging of the bone marrow: an adjunct tool for the diagnosis of a diffuse MR imaging pattern in patients with multiple myeloma. Radiology 282:484–493

Koutoulidis V, Terpos E, Papanikolaou N et al (2022) Comparison of MRI features of fat fraction and ADC for early treatment response assessment in participants with multiple myeloma. Radiology 304:137–144

Kubo T, Furuta T, Jahan MP et al (2016) Percent slope analysis of dynamic magnetic resonance imaging for assessment of chemotherapy response of osteosarcoma or Ewing sarcoma. Systematic review and meta-analysis. Skeletal Radiol 45:1235–1288

Kubo T, Furuta T, Johan MP et al (2017) Value of diffusion-weighted imaging for evaluating chemotherapy response in osteosarcoma: a meta-analysis. Mol Clin Oncol 7:88–92

Latifoltojar A, Hall-Craggs M, Bainbrigde A et al (2017) Whole-body MRI quantitative biomarkers are associated significantly with treatment response in patients with newly diagnosed symptomatic multiple myeloma following bortezomib induction. Eur Radiol 27:5325–5336

Laux CJ, Brzaczy G, Weber M et al (2015) Tumor response of osteosarcoma to neoadjuvant chemotherapy evaluated by magnetic resonance imaging as prognostic factor for outcome. Int Orthop 39:97–104

Lecouvet FE, Vekemans MC, Van Den Berghe T et al (2022) Imaging of treatment response and minimal residual disease in multiple myeloma: state of the art WB-MRI and PET/CT. Skeletal Radiol 51(1):59–80

Ledermann HP, Schweitzer ME, Morrison ME (2002) Nonenhancing tissue on MR imaging of pedal infection: characterization of necrotic tissue and associated limitations for diagnosis of osteomyelitis and abscess. AJR Am J Roentgenol 178(1):215–222

Lee J, Yoo YH, Lee S et al (2018) Gelatinous transformation of bone marrow mimicking malignant marrow-replacing lesion on magnetic resonance imaging in a patient without underlying devastating disease. iMRI 22:50–55

Lee SH, Kwok KY, Wong SM et al (2022) Chordoma at the skull base, spine and sacrum: a pictorial essay. J Clin Imaging Sci 12:44

Lejoly M, Van Den Berghe T, Creytens D et al (2024) Diagnosis and monitoring denosumab therapy of giant cell tumors of bone: radiologic-pathologic correlation. Skeletal Radiol 53(2):353–364

Li Z, Guo L, Zhang P et al (2023) A systematic review of perioperative complications in en bloc resection of spinal tumors. Global Spine J 13:812

Lim CY, Ong KO (2013) Imaging of musculoskeletal lymphoma. Cancer Imaging 14:448–457

Lin E, Scognamiglio T, Zhao Y et al (2018) Prognostic implications of gadolinium enhancement of skull base chordomas. AJNR Am J Neuroradiol 39(8):1509–1514

Liu X, Duan Z, Fang S, Wang S (2024) Imaging assessment of the efficacy of chemotherapy in primary malignant bone tumors: recent advances in qualitative and quantitative magnetic resonance imaging and radiomics. J Magn Reson Imaging 59(1):7–31

Matsumoto Y, Fukumitsu N, Ishikawa H, Nakai K, Sakurai H (2021) A critical review of radiation therapy: from particle beam therapy (proton, carbon and BNCT) to beyond. J Pers Med 11:825

Mayerhoefer ME, Archibald SJ, Messiou C et al (2020) MRI and PET/MRI in hematologic malignancies. J Magn Reson Imaging 51:1325–1335

Meixel AJ, Hauswald H, Delorme S, Jobke B (2018) From radiation osteitis to osteoradionecrosis: incidence and MR morphology of radiation-induced sacral pathologies following pelvic radiotherapy. Eur Radiol 28:3550–3559

Mule S, Reizine E, Blanc-Durand P et al (2020) Whole-body functional MRI and PET/MRI in multiple myeloma. Cancers 12:3155

National Institute for Health and Care Excellence NICE Myeloma (2016) Diagnosis and management. https://www.nice.org.uk/guidance/ng35/chapter/Recommendations

Noebauer-Huhmann IM, Chaudhary SR, Papakonstantinou O et al (2020) Soft tissue sarcoma follow-up imaging: strategies to distinguish post-treatment changes from recurrence. Semin Musculoskelet Radiol 24:627–644

O'Sallivan B, Davis AM, Turcotte R et al (2002) Preoperative versus postoperative radiotherapy in soft tissue sarcoma of the limbs: a randomized trial. Lancet 29(359):2235–2241

Oguro S, Okuda S, Sugiura H et al (2018) Giant cell tumor of the bone: change in image features after denosumab administration. Magn Reson Med Sci 17:325–333

Oka K, Yakushiji T, Sato H et al (2010) The value of diffusion-weighted imaging for monitoring the chemotherapeutic response of osteosarcoma: a comparison between average apparent diffusion coefficient and minimum apparent diffusion coefficient. Skeletal Radiol 39:141–146

Ollivier L, Leclere J, Vanel D et al (1991) Femoral infarction following intraarterial chemotherapy for osteosarcoma of the leg: a possible pitfall in magnetic resonance imaging. Skeletal Radiol 20:329–332

Ollivier L, Gerber S, Vanel D, Brisse H, Leclere J (2006) Improving the interpretation of bone marrow imaging in cancer patients. Cancer Imaging 6:194–198

Papakonstantinou O, Isaac A, Dalili D, Noebauer-Huhmann IM (2019) T2 hypointense tumors and tumor like lesions. Semin Musculoskelet Radiol 23:58–75

Parmeggiani A, Miceli M, Errani C, Facchini G (2021) State of the art and new concepts in giant cell tumor of the bone: imaging features and tumor characteristics. Cancers 13:6298

Patel SR (2000) Radiation-induced sarcoma. Curr Treat Options Oncol 1:258–261

Radcliff K, Morrison WB, Kepler C et al (2016) Distinguishing pseudomeningocele, epidural hematoma and postoperative infection on postoperative MRI. Clin Spine Surg 29:E471

Rahmouni A, Meigan M, Diine M et al (2003) MRI and PET of bone lymphoproliferative diseases. Cancer Imaging 3:122–125

Reinert CP, Krieg EM, Bosmuller H, Horger M (2020) Mid-term response assessment in multiple myeloma using a texture analysis approach on dual energy-CT-derived bone marrow images—a proof of principle study. Eur J Radiol 131:109214

Richardson ML, Zink-Brody GC, Patten RM et al (1996) MR characterization of post-irradiation soft tissue edema. Skeletal Radiol 25:537–543

Roberge D, Skamene T, Nahal A et al (2010) Radiological and pathological response following pre-operative radiotherapy for soft-tissue sarcoma. Radiother Oncol 97:404–440

Rodallec MH, Feydy A, Larousserie F et al (2008) Diagnostic imaging of solitary tumors of the spine: what to do and say. Radiographics 28:1019–1041

Saleh MM, Abdelrahman TM, Madney Y et al (2020) Multiparametric MRI with diffusion-weighted imaging in predicting response to chemotherapy in cases of osteosarcoma and Ewing's sarcoma. Br J Radiol 93(1115):20200257

Santos P, Peck KK, Arevalo-Perez J et al (2017) T1-weighted dynamic contrast-enhanced MR perfusion imaging characterizes tumor response to radiation therapy in chordoma. Am J Neuroradiol 38:2210–2216

Sasaki T, Moritani T, Belay A et al (2018) Role of apparent diffusion coefficient as a predictor of tumor progression in patients with chordoma. Am J Neuroradiol 39:1316–1321

Schilling AT, Ehresman J, Huq S et al (2020) Risk factors for wound related complications after surgery for primary and metastatic spine tumors: a systematic review and metaanalysis. World Neurosurg 141:467–478

Schultheiss TE (2008) The radiation dose-response of the human spinal cord. Int J Radiat Oncol Biol Phys 71:1455–1459

Schulze M, Weisel K, Grandjean C et al (2014) Increasing bone sclerosis during bortezomib therapy in multiple myeloma patients: results of a reduced-dose whole-body MDCT study. AJR Am J Roentgenol 202(1):170–179

Seam P, Juweid ME, Cheson BD (2007) The role of FDG-PET scans in patients with lymphoma. Blood 110:3507–35016

Shapeero LG, De Visschere PJ, Verstraete KL et al (2008) Post-treatment complications of soft tissue tumors. Eur J Radiol 69(2):209–221

Sheppard DG, Libshitz HI (2001) Post-radiation sarcomas: a review of the clinical and imaging features in 63 cases. Clin Radiol 56:22–29

Son HM, Yoo HJ, Hong SH et al (2022) Detection of soft tissue sarcoma recurrence: feasibility of ultrafast 3D Gradient-echo sequence in additional to contrast enhanced MRI to provide early-phase post contrast information. J Belg Soc Radiol 106(51):1–9

Subhawong TK, Jacobs MA, Fayad LM (2014) Diffusion-weighted imaging for characterizing musculoskeletal lesions. Radiographics 34(5):1163–1177

Uhl M, Saueressig U, Koehler G et al (2006) Evaluation of tumor necrosis during chemotherapy with diffusion-weighted MR imaging: preliminary results in osteosarcomas. Pediatr Radiol 36:1306–1311

Verstraete K (2009) Assessment of response to chemotherapy and radiotherapy. In: Davies AM, Sundaram M, James SLJ (eds) Imaging of bone tumors and tumor-like lesions. Techniques and applications. Springer, Berlin

Vilanova JC, Baleato-Gonzalez S, Romero M et al (2016) Assessment of musculoskeletal malignancies with functional MR imaging. Magn Reson Imaging Clin N Am 24:239–259

Wahl RL, Jacene H, Kasamon Y et al (2009) From RECIST to PERCIST: evolving considerations for PET response criteria in solid tumors. J Nucl Med 50:122S–150S

Wang CS, Du LJ, Si MJ et al (2013) Noninvasive assessment of response to neoadjuvant chemotherapy in osteosarcoma of long bones with diffusion-weighted imaging: an initial in vivo study. PloS One 26:72679

Wardelmann E, Haas RL, Bovee JVMG et al (2016) Evaluation of response after neoadjuvant treatment in soft tissue sarcomas; the European Organization for Research and Treatment of Cancer-Soft Tissue and Bone Sarcoma Group (EORTC-STBSG) recommendations for pathological examination and reporting. Eur J Cancer 53:84–95

Yamamoto Y, Taoka T, Nakamine H (2009) Superior clinical impact of FDG-PET compared to MRI for the follow-up of a patient with sacral lymphoma. J Clin Exp Hematopathol 49:109–115

Yamazaki T, McLoughlin GS, Patel S et al (2009) Feasibility and safety of en bloc resection for primary spine tumors: a systematic review by the spine oncology group. Spine (Phila Pa 1976) 34(22 Suppl):S31

Yeom KW, Lober RM, Mobley BC et al (2013) Diffusion-weighted MRI: distinction of skull base chordoma from chondrosarcoma. Am J Neuroradiol 34:1056–1061

Young PM, Berquist TH, Bancroft LW, Peterson JJ (2007) Complications of spinal instrumentation. Radiographics 27(3):775–789

Zeng YN, Zhang BT, Song T et al (2022) The clinical value of dynamic contrast-enhanced magnetic resonance imaging (DCE-MRI) semi-quantitative parameters in monitoring neoadjuvant chemotherapy response of osteosarcoma. Acta Radiol 63:1077–1085

Printed in the USA
CPSIA information can be obtained
at www.ICGtesting.com
LVHW082154150724
785622LV00005B/22